Second Edition

A SURVEY OF ADULT APHASIA AND RELATED LANGUAGE DISORDERS

G. ALBYN DAVIS
University of Massachusetts at Amherst

PRENTICE HALL, Englewood Cliffs, New Jersey 07632

Library of Congress Cataloging-in-Publication Data

Davis, G. Albyn (George Albyn)
    A survey of adult aphasia and related language disorders / G.
Albyn Davis. — 2nd ed.
        p.   cm.
    Rev. ed. of: A survey of adult aphasia / G. Albyn Davis. c1983.
    Includes bibliographical references and index.
    ISBN 0-13-878018-8
    1. Aphasia. I. Davis, G. Albyn (George Albyn) Survey of
adult aphasia. II. Title.
    [DNLM: 1. Aphasia — in adulthood. 2. Language Disorders. WL
340.5 D261a]
RC425.D38 1993
616.85'52 — dc20
DNLM/DLC
for Library of Congress   92-49840
                                                          CIP

Editorial/production supervision
    and interior design: *Mary Kathryn L. Bsales*
Acquisitions editor: *Julie Berrisford*
Editorial assistant: *Nicole Signoretti*
Prepress buyer: *Kelly Behr*
Manufacturing buyer: *Mary Ann Gloriande*
Cover design: *Joe DiDomenico*
Copy editor: *Eleanor Ode Walter*

© 1993, 1983 by Prentice-Hall, Inc.
A Paramount Communications Company
Englewood Cliffs, New Jersey 07632

Printed in the United States of America
10 9 8 7 6 5 4 3

ISBN 0-13-878018-8

Prentice-Hall International (UK) Limited, *London*
Prentice-Hall of Australia Pty. Limited, *Sydney*
Prentice-Hall Canada Inc., *Toronto*
Prentice-Hall Hispanoamericana, S.A., *Mexico*
Prentice-Hall of India Private Limited, *New Delhi*
Prentice-Hall of Japan, Inc., *Tokyo*
Simon & Schuster Asia Pte. Ltd., *Singapore*
Editora Prentice-Hall do Brasil, Ltda., *Rio de Janeiro*

CONTENTS

PREFACE

This book is a comprehensive reconstruction of the original A *Survey of Adult Aphasia* (1983). The new version maintains the original assumption that speech-language pathologists are empowered at the core by knowledge of their domain. Substantial modifications were motivated by two intersecting developments during the 1980s. One development has been the widening scope of clinically managed communicative impairments to include outcomes of traumatic brain injury and right hemisphere stroke. The other development has been the budding of cognitive psychology as the basis for conceptualizing and investigating language dysfunctions as mental phenomena. This text should not be interpreted as representing a peculiar alternative viewpoint. Instead, it is an attempt to represent the emerging alignment of clinical aphasiology with the science of language functions, namely, the specialty of psycholinguistics in cognitive psychology. The principles for studying attention, perception, and memory are being applied to the study of language comprehension and formulation, and vice versa. This "work in progress" is reaching basic research on language disorders before intervening convincingly in clinical management.

Beginning in the first chapter, the text contains periodic acknowledgment of cross-linguistic research and aphasia in bilingual persons. Further modifications include the addition of chapters on the cognitive bases of language functions (Chapter 3), right hemisphere dysfunction (Chapter 7), and pragmatics and discourse (Chapter 8). The study of aphasia is expanded into two chapters that distinguish general investigation from the controversial study of syndromes (Chapters 4 and 5). Basic information on closed head injury and Alzheimer's dementia is expanded into a new chapter (Chapter 6). The original chapters on diagnostic methods are updated partly because of current movements to make assessment more efficient and functional (Chapters 9 and 10). An introduction to single-subject experimental design accompanies discussion of treatment efficacy in Chapter 11. The two chapters on treatment approaches are reorganized and updated by several influences that include pragmatics and microcomputers (Chapters 12 and 13). The original chapter on psychosocial considerations is eliminated, but much of this information is integrated into discussions of pragmatic treatment that fosters generalization. A desire to teach hopefully has overcome a desire to cite all available references. This emphasis may be partly responsible for the omission of some important bodies of research pertaining to reading and writing, perseveration, and speech automatisms. It is hoped that instructors using this text will make up for these and other deficiencies.

I am still inspired by the generous understanding and encouragement for the first text that was provided by friends and colleagues in Memphis. The atmosphere at Memphis State University was electrified by people supporting each other. I continue to be grateful for my parents' love and patience. Moreover, the patience of editors at Prentice Hall has been astounding. Laura Silk, at the University of Massachusetts, provided a year of valuable student assistance in keeping track of details. I received valued support and advice from Therese O'Neil at Spaulding Rehabilitation Hospital in Boston. Harry Seymour of UMass provided some helpful feedback, and Mick McNeil at the University of Wisconsin challenged my thinking scrawled in manuscripts related to this work. Susan Fryburg came to the rescue with some important clinical information. Several students assisted through projects, namely, Kate Dimitry, Marie Dolan, Elise Katz, Randee Lopate, Rebecca Loveland, Susan Savoy, and Diane Susi. I would like to thank Rosemary Lubinski of SUNY at Buffalo and Donald Robin of the University of Iowa for reviewing the manuscript. I want to thank friends and colleagues, especially Kevin Kearns at Northeastern University, who occasionally asked how it was going or who, at least, wondered what I was up to.

G. Albyn Davis

1

INTRODUCTION TO APHASIA AND RELATED DISORDERS

A person who suffers a stroke may experience a lasting dysfunction called aphasia. Whenever the individual has a message to convey, he or she is likely to say, "I know what it is, I just can't think of the word." It's like having a name on the tip of the tongue. All of us experience being unable to think of a word; but, for someone with aphasia, saying any word to anyone at any time can be like reaching for a distant fruit on a tree. Despite their difficulty in finding words, aphasic people remember their past, follow schedules, and find their way around town. Phineas Gage, a railroad worker in Vermont, suffered another kind of injury. In 1848 an explosion propelled a tamping iron through the front of his brain. His friends were astonished that he survived and could tell the tale of his ordeal. Yet, on returning to his job as a foreman, he could not stick to a plan as before. He was no longer himself, having become irreverent and

impatient. He wandered about the United States until he died in San Francisco in 1861 (Macmillan, 1986). Many kinds of impairment occur because of the location and type of brain injury.

Many disciplines are involved in the study of aphasia for different reasons. Some of these fields, such as the neurosciences, are involved in discovering how the brain works. This book is directed mainly to clinical study of language disorders with the objective of providing rehabilitation based on the best knowledge of the disorders. In the United States, speech-language pathology was organized as a profession in 1925 mainly to provide "speech correction" in public schools, but the two world wars dramatized the effects of brain injury in adults. Responding to that need, speech-language pathologists and psychologists created rehabilitation programs in military hospitals throughout the world.

Ideas for therapy came from diction, speech correction, classroom teaching, and psychotherapy. Since then, much has been learned about the unique needs of people with brain injury, and research has shown that brain injuries are more varied, complex, and mysterious than they seemed to be 50 years ago. Many speech-language pathologists acquired a respect for the challenges presented by neuropathologies, and clinical aphasiologists emerged to specialize in the management of language dysfunctions in medical settings. These specialists embrace knowledge from many disciplines, mix in their own discoveries, and direct this expertise toward maximizing the communicative capabilities of brain-damaged individuals.

THE DOMAINS OF APHASIOLOGY

Speech-language pathologists may refer to aphasia as a linguistic, neurogenic, or cognitive disorder. These classifications point to domains of the universe in which aphasia is thought to occur and, thus, point to the prerequisite sciences that might be presented in the training of a clinical aphasiologist. This chapter introduces the study of aphasia and related disorders with the idea that aphasiology lies in the intersection of studies that can be focused on language behavior, the brain, or the mind. Understanding aphasia and related language disorders entails a grasp of relationships among these three domains.

Clinical Behavior

Speech-language pathologists usually ask clients to tell what happened to cause their hospitalization. One client may think about it and then take about 60 seconds to say, "Sleeping ... um ... bathroom ... fall down ... um ... wife ... um ... hospital." Gardner (1974) asked another patient to talk about what brought him to the hospital, and the following is part of what this patient said:

"Oh sure, go ahead, any old think you want. If I could I would. Oh, I'm taking the word the wrong way to say, all of the barbers here whenever they stop you it's going around and around, if you know what I mean, that is tying and tying for repucer, repuceration, well, we were trying the best that we could while another time it was with the beds over there the same thing. ..." (p. 68).

These samples are routine observations for clinicians, and each sample is an example of aphasia. Aphasia appears in different forms. One response to the question contained few words and much hesitation. Gardner's patient generated sentences easily but seemed to create new words and did not appear to be answering the question or making much sense at all.

In order to analyze our observations of aphasia, we present patients with numerous tasks in a controlled manner. We achieve control by selecting a task that focuses the type of stimulus and the type of response. We can compare writing under two stimulus conditions by asking someone to copy a sentence and write it to dictation. In Constance Cummings' portrayal of aphasia in Arthur Kopit's play *Wings*, she clutched a toothbrush and called it a "toobridge." If we were to put a few more objects in her hand, then we may find out that she has frequent difficulty producing names when looking at objects. Moreover, when we realize that she was looking and touching, we might decide to compare naming under two stimulus conditions. By presenting the object through sight alone and then only through touch, we could determine if the naming problem is related to a particular stimulus modality.

In traditional behavioral psychology, a person's environment provided explanation of behavior. Behaviorists had insisted that little is gained by appealing to forces that Mowrer (1982) likened to the magic of alchemy and divination. Accordingly, laws of cause and effect were constructed from "a functional relationship between stimulus events (S) and response events (R) .... If a response always varies directly with the manipulation of a stimulus, we must conclude the stimulus causes the response" (Mowrer. 1982, p. 40). Regarding speech disorders, Sloane and Mac-

Aulay (1968) explained that "behavior modification approaches consider the speech defect the problem itself, rather than a symptom of some 'underlying' difficulty" (p. 4). They rejected therapies based on neurological phenomena or "mentalistic hypothetical constructs such as 'anxiety'" (p. 4).

Basing clinical decisions solely on behavioral observation is often advertised as the objective approach. This may be called the **fallacy of objectivity.** A physicist argued that there is no such thing as a science coldly separated from human influence; he wrote that "the celebrated ability to quantify the world is no guarantee of objectivity and that measurement itself is a value judgment created by the human mind" (Jones, 1982, p. 11). A point of view selects behaviors thought to be important, such as tasks that should be indicative of aphasia or recovery. Response is recorded through the filter of perception. Because of the variability of behavior, statistics uncover only the probability of effects. Scientists can only minimize the inevitable influence of subjectivity when making judgments, such as concluding that word struggle and fluent vagary are both examples of aphasia.

The Brain

When neurosurgeons used tiny electrodes to stimulate surfaces of their patients' brains, patients reported hearing an orchestra or a choir although neither was present in the room (Penfield and Perot, 1963). The whole story of function does not reside in clinically observable phenomena. When someone suffers brain damage, a change inside the person's head is causing him or her to behave in a new way. Long ago, we turned to neurology for explaining what goes wrong between a stimulus and the patient's attempt at response. Denes and Pinson's (1963) "speech chain" located communicative transactions in human neuroanatomy (Figure 1-1). According to the logic of neurodiagnosis, behavior signifies the presence of a neuropathology. Porch (1986), a clinical aphasiologist, argued that aphasia tests should reveal "the relative efficiency of various 'brain circuits'" (p. 295). Inferring the nature of hidden conditions can be consistent with behaviorism. The focus on observation "does not mean that all behavior must be visible to the naked eye" (Sloane and MacAulay, 1968, p. 4). Indeed, modern tech-

FIGURE 1-1 A representation of physical mechanisms as the inner basis for communication. (Reprinted by permission from Denes, P.B. & Pinson, E.N., *The speech chain.* New York: Anchor Press, 1963, p. 5. Doubleday, publisher.)

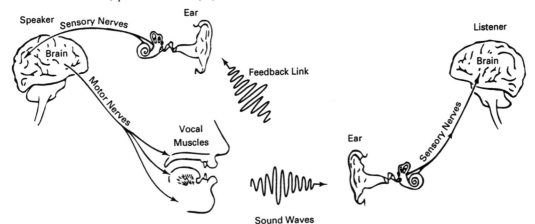

nology exposes cerebral conditions and events to the naked eye, and this research allows us to assume that a stroke is a stimulus causing changes in behavior.

Damaged tissue is called a **lesion.** Aphasia is caused by a lesion in the cerebral cortex. A few neuropathologies destroy a small part of the brain, and such localized damage is called a **focal** lesion. Focal lesions are caused by stroke, a disruption of blood flow to the brain. Also, small areas of the brain can be scraped during life-saving surgery. A client may have multiple lesions incurred by suffering several strokes through the years. This **multifocal** pattern also shows up in slowly progressing pathologies such as Alzheimer's disease. A **diffuse** lesion is spread throughout the brain. Head trauma in World War II was described as "a cleanly punched out defect in a cerebrum" (Luria, 1970b, p. 2). Yet, traffic collisions and modern firearms inflict more complex damage that seems to be multifocal and diffuse. Stroke and head injury are likely to produce quite different clinical problems.

Thus, study of the nervous system has been a traditional prerequisite for coming to grips with the nature of aphasia. The nervous system provides a basis for explaining why some stroke victims have aphasia and others do not, or why some persons with aphasia have good comprehension and others have very poor comprehension. Different disorders occur because the central nervous system is divided into regions of differing functional significance, which Luria (1970a) indicated with his diagram shown in Figure 1–2. Luria divided the central nervous system (CNS) into three functional levels. The first level includes deep cerebral nuclei (e.g., hypothalamus) and the reticular formation through the brainstem. The **reticular activating system** (RAS), in particular, distributes nerve impulses to all areas of cerebral cortex. In effect, the RAS turns on the complex systems of the cortex and maintains alertness to stimuli from the outside world. The second level is **posterior cortex,** which perceives, recognizes, and integrates sensory information. The third level is **anterior cortex,** which generates volitional response. Thus, damage

to anterior cortex causes serious difficulty with some functions and leaves other functions in much better condition.

Aphasiologists have been most familiar with the macrostructural level of neuroanatomy depicted in Figure 1–2. We see the surface of cortex, which is 2 to 2½ square feet of neural circuits folded into wormy convolutions within the skull. Four lobes provide a frame of reference for locating a region of cerebral cortex. The frontal lobe coincides with anterior cortex. Posterior cortex receives sensory input of audition (temporal lobe), vision (occipital lobe), and touch (parietal lobe). However, neural activity takes place at a level that cannot be seen with the naked eye. Requiring powerful microscopes for observation, the microstructure of neuroanatomy contains 30 billion neurons delicately networked within the cortex. These cortical cells are stacked in a thickness of less than two typewriter spaces (Calvin and Ojemann, 1980). **Architectonics** is "the study of the arrangement of cells and other units in the nervous system as seen under lower-power microscope magnification" (Galaburda, 1984, p. 292).

The Mind

Aphasic people experience the aftermath of brain damage as problems of comprehending utterances and finding words. Rehabilitation addresses phenomena that we refer to as comprehension and formulation. In the 1950s, speech-language pathologists relied on a theory of communication to depict what happens inside our heads as comprehension and formulation of language. The theory was conceived in studies of radio signal transmission between air-traffic controllers and pilots. This "message model" is illustrated in Figure 1–3. When "encoding," speakers translate an idea or message into a linguistic code and then into a speech signal. Listeners "decode" an acoustic signal into a message. Wepman tried to characterize the nature of aphasic dysfunction hidden between sensory and motor channels (Wepman and van Pelt, 1955). Aphasia was identified with such things as

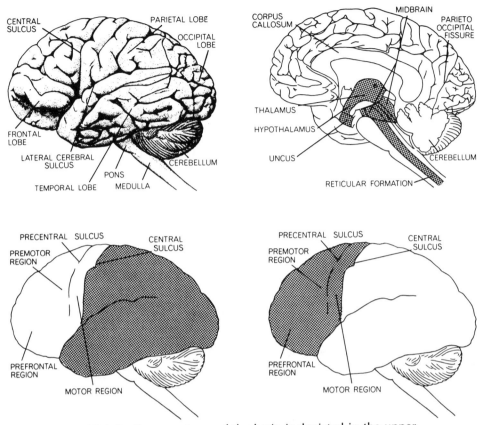

FIGURE 1-2 Gross anatomy of the brain is depicted in the upper left (lateral view) and upper right (medial view). The shaded regions represent Luria's three functional levels or "blocks": reticular formation, posterior cortex, and anterior cortex. (Reprinted by permission from Luria, A. R., The functional organization of the brain. Scientific American, 222(3), 66–78, 1970. Copyright © 1970 by Scientific American, Inc. All rights reserved.)

integration, symbolic formulation, and recall (Figure 1-4). However, the message model and Wepman's prosaic box seemed to be feeble accounts of the inner workings of linguistic communication when compared with the speech chain's neurology.

The aphasic person is now thought to be a faulty information processor (Brookshire, 1978a). In the discipline of cognitive psychology, information processing is considered to be the activity of the human mind; and **cognition** is the formal term used to refer to the mind. Cognition is defined as "human infor-

mation processing . . . information we have in our memories and the processes involved in acquiring, retaining, and using that information" (Wessells, 1982, pp. 1–2). Language comprehension, for example, is a system for using information and is studied as a cognitive function. The study of cognition became a science when psychologists acquired millisecond timers for measuring duration of human information processing. Like modeling an ancient city from archaeological observations, experimental psychologists construct hypothetical models of the functional "archi-

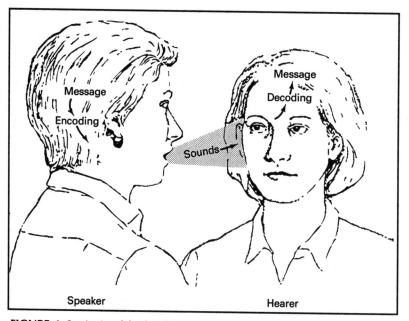

FIGURE 1-3 A simplified indication of psychological or "mental" mechanisms of communication. (Reprinted by permission from Akmajian, A., Demers, R.A., & Harnish, R.M., *Linguistics: An introduction to language and communication* (Second Edition). Cambridge, MA: MIT Press, 1984, p. 393.)

tecture" of the mind (Anderson, 1983). Behavior patterns and response latency are the fractured pottery and carved stone of cognitive psychology.

We examine two broad aspects of cognition. One is **knowledge,** which is a person's store of information. The knowledge of language, or *linguistic competence,* contains information about sound structure (phonology), word structure (morphology), sentence structure (syntax), and the meaning of linguistic forms (semantics). The other feature of cognition is **processing,** which is harmonious with the notion of *linguistic performance.* Knowledge is passive and stable, but processing is dynamic and fleeting. Key questions in cognitive psychology address **representation,** or the form of information in the mind. That is, while someone is reading, the mind may automatically translate graphemic representation of words into a phonemic representation. Mental representation is a mystery with respect to the nature of knowledge

and the nature of information in a state of active processing. A cognitive function depends on both knowledge and processes, and a common question for research and diagnosis is whether a disorder lies in knowledge/competence or processing/performance.

Cognition and the Brain

Medieval clergy insisted that the earth is the center of the universe and that spiritual and material phenomena do not cohabitate. In medical schools anatomic dissection was frowned upon, and dissecting sex organs and the brain was forbidden. It was comfortable to think that the mind or soul inhabits the spaces of the lateral and third ventricles in the core of the brain. In 1504, Gregor Reisch illustrated a thousand-year belief that three mental functions reside in these adjoining caverns: sensations converge in the first ventricle; thinking occurs in the second; and memories are stored in the third. During the

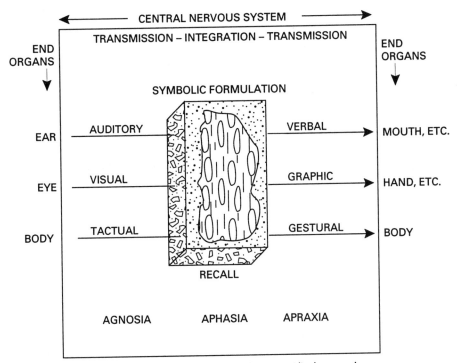

FIGURE 1–4 A classical positioning of unspecified central integrative processes between receptive and expressive modalities. (Reprinted by permission from Wepman, J.M. & Van Pelt, D., A theory of cerebral language disorders based on therapy, *Folia Phoniatrica, 7,* 1955, p. 225. International Association of Logopedics and Phoniatrics, publisher.)

Renaissance, this tripartite view was reflected in anatomic drawings by Leonardo da Vinci. A philosophical dualism stated that the mind and brain are legitimate but separate entities.

A century of discoveries linking gray matter to the mind has pervaded our consciousness such that the general public speaks of the mind and brain interchangeably. *USA Today* ran a front-page story on "Sex and the Brain," and it started with reports that "men have better spatial abilities; women have better language skills." The Public Broadcasting System aired a show called "Fires of the Mind," and it was mostly about the brain. An anatomist put it this way: "The clinical evidence gives no support for the idea that there is some entity or spirit that can exist apart from the brain. . . . That we have conscious minds seems to me to be indisputable, but

mind is an aspect of the functioning of the brain, not something that can exist apart from the brain. . . . We might say that mind is a property of the brain as rotation is a property of a wheel, or calculation of a computer" (Young, 1986, p. 2). A **doctrine of reductionism** is "a unified theory of the mind-brain, wherein psychological states and processes are explained in terms of neuronal states and processes" (Churchland, 1986, p. 278).

On the other hand, a **doctrine of functionalism** states that "the mind can be studied independently from the brain" (Johnson-Laird, 1983, p. 9); "it is perfectly legitimate to talk of mental events, to posit one mental event as causing another, and to do so without taking a position on whether only brain events have the properties to define mental states" (Gardner, 1985, p. 79). Computers have provided an analogy: "Once you know the way in which a computer program works, your understanding of it is in no way improved by learning about the particular machine on which it runs on this occasion or that" (Johnson-Laird, 1983, p. 9). The position is that the mind can be *studied* apart from the brain, but "many working psychologists" do not think that the mind *exists* apart from the brain (Hatfield, 1988). Many psychologists are reluctant to constrain models of the mind with a neurology that fails to explain remembering, reasoning, and communicating. The view "that psychological processes are localised in the brain is apt to impede scientific progress by prematurely limiting the search for the appropriate elements that might ultimately enter onto the neurophysiological substrate" (Mehler, Morton, and Jusczyk, 1984, p. 84). "My own recommendation is that psychologists and neuroscientists drop the language of reduction, and replace it with the reduction-neutral language of psychological function and neural implementation or realization" (Hatfield, 1988, p. 744).

Disciplines

A discipline follows particular strategies for answering questions about a domain. Many disciplines have something to say about behavior, the brain, and cognition. They include neuroscience (Thompson, 1985), cognitive psychology (Eysenck and Keane, 1990; Reed, 1992), clinical neuropsychology (Heilman and Valenstein, 1985; Lezak, 1983), psycholinguistics (Garnham, 1985), neurolinguistics (Caplan, 1987b), and cognitive neuropsychology (Ellis and Young, 1988). The medical profession, especially neurology, established a foothold at the beginning of aphasiology with models of brain centers for language functions. In the early 1900s, behaviorism gripped psychology and, later, speech-language pathology. Psychology started to free itself "in the critical year of 1956" with the birth of cognitive psychology (Eysenck and Keane, 1990). Psycholinguists began to study the "psychological reality" of linguistic theory. A decade later, Neisser

(1967) wrote a book that became the first general text on cognitive psychology (Eysenck and Keane, 1990). The transformations in psychology were punctuated when the *Journal of Verbal Learning and Verbal Behavior* was retitled in 1985 to become the *Journal of Memory and Language*.

Therefore, the formal study of cognition is relatively new, as "the term *cognitive science* first began to be bandied about in the early 1970s" (Gardner, 1985, p. 5). Cognitive science is "the science of the mind" and is an umbrella for many disciplines, including artificial intelligence and cognitive psychology (Stillings, Feinstein, Garfield, Rissland, Rosenbaum, Weisler, and Baker-Ward, 1987). Most of these disciplines are involved in studying aphasia, because aphasia provides clues to the nature of cognition. However, the aphasia laboratory has become like a kitchen crowded with many chefs, each with a particular approach to making an omelet.

Disciplines differ in origin, method, and terminology; aphasiology must contend with this occasionally discordant variability. Two disciplines may be oblivious to each other's accomplishments, even though they deal with the same domain. One result is that one term means different things to different experts. For example, "short-term memory" lasts a few seconds in cognitive psychology, but a few hours in traditional clinical neuropsychology. "Semantics" (e.g., "semantic memory," "semantic system") is another concept suffering from multidisciplinary variation. Followers of a disciplinary tradition may occasionally appear to be defensive and competitive instead of receptive and cooperative. Johnson (1991) attended a conference and found those who study memory to be like warring tribes suspicious of each other's customs. Squire (1987) noted that "cognitive psychology and neuroscience can clearly work together . . . although some have regarded these disciplines as independent or irrelevant to each other" (p. 174). LeDoux and Hirst (1986) edited a book in which neuroscientists and cognitive psychologists took turns writing about perception, attention, memory, and emotion. The book was promoted on its jacket as "a pioneering attempt . . . to force scientists who are working on the same problem but from different perspectives to address each other."

THE NOTION OF APHASIA

With the crowded kitchen of aphasiology, it should not be surprising that we find disagreement as to the diagnosis of aphasia. When there is agreement about diagnosis, there is disagreement about the manner in which aphasia should be defined, partly because of the different disciplinary orientations taken by aphasiologists. While this situation is perplexing, a comprehensive approach to the study of aphasia sometimes involves contending with disagreements when the truth is that there are no clear answers.

Disagreements and a Reorientation

There has been an ongoing debate over "when is aphasia aphasia" (e.g., Rosenbek, 1982). Benson (1979a) defined aphasia as "loss or impairment of language caused by brain damage" (p. 1) and wrote of "aphasia of Alzheimer dementia" (p. 169). The generality of Benson's definition is reflected in considering "*any* language disorder that results from brain damage as a form of aphasia, even though these various language disorders may differ from classical aphasic syndromes caused by focal, vascular insults" (Au, Albert, and Obler, 1988, p. 164). On the other hand, Darley (1982) defined aphasia as a language impairment that is "disproportionate to impairment of other intellective functions" and is "not attributable to dementia, confusion, sensory loss, or motor dysfunction" (p. 42). This aphasia is associated with a focal lesion, usually in left cerebral cortex. Bayles (1986) added that "the majority of speech-language pathologists do not believe the linguistic impairment associated with dementia should be called aphasia" (p. 465). Thus, one view is that any language disorder caused by brain damage should be called aphasia. The other posi-

tion is that only a subset of these language disorders is aphasia.

Benson (1979a) suggested that "the difficulty and controversy stem from what is meant by the word *language*" (p. 1). Language disorder seems to be identified with deficient performance on simple language tasks. In this regard, "language" may refer to verbal as opposed to nonverbal behavior. However, disorder may also be identified as dysfunction of inferred mental mechanisms, and "language" may refer to hidden systems of comprehension and formulation. Moreover, language disorder may be discussed as an impaired linguistic code, but there is a question as to whether a linguistic theory actually depicts knowledge or processes used in the mind when people are comprehending and formulating sentences. People with traumatic head injury, Alzheimer's disease, and right-hemisphere stroke make errors on so-called tests of aphasia or language; but some are diagnosed as having aphasia, and others escape being labeled as even having a language disorder. It may be apparent that simply identifying problems in behavior is not sufficient to diagnose a disorder associated with functioning of the brain. A decision has to be made as to the status of underlying mechanisms. Our ability to make such decisions has been hampered by neurological theory that is too simple and cognitive theory that is too recent to be adequate in accounting for the complexities of behavior.

The ambiguity of "language" coincides with a prevalent separation of language and cognition into independent categories (e.g., Gazzaniga and Smylie, 1984). Clinicians speak of assessing language with some tasks and cognition with others. Rosenbek (1982) concluded that "most traditional aphasiologists would like to separate cognition and language and leave cognitive deficit out of the definition of when aphasia is aphasia" (p. 364). Martin (1981) proposed a daring definition in which aphasia is an impairment of cognition; but Rosenbek (1982) responded that Martin is "among those who would have us believe that aphasia is a cognitive deficit" (p. 363). This skepticism reappeared with the remark that "this portrayal of language's relationship to cognition is also especially felicitous for those . . . who would have aphasiologists spurn specific drills of specific linguistic stimuli" (Rosenbek, LaPointe, and Wertz, 1989, p. 10).

Why has "cognition" not been used as a label for language processes? In some circles of speech-language pathology, cognition seems to have been identified with conscious faculties of thinking, imagining, or the so-called "other intellective functions." Everyday language use is different because it tends to occur without thinking. Word retrieval just happens. However, contemporary cognitive psychology teaches that mental activity occurs at different levels of awareness. At one level, **automatic processing** happens without conscious awareness; but at another level, **strategic processing** occurs consciously and is said to be effortful. In general, one function can be carried out at automatic or strategic levels. Language functions are effortful in "metalinguistic" tasks such as sorting words or editing a manuscript. Separating cognition and language simply makes no sense when "language" is used to refer to mental functions of comprehension and word-finding.

Defining and Diagnosing Aphasia

The notion of aphasia to be surveyed in this text is consistent with the diagnosis that has been traditional in speech-language pathology, although the wording of the definition is aligned with cognitive psychology. **Aphasia** is defined here as follows:

Aphasia is an acquired impairment of the cognitive system for comprehending and formulating language, leaving other cognitive capacities relatively intact.

Acquired disorder is contrasted with congenital disorder in that the former occurs after birth and usually after a period of normal development, whereas the latter is present at birth and impedes development. In this text, we shall be dealing mainly with disorders acquired in adulthood. Also, aphasia is the dysfunction of a specific **cognitive system.** A system contains knowledge and processes specialized for a complex ability, such as musical or visuospatial skills. The **language system** is the storage and manipulation of a linguistic code used for comprehension and formulation. The definition indicates that aphasia is a "language-specific" disorder. The definition also indicates that diagnosis of aphasia is based on comparison of cognitive systems. In order for this idea to be useful for clinical diagnosis, there must be a basis upon which cognitive systems can be compared through what a clinician can observe.

The current definition also differs from previous ones in that it omits reference to etiology. The following is an example of previous definition:

Aphasia is "an acquired impairment of language processes underlying receptive and expressive modalities and caused by damage to areas of the brain which are primarily responsible for the language function" (Davis, 1983, p. 1).

Other definitions refer to etiology similarly (e.g., Goodglass and Kaplan, 1983). Etiology is omitted in the current definition on the logical grounds that the cause of a dysfunction does not comprise the dysfunction. Also, aphasia is a cognitive phenomenon, whereas stroke and traumatic brain injury are neurological phenomena. It is up to research to discover the site and type of neuropathology causing a dysfunction. Because aphasia is associated with focal lesion, etiology is a useful clue for confirming diagnosis of dysfunction but is not inherent to defining or diagnosing the dysfunction. A clinician assumes the burden of demonstrating language-specific disorder through examination of behavior.

Aphasia and Bilingualism

Half the people of the world use at least two languages. A florist in the United States may converse with family and friends in Spanish and, across town, speak with colleagues and customers in English. One day she suffers a stroke, and in the hospital her family discovers to their dismay that she can speak only English. How often does this happen? While many people are multilingual, let us make the topic more manageable by focusing on bilingualism (Grosjean, 1982; Hakuta, 1986).

Grosjean (1989) defined bilinguals as "those people who use two or more languages in their everyday lives" (p. 4). Grosjean objected to an apparent *monolingual* (or *fractional*) *view* that treats bilingualism as an exception and considers bilinguals to be like "two monolinguals in one person and that they can therefore be studied like any other monolingual" (p. 3). A legacy of this view is a tendency to classify speakers by comparing abilities in the two languages. A *bilingual* (or *wholistic*) *view* is that a bilingual person "cannot be decomposed into two separate parts. . . . Rather, he or she has a unique and specific linguistic configuration" (Grosjean, 1989, p. 6).

The language behavior of a "stable bilingual" varies according to the situation. When bilingual speakers converse with monolingual persons, bilinguals enter a **monolingual mode,** in which they deactivate the language not known by the monolinguals. When conversing bilinguals share the same two languages, the conversants enter a **bilingual mode,** in which they activate both languages and mix them in various ways (e.g., code-switching). An aphasic bilingual is likely to display different behaviors depending on the interactional mode necessitated by a clinician's linguistic status. Failure to consider the conditions in which multiple languages are evaluated has been one weakness in the study of aphasia's intrusion on the bilingual's linguistic skill.

Would aphasia not impair the use of all languages? Neurolinguists have struggled to piece together a picture of aphasia in bilinguals by reviewing cases reported over several decades. Albert and Obler (1978) acknowledged the extensive flaws in their retrospective and suggested that their data "cannot be taken to represent that which would be seen in a systematically tested population of polyglot aphasics" (p. 141). The data was published anyway. Each language seemed to be impaired, but the two languages appeared to differ in severity of aphasia in 80 percent of the cases. Albert and Obler were skeptical "because cases representing discrepancy are the more interesting to report" (p. 141). From another retrospective study, Paradis (1977) found that 41 percent of aphasic bilinguals seemed to have aphasia equally between the two languages spoken, which was twice the proportion reported by Albert and Obler. Paradis noted other studies reporting as high as 90 percent of patients having similar deficit across two languages. These studies have been characterized as being "primitive" (e.g., Solin, 1989; Zatorre, 1989), making it difficult to substantiate compelling conclusions about functional organization in the brain (Chapter 2), aphasia in the two languages (Chapter 4), and relative recovery of languages (Chapter 11).

Aphasia and Anglocentrism

Because the brain is a universal structure and strokes are probably the same across cultures, aphasia should be understood with respect to universal characteristics. However, aphasiology in the United States, which has been influential throughout the world, has been built upon what Bates and Wulfeck (1989) called an anglocentrism in which aphasia is understood with respect to its manifestation in English. Beginning in the 1980s, **cross-linguistic research** (or comparative aphasiology) has demonstrated that observations of aphasia differ depending on the language studied. Universal mechanisms of aphasia are determined through the comparison of languages.

Let us consider why aphasia could appear to differ according to the language impaired. In considering these differences, we begin to consider the nature of language use per se. A linguistic code enables a speaker to convey basic concepts, such as "who is doing what to whom." These concepts, called thematic roles, are conveyed through linguistic cues, such as word order, and grammatical morphemes, such as articles and inflectional endings attached to root words. A linguistic awareness leads a clinician to look for particular deficits in the use of word order or grammatical morphemes. English speakers rely a great deal on word order to signify the agent of an action, whereas other Indo-European languages rely on a much more intricate system of grammatical morphemes for constructing phrases and signaling thematic role. French distinguishes articles according to gender, whereas English does not. Italian and many other languages signify thematic role with the inflectional case-marking of nouns, such as accusative (i.e., object or recipient role) and dative (i.e., indirect object or goal). Abilities with grammatical inflection may be manifested differently in behavior due to differences among languages instead of differences among aphasias. The relatively recent emergence of cross-linguistic research may lead us to a deeper understanding of aphasia than has been attained by concentrating on one language (Bates, Wulfeck, and MacWhinney, 1991).

RELATED COMMUNICATION DISORDERS

The limited information in a definition can be expanded so that aphasia is more easily differentiated from other communicative disorders. Some of these other disorders involve language impairments that may not be diagnosed as aphasia. Any definition can be misleading regarding the realities of diagnosing many patients. As Brookshire (1986) observed, there are shades of gray in which aphasia does not always manifest itself as a demonstrable separation of one cognitive system from others.

Propositional Disorder

Aphasic persons may struggle to produce a word in conversation but can fluently say, "Whew! I can't say that one." The patient may produce an unwavering "eleven" when counting but cannot answer, "How many players are on a football team?" Unable to converse at all, patients still may curse when frustrated, offending nearby family until they understand that the profane eruption is unintended and driven by the forces of injury. The paradox of occasional fluency amidst aphasic inhibition has been noticed for over a century. It indicated that a lesion does not erase words from storage but, instead, is a problem with the manner of using the words that are stored.

The damage has been said to occur in the propositional or volitional use of language. Eisenson (1984) defined **propositional language** as "a creative formulation of words with specific and appropriate regard to the situation," as opposed to subpropositional forms, which "come 'ready made' or preformulated for the speaker" (p. 6). Aphasia allows for production of subpropositional or nonvolitional forms, including *automized sequences,* such as days of the week; *memorized sequences,* such as a prayer or song; *recurrent social speech,* such as, "How are you?" or "I'm fine"; and *emotional speech,* such as profanity embedded in an emotional outburst. Propositional deficit distinguishes aphasia from paralysis or other neuromuscular impairments affecting the speech musculature. The speech impairment, called **dysarthria,** impedes the mechanics used for subpropositional and propositional levels of language production.

Multimodality Disorder

When someone's name is just on the tips of our tongues, it is also just on the tips of our fingers. Similarly, aphasic difficulty with finding words is manifested through speech and writing, and the same patient has problems comprehending language through audition and vision. The aphasic person usually has clear difficulty in listening, reading, speaking, and writing. This feature of aphasia has been quite salient in the diagnostic criteria of speech-language pathologists, based on evidence from several studies employing comprehensive batteries of tests that assess each of the four modalities (Basso, Taborelli, and Vignolo, 1978; Duffy and Ulrich, 1976;

Schuell and Jenkins, 1961b; Smith, 1971). The multimodality deficit distinguishes aphasia from disorders specific to a sensory or motor channel, as suggested by Wepman's diagram (Figure 1-4).

Without sensory impairment, an aphasic person can hear speech and see print but may not understand either. This differs from **sensory disorders,** such as hearing loss, caused by damage anywhere along the sensory nerves to cerebral cortex (Figure 1-1). Other modality-specific disorders can occur without loss of sensation. These include disorders of stimulus recognition, a level of cognitive processing in which someone indicates that a stimulus is familiar. Impaired stimulus recognition is called **agnosia.** *Auditory agnosia* often refers to impaired recognition of nonverbal sounds (e.g., car horn, running water). *Visual agnosia* is impaired recognition through sight, in spite of an ability to see the stimulus. The possibility that a patient has visual object agnosia is a concern when testing object naming ability. *Tactile agnosia*, also called astereognosis, is the inability to recognize an object through the sense of touch and cannot be attributed to hemianesthesia (i.e., unilateral sensory loss). Diagnosis becomes demanding when a patient has aphasia plus modality-specific impairments of sensation or recognition.

Even when an aphasic person produces the wrong word or a confusing sentence, speech is often fluid and well-articulated. Aphasia may not be accompanied by **motor disorders,** caused by damage along neural pathways from cerebral cortex to the muscles used for speech and gesture (Figure 1-1). **Dysarthrias** are neuromuscular impairments of speech involving weakness or rigidity of movement. Speech may be slowed or slurred. Impaired programming of movement, called **apraxia,** can occur without neuromuscular deficit. *Limb apraxia* is an inability to perform an action on command when the movement can be performed spontaneously. That is, a patient fails to manipulate a knife and fork when instructed to do so but later uses them easily when eating. Limb movement is especially important when we consider gestural communicative capacities. *Apraxia of speech* impairs the organization of movement for speaking in spite of an intact neuromuscular system. The co-occurrence of language and speech symptoms does not mean that both are part of the same disorder. Because of site of damage, a client may have aphasia *and* dysarthria or aphasia *and* apraxia of speech.

Multimodality deficit permits some general conclusions about the inner workings of aphasia. An early suggestion was that aphasia is a disruption of something "central" to modalities, so aphasia is often called a **central disorder.** Linguistic components provide a means of identifying centralized functions. Wepman suggested that aphasia occurs "in the arousal of a meaningful state, in the semantic process of word selection, or in the syntactic processes" (Wepman, Jones, Bock, and Van Pelt, 1960, p. 328). We rely on the same syntax for listening, reading, and speaking. Most aphasic persons have deficient comprehension *and* formulation, but investigators have started to wonder whether this depth of centrality is inherent to aphasia or present in all cases of aphasia. *Shallow centrality* of processes may exist across the receptive modalities *or* the expressive modalities. That is, some central processes may be used in formulation but not comprehension, so that an aphasic impairment could be isolated in formulation across speaking and writing. *Deep centrality* applies to any component that may underlie both receptive *and* expressive modalities. An aphasic person could have difficulties across the four modalities because of damage to a single deep mechanism or to multiple shallow mechanisms.

Sometimes uncommon cases provide key pieces to the puzzles of cerebral and cognitive function, and one remarkable group addresses the notion of central impairment. Researchers examined a small group of deaf persons who had suffered single strokes in the left or right cerebral hemisphere (Poizner, Klima, and Bellugi, 1987). These subjects were communicating with American Sign Language (ASL), which is expressed in a visuospatial mode and possesses grammatical features akin to spoken languages. We would figure that stroke in deaf persons does not differ from stroke in hearing persons; and the same may be said for some essential aspects of cognitive dysfunction. Subjects with left-hemisphere damage had disorders similar to the aphasias observed in spoken languages (e.g., lexical and grammatical deficits). Those with right-hemisphere damage did not exhibit language problems. The investigators concluded that "the left cerebral hemisphere in humans may have an innate predisposition for the central components of language, independent of language modality" (Poizner, et al., 1987, p. 212). The nature of aphasia should be compatible with language-specific impairment in ASL users and, thus, should be specified with a theory of cognition that can be compatible with transmission modes of any type.

A System-Specific Disorder

The centrality of deficit distinguishes aphasia from modality-specific disorders. Yet, there are other so-called central disorders. Someone can have a faulty memory for events that is revealed in speaking and writing. In thinking of memory, we could begin thinking about features of cognition besides the language system. The **assumption of modularity** proposes that cognition consists of somewhat independent large functional systems, such as a music system and a visuospatial system. Like the language system, these systems contain a specialized knowledge base and peculiar processes; and the fact that brain damage can impair one system but not others is evidence that modularity is a valid assumption (Fodor, 1983; Jackendoff, 1987). Clinical aphasiologists have distinguished between *verbal* and *nonverbal* behavior when characterizing different cognitive disorders. This broad distinction may correspond to differences among cognitive systems. The visuospatial system deals with objects, and the language system deals with words. Moreover, **generalized features of cognition** contribute to all of these systems, such as the ability to focus attention on information of any type or abilities to acquire and

retain information of any type. Theories of general and modular features of cognition provide the basis for understanding what "language-specific disorder" means as a definition of aphasia.

With a lesion in the right cerebral hemisphere, nonverbal functions seem to be impaired while verbal functions are spared. Deficits in spatial and musical abilities occur with **right-hemisphere dysfunction,** affecting artistic expression as well as orientation to everyday sights and sounds. A nonartist may not tolerate music on the radio. For a long time, physicians did not refer these patients to speech-language pathologists, because patients exhibit impressive language skills, especially in the lexical and syntactic features of sentence production. Because "language" has been associated with words and sentence structure, diagnosis is seldom language disorder after right-hemisphere stroke. Yet, some of these patients "miss the point" of metaphors, proverbs, and jokes; and they "wander from the point" when telling a story. These examples of language behavior have been associated with the *pragmatics* of language use and the *discourse* level of language. Researchers have become quite curious about the impression that damage of nonverbal systems can lead to deviations of language behavior.

Some neuropathologies seem to impair generalized cognitive functions such as attention and memory. An immediate effect of **traumatic brain injury** (TBI) is a loss of consciousness for an hour or perhaps a month. Coma is considered to be the most severe form of impaired awareness or attention. Some persons with TBI are severely paralyzed and cannot talk. Others are nimble talkers who do not recall what happened in the morning and may be wildly distracted and fiercely agitated. Other neuropathologies sneak up on a person and gradually become worse over time. One of these is **Alzheimer's disease,** a progressive illness causing a range of changes in memory, reasoning, and personality known as *dementia*. A woman with this disease may not remember her husband's name but, unlike an aphasic victim of stroke, may not recognize him either. Earlier, this text noted disagreement over whether language behavior in dementia should be put into the category of "aphasia," and similar controversy accompanies the study of traumatic injury (e.g., Holland, 1982b). Analyzing dysfunction according to the verbal-nonverbal distinction has not been given enough conceptual foundation for us to understand the complexities of various neurogenic dysfunctions.

SYMPTOMS OF APHASIA

Aphasia is evident in verbal expression, and symptoms are delineated with respect to the units of language within sentences. We hear symptoms of *omission* and symptoms of *commission*, in which incorrect units are produced (e.g., substitution, addition). Another general classification reflects the underlying dynamics of a brain struggling with damage to one of its parts. *Negative symptoms* indicate that something is not working; an omission would be an example. *Positive symptoms* are assumed to arise from spared processes. These orientations to symptoms may be illustrated by the general category of **anomia** (also, *dysnomia*), which is a deficit in finding words and is the most consistent feature of aphasia. A patient may be just unusually slow coming up with words but occasionally does not produce the word. A symptom of commission occurs when a patient calls a watch a "clock." **Circumlocution** is a positive symptom of anomia in which, upon failure to retrieve a word, a patient talks around the word by defining it, describing a referent, or even making sound effects. Pointing to his wrist, a patient might say, "I wear it right here, and I tell time with it; mine goes tick, tick." Anomia is a vague notion, because word-finding problems appear in different ways.

Word-Finding Errors

Word substitution errors are called **paraphasias**. They are produced unintentionally, and patients may be surprised upon hearing these mistakes. Paraphasias differ according to their relationships to the intended word, but identifying the target can be difficult in discourse. Context may help, but types of paraphasia are revealed best when a clinician already knows the required word, such as when a patient is naming objects or reading aloud. A tendency to produce one type of error in these restricted conditions may be the basis for judgments about paraphasias in conversation.

The types of paraphasia introduce an analytical orientation to the examination of expressive behavior. **Phonemic paraphasias** (also *literal paraphasias*) sound like the correct word. Sounds are substituted, added, or rearranged. Goodglass and Kaplan's (1983) criterion is that more than half of the correct word is preserved. The error may be a "dictionary word" from the patient's language (e.g., "pike" for *pipe*) or a nonword (e.g., "kipe" for *pipe*) (Lecours and Vanier-Clement, 1976). These errors are produced in fluent sentences and are not the same phenomenon as substitutions from motor speech disorders: "the distorted pronunciation of patients with poor articulation does *not* come under this heading" (Goodglass and Kaplan, 1983, p. 8). **Semantic paraphasias** are real words but are similar to the target in meaning, such as "chair" for *sofa*, "sister" for *wife*, or "see the odor" instead of *smell the odor*. When there is no apparent semantic relationship to the correct word, the errors are called **unrelated paraphasias** (or *random paraphasias*). A patient speaks of "turnips" in the laundry. The strangest error is the **neologism**, which is not a recognizable word from a patient's language. We can recognize a neologism most easily when it does not bear a phonemic similarity to the correct word. A patient asks for a "pinwad" or a "ferbish." Someone may call a comb a "planker" and even insist by spelling "p-l-a-n-k-e-r!" A neologism may strike us as an invention, but it is not produced with the intentionality of invention.

The nature of errors is one type of observation that leads to making an hypothesis about the cognitive impairment, but monosyllabic words can be especially ambiguous in this regard. Should an error be called a phonemic or unrelated paraphasia (e.g., "pike" for *pipe*)? The label is important because it carries implications for whether the disorder is identified with phonological or semantic processes. One of Goodglass and Kaplan's patients said "hike" and then "pike" on the way to saying *pipe,* which seemed to be a resolving phonological process. We may be quite properly ambivalent about whether one particular error is phonemic or neologistic. Someone might say "spork" for *spoon* and *fork,* an error that Eisenson (1973) called a neologism but one that Lecours and Vanier-Clement (1976) would have called a "phonemic telescopage." The ambiguities are perplexing, but clinicians rarely rely on single instances for making generalizations about a patient's expression. A paraphasia usually occurs with others, and a tendency to produce one type of error may lead to a decision about the ambiguous ones.

Problems with Sentence Production

Some symptoms can be observed only when a patient tries to produce a sentence so that we can evaluate linguistic features pertaining to grammar. In a category of omissions called **agrammatism,** certain types of words drop out of an utterance. A sentence such as *The girl was chasing a boy into the house* becomes "Girl chase boy house." Because English listeners use word order to figure out who does what to whom, they are likely to assume that the girl is chasing. The omitted words are **grammatical morphemes,** and these morphemes include closed class or function words (e.g., articles and verb auxiliaries) and inflectional endings such as *-ing.* Content or open class words are produced so that utterances sound like a telegram or "telegramese" (Gardner, 1974). Linguists are fascinated by this assault on syntax, and worldwide investigation includes cross-linguistic studies that are forcing modification of the traditional view of agrammatism. In highly inflected languages (e.g., Italian, German), a problem with grammatical morphemes is manifested in substantial substitution errors, not just omissions. Also, articles in German carry more information than articles in English; and this seems to be a reason for a 70 percent omission rate in English but only a 15 percent rate of omission in German (Bates, Friederici, Wulfeck, and Juarez, 1988). Thus, agrammatism appears to be a problem in producing grammatical morphemes, but the nature of this problem varies with the language.

Jargon makes little sense. Its flow, length, and structure have the appearance of normal prosody and grammar; but it is detached from meaning in a way not heard in agrammatic utterance. Jargon is stocked with paraphasias and is informally portrayed as word salad or gibberish. It seems to be the opposite of agrammatism (Table 1–1). Two kinds of jargon are recognized based on the paraphasias dominating utterances. A predominance of verbal paraphasias is called *semantic jargon,* sounding like a confused version of the speaker's language. With respect to content words, *neologistic jargon* sounds like an idiosyncratic new language. Semantic jargon is thought to be a less severe deficit because of the predominance of dictionary words. In the response of Gardner's patient early in this chapter, we see a semantic jargon with occasional neologisms. **Paragrammatism,** or grammatical morpheme errors, is thought to be a feature of jargon. For example, between editions of their aphasia test, Goodglass and Kaplan (1983) changed terms from "extended English jargon" to "paragrammatism" and from "extended neologistic jargon" to "neologistic paragrammatism." However, omission and error may not be a valid differentiation of grammatical disorders. Lesser (1986) recommended that the agrammatic-paragrammatic dichotomy be suspended until linguistic analyses determine what is what. Others have argued that a paragrammatism does not exist apart from agrammatism (e.g., Bates, et al., 1991; Heeschen, 1985). In the late 1980s, notions about grammatical difficulties in aphasia were entering a period of transition.

TABLE 1-1 Traditional contrasting features of agrammatism and jargon.

	Agrammatism	*Jargon*
Utterance length	Reduced	Normal or increased
Content words	On target	Paraphasic substitutions
Grammatical morphemes	Omissions or errors	Occasional substitutions
Initiation and flow	Hesitant	Smooth
Prosody	Reduced	Seemingly normal

Other Attributes of Verbal Behavior

Sometimes the most severely impaired aphasic persons seem unable to say anything except for **stereotypic utterances.** These restricted forms come out involuntarily and are thought of as subpropositional. They may appear in any attempt to respond, as if they were the only language forms available. Stereotypes occur at the onset of aphasia and may persist for months "without apparent modification of their structure" (Alajouanine, 1956). A patient may produce a recurrent syllable, called *iterative stereotype* (e.g., "dee, dee, dee") or a *jargonized* or *neologistic stereotype.* A neologistic version was heard by the nineteenth-century neurologist Hughlings Jackson during a boyhood experience, sparking his interest in aphasia:

When quite a child on a seaside holiday, he lodged at a house where the landlady—as he discovered to his wonderment and awe—could say nothing but "watty." This unlikely disyllable was articulated with such a range of cadence that it could express a variety of emotions. Her laugh was merry and ringing, and when anything amused her she would say: "Watty, watty, watty" (Critchley, 1960, p. 8).

When stereotypy consists of dictionary words, a common example is the use of "yes" and "no" (often incorrectly) as the only verbalization. Another example is a phrase such as "down the hatch" or a vulgarity like "shit." Ask a patient his name, and he will reply with a vulgarity that clinicians become used to and family members learn to tolerate with understanding.

Perseveration is a common symptom of brain damage, defined as "the recurrence, out of context and in the absence of the original stimulus, of some behavioral act" (Buckingham, Whitaker, and Whitaker, 1979, p. 329). A behavior is repeated involuntarily and seems to occur particularly when a patient is fatigued or frustrated. In verbal behavior such as naming a series of objects, an object may be named correctly as "pencil," but then a cup is called a "pencil," a fork is called a "pencil," and so on. The patient seems to be stuck on a particular response.

VARIATION OF APHASIA

A brain is as unique as a fingerprint, and lesions vary widely in type, size, and location. This combination produces unique problems. Clinicians approach a language-impaired client as an individual with problems that have not been dealt with before. However, we tend to manage this variability by classifying individuals into groups, especially when clients share general features of impairment. Classification relies on measuring severity of deficit and identifying type of linguistic deficit.

Severity of Deficit

Severity of deficit is usually divided into three categories. In **mild** aphasia, comprehension deficit may be detected only with careful testing. A patient converses well, but an anomia still may annoy the most charitable listener. Expressive deficits may be so subtle that they are also hard to detect. Language disorder is conspicuous in **moderate** aphasia. A patient comprehends fairly well but does not retrieve many words and may produce telegraphic sentences. In **severe** aphasia, the deficit is pronounced in all modalities. Propositional expression is incomprehensible or nonexistent. A large brain lesion may leave a 55-year-old attorney able to say only "dee dee dee." Severity of deficit is usually compared among listening, reading, speaking, and writing. Each modality is tested with tasks at different levels (i.e., words, sentences, and paragraphs), and then proportion of errors may be used as a measure. In aphasia, modalities are impaired in a rank order that is familiar to clinicians. Expressive modes are more impaired than receptive modes. Graphic modes usually involve more errors than auditory-oral modes; that is, reading is more deficient than listening. When a suspected mild aphasia is not readily apparent in speech, it is likely to be evident in writing.

Type of Deficit

For over a century, aphasia has been subdivided into types of language-specific disorder because of impressions that patients can be grouped with respect to particular symptoms. Two broad forms are diagnosed according to parameters of verbal expression. In **nonfluent aphasias,** utterances are grammatically sparse, as in English agrammatism. Production may be quite effortful. **Fluent aphasias** present a seemingly normal utterance length and grammaticality. Words flow easily. Nouns are replaced by vague terms, circumlocution, or paraphasias. Lesions in an anterior region of the brain produce nonfluent aphasia, and posterior lesions produce fluent aphasias (see Figure 1–2). Taking a neurological perspective, some researchers speak of **anterior aphasia** and **posterior aphasia.** This "neoclassical" dichotomy differs from a traditional division of aphasias into sensory/receptive and motor/expressive forms. This input-output terminology has shifted to a division based on utterance char-

acteristics, partly because speech-language pathologists have long presumed that all aphasias involve receptive and expressive impairments (e.g., Schuell and Jenkins, 1959). Moreover, "motor" and "sensory" imply transmission disorder rather than a central disorder.

Clinical Syndromes of Aphasia

A recurring pattern of symptoms is called a **syndrome,** and the history of aphasiology is cluttered with systems for labeling patterns of aphasia. Benson (1979a) noted that "the resulting aphasic syndromes represent one of the most confusing aspects of the complex topic of language disturbance" (p. 57). The most common classification system in contemporary investigation is attributed to a research group in Boston (e.g., Goodglass and Kaplan, 1983). This system fits within the nonfluent/anterior-fluent/posterior dichotomy, and the syndromes are identified especially according to three key areas: comprehension, spontaneous verbal expression, and repetition when compared with spontaneous expression (Table 1–2). A syndrome may also be identified with respect to a key symptom. Some groups are now labeled in terms of the symptom being studied (e.g., **agrammatic aphasia**).

Amount of verbalization is reduced in nonfluent/anterior aphasias. In **Broca's aphasia,** named for a nineteenth-century French physician, agrammatism is the dominant feature. Auditory comprehension is slightly impaired, much less so than expression when linguistic levels are compared. This patient may also have the clumsiness in apraxia of speech intermingled with agrammatism. The patient is often a successful communicator because the few words produced represent some of the message, and our guesses about the message are within the patient's comprehension ability. **Global aphasia** is severe depression of language ability in all modalities. Patients can be alert and aware of their surroundings, and they can express feelings and thoughts through facial, vocal, and manual gesture. Speech may appear as verbal stereo-

TABLE 1–2 Syndromes according to the Boston classification system, with repetition compared with spontaneous verbal expression. (Salient features are in boldface.)

	Comprehension	Verbal Expression	Repetition	Other Names
		Nonfluent		
BROCA	Mild to moderate	**Agrammatic**	Agrammatic but better	Motor Expressive Syntactic
GLOBAL	Severe	Minimal Stereotypic	Equally impaired	
TRANSCORTICAL MOTOR	Mild to moderate	Nonfluent	**Less impaired**	Dynamic
		Fluent		
WERNICKE	Severe	Paraphasic **(jargon)**	Equally impaired	Sensory Receptive Semantic
CONDUCTION	Mild to moderate	**Phonemic paraphasia**	**More impaired**	
ANOMIC	Mild	Vague, **circumlocution**	Spared	Amnesic Nominal
TRANSCORTICAL SENSORY	Severe	Paraphasic	**Less impaired** (echolalia)	Isolation syndrome

types. **Transcortical motor aphasia** is a rare syndrome similar to Broca's aphasia except for a startling ability to repeat. The patient has "a stumbling, repetitive, even stuttering spontaneous output" (Benson, 1979a, p. 84). The patient may struggle to answer a question but repeat a 15-word sentence without missing a beat.

The fluent/posterior aphasias are a diverse collection of syndromes. The most severe form was named for Carl Wernicke, a nineteenth-century German physician. Wernicke's aphasia has been known by many other names, such as sensory aphasia, receptive aphasia, and jargon aphasia. The patient has poor language comprehension, produces jargon, and often lacks awareness of semantic or neologistic paraphasias. A patient may continue his muddled talking when it is his turn to listen. This apparent drive to talk is

called *press for speech.* Sparks (1978) described people with Wernicke's aphasia as having poor "therapeutic set," because they do not realize why they are in the presence of a speech-language pathologist.

Conduction aphasia is characterized by an impairment of repetition that is disproportionately severe relative to comprehension and spontaneous speech. Verbal expression is communicative but hampered by word-finding problems and, especially, phonemic paraphasias. Repetition can be good with single words and short, familiar phrases. With stimuli of increasing length and decreasing familiarity, repetition may collapse into a jumble that is never heard in conversation.

Anomic aphasia (or "amnesic aphasia") consists of mildly impaired language comprehension and fluent, syntactically coherent utterances that are weakened in communicative power by a word-retrieval deficit. Utterances are vacuous, with indefinite nouns and pronouns filling the void of content words. For example, an automobile buff explains how to drive a car:

When you get into the car, close your door. Put your feet on those two things on the floor. So, all I have to do is pull ... I have to put my ... I'm just gonna do it the way I'm thinking of right now. You just put your thing which I know of which I cannot say right now, but I can make a picture of it ... you put it in ... on your ... inside the thing that turns the car on. You put your foot on the thing that makes the, uh, stuff come on. It's called the, uh. ...

Ambiguities can be resolved with situational context and knowledge of the topic. When naming objects, these patients retrieve some words quickly or engage in elaborate circumlocution while trying to think of names for other objects. While comprehension is quite good, word recognition difficulties can be detected. The patient may retrieve a word and then for a moment fail to recognize that the word is correct. It might be helpful to keep in mind that all aphasic persons have "anomia" of some kind (the symptom), while only some have "anomic aphasia" (the syndrome).

In a sense, **transcortical sensory aphasia** is to Wernicke's aphasia what transcortical motor aphasia is to Broca's aphasia; it includes features of Wernicke's aphasia but also a remarkable ability to repeat. Echolalia, in which a person repeats a question instead of answering it, is a prominent feature. It is as if intact mechanisms of speech recognition and production have been "isolated" from intentions and meanings generated in the rest of the brain (Goodglass and Kaplan, 1983). Benson (1979a) and Kertesz (1979) considered *isolation syndrome* to be a separate disorder that is, according to Benson, a "mixed transcortical aphasia."

SUMMARY AND IMPLICATIONS

Speech-language pathologists deal with a wider variety of neurological impairments than they did a couple of decades ago. Dysfunction with head trauma, for example, often differs from the aphasic disturbances addressed in traditional speech-language pathology texts. The number of disciplines studying language disorder has expanded the nature of theory and research. Thus, we should not expect simple questions and simple answers if we take a comprehensive approach to the study of aphasia and related disorders. In wading through the clutter of terminology, we should remind ourselves of the basic domains in the arena of neurogenic communicative disorders. In the clinic, we can observe *behavior,* and we may wonder about underlying causes. We have focused on *neurological phenomena* to explain why a patient does this or that. We also wonder, whether we realize it or not, about the status of the mind or *cognitive phenomena* when we think someone has a problem with comprehension as well as attention and memory. When confronted with an investigator's brand of jargon, we should at least try to figure out when he or she is talking about behavior, the brain, or cognition.

Aphasia is an acquired disorder of the portion of the cognitive system responsible for language comprehension and production. An aphasic patient understands and remembers what he or she had for breakfast but has a hard time telling us about it. Neurologists use the presence of aphasia to diagnose injury in the language areas of the brain (Chapter 2). Symptoms are also indicative of disorders identified with respect to the cognitive bases for language functions (Chapter 3). Some patients have more problems retrieving nouns than producing sentences. Others have more difficulty producing sentences than retrieving nouns. Cognitive neuropsychologists use the presence of a symptom pattern to diagnose injury in a component of the language system or another cognitive system (chapters 4, 5, 6, and 7). Diagnosis has always been an inferential process. In modern clinical research, there is an increasing reliance on a theoretically explicit and empirically supported basis for determining behavior-cognition relationships, rather than relying on a common sense of what language comprehension or formulation might be like.

CHAPTER

2

FOCAL ETIOLOGY
AND LOCALIZATION
OF DYSFUNCTION

Why can a person have language abilities impaired with many aspects of cognition seemingly spared? Isolated dysfunction, called a dissociation, is possible because a focal lesion impairs a brain that is organized into functionally specialized regions. With aphasia, the lesion has occurred in the region specialized for language functions; eventually we should come to understand why a person can have much greater problems producing little function words than producing substantive nouns and adjectives. We should understand the relationship between two factors: *neuropathologies* that strike specific regions of the brain and the *functional specializations* of regions in the cerebrum.

STROKE

I was sleeping on a couch in the dining room, and I got up to go to the bathroom, and I had to come out one door and then sorta go around the kitchen stove to get into the bathroom. The bathroom was on the first floor. So when I was through going to the toilet, I went to get up and fell backwards. I don't know why, but I just did. Oh, previous to that, I mean going into the bathroom, I was sorta limping, that I had lost control of my left side. And my wife noticed it. Then when I fell backwards, she called the police station, and they came down and took me to Norwood Hospital.

A stroke or **cerebrovascular accident** (CVA) disrupts the flow of blood to the brain. CVA has been the third most common cause of death of people over age 45 in the United States, but several surveys have indicated that incidence of stroke has been declining due to preventive measures and lifestyle changes (Posner, Gorman, and Woldow, 1984). Nevertheless, in the United States, 250,000 to 500,000 persons annually will suffer a stroke, and about 1 million will be living with the effects of a stroke at a given time; "incidence of stroke increases geometrically with age and is primarily a disorder of aging" (Metter, 1986, p. 141). Surveys indicate that 20 to 33 percent of stroke survivors have aphasia shortly after their stroke, and 10 to 18 percent still have aphasia months later (Wade, Hewer, David, and Enderby, 1986). These figures allow us to estimate 50,000 to 100,000 new cases of aphasia resulting from CVA each year in the United States.

Blood Supply

The health of neurons is maintained by **metabolism,** the exchange of nutrients and "digestive" waste products between the circulatory system and neural tissue. The nutrients, including oxygen and glucose, are transported by arteries to the brain, and the brain's appetite is indicated by the fact that it uses 15 to 20 percent of the body's blood while taking up about 2 percent of body weight (Metter, 1986). Oxygen and glucose pass through the capillary membrane, cross an extracellular space, and then pass through the membrane of neurons. The cell transforms the nutrients into waste products, which are carried away through venous drainage. The capillary membrane (i.e., *blood-brain barrier*) is impermeable to many substances, which is of interest to pharmacologists who want medications to get to neurons through the arterial system.

Different degrees and patterns of deficit are related to site of damage in the circulatory system. The arterial system can be viewed with respect to three structural levels: cerebral arteries on the surface of the cortex, the origin of these arteries at the base of the brain, and arteries in the neck through which blood is pumped from the heart to the base of the brain. In the neck, the left and right common carotid arteries course upward and divide near the larynx, creating the internal and external carotids. The left and right **internal carotid arteries** proceed to the base of the brain where they are continuous with one of the arteries supplying nutrients to cerebral cortex (Figure 2–1). The left and right **vertebral arteries** are behind the carotids. They are held in place along the vertebral column and come together at the medulla where they

become the **basilar artery.** Branches of the basilar artery supply the brainstem and cerebellum.

The cerebral arteries originate in an arrangement at the base of the brain, anterior to the brain stem and called the **Circle of Willis** (Figure 2–1). It consists of small **communicating arteries** between the cerebral arteries. Central branches of the communicating arteries and main vessels of the cerebral arteries supply the posterior and anterior nuclei of the thalamus. Three cerebral arteries supply the cortical surface for each hemisphere, and their general location is sketched in Figure 2–2. The main vessel of the **middle cerebral artery** (MCA) runs along the Sylvian fissure and branches to most of the lateral cortical convexity (Figure 2–2a). A close look at Figure 2–1 shows that the MCA is continuous with the internal carotids at the Circle of Willis, just as the name of a street suddenly changes. The left hemisphere's MCA (or LMCA) nourishes regions essential for speech and language. The **anterior cerebral artery** is distributed mostly throughout medial frontal and parietal regions (Figure 2–2b). The **posterior cerebral artery** covers the medial surface of the occipital lobe and the base of the temporal lobe. It can be seen in the lateral view as reaching around the posterior portion of the occipital region (Figure 2–2a).

Ischemic Stroke

An **ischemic stroke** is an occlusion of an artery causing a reduction or cessation of blood flow. Aphasia is most likely to occur from occlusion of the middle cerebral artery or the internal carotid artery. The most common cause of occlusion is *atherosclerosis,* a proliferation of cells (i.e., blood platelets) along arterial walls and an accumulation of fatty substances (i.e., lipids) within associated connective tissue (Metter, 1986). Another factor that could lead to ischemic stroke is high cholesterol, which is too much fat in the blood (Shimberg, 1990). Atherosclerosis is an untreatable, "fixed" risk factor, whereas high cholesterol is a treatable risk factor.

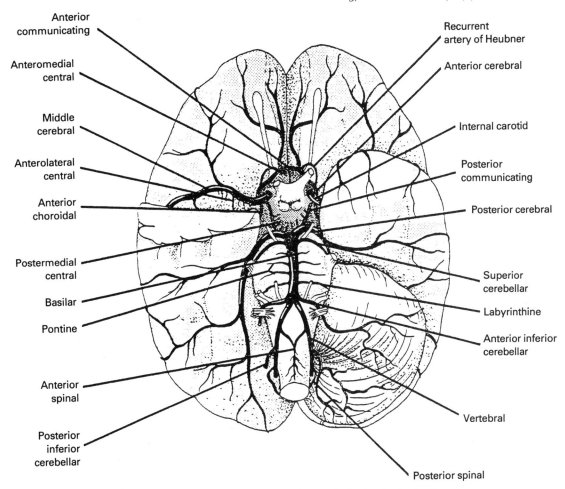

Anterior communicating

Anteromedial central

Middle cerebral

Anterolateral central

Anterior choroidal

Postermedial central

Basilar

Pontine

Anterior spinal

Posterior inferior cerebellar

Recurrent artery of Heubner

Anterior cerebral

Internal carotid

Posterior communicating

Posterior cerebral

Superior cerebellar

Labyrinthine

Anterior inferior cerebellar

Vertebral

Posterior spinal

FIGURE 2–1 The blood supply at the base of the brain, including the Circle of Willis. (Reprinted by permission from Barr, M.L. & Kiernan, J.A., *The human nervous system* (Fourth Edition). Philadelphia: Harper & Row, 1983, p. 362.)

Types of Ischemia. Two types of ischemic CVA produce similar clinical characteristics but result from somewhat different processes. Most strokes are a **thrombosis,** which occurs from accumulation of atherosclerotic platelets and fatty plaque on the vessel wall *at the site of occlusion.* Thrombus formation may take minutes or weeks to clog an artery. Dysfunction arises suddenly and increases in severity over minutes, hours, or even days during the final stages of accumulation. This *stroke-in-evolution* (or "progressing stroke")

may proceed in a step-wise fashion, and maximum deficit is referred to as *completed stroke.* There is higher incidence of thrombosis among people with diabetes mellitus and hypertension (or high blood pressure) than in the general population.

A frequent signal of impending thrombosis is the *transient ischemic attack* (TIA), or "little stroke." TIAs are temporary disruptions of blood flow that produce transient neurological signs indicating that platelet formation is underway, generally in the internal

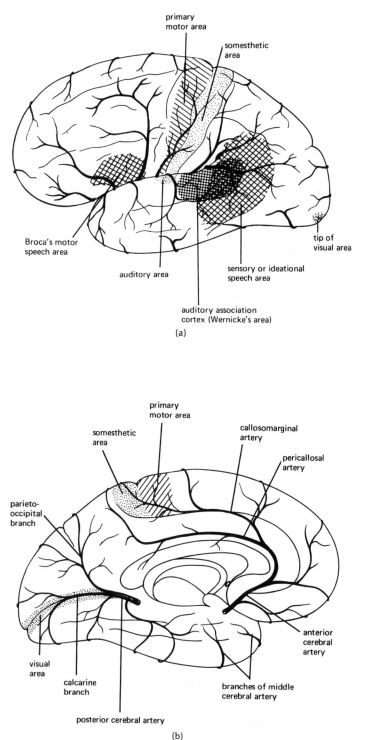

(a)

(b)

FIGURE 2–2 Distribution of the three cerebral arteries to the (a) lateral and (b) medial surfaces of the brain are shown relative to functional areas for speech and language (also see Figure 3–1). The lateral view primarily depicts the middle cerebral artery. (Reprinted by permission from Barr, M.L., *The human nervous system.* Hagerstown, Md.: Harper & Row, 1974)

carotid artery. A TIA is experienced as blurring of vision, numbness or weakness on one side, speech difficulty, imbalance or unsteadiness of gait, or a combination of these. The event frequently lasts a few minutes, usually less than an hour, but is defined as completed within 24 hours. There is about a 20 percent chance of suffering a stroke during the first year after TIAs begin and a 30 to 60 percent chance within five years (Metter, 1986). Thrombosis can be delayed or avoided with anticoagulants prescribed judiciously. Surgery to clear a carotid artery (i.e., endarterectomy) may be performed as a preventive measure, but its effectiveness has been questioned.

Whereas sites of origin and occlusion are the same in thrombosis, these sites differ with an **embolism.** With embolism, platelets and fatty plaque break off a vessel wall and then travel until they become stuck in a smaller cerebral artery. The heart is the most common source of embolic material, and medical history is likely to include cardiac disease. Embolism may also be a secondary effect of trauma. Clinical onset differs from thrombosis because time for occlusion is quicker or more abrupt, resulting in time to maximum deficit taking seconds or minutes. Thus, stroke-in-evolution is less frequent. There are usually no warnings, although TIAs may occur when an embolus originates in arteries of the neck. Often, however, physicians are unable to determine whether ischemia is thrombotic or embolic, so that they may refer to *thromboembolic* CVA in a medical report.

Infarction. When metabolism is prohibited for about two minutes, the result is death (**necrosis**) of neural tissue. The necrotic tissue is called an **infarct,** and a physician may refer to this effect of ischemia as a "thromboembolic infarction." Damaged tissue softens and liquefies; this waste is removed, probably by the astroglial cells that are supportive of neurons. Waste removal is called *gliosis,* which leaves a cavity in cortex looking like a crater on the moon. Astrocytes form a rim of scar tissue around the cavity. An in-

farct may be avoided by a *collateral circulation,* which redistributes blood through alternate routes, especially in the Circle of Willis (Figure 2–1). However, this possibility is often prohibited in persons with communicating arteries narrowed by vascular disease.

Clinical and Physiologic Phases. A speech-language pathologist's first contact with a thromboembolic patient may be at bedside soon after admission to the hospital. During this **acute phase,** the physician's main concern is the patient's survival. The patient is confined to bed with feet slightly elevated for a few days to avoid rapid lowering of blood pressure during stroke-in-evolution. Patients with swallowing problems are nourished with intravenous fluids. Within 24 to 48 hours after completed stroke, physical exercises are started a few times per day to prevent muscle contractures. Self-care activities are started for psychological and physical well-being. Anticoagulants may be administered to prevent another episode. Inside a patient's head during the acute period, a swelling of surrounding tissue develops because of accumulation of water. This *edema* takes a few days to reach its peak and takes one or two more weeks to subside. Also, a *reduction of blood flow* (or **hypoperfusion**) occurs in both hemispheres following a single occlusion. Flow to the uninfarcted side was found to improve dramatically within two or three weeks after onset (Meyer, Shinohara, Kanda, Fukuuchi, Ericsson, and Kok, 1970). Edema and reduced blood flow are likely to cause severe generalized deficits for most patients. This temporary suspension of functions that depend on structures remote from the infarct has been called *diaschisis.*

After three weeks or so, the pattern of dysfunction attributed to the infarction begins to emerge from the haze of edema and blood flow reduction. At this point, the **chronic phase** begins, and long-term rehabilitation is planned. Speech-language pathologists often delay their first comprehensive examination until medical stability is established and the specific disorder is apparent. Because neural tissue in the cortex does not regenerate, the infarct presents a permanent neurological condition. For a long time, we figured that dysfunction is caused by the size and location of infarction, but we suspected that damaged tissue would reduce the efficiency of nearby regions. Studies of cerebral metabolism support a more complex picture of ischemic pathophysiology because of **remote effects** some distance from infarction (Metter, 1986, 1987). For years beyond the period of diaschisis, reductions of metabolism (called *hypometabolism*) remained in regions where blood still flowed. For example, with an infarct in left cortex around the Sylvian fissure, hypometabolism was detected in adjacent and distant cortex of the same hemisphere and in subcortical regions. Hypometabolism is indicative of extensive hypoperfusion of blood flow, creating what is called an *ischemic penumbra*, or a flow that is insufficient for normal operation of structurally intact neurons (e.g., Olsen, Bruhn, and Oberg, 1986). A patient's chronic symptom pattern may be attributed to tissue damage and these remote effects.

Hemorrhage

Dr. K. begins to talk, I hear almost nothing after the words "brain hemorrhage." . . . My mouth hangs open, and my respiration comes in percussive bursts, like a cap gun. Each breath pokes the fingertip of this new danger into my ribs, and hurts. My eyes work the shadows, I can't meet Dr. K.'s gaze. . . . I imagine a navy-blue baseball jacket with a gold team patch, the one I wore as a clumsy teen to make me feel pride. This isn't like me to be so sick . . . (Fishman, 1988, pp. 65–66).

While in a hotel lobby in Nicaragua, journalist Steve Fishman's vision suddenly became fuzzy and undulating, and then an arcing pain pounded in his head with each heartbeat. Later he wrote a book about his experiences, including his neurological evaluations and neurosurgery. In mechanical terms, a hemorrhage is a bursting artery that causes blood to flood the brain's surface or invade brain tissue. The accumulation, called a *hematoma,* is a rapidly expanding mass that displaces and compresses adjacent structures. Common early symptoms include excruciating headache, nausea, and vomiting, which may precede loss of consciousness or cognitive impairment. Hemorrhage is associated with hypertension, aneurysm, or arteriovenous malformation; it also accompanies traumatic brain injury.

Typology is established with respect to location. An **intracerebral hemorrhage** invades regions of the thalamus, internal capsule, and lenticular nuclei (Figure 2–3). About half of these cases lose consciousness in minutes to hours after rupture, which may be precipitated by a sudden increase of blood pressure during physical activity or emotional stress. Branches of the Circle of Willis and basilar artery are most susceptible. Medication reduces edema and blood pressure, and surgical evacuation of the hematoma is possible in some areas. **Subarachnoid hemorrhage** occurs in the pia-arachnoid space surrounding the brain and can be caused by a ruptured aneurysm near the Circle of Willis. An **aneurysm** is a dilated blood vessel, ranging in size from that of a pea to an orange, that stretches and weakens the vessel wall (Chusid, 1979). Rupture of an aneurysm may be provoked by sudden physical exertion but can be prevented by surgery when the dilation is accessible. Procedures include "trapping" the reservoir by applying clips on both sides, clipping the neck of the bulge, or packing muscle around the aneurysm. Plastics may be sprayed on the dilation and surrounding vessels.

Arterial walls are also weakened in the condition of **arteriovenous malformation** (AVM), in which the capillary network between arteries and veins is absent. Vessels are twisted and tangled. It may occupy a tiny area or an entire hemisphere. Presumably a congenital condition, presence of AVM may not be signaled until hemorrhage or seizures occur in adulthood. Bleeding occurs in the subarachnoid space. A hemorrhaging AVM is usually less damaging than a bursting aneurysm.

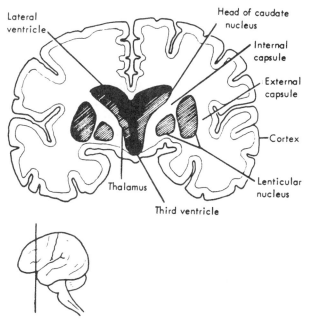

Lateral ventricle

Head of caudate nucleus

Internal capsule

External capsule

Cortex

Thalamus

Lenticular nucleus

Third ventricle

FIGURE 2–3 Frontal (coronal) section of the cerebrum shows location of the layer of cortex and certain interior structures. (From Willard R. Zemlin, *SPEECH AND HEARING SCIENCE: Anatomy and Physiology,* ©1968, pp. 466, 469. Reprinted by permission of Prentice-Hall, Inc., Englewood Cliffs, N.J.)

TUMOR

A **tumor** (neoplasm) is an abnormal mass of tissue. Benign tumors do not spread to other parts of the body and are not recurrent. Malignant tumors expand uncontrollably and are resistant to treatment. They not only press against adjacent tissue but also invade and destroy surrounding tissue and may obstruct circulation. Cancerous cells may infiltrate widely before destroying a vital region of brain tissue, and early symptoms of malignant neoplasms usually are quite general reductions of function. Headache is one of the earliest signs, precipitated by stopping, straining, or exercising. Nausea and vomiting are common. Sensory impairments and dulled mental function may occur; and, if the tumor is allowed to enlarge, impairment may evolve to stupor and coma. Specific dysfunctions depend on location of the tumor and may include loss of vision and hearing when there is pressure on the optic and acoustic cranial nerves. Neoplasms are classified according to their tissue origin.

A common source of neoplasm is supportive cells throughout the CNS. Called **glial** cells, or neuroglia, they are attached to nerve cells and axons but are not involved directly in the transmission of neural impulses. Cited in discussion of metabolism, star-shaped *astroglia* (astrocytes) hold neurons in place in addition to their housekeeping function. *Oligodendroglia* are responsible for producing and maintaining a myelin sheath that surrounds many axons. **Astrocytomas** originate in astroglia, and several grades of malignancy can be determined based on rate of cell growth, differentiation of cell types, and number of abnormal cells. *Astrocytoma grades 3–4* (also, *glioblastoma multiforme* or malignant glioma) is the most common primary brain tumor in adults. Peak incidence is between 45 and 55 years. A **glioma** is a rapidly growing mass likely to infiltrate both hemispheres through the commissures. Survival is about one year. Surgeons may report "gross total removal of the tumor," but it will usually recur in months (Weiss, 1982). *Astrocytoma grades 1–2* (low-grade astrocytoma) and *oligodendrogliomas* are much less common but have a more favorable prognosis. They expand slowly, and symptoms may appear years before the tumor is discovered. The preferred treatment is surgery: craniotomy (i.e., opening the skull) followed by the resection of tissue. Complete removal is seldom accomplished. However, repeated surgery can be beneficial when the neoplasm is accessible. Prognosis after surgery has been reported variably at three to six years.

Meningioma is a benign tumor arising from the arachnoid tissue covering the brain. After glioblastoma, it is the second most common primary brain tumor in adulthood, with peak incidence in the 30s and 40s. Unlike other tumors, it occurs more frequently in women than men. Fifty percent occur over the lateral surfaces, and 40 percent occur at the base of the brain. Meningiomas grow slowly and usually do not invade cortex. Complete removal is often possible. This makes prognosis generally favorable, with prolonged survival being a frequent outcome of surgery. Recurrence is possible in a small proportion of cases.

PROGRESSIVE ETIOLOGY

Malignant neoplasm does not have the sudden impact of an embolism, but the traditional view of focal etiology for language-specific disorder is expressed in the following remark: "we believe aphasia in adults does not creep, it erupts" (Rosenbek, et al., 1989, p. 53). However, discovery of a so-called **progressive aphasia** indicates that a creeping aphasia may occur (Duffy and Peterson, 1992). Having associated progressive neuropathology with dementia, speech-language pathologists wonder if aphasia is being diagnosed when language is not the only area of deficit (i.e., the broad definition discussed in Chapter 1). Yet, a few patients have a language-specific disorder that is first observed as a mild and specific deficit that deteriorates and expands to additional language functions. These cases are labeled as having aphasia without dementia (e.g., Kirshner, Tanridag, Thurman, and Whetsell, 1987). One of these cases was described by Northen, Hopcutt, and Griffiths (1990). The patient started with effortful spontaneous speech and 51/60

on a naming test and then evolved over two years into a person with deficits of comprehension and very limited verbal expression. Nonverbal capacities were intact. Brain imaging showed increasing atrophy of structures in the left hemisphere along with dilation of left ventricles. Two years after initial diagnosis, metabolic studies revealed reductions in the left hemisphere and normal uptake in the right hemisphere. Several months later, brain imaging began to expose changes in the right side. The neuropathology was unknown. Unilateral atrophy has been seen regularly in the cases reported.

NEUROLOGICAL DIAGNOSIS

The neurologist can examine the basic status of sensory, motor, and cognitive systems in about 30 minutes. In addition to determining if someone's problems are caused by neurological dysfunction, the physician wants to determine the nature and site of damage. Radiological tests may confirm and elaborate preliminary diagnosis based on the neurologist's quick examination. Then, the neurologist orders referrals to rehabilitative specialists so that impairments can be evaluated more thoroughly.

Neurological Examination

A patient's alertness indicates the status of the reticular activating system. An initial interview yields clues about cognition. A stethoscope is pressed lightly to each temple in an examination of circulation called *auscultation*. The neurologist listens for unusual sounds in the arteries, which are called *bruits*. Systematic examination begins with motor and sensory systems at different functional levels to assess the peripheral and central nervous systems. Simple reflexes are tapped from head to toe, with *hypoactivity* indicating peripheral damage and *hyperactivity* indicating central damage. Balance and coordination are indicative of cerebellar function. Loss of sensation on one side is called *hemianesthesia,* and paralysis on one side is called *hemiplegia*. Left and right sides are compared, with the normal side being a standard for estimating severity of unilateral impairment. Motor and/or sensory impairment of one side signifies damage to the contralateral cerebral hemisphere, and deficits of specific body parts reflect damage to particular locations along pre- and postcentral gyri.

Brain Imaging

Scientists have been amazing us with the development of increasingly safe, efficient, and accurate means of viewing someone's brain to determine the site and nature of damage. The results of a radiologist's examination can be found in a section of a patient's medical chart. Two techniques were used extensively in the 1960s and 1970s. **Angiography,** or *arteriography*, is an X-ray procedure for observing arteries in the head and neck. An invasive approach, it entails injecting a foreign substance into the arterial system. An iodinated opaque fluid is used so that the arteries can be seen on X-ray film. With an ischemic stroke, vessels cannot be seen beyond the point of an occlusion. Tumors or other space-occupying lesions are inferred from distortion of the arterial pattern. **Radioisotopic scanning,** or the *brain scan,* was used more frequently as a research and

diagnostic tool (Kertesz, 1979). Other names for this procedure included *isotope scanning, radionuclide scanning,* and *cerebral scintigraphy.* Though invasive, the brain scan was relatively safe; however, images did not provide a very precise rendering of lesion location.

Computerized tomography (CT scan) permits detailed imaging of cerebral structures through computerized reconstruction (Murdoch, 1988; Patronas, Deveikis, and Schellinger, 1987). First developed in England and announced in 1972, it "permits the clinician to perform a gross brain autopsy at any time during the course of an illness" (Oldendorf, 1978, p. 531). Scanners have undergone stages or generations of development, and a fourth-generation scanner is sketched in Figure 2–4. CT scan is relatively accurate and is safe and easy to administer. It uses narrow beams of X-rays on a single plane from a scanner that rotates around the head. Intensity of the X-rays is detected and sent to a computer, which transforms the data into absorption coefficients indicative of tissue densities. Results are displayed as tiny blocks of tissue, a "reconstruction" of the structures in a particular plane of the cerebrum. Images of several planes are obtained in about 30 minutes. Figure 2–5 shows locations of infarct as they might be found in a horizontal plane: **anterior** to the central sulcus (includ-

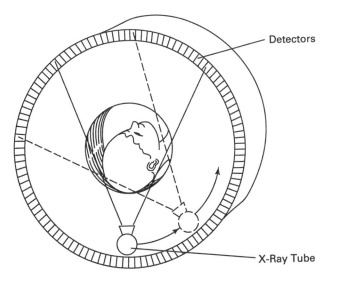

FIGURE 2–4 Schematic representation of a fourth generation CT scanner. An X-ray tube revolves around the body while emitting a beam wide enough to encompass the width of a patient. Stationary detectors measure the activity penetrating the body. (Reprinted by permission from Patronas, N.J., Deveikis, J.P., & Schellinger, D., The use of computed tomography in studying the brain. In H.G. Mueller & V.C. Geoffrey (Eds.), *Communication disorders in aging: Assessment and management.* Washington, D.C.: Gallaudet University Press, 1987, p. 110.)

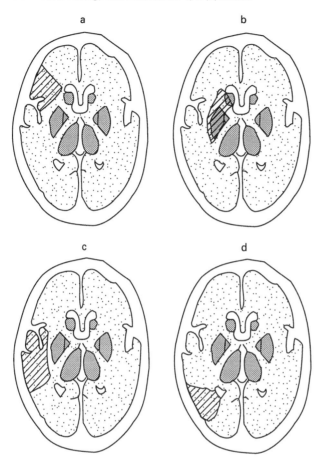

FIGURE 2–5 Four areas of infarction within the territory of the middle cerebral artery: (a) anterior, (b) deep, (c) medial, and (d) posterior. (Reprinted by permission from Habib, M., Ali-Cherif, A., Poncet, M., & Salamon, G., Age-related changes in aphasia type and stroke location. *Brain and Language,* 31, 1987, p. 247. Academic Press, publisher.)

ing the insula), **deep** in lenticular nuclei, **medial** (including posterior insula) and **posterior** invading the occipital lobe. Simple anterior-posterior classification may include this medial infarction in the posterior category.

The clinical value of CT scan lies in power of resolution of a lesion and detection of longstanding CVAs. Pathology is indicated by alterations in the normally expected densities of different brain structures. Infarct is shown as decreased tissue density, and hemorrhage is shown as increased density. Identifying an infarction can be improved with injection of a contrast material. Research showed that CT scan is particularly good at distinguishing between infarct and intracerebral hemorrhage (Gado, Coleman, Merlis, Alderson, and Lee, 1976). Methods for calculating lesion size and tissue density were detailed in CT studies of aphasia (Naeser, Hayward, Laughlin, and Zatz, 1981). Mazzocchi and Vignolo (1978) described a procedure for mapping lesions onto a standard lateral diagram of the brain and found satisfactory reliability among three clinicians. Sources of variability included standard diagrams that do not take into account the individual differences among human brains and clinicians' differing in their criteria for outlining an area of damage. Diagramming has been illustrated with aphasic subjects (e.g., Basso, Lecours, Moraschini, and Vanier, 1985).

So far, the clearest image of brain structure is achieved with **magnetic resonance imaging** (MRI), also known as nuclear magnetic resonance (NMR). This noninvasive procedure capitalizes on areas of high water density, such as the brain's white and gray matter. MRI cannot expose teeth and bones. The procedure is based on something called the "spin" of molecules within the nucleus of an atom. First, the body is placed in an area surrounded by a large electromagnet (meaning that persons with metallic implants cannot be assessed). It manipulates the spin of hydrogen molecules with the magnetic field and radio waves. Then, a computer creates a picture of the brain from the electromagnetic signals generated by this manipulation (see *National Geographic*, January 1987). The image shows sharp contrast between gray and white matter and detects a variety of defects. MRI is superior to CT scans in its sensitivity to subtle neuropathologies and its potential for early detection of diseases involving physiological changes.

FUNCTIONAL ASYMMETRY

At the start of this chapter, it was stated that someone can have a language-specific disorder partly because of the functional specializations of regions of the brain. Aphasia occurs because, for most people, one half of the brain is responsible for language functions. Aphasia, in turn, has provided evidence for this responsibility. Before 1965, researchers thought in terms of the "dominance" of the hemisphere that controls language. The left hemisphere (**LH**) was found to be "dominant" for most people, and the right hemisphere (**RH**) was considered to be "just a rather stupid spare for the left" (Galin, 1976). After 1965, the idea of dominance was replaced with an appreciation for each side's talents, a perspective conveyed in the more neutral terms of "specialization" or "asymmetry" (e.g., Beaton, 1985; Springer and Deutsch, 1989). The asymmetry has been viewed with respect to preferences for dealing with types of stimuli or types of response, and the difference between the LH and RH has been associated with a difference between verbal and nonverbal abilities. Many types of evidence have been brought to bear on ques-

tions of functional asymmetry, and one of the best known of these is the study of "split-brain" persons. Yet, no single method can provide definitive information because of the limitations of each, so investigators rely on accumulating *converging evidence* from many sources.

Some Sources of Evidence

The busiest experiment in neuropsychology is comparison between groups defined as left-hemisphere damaged (LHD) and right-hemisphere damaged (RHD). This is one example of the **lesion-deficit method** for determining normal cerebral function. The reasoning has been this: if a dysfunction is caused by damage to one place, then that site is responsible for that function in the normal brain. The dysfunction is identified as a **dissociation**, which is an impairment of one function while others remain intact or clearly less impaired. It is as if one function is separated from others indicating that the function is an independent system. Aphasia is said to be a dissociation of language functions from other abilities. This is the basic idea behind lesion-deficit studies of normal function.

Let us think some more about the notion of dissociation by supposing that RHD impairs drawing but not writing, tempting us to conclude that the RH is responsible for drawing as an independent function. This conclusion is flawed, however, because the evidence does not rule out the possibility that the LH also participates in drawing. What if damage to the LH causes a drawing disorder, too, or drawing and writing disorders? To examine this possibility, LHD is compared with RHD for drawing and writing. A **double dissociation** is thought to be a minimal requirement for localizing functions based on dysfunction (Glassman, 1978). A double dissociation is shown when damage to one region (e.g., LH) produces a deficit in one ability along with minimal difficulty in another ability, and damage to another region (e.g., RH) has the opposite effect. Let us suppose that RHD produces the deficit in drawing but not writing, and LHD produces a deficit in writing but not drawing. We may infer that the RH is responsible for an independent drawing function and that the LH is responsible for writing as a function that is independent of drawing.

A couple of other methods are employed less frequently. Neurosurgeons want to determine the side of language function before they perform surgery, and the **Wada test** is used for this purpose. An anesthetic, called sodium amytal, is injected into the left or right carotid artery, causing temporary "paralysis" of one hemisphere. Following the injection, a patient is asked to count, say days of the week, and name objects. Talking is impeded if the drug immobilized the speech hemisphere. Some patients have surgery to avoid brain damage, and study of the neurologically intact brain is a vital source of converging evidence for normal function, to say the least. An approach to functional asymmetry involves the use of *electroencephalography* (EEG), a record of electrical activity of the brain taken from the scalp. The *alpha-rhythm* is a component of the multi-rhythmic EEG and is dominant during quiet times such as sleep. It is attenuated during activity, and detecting **alpha suppression** became a crude means of comparing regions of neural activity while someone is doing something (Ornstein, Johnstone, Herron, and Swencionis, 1980).

Auditory Asymmetries: Speech and Music

Sounds are perceived in the primary auditory area of the temporal lobes (Figure 2–2). Regions surrounding primary sensory areas are associated with relating the stimulus to previously stored information (i.e., recognition). Differences between the hemispheres are seen when language is compared with music. Milner (1967) compared patients before and after temporal lobectomy, or removal of a portion of the lobe. Left temporal lobectomy resulted in reduced verbal recall and sparing of musical tone discrimination, whereas right lobectomy resulted in reduced

music discrimination and spared verbal recall. Sidtis and Volpe (1988) detected a double dissociation between RHDs and mildly aphasic LHDs. RHDs were impaired in pitch pattern perception but not speech perception, whereas aphasic subjects had difficulty with speech but not tones. In an earlier study, RHDs did worse than LHDs in recognizing music without commonly known lyrics, such as "Hail to the Chief" (Gardner and Denes, 1973). RHDs did worse than LHDs in detecting rhythmic errors in familiar musical pieces (Shapiro, Grossman, and Gardner, 1981). Eleven subjects, who imagined orchestras and choirs when the right temporal gyrus was probed with electrical stimulation, heard songs such as "White Christmas" and "Hush-a-Bye Baby" (Penfield and Perot, 1963). In a study of EEG alpha-suppression, the RH was more active for recognizing a Bach concerto than for reading the *Congressional Record* (McKee, Humphrey, and McAdam, 1973).

In **dichotic listening**, stimulus pairs are presented to neurologically intact adults through headphones, one item to each ear simultaneously. A subject may perceive stimuli in one ear better than the other, called a right-ear advantage (**REA**) or left-ear advantage (**LEA**). These effects are used to indicate that the contralateral hemisphere is favoring the type of stimulus presented. An REA has been observed for digits (Kimura, 1961), indicative of LH preference for language. The REA occurs most clearly and consistently in right-handers with pairs of stop-consonant CV syllables (Bloch and Hellige, 1989). LEAs (RH) have been obtained for chamber music (Kimura, 1964) and environmental noises (Piazza, 1980). Such results have been unreliable with repeated testing. One source of variability is an attentional bias caused by task instructions, an artifact that makes it difficult for the researcher to attribute an asymmetric result to dominant activation of a hemisphere (Bloch and Hellige, 1989). Dichotic listening also underestimates the high incidence of LH control of language in right-handed clinical cases (Springer and Deutsch, 1989).

Visual Asymmetries: Names and Faces

The visual system is not built in a contralateral relationship between sense organs and occipital lobes. Instead, contralaterality exists between fields of vision and the hemispheres (Figure 2–6). The system is understood with respect to relationships among the visual fields, the concavity of each retina, and pathways to primary cortex of each occipital lobe. The portions of each retina are designated as nasal (inner) and temporal (outer) retinae. Figure 2–6 shows that the left temporal and

FIGURE 2–6 The arrangement of the nerve tracts between the eyes and visual cortex of the brain, showing the basis for the contralateral relationship between visual fields and visual cortex. Information is also shared across commissural fibers. (Reprinted by permission from Ashcraft, M.H., *Human memory and cognition.* Glenview, IL: Scott, Foresman, and Company, 1989, p. 673.)

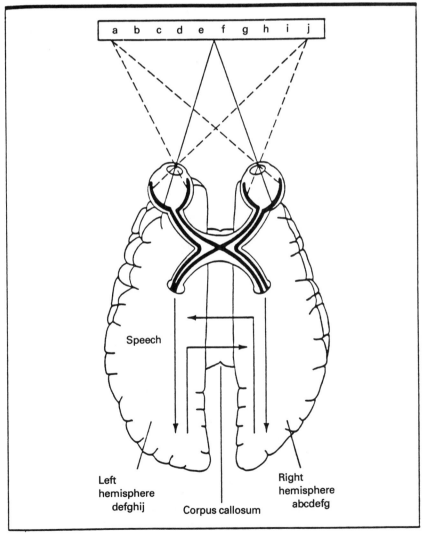

right nasal retinae "see" mainly the right visual field (RVF). The optic tracts from these retinae proceed to the left occipital lobe. The nasal tracts cross at the *optic chiasm,* and the temporal tracts proceed ipsalaterally beside the chiasm. Tracts proceed by wrapping around the brain stem, synapsing in the thalamus, and radiating to the cortex. Thus, the LH perceives *defghij* from the right field. Visual deficits are informative regarding site of neuropathology. Damage to the left optic tract between the left retina and the optic chiasm produces blindness of the left eye, leaving the right eye able to see both fields. Damage to the optic tract between the chiasm and the left occipital lobe causes blindness of the RVF. Unilateral loss of a field of vision is called **homonomous hemianopia.** Loss of vision in the RVF can occur with aphasia, because the optic radiation traverses the parietal and temporal lobes.

Study of "split-brain" persons takes advantage of the structure of the visual system (Gazzaniga, 1970). When medicine fails to manage seizures, a **commissurotomy** may be performed to separate the hemispheres so that seizure activity is confined to one side. Each side of the brain can be studied somewhat independently. A stimulus, such as a word or object, is sent to the LH or RH by presenting it to the contralateral visual field or tactile modality. The optic tracts are intact; the hemispheres are separated by a cut through commissural fibers such as the corpus callosum (Figures 2–6, 1–2). Through the 1960s, only single words could be presented to each field, because very brief exposure durations were used so that lateral eye movement would not confound results. Subjects were also asked to focus on a centered spot. Then, Zaidel (1975) developed an apparatus called the "Z-lens" which permitted presentation of stimuli for much longer durations and study of language at the sentence level. Results of studies over the years showed that the LH has superior comprehension of language but the RH can comprehend common nouns and verbs and sentences at the level of a four-year-old child. The LH was still better in processing words, and the RH

showed a preference for dealing with nonverbal visuospatial stimuli including recognition of unfamiliar faces (Levy, Trevarthen, and Sperry, 1972).

Neurologically intact subjects are studied with **hemifield presentation** (also *visual half-field paradigm* or *lateral tachistoscopic presentation*). Psychologists employed the "T-scope" widely to study visual processes, and Marzi (1986) believed that it became "wildly" used. Basically, a subject fixates on a central point, and a stimulus is shown to the left or right. Central fixation maximizes reception in peripheral regions of the retina. A confound from eye movement is minimized with a quick stimulus exposure of no more than 150 to 180 milliseconds. When as much as 800 milliseconds is used for increased stimulus complexity, eye movement is monitored. Stimuli are presented unilaterally or bilaterally, and different methods are employed for maximizing central gaze fixation. One risk is that an asymmetry in results may reflect an early retinal stage of processing rather than the cortical levels presumed to be studied (Sergent and Hellige, 1986). Another concern pertains to whether a person's **characteristic hemispheric arousal** may also make results appear to reflect preference for a specific verbal or nonverbal skill when actually the results come from an individual's tendency to orient attention (Levine, Banich, and Koch-Weser, 1988). Corballis (1986) remarked, "Studying hemispheric specialization with a tachistoscope may therefore be rather like exploring the ocean depths wearing snorkel and goggles" (p. 242).

The lesion-deficit data presented by aphasic clients showed that the comprehension of words could be impaired while object recognition remains intact. Aphasic people still recognize family and new acquaintances such as hospital personnel and fellow patients. This retained ability is attributed to sparing the RH. Hemifield presentation to normal adults has reinforced split-brain studies regarding RH-superiority for recognizing unfamiliar faces. Findings have been mixed with respect to familiar or famous faces (Levine, et al., 1988). Associating the

RH with visuospatial skills has become problematic, however. An expected left visual field (LVF) advantage for face classification occurred when a stimulus was exposed for 40 milliseconds, but there was no preference at 120 milliseconds, and an RVF (LH) preference at 200 milliseconds (Sergent, 1982). The LVF (RH) preference has occurred for upright faces and houses but not for inverted faces and houses. Moreover, this asymmetry occurred only for right-handers with a hemispheric arousal orientation to the RH anyway (Levine, et al., 1988). The idea of relating each hemisphere to simple categories of stimuli began to collapse. Later, let us reconsider the identification of abilities that distinguish the two sides of the brain.

Individual Differences

The lateralization of language-specific skills to one side of the brain is a well-established fact accounting for disorders and retained capacities of people with focal damage to one hemisphere. For most people, language is managed by the left hemisphere. For some, language function is managed by the right hemisphere, and for others, it may be managed bilaterally. Factors related to individual differences lead to improved controls in studies of normal cerebral function. In particular, researchers wonder if people who are left-handed, female, young, or bilingual possess bilateral distribution of abilities.

Handedness and Crossed Aphasia. There has been a sad mythology about a link between handedness and the lateralization of language functions. The myth motivated some teachers to rap the knuckles of left-handed students to force them to become right-handed. Left-handedness or "sinistrality" was considered to be bad if not pathological, whereas right-handed "dexterity" was thought to reflect a normal "dominance" of the left hemisphere (Springer and Deutsch, 1989). The laterality of language was believed to be so tied to handedness that pushing a left-hander to become right-handed was thought to lead to a reorganization of the brain into a "proper" asymmetry.

These beliefs have not been supported by the investigation of aphasia in relation to side of lesion and handedness of patients. Handedness is not directly linked to laterality of language in the sense that LH dominance causes right-handedness. With Wada testing, most right-handers have displayed language function restricted to the LH (95 percent), but left-handers displayed a varied asymmetry that did not even favor the RH. In fact, 70 percent of left-handers displayed LH dominance for language, with 15 percent having bilateral language and only 15 percent having contralateral RH representation (Rasmussen and Milner, cited in Springer and Deutsch, 1989). The 70 percent estimate for left-handers was substantiated by the proportion having aphasia after surgery in the LH (Penfield and Roberts, 1959). Ambidextrous persons are also a heterogeneous group. Many left-handers have aphasia after LH lesion, indicating that their language is in the LH anyway. Because there are more right-handed people, most clients with aphasia will have suffered LH damage. Left-handed people are more likely to have a different cerebral organization, and handedness may be a small clue in developing a prognosis, although the proportion of left-handers with bilateral representation of language abilities is rather small.

Right-handed aphasic persons are expected to have had a stroke in the left hemisphere. However, less than 4 percent of right-handed aphasic persons have **crossed aphasia**, in which lesion is in the ipsilateral or right hemisphere. Researchers wonder if these cases are indicative of either a *mirror organization*, which is a reversal of the usual asymmetry, or a more unusual functional organization (Brown and Code, 1987). Reviews of reported cases indicate that most classical syndromes are possible, which reflects a mirrored lateralization of language (Alexander, Fischette, and Fischer, 1989; Castro-Caldas, Confraria, and Poppe, 1987). A reversal of asymmetry for language was suggested by a CT and metabolic study of one case in which latent abnormality of the LH could not be found to account for aphasia with RH damage (Schweizer, Wechsler, and Mazziotta,

1987). Mirror aphasias and anomalous cases are possible, but the anomaly seems to occur with respect to disorders accompanying aphasia. Castro-Caldas found a higher incidence of nonverbal problems that usually result from RH damage in persons with LH language. These disorders include left-neglect and deficits in drawing that occur with constructional apraxia (see Chapter 7). On the other hand, the incidence of limb apraxia and oral apraxia was comparable to aphasia after LH damage. Thus, crossed aphasia indicates that rare reversal of language responsibility does not necessarily reflect a mirrored reversal of all cognitive functions. The RH still may possess some of its usual capacities.

Gender. Do women and men differ in the functional organization of their brains? The possibility that a difference exists has been supported mainly by comparisons of abilities that have been thought to be directed by one side of the brain or the other. Women have been measured to be superior in language skills, whereas men have been tested to be superior in spatial tasks (Springer and Deutsch, 1989). We can choose from two explanations. Is there a biological/neurological difference between men and women, or does the difference in abilities reflect a difference of environment (i.e., socialization)? Different brain organization was suspected when McGlone (1977) discovered aphasia occurring three times more often in males than females after LH stroke, but performance on nonverbal tests did not differ. The greater occurrence of aphasia in males was supported by Kimura (1983) but not in two other studies (DeRenzi, Faglioni, and Farrari, 1980; Kertesz and Sheppard, 1981). McGlone's study fostered a widely publicized theory of biological difference stating that language and spatial abilities are represented more bilaterally in females and, thus, are more lateralized to each hemisphere in males. This theory does not readily account for the difference in verbal and spatial abilities. An environmental theorist would argue that females are brought up to be more verbal, and males are brought up to be more spatial.

Dichotic listening, hemifield presentation, and brain wave measurement have been brought to bear on the question of neurological difference. Of course, bilateral stimulus presentations permit only inference about whether the brain is responsible for asymmetric behavior. Not mentioning DeRenzi's and Kertesz's studies, Springer and Deutsch's (1989) review of research led them to conclude that the hypothesized differences of lateralization are quite likely to be true. The verbal-spatial asymmetry emphasized so far in this text may actually be a peculiarity of maleness. In a study of specific EEG responses during word-reading and figure-matching, females differed from males but not in a way that suggests a less differentiated organization for females (Van Strein, Licht, Buoma, and Bakker, 1989). In consideration that other factors might be at work besides gender, the visuospatial skills of right-handed women were studied. Casey and Brabeck (1990) divided subjects into groups to examine two variables; namely, experience with spatial tasks and genetic predisposition for spatial ability estimated by familial handedness. Women with spatial experience and a genetic predisposition did significantly better than women without these attributes, indicating that both factors are important in determining spatial skill.

Age. Clinicians anticipate exceptions to LH language in persons who are left-handed or female. Variation in the distribution of cerebral functions may also be related to age. We can begin thinking about this factor with respect to development of functional specialization from birth. Lenneberg (1967) proposed that the cerebral hemispheres are equally capable of assuming language functions at birth and that one side gradually acquires control of these functions as children mature. Language functions were thought to settle into one hemisphere by puberty. This proposal was used to account for the rapid recovery of language by young children suffering focal injury to one side of the brain, assuming that the undamaged hemisphere is capable of taking on the language function.

This *plasticity* for assuming functions at an early age coincides with the general notion of a **critical period** in which a neural structure is susceptible to modification by certain environmental stimuli (Thompson, 1985). There may be a crucial period during which learning language, including a second language, is easier and faster. However, the idea of a critical period for second-language learning has been seriously questioned (Zatorre, 1989).

A level of specialization for language in one hemisphere may be present at an early age and may even be innate. At five months, infants have left-hemisphere EEG responses to speech (Molfese, 1977). REAs for speech in dichotic listening have been found in children at three years (Kinsbourne and Hiscock, 1977). Early lateralization was investigated with children who underwent cerebral hemispherectomy during infancy (Goodman and Whitaker, 1985). To manage epilepsy and severe behavioral disorder, the cortex of one hemisphere was removed at as early as one month of age, leaving the other hemisphere to develop cognitive capacities needed for adulthood. Dennis (1980a, 1980b) followed a few cases indicating that, by at least nine years of age, the RH developed equally with the LH in phonemic and semantic aspects of language use, but the RH was unable to assume syntactic abilities as well as the LH. These cases indicated that an infant RH can develop language that later achieves a verbal IQ over 90. They also indicated that lateralization for syntactic processing is present in early infancy and may actually be genetically wired into the brain. In another study, children with left or right congenital brain damage were compared with respect to later verbal and performance IQ scores, and pattern of deficit differed (Nass, deCoudres, Peterson, and Koch, 1989). RH lesions lowered verbal and performance IQ, but LH lesions depressed only performance IQ. This is difficult to explain with an innate lateralization of language capacity to the left.

Comparisons of aphasic syndromes in adults encouraged a **continuing lateralization hypothesis,** which stated that intrahemispheric specialization of specific language functions does not stop at puberty and evolves through adulthood (Brown and Jaffe, 1975). Frontal lobe location of formulation processes that are impaired in Broca's aphasia may be completed well before lateralization and concentration of the comprehension processes impaired in fluent, Wernicke's aphasia. This notion was supported by studies showing that persons with Wernicke's aphasia (mean age in 60s) were significantly older than persons with Broca's aphasia (mean age in 50s) (DeRenzi, Faglioni, and Ferrari, 1980; Harasymiw, Halper, and Sutherland, 1981; Obler, Albert, Goodglass, and Benson, 1978). A similar significant difference was found in a comparison between fluent and nonfluent aphasias (Code and Rowley, 1987). Focusing on patients examined within 48 days post onset, Kertesz and Sheppard (1981) did not find age differences among syndromes. Coppens (1991) reviewed this research and concluded that differences do not exist at one month post onset.

Multilingualism. An impression of differential language impairment in multilingual individuals fueled speculation that their lateralization of language differs from that of monolinguals. Languages could be stored in different locations, making one language less susceptible to a focal injury than another. From one retrospective survey (Chapter 1), Albert and Obler (1978) proposed that multilinguals possess a more bilateral representation of language function and, thus, greater involvement of the right hemisphere. Evidence included reports of incidence of aphasia after right-hemisphere damage that is higher in bilinguals than monolinguals and higher incidence of crossed aphasia in bilinguals. However, the evidence has been judged to be contradictory and based on selection biases (Karanth and Rangamani, 1988). Solin (1989) showed that researchers have misrepresented data on crossed aphasia to support theory of RH language in bilingualism.

Contradictions occur across experiments with normal subjects such as dichotic listening and hemifield stimulation (Vaid, 1983).

Inconsistencies "have been shown to be almost certainly the results of methodological, analytical, and conceptual shortcomings" (Zatorre, 1989, p. 143). The prevailing opinion is that languages of bilinguals are maintained in the LH and, thus, the RH does not support the use of language in any way that differs from monolinguals (Mendelsohn, 1988; Paradis, 1990). When the Wada test was given to bilinguals prior to neurosurgery, a brief "aphasia" followed amytal injection to the LH but not the RH (Bertheir, Starkstein, Lylyk, and Leiguarda, 1990; Rapport, Tan, and Whitaker, 1983). However, the languages "recovered" differently during the minutes after injection, indicating that languages may be positioned somewhat differently within the LH. Springer and Deutsch (1989) concluded that "the nature of the relationship between hemispheric asymmetry and bilingualism is clearly complex. As a result, the controversy surrounding this issue is likely to continue until reasons for the variation from study to study are identified and explained" (p. 246).

LOCALIZATION FOR APHASIAS AND LANGUAGE FUNCTIONS

In discussing lateralization of function, this chapter has dealt with language as one monolithic function. Yet, language use involves several skills, such as listening, reading, speaking, and writing. Now let us turn to the problem of localizing more specific functions within a hemisphere, and let us bow to the majority by thinking of language as being represented in the left hemisphere. We shall begin with site of lesions responsible for aphasic syndromes. Lesion-deficit logic utilizes syndromes and CT scans for inferring sites of functions in the undamaged brain. Then, additional new methods will be introduced as we consider detection of cortical activation with PET scans while a neurologically intact person performs a task. The convergence of these sources of evidence should be of interest. The lesion-deficit method, in particular, began long ago when

investigators thought of "faculties" rather than functions.

Historical Perspective

Distribution of faculties in the brain was contemplated when even the appearance of materialistic explanation of the human spirit was rejected by church-guided authorities (Chapter 1). Early in the 1800s, Franz Gall traveled to a tolerant Paris to escape the Austrian Kaiser's wrath, because Gall was relating traits such as pugnacity and love of wine to areas of the brain. People with a quarrelsome disposition were assumed to have large pugnacity cortex. Based on a "science" called *phrenology*, Gall would detect the most enthusiastic wine lovers or those with strong "alimentariness" by feeling bumps on their skulls. Physicians, however, were looking forward to serious proof that human faculties could be localized in cerebral matter.

In an incident reported in 1861, Paul Broca performed an autopsy on a patient with a dissociated speech disorder and discovered a lesion in a frontal region of left cerebral cortex (Broca, 1960). Broca's discovery was enthusiastically received by the medical community. In 1874, Carl Wernicke wrote of someone with severe comprehension deficit and a lesion in left temporal cortex (Wernicke, 1977). Medical journals filled with descriptions of specific disorders linked to sites of damaged brain. Physicians were convinced that these relationships indicated sites of normal functions. Journals published diagrams portraying cortical "centers" in which auditory, visual, spoken, and written images of words are maintained (Figure 2–7). Diagrams were used to predict the type of disorder resulting from an impaired center or connection, and this was the first basis for aphasia classification (e.g., Lichtheim, 1885). Bramwell's (1906) nomenclature for four types of aphasia corresponds to his word storage centers in Figure 2–7 (i.e., two sensory aphasias, auditory and visual; and two motor aphasias, vocal and graphic).

This approach did not escape argument. John Hughlings Jackson (1879), a British neu-

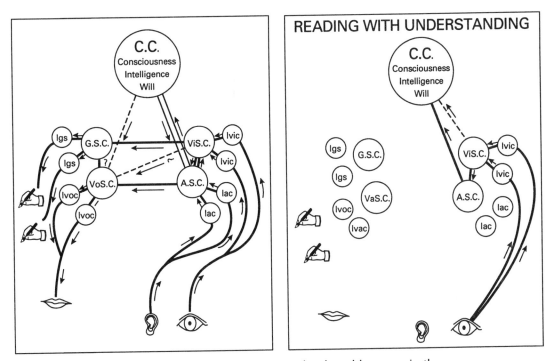

FIGURE 2–7 An example of diagrams developed by many in the late 1800s in order to portray hypothetical functional centers of the brain and connections between them. Bramwell drew several diagrams focusing on specific functions in which modality-defined information is related to higher cognitive functions such as "intelligence." (Reprinted by permission from Bramwell, B., A series of lectures on aphasia. *The Lancet,* 1, 1906, pp. 78, 354.)

rologist, wrote extensively that it was premature to locate poorly understood functions in a poorly understood brain. Yet, Jackson was largely ignored. Henry Head (1920) referred to "a veritable mania" by the "diagram-makers." Head's (1926) and Kurt Goldstein's (1948) clinical studies led them to conclude that damage to one function must affect other functions because of the interconnectedness of regions of the brain. Thus, it should be difficult to relate dysfunction to normal function in a straightforward manner. Diagram-makers were scolded for sloppy methodology, because they reported incomplete observations and focused on behavior selected to promote a theory. According to Goldstein (1948), a symptom pattern arises from the whole organism's adjustment to a deficient part. To simplify things for the textbooks, Goldstein's view was put into a holistic or antilocalization category. Camps "for or against" localization formed the landscape of aphasiology through the 1960s.

Locating the Causes of Aphasic Syndromes

Lesion-deficit method through the 1970s was modernized through improved imaging of lesions that could be identified near the time of comprehensive and standardized evaluation of behavior. The brain is clearly arranged into posterior sensory-integrative areas and anterior areas that direct motor pathways. In the left hemisphere, damage to these regions produces fluent and nonfluent aphasias, respectively (Mazzocchi and Vignolo, 1979; Naeser and Hayward, 1978; Yarnell, Monroe, and Sobel, 1976). The more specific syndromes of aphasia (Table 1–2) are assumed to be caused by focal LH lesions, and only a few of these syndromes are discussed in this section.

The Perisylvian Region and Global Aphasia. Only a portion of the LH is involved in language-specific functions, as shown with **cortical mapping** during surgery. Tiny electrodes are inserted into spots of cortex, and effects of electrical stimulation are observed while the conscious patient performs a task (Penfield and Perot, 1963; Penfield and Roberts, 1959). Stimulation has varied effects. For example, probing interferes with verbal behavior by acting "like a temporary, reversible lesion" (Ojemann, 1983) but it may also elicit a "sustained or interrupted cry" (Beaton, 1985). The procedure showed that language functions are concentrated around the Sylvian fissure or perisylvian region, excluding the precentral and postcentral gyri (Figure 2–8). The figure illustrates a shaded Broca's area and a posterior region that includes Wernicke's area as well

as other temporal and inferior parietal regions related to language. With cortical mapping, naming errors were elicited in Broca's area and posterior perisylvian areas (Ojemann and Whitaker, 1978).

When a CVA causes the severe deficits of global aphasia, brain scans and CT scans usually expose lesions covering the entire perisylvian region, including Broca's and Wernicke's areas (Kertesz, 1979; Mazzocchi and Vignolo, 1979; Murdoch, Afford, Ling, and Ganguley, 1986; Naeser and Hayward, 1978). Many of these lesions reach deep into white matter beneath cortex. A few cases have lesions confined to deep structures including the insula, lenticular nuclei, and internal capsule (Figure 2–3). An exception to pervasive perisylvian damage is an occasional global aphasia with Wernicke's area spared (Basso, Lecours, Maraschini, and Vanier, 1985; Cappa and Vignolo, 1988; Vignolo, Boccardi, and Caverni, 1986).

Broca's Aphasia. Area 44 in the Brodmann numerical system, or Broca's area, is located in the third frontal convolution immediately anterior to the precentral gyrus for distribution of impulses to the muscles.

SPEECH AREAS
EVIDENCE FROM STIMULATION

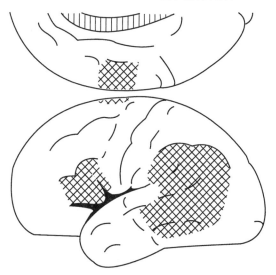

FIGURE 2–8 Areas of left cerebral cortex that are involved in verbal expression, as determined by electrical stimulation. Damage to these areas produces aphasia and/or apraxia of speech. (Reprinted by permission from Penfield, W., & Roberts, L. *Speech and brain mechanisms.* New York: Atheneum, 1959, p. 135. Macmillan, publisher.)

Partly because of its name, it was common to associate Broca's aphasia with damage to Broca's area. However, starting with Mohr's extensive literature review, it became evident that damage to area 44 and immediate surroundings produces apraxia of speech or "Broca's area infarction syndrome" (Mohr, Pessin, Finkelstein, Funkenstein, Duncan, and Davis, 1978). Chronic agrammatic aphasia is produced by lesions extending from Broca's area to the anterior insula and neighboring anterior temporal and inferior parietal areas. Small lesions restricted to area 44 can cause an acute Broca's aphasia that may resolve quickly into something else (Kertesz, 1979). Three cases were studied two days after onset, and lesions included insula and lenticular nuclei without much damage to area 44 (Murdoch, et al., 1986). Chronic Broca's aphasia usually involves damage to cortex and these deep nuclei, but sometimes this disorder appears to occur only with deep lesions (Mazzocchi and Vignolo, 1979). Kertesz (1979) stated "there is a spectrum of syndromes produced by Broca's area infarct. . . . The larger lesions produce the full-blown symptom complex of Broca's aphasia" (p. 187).

Wernicke's Aphasia. The syndrome of severe comprehension deficit and fluent jargon can be found with damage to Wernicke's area (posterior area 22) and neighboring temporal and parietal regions (Kertesz, 1979; Naeser and Hayward, 1978). On a CT scan, damage may look like the medial or posterior lesions of Figure 2–5 (Kirshner, Casey, Henson, and Heinrich, 1989). Often the posterior insula is involved (Mazzocchi and Vignolo, 1979), and in eight of 77 cases, some "pre-Rolandic" (i.e., frontal lobe) damage made the lesions look as if they should have caused global aphasia (Basso, et al., 1985; Kirshner, et al., 1989). Some researchers tried to distinguish among the expressive symptoms that may dominate in forms of Wernicke's aphasia (Chapter 5). A predominance of fluent phonemic paraphasias was related to damage in Wernicke's area and the inferior parietal area above, whereas verbal paraphasias were related to

damage in the more posterior angular gyrus and occipital area 19 (Cappa, Cavalotti, and Vignolo, 1981). Lesions causing neologistic jargon extended more posteriorly than lesions producing semantic jargon (Kertesz, 1981).

Conduction Aphasia. The idea of a "disconnection syndrome" is that a dysfunction need not result from a damaged functional center but can result from an impaired connection between structurally intact centers (Geschwind, 1965). **Association tracts** are white axonal fibers running beneath cortex and connecting one cortical region to another within a hemisphere. The **arcuate fasciculus** is the tract that sends impulses from Wernicke's area to Broca's area. This connection enables us to repeat and is thought to be damaged in conduction aphasia. CT scans of individuals with this repetition disorder show damage to posterior superior temporal cortex and inferior parietal cortex (i.e., supramarginal gyrus) along with infarction of deep white matter consistent with prediction of damage to the arcuate fasciculus (Damasio and Damasio, 1980; Murdoch, et al., 1986). As predicted by the disconnection theory, the posterior temporal damage does not usually impair Wernicke's area (Naeser and Hayward, 1978). Often the insula is damaged, too. Exceptions were noted by Mendez and Benson (1985), who examined three patients without lesions beneath cortex. Also, Kertesz (1979) speculated that two forms of conduction aphasia may arise, depending on whether the lesion is more anterior (a less fluent "efferent conduction aphasia") or more posterior (a more fluent "afferent conduction aphasia").

Inferring Normal Brain Function. Other aphasias have not contributed as succinctly to theory of brain function. When using the clinical syndromes as evidence for the distribution of function, researchers tend to identify a syndrome with a particular language function. That is, Broca's aphasia emphasizes deficient production so that the site of damage may be thought to be specialized for this function (Kertesz, 1991). Production is said to be somewhat separated from comprehension.

Pronounced receptive deficit and fluent speech implicates Wernicke's area for carrying out auditory language comprehension. With these areas connected by the arcuate fasciculus, Geschwind (1979) imagined a neural model of language production: "The underlying structure of an utterance arises in Wernicke's area. It is then transferred through the arcuate fasciculus to Broca's area, where it evokes a detailed and coordinated program for vocalization" (p. 187).

A linguistic version of specific faculties has associated agrammatism of Broca's aphasia with a "syntactic function" and paraphasias of Wernicke's aphasia with a "semantic function" (Chapter 5). Thus, comparison of Broca's aphasia and Wernicke's or fluent aphasia has been considered to be a means of investigating the possibility of a double dissociation between syntax and semantics that would assign each to its own cortical territory. Anterior and posterior sites in the LH have been compared. Broca's aphasia has represented a syntactic disorder that is much greater than any problem with semantics, whereas Wernicke's aphasia has represented the reversed problem. As a review of cerebral specializations discussed so far, characterizations of double dissociations are shown in Table 2-1.

Subcortical Aphasias. The CT scan studies indicated that infarction often extends from cortex to deep structures such as the lenticular nuclei (Mazzocchi and Vignolo, 1979). Less frequently, classical aphasia syndromes appeared to be caused by lesions exclusively beneath cortex and in the area of lenticular nuclei (Figure 2–3). The notion of subcortial aphasia arose out of these findings. Damage is found in different parts of this region, and researchers refer to the same parts in different ways. There is a passage for motor and sensory fiber tracts called the internal capsule, which is squeezed between the thalamus and lenticular nuclei. The lenticular nuclei are the putamen and globus pallidus; and both may be referred to as the striatum along with the caudate nucleus. These nuclei also comprise a substantial part of the basal ganglia in the extrapyramidal motor system. In the literature on subcortical aphasia, an infarct may be identified generally in the basal ganglia or specifically in the putamen.

Language deficit has been diagnosed after ischemia or hemorrhage in the following locations within the left cerebral hemisphere:

— *Thalamus* (Cappa and Vignolo, 1979; Crosson, Parker, Kim, Warren, Kepes, and Tulby, 1986;

TABLE 2–1 The criterion of double dissociation in localization research (Glassman, 1978) is related to some common double dissociations which have been suggested in various investigations. A single dissociation occurs when a lesion site X yields a deficit A which is greater than a deficit B.

| Lesion Site X | → | Deficit A | > | Deficit B |
Lesion Site Y	→	Deficit B	>	Deficit A
Left hemisphere (LH)	→	Verbal tasks	>	Nonverbal tasks
Right hemisphere (RH)	→	Nonverbal tasks	>	Verbal tasks
Temporal LH	→	Language	>	Music
Temporal RH	→	Music	>	Language
Anterior LH	→	Speech fluency	>	Comprehension
Posterior LH	→	Comprehension	>	Speech fluency
Anterior LH	→	Syntax	>	Semantics
Posterior LH	→	Semantics	>	Syntax

Gorelick, Hier, Benevento, Levitt, and Tan, 1984; Kennedy and Murdoch, 1989; Robin and Schienberg, 1990);

—*Basal ganglia* (Kennedy and Murdoch, 1989; Robin and Schienberg, 1990; Wallesch, 1985);

—Internal capsule and proximal striatal structures identified as the *capsulostriatum* (Tanridag and Kirshner, 1987), "striato-capsular lesion" (Murdoch, 1988), or, more specifically, "capsular/putaminal" lesion (Alexander, Naeser, and Palumbo, 1987);

—*White matter,* including the internal capsule and other sensory or motor projection fibers (Naeser, 1988; Naeser, Palumbo, Helm-Estabrooks, Stiassny-Eder, and Albert, 1989).

The issue of "when is aphasia aphasia" plagues claims about subcortical aphasia. Moreover, if these are genuine aphasias, the peculiar anatomical classification raises the question of whether these aphasias differ from the aphasias classified as Broca's, Wernicke's, conduction, and so on. Helm-Estabrooks and Albert (1991), in their *Manual of Aphasia Therapy,* claimed that there are "subcortical syndromes" called anterior, posterior, and global "capsular/putaminal aphasias." One reason for skepticism involves the speech disturbances accompanying many of these disorders and the suspicion that apraxia of speech is being equated with aphasia. Thus, researchers may be equating speech with language. For example, in reviewing reports of subcortical aphasia, Alexander and others (1987) looked for "components of aphasic syndromes" that include "ease of speech initiation, articulation, and voice volume" (p. 961). According to Naeser (1988), anterior capsular-putaminal aphasias are like Broca's aphasia because "they have slow, poorly articulated speech output," and are unlike Broca's aphasia "because they have intact grammatical form . . ." (p. 365). Yet, it is the grammatical impairment that makes the aphasia an aphasia. On the other hand, Naeser's posterior capsular-putaminal syndrome is very much like Wernicke's aphasia.

Thalamic lesions may produce a language disorder with good comprehension and fluent semantic paraphasias and neologisms. Cases are compared to transcortical aphasias

(Cappa and Vignolo, 1979; McFarling, Rothi, and Heilman, 1982). A transcortical-like sparing of repetition is reported as being characteristic of thalamic language disturbance (Murdoch, 1988). However, Robin and Schienberg (1990) found exceptions. Kennedy and Murdoch (1988) observed semantic paraphasias in their cases of lesion in the thalamus and basal ganglia, and each case had dysarthric speech. Like many other investigators, they considered their cases to be "atypical" with respect to classical forms of aphasia.

Subcortical lesion may cause aphasia in two ways. One explanation supposes that the thalamus and parts of the basal ganglia have a direct role in language functioning so that the lesion impairs that role (Crosson, 1985; Robin and Schienberg, 1990). The other explanation need not assume a direct role of subcortical structures in language functions. The thalamus contains many nuclei connected with sensory, motor, and association areas of cortex. Studies of blood flow and metabolism indicate that subcortical lesion is accompanied by remote hypoperfusion, creating a penumbral insufficiency for the left perisylvian cortical regions responsible for language functions (Metter, Riege, Hanson, Kuhl, Phelps, Squire, Wasterlain, and Benson, 1983; Olsen, Bruhn, and Oberg, 1986).

Locating Focal Activation in the Normal Brain

Activation of cortical regions in the normal brain can be inferred from measures of **regional cerebral blood flow (rCBF)**. The procedure capitalizes on an increase of activity in a cortical region, causing an increased demand for nourishment and, thus, an increased rate of delivery. Early researchers produced dramatic views of multiple-region activity in the left hemisphere during speaking and reading (Lassen, Ingvar, and Skinhoj, 1978). Colorful displays showed busy regions as red and yellow in a background of blue and green (for minimal activity). Less expensive and colorful methods, which are noninvasive, were developed in the United States (Stump and Williams, 1980). However, rCBF is only an indirect measure of metabolism in a nerve cell.

Position emission tomography (PET scan) is a direct measure of metabolism and is more responsive to rapid variations of activity than rCBF. Extensive studies have been conducted by Metter, Riege, and their colleagues in Los Angeles. Metter (1987) classified PET as operating on a principle of *emission*; namely, images are derived from an energy source within the body. This contrasts with *transmission* methods, in which the energy source is external (i.e., X-rays). With PET, radioactive tracers, called positron-emitting isotopes (e.g., fluorodeoxyglucose, or **18-FDG**), are combined with oxygen or glucose and injected into arteries. After 50 minutes, a rotating scanner detects the rate at which tissue utilizes the radioactive nutrients. Metter (1987) noted that "the primary limitation for its widespread use is the short half-life of the radionuclides which require the presence of a readily available cyclotron for isotope production" (p. 7). In detecting cortical activation, PET studies show that "the brain continues to work even during the non-specific stimulation that occurs during resting" (p. 11). Thus, cortical activity during task performance may be an increase of activation that must be compared against activation during rest.

Measurements of blood flow and metabolism have provided an enormous opportunity to discover the location of areas that may be especially active while a subject engages in a task. If a holistic theory of brain function were true, then the whole brain should activate while someone is talking or reading. If these language functions are lateralized to the LH, then only the LH should increase its energy level when we talk and read. If functions delineated as reading or talking reside in their own centers, then only one region should activate as someone performs one of these functions. These predictions are compatible with various theories of cerebral function, but rCBF and PET scans have indicated that none of these theories present the complete story. When we hear or see a word,

metabolism is enhanced bilaterally, with more differentiated activation of areas in the LH (Peterson, Fox, Posner, Minton, and Raichle, 1988). Reading occupies areas in the occipital, temporal, and frontal lobes of the LH. Listening to a story about Sherlock Holmes raises activity in multiple regions of both hemispheres, but more so in the LH than the RH (Mazziotta, Phelps, Carson, and Kuhl, 1982). Musical chords evoke right temporal and bilateral inferior parietal activity. Task difficulty may determine the degree to which the "other hemisphere" participates (Metter, 1987). The main point is that multiple regions are activated, which indicates that simple functions are "located" in multiple centers operating in relationship to each other.

REORIENTATION TO BRAIN FUNCTION

If language function is not completely lateralized to the LH, does this mean that the LH and RH are not specialized for anything? If multiple areas of cerebral cortex activate while performing a simple task, what can we say is done by each of these areas? Strategies for answering these questions are appearing as many investigators become reoriented as to the basis upon which hypotheses about cerebral function are formulated.

Lateralization of Cognition

With the unilateral presentation of verbal and nonverbal stimuli, asymmetrical response has too often been inconsistent or insignificant. As indicated earlier, the idea of identifying hemispheric specialization with general categories of stimulus and response began to collapse. For example, the LH dominated in some nonverbal activities. LH activity increased when difficulty of block design tasks increased (Galin, Johnstone, and Herron, 1978) and when visuospatial tasks involved responding to a rotated figure (Ornstein, et al., 1980). An REA (LH) occurred for rhythmic features of music (Gates and

Bradshaw, 1977). Conversely, the RH activated for verbal stimuli in other research. Lateralization of speech perception varied according to the acoustic feature being processed. The LH processed place of articulation and related formant transitions. Voicing contrasts elicited RH responses. Vowels were processed by both hemispheres. Molfese, Molfese, and Parsons (1983) concluded that "each cue is processed by a number of distinct mechanisms, some of which are bilaterally represented, and some of which are lateralized to one cortical region. . . . There is some degree of redundancy in the cortical mechanisms involved in speech perception" (p. 46).

Lesion-deficit evidence also caused difficulty for the classical theory of asymmetry. LH damage impaired perception of sequences of tones, clicks, and lights more than RHD (Carmon and Nachson, 1971; Lackner and Teuber, 1973). In a study of music recognition, LH damage caused more problems than RH damage when music with familiar lyrics was presented (Gardner and Denes, 1973). Effects of LH stroke on deaf users of American Sign Language are excellent examples of the paradox that the LH is needed for a visuospatial activity. Moreover, RH damage spares certain aspects of manual sign use. Syntax is expressed with varied spatial relationships. Three RH-damaged signers were impaired in comprehension of spatially organized syntax but were unimpaired in comprehending other components of ASL. They were "flawless" in production of syntactic and other features of ASL (Poizner, et al., 1987).

Some of these studies pointed to key modifications in the depiction of lateralized function. The most basic modification was that each hemisphere could be identified with an aspect of cognition rather than with types of stimuli, response, or general reference to ability, capacity, or function. For example, an LH response to music with familiar lyrics indicates that the LH was engaged in linguistic *encoding* of the nonverbal stimulus. Effects of LH damage on nonverbal sequences indicates that it might be the sequential feature of the stimulus that determines lateralization

of response inside someone's head. Propensities of each hemisphere may have more to do with the manner of *processing* rather than the type of stimulus per se. There is a massive body of evidence converging on the belief that each hemisphere is specialized for something, but what is lateralized is what a person is doing mentally rather than a vague notion of function or ability. In 1802, Cabanis figured that "the brain secretes thought as the liver bile" (Berlin, 1956, p. 269), and now sense is being made of seemingly contradictory evidence when questions pertain to the manner in which the brain secretes cognition.

The initial reformulation of functional asymmetry appealed to general types of **cognitive style**. The hemispheres were believed to differ according to attributes in Table 2–2. The hypothesis of cognitive asymmetry states that the LH is more active than the RH for verbal encoding and sequential-analytic processing, and the RH is more active for imagistic encoding and simultaneous-holistic processing. Thus, a verbal-nonverbal distinction is retained with respect to assumptions about the mental representation of information when performing a task. In recalling tone sequences, aphasic subjects improved with increasing length of sequence, but subjects with RH damage did worse as sequences got longer; Brookshire (1975) concluded that RH damage impairs the ability to deal with long sequences as if they were music, whereas persons with LH damage can use this strategy with their intact RH. In a study of normal adults recalling tonal sequences, PET scan-

TABLE 2–2 Contrasting cognitive styles have been attributed to the two cerebral hemispheres

Left Hemisphere (LH)	Right Hemisphere (RH)
Temporal	Spatial
Sequential	Simultaneous
Successive	Parallel
Linear	
Analytic	Holistic
Rational	Intuitive
Logical	Emotional

ning detected more left posterior temporal activation in those using analytical strategies and more right posterior activation in those using nonanalytical strategies (Mazziotta, et al., 1982).

Galin (1976) worried about oversimplified distinctions that he called "dichotomania." He wrote that "the specialization of the two halves of the brain is being offered as the mechanism underlying everybody's favorite pair of polar opposites" (p. 46). Broad cognitive asymmetry is being used to explain the conscious and subconscious, the masculine and the feminine, and classroom performances of the middle class and urban poor. Watzlawick (1978) saw psychotherapy as a process of unleashing emotion and fantasy that we imprison in the RH by our excessive reliance on the rational LH. Drawing from the right side of the brain is taught as a "shift from the ordinary verbal, analytic state to the spatial, nonverbal state" (Edwards, 1989, p. 46). We can improve ourselves with "the right brain experience: an intimate program to free the powers of your imagination" (Zdenek, 1983). We can learn "whole-brain thinking" for peak job performance (Wonder and Donovan, 1984). We can try "whole-brained investing" (Goodspeed, 1983). Harris (1985) noted that Edwards' drawing exercises "are mostly old hat, having been used by art teachers for many years" (p. 265). After reviewing many educational "fads," Harris recommended that "if educators are unsatisfied with the educational *curriculum*, they ought to present the case for change on its *own* merits, and not seek to win scientific respectability for their arguments by cloaking them in neuropsychological jargon" (p. 267).

Focusing on Cognitive Processes

In addition to the problems with relating a hemisphere to stimuli or responses, there have also been problems in relating a side of the brain to a single characterization of a task such as "language-comprehension task" or "object-naming task." Speech-language pathologists think of object-naming as a test of word-finding, but cognitive psychologists use

the task as a test of object recognition (see Chapter 7). These two orientations indicate that there are two aspects of object-naming that may bring each hemisphere to bear on the task. Springer and Deutsch (1989) said "there is little to support the notion that either one or the other hemisphere turns on to perform a specific task all by itself" (p.126). A group of researchers concluded that "both hemispheres of the brain participate actively in many, if not most, tasks which have been viewed in clinical neurology as focal" (Halsey, Blauenstein, Wilson, and Wills, 1980, p. 59).

Fischer and Pellegrino (1988) presented pairs of figures to a visual field of normal subjects asked to decide whether the figures matched. The figures did not have quite the same orientation. Matching figures in different orientation was assumed to require an imagistic process called *mental rotation*, so the task is often called a test of visual imagery or mental rotation. Yet, there was a consistent right-field effect indicating an LH preference for the task. Why would the LH do better than the RH with a task assumed to assess visual imagery? Fischer and Pellegrino figured that the task required multiple processes, beginning with stimulus perception and concluding with making a response. Mental rotation is likely to be only one cognitive step in performing the task. The investigators concluded that the LH dominated for steps other than mental rotation. Considering the mental steps between stimulus and response makes room for the possibility that the LH does one part of an imagery task and the RH does another (Kosslyn, 1987).

The **distinction between task and process** influences rehabilitation as well as the study of cerebral function. In basic research, an investigator makes explicit assumptions about the processing components of a task. Such components are introduced here for a spatial task. Tests of visuospatial skills have a stimulus perception component, an interpretation component, and a response component (Morrow, Ratcliff, and Johnston, 1985). Sometimes the response requires constructional skills that are exhibited, for example, in drawing. Grossi, Orsini, and Modafferi (1986) discovered a dissociation in drawing by a patient with a left occipital lesion. The patient could not draw an object on command (without a model) but was able to copy or draw with a model present. In order to diagnose an impaired mental process, the investigators proposed a model of the processes involved in *the task that exposed impairment* (Figure 2–9). The model begins with perceiving a command and takes us through cognitive steps leading to constructing a response. At least two steps are probably not needed for copying, which the patient was able to do. When shown the object to copy, a patient does not need to comprehend the noun in a command and does not need to activate an internal representation of the object. The patient in the study could comprehend words and sentences, so the disorder was diagnosed as a dissociation of visuospatial imagery, not as impaired drawing ability. The study indicates how researchers might develop hypotheses about the functions engaged by each of the multiple areas of activation on a PET scan.

Problems
for Intrahemispheric Localization

The same considerations apply to determining how the left hemisphere contributes to language functioning. Contemporary worries are consistent with Hughlings Jackson's concerns over a century ago when he argued that it was premature to relate poorly understood functions to a poorly understood material mechanism. Localization has been a question of *what* goes *where*; and it has become evident that those who study the brain have had trouble conceptualizing what they want to localize. Locating "language," reading, or syntax seems vague. Discussing the use of Broca's aphasia for inferring normal function, Kertesz (1991) noted that "many identifiable, even dissociable, central processes contribute to the syndrome, but, so far, none of these has a reliable localization, only the syndrome as a whole" (p. 219). Also, articulation has been strangely identified with language and, thus, aphasia. Murdoch (1988) suggested that "a crucial linguistic role for the

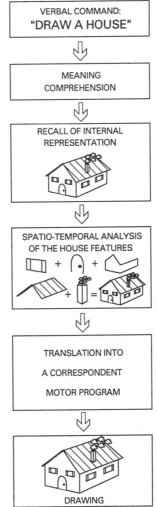

FIGURE 2–9 A model of cognitive processes when drawing on command. Such models specify mental events occurring between a stimulus and response for a task. Localization of function is now assumed to be a matter of relating such events (or components) to areas of the brain; and, similarly, diagnosis entails determining the impaired component that is responsible for difficulty with a task. (Reprinted by permission from Grossi, D., Orsini, A., & Modafferi, A., Visuoimaginal constructional apraxia: On a case of selective deficit of imagery. *Brain and Cognition, 5,* 1986, p. 265. Academic Press, publisher.)

precentral gyrus appears likely" because others (who studied dysarthria) "proposed that injury to the left precentral gyrus causes an articulatory disturbance comparable to that usually seen with Broca's aphasia" (p. 446). This notion should be countered with the realization that the common co-occurrence of two impairments does not mean that they are the same disorder.

Localization theory has been strained by the absence of a theory for what is to be localized. With the emergence of psycholinguistics, the problem became inattention to such theory. Neurological models of language functioning are published without references from psycholinguistics (e.g., Crosson, 1985). Caramazza and Berndt (1978) noted that "historically, the study of language dissolution has been almost exclusively the province of neurologists, whose concerns were not so much with the normal organization of language processes as with the correlation between brain structures and specific language behaviors" (p. 898). Later, Caramazza (1988) added that "classical neuropsychological research operated within a medical model framework mostly uninformed by cognitive or linguistic theory" (p. 397).

There is also a question as to "where" cognitive processes should be located. When an infarct has effects on areas remote to the lesion, lesion-deficit methodology suffers from the problem of locating the malfunctioning part of the brain. Also, Caplan (1981) said that the most widespread approach, which he called "convolutional," identifies functional sites at a level of "gross neuroanatomy." "Working at this level of neural description cannot, in the face of what we know about nervous function, allow us to frame the most important questions about language-brain relations in ways amenable to investigation" (p. 129). Now neuroscientists are turning to the microscopic level of neural structure.

Finally, researchers may have restricted the type of relationships that are possible by thinking of mind-brain relations mainly as a localization problem. Caplan (1981) wrote that "given a psychology of language which is

'informational' and 'computational' ... we cannot relate it causally to a neurological analysis which does not provide for the representation and processing of information" (p. 133). Assumptions about mental events may correspond to assumptions about neural events occurring between a stimulus and response, or what Caplan (1984) called a "physiology of language." Thus, exploration for sites of functions should be supplemented by figuring out *how* the functions are carried out, perhaps with respect to measuring duration of neural events (Chapter 3). As we survey the past, we may conclude that localizing pugnacity was farfetched. Finding a site for reading was more reasonable. Now, the problem is one of linking a cognitive system for reading to anatomy and physiology.

SUMMARY AND IMPLICATIONS

Aphasia occurs because some neuropathologies strike a region of the brain that is responsible for psycholinguistic functions. The causes of aphasia include ischemic and hemorrhagic stroke and tumors and may include mysterious progressive pathologies. Speech-language pathologists are most familiar with the impact of relatively sudden infarction. Reasons for this or that problem are often requested by family members who were probably in a state of shock when their doctor explained the problems to them. Why is my wife's problem worse than his? Why can she produce sentences but my husband cannot say more than a word at a time? We recall the medical report, and we think of how locations of occlusion can cause different amounts and kinds of impairment. The cerebral vascular system has a geography of big rivers and small branches nourishing states and counties with unique characteristics. Blocking the big river at its source causes wider damage than blocking the small rivers and streams. Our expertise on functional specializations of the brain in relation to site of lesion engenders confidence in our ability to help and encourages clients to do what we ask them to do.

Physicians treat physiological disruptions

and preserve life, and they turn their patients over to rehabilitation specialists for evaluation and treatment of associated dysfunctions. Having read the results of a CT scan and neurological evaluation, we know that the patient has damage in the left or right hemisphere. Knowledge of functional asymmetry allows us to predict negative and positive symptoms that will be revealed in our first visit with the patient. Treatment will be motivated by the desire to repair cognitive processes underlying negative symptoms and expand the communicative value of spared processes underlying positive symptoms. Our predictions may be modified slightly with knowledge of a patient's handedness and age. We may anticipate the need to evaluate dysfunction in more than one language. Our approach to evaluation has historically been modeled after approaches to studying the functional organization of the brain. As clinicians, we too are looking for dissociations. Clinical disciplines are challenged by the same modifications of paradigm that have badgered traditional science.

3

COGNITIVE FOUNDATIONS
OF LANGUAGE FUNCTIONS

Clinical aphasiologists assess and treat problems in the comprehension and formulation of language. We also deal with these problems as they occur in the context of disorders of attention, memory, and orientation. We do not usurp the physician's responsibility for treating the brain. We focus on what Luria (1966) called "higher cortical functions" comprising various features of cognition. Speech-language pathologists have a tradition of understanding communicative disorders according to contemporary theory and method of basic sciences, and this chapter presents the adolescence of a few cognitive sciences. It draws mainly on the field of cognitive psychology and its specialization in psycholinguistics. Taking time to think about the examples in the next three chapters should train us to be sensitive to the nuances of psycholinguistic dysfunction. Also, this chapter elaborates on cerebral function in terms of theory of cognition.

THE DISCIPLINES

The first chapter focused attention on the difference between domains and disciplines. Clinicians are familiar with "neuropsychology" as part of the name of the discipline of clinical neuropsychology, but the term also refers to relationships between neural and psychological phenomena that are studied by many disciplines. The division between "language" and cognition discussed in Chapter 1 has been used to identify domains of speech-language pathology and clinical neuropsychology. Yet, when we think of comprehension and word-finding as cognition, rearrangement of clinical disciplines is not the logical consequence. Instead, we may be rearranging the way we talk about the interrelated domains of clinical disciplines. This section introduces some of the disciplines involved in studying cognition.

Cognitive Psychology

Cognitive psychology stands on the doctrine of functionalism, which states that the mind can be studied independently of the brain (Chapter 1). Notions about the mind are called frameworks, theories, and models. Architecture is a common metaphor. By sharpening distinctions among these terms, Eysenck and Keane (1990) differentiated levels in cognitive psychology's portrayal of the mind. A *framework* (or "approach" or "paradigm") is a set of general assumptions that forge the foundation of a discipline. Research is based on three assumptions: "(1) that mental processes exist; (2) that people are active information processors; and (3) that mental processes and structures can be revealed by time and accuracy measures" (Ashcraft, 1989, p. 31). A *theory* specifies features of cognition that account for general phenomena such as language comprehension. A *model* is theory applied to a situation and is often seen as an account of mechanisms employed in a specific task, such as drawing on command (Figure 2–9). A *cognitive architecture* is an integration of theories. It might show how knowledge, comprehension, and attention are interrelated. Throughout the rest of this book, these terms will be used somewhat interchangeably as they usually are in the literature.

Psycholinguistics is an examination of processes used in the recall, comprehension, and formulation of language. It may also include the study of knowledge used in carrying out these processes (Garnham, 1985). Modern psycholinguistics was motivated by a revolution in linguistics in the 1960s; many linguists include psycholinguistics in the domain of linguistics (e.g., Akmajian, et al., 1984). A psycholinguistic aphasiology applies what is called "on-line" methodology to determine what is happening in the mind while an aphasic person is comprehending a sentence (e.g., Friederici, 1988; Swinney, Zurif, and Nicol, 1989; Tyler, 1987). It also entails interpreting patterns of linguistic expression with respect to cognitive disorders that could produce the behavior (e.g., Schwartz, 1987).

Cognitive Neuropsychology

Cognitive psychology and cognitive neuropsychology have the same goal: namely, to determine the nature of normal cognition. Cognitive psychology relies on neurologically intact subjects, and cognitive neuropsychology relies on neurologically impaired subjects. Some other differences have created divisions within cognitive neuropsychology. Some investigators prefer the study of single cases (Caramazza, 1991; Ellis and Young, 1988); others prefer groups in a manner that is more characteristic of cognitive psychology (e.g., Bates, McDonald, MacWhinney, and Applebaum, 1991; Zurif, Swinney, and Fodor, 1991). A single case is usually used to test a **process model,** which is a "hypothesis about the specific mental processes that take place when a particular task is performed" (Ashcraft, 1989, p. 58). The case with drawing problems at the end of Chapter 2 is an example of these studies. The process model, with its boxes and arrows, is found much more in the literature of cognitive neuropsychology than the literature of cognitive psychology, which relies more on detailed statements about the nature of a cognitive structure or process.

Emerging from experimental psychology, cognitive neuropsychology should be distinguished from **clinical neuropsychology.** Clinical neuropsychologists provide behavioral assessment services in rehabilitation settings, and the discipline grew from "its parent disciplines of neurology and psychology" and began to "develop an identity of its own in the 1940's" (Lezak, 1983, p. 3). Neuropsychological assessment has been mainly an application of tests that were already being used for the evaluation of intelligence, memory, and personality. In establishing ties with neurology, clinical neuropsychology took a path that differed somewhat from the strains of thought developing later in cognitive psychology. Clinical neuropsychology has been focused primarily on relating tasks or test scores to regions of the brain.

Caramazza has been critical of clinical neuropsychology and has written several essays on the different assumptions underlying modern cognitive neuropsychology: "We are interested not in *brain/behavior* relationships, but in *brain/cognitive-mechanism* relationships. That is, what we want to know is not how impairment on a particular task is related to the loci of brain lesions, but rather how damage to a particular cognitive mechanism is related to lesion site" (McCloskey and Caramazza, 1988, p. 612). His **transparency assumption** states "that the cognitive system of a brain-damaged patient is fundamentally the same as that of a normal subject except for a 'local' modification of the system" (Caramazza, 1986, p. 52). The goal is to figure out the local modification, which is sometimes called a "functional lesion." The remote effects of a local infarction may create problems for the transparency assumption, but clinicians are thinking about the clinical implications of this strategy. Howard and Patterson (1989) said that the objective for diagnosing an aphasic patient is "to determine which components of the patient's language system are impaired and which are operating with at least partial efficiency" (p. 41). The strategies of cognitive neuropsychology will be more evident in subsequent chapters.

Linguistics and Linguistic Theory

Speech-language pathologists have tended to receive more training in linguistics than in cognitive psychology. Linguistics is the study of the structure of language through the logical examination of relationships among words, sentences, and meaning (e.g., Fromkin and Rodman, 1988). Linguistics makes us sensitive to nuances of aphasic expression and stimuli presented to aphasic people. Garnham (1985) noted that "the nature of linguistics is a matter of debate, even among its own practitioners" (p. 16). A traditional linguist may study sentences, leaving psycholinguists to study people using sentences. However, since Chomsky (1968) wrote that a grammar depicts intuitions about language and is a window to the mind, linguistics has influenced cognitive theory. In aphasiology, a few investigators claim that linguistic theory

depicts "syntactic representations" that might be impaired (e.g., Caplan, 1987b; Grodzinsky, 1989). "One hope for psycholinguistics is that linguists' descriptions of language correspond to the information that is stored in the mind of the language user" (Garnham, 1985, p. 11). Yet, Garnham (1985) explained that for a grammar to be a theory of knowledge, it must be tested in a laboratory of subjects recalling and comprehending sentences on the basis of features that are unique to the grammar. He added that "a grammar is not an account of how speakers produce utterances when they talk, and it may not even reflect the way that linguistic knowledge is organized" (p. 27).

DIMENSIONS OF MEMORY

Everyday memory means remembering a teacher from childhood or where we parked the car. We can achieve great feats, such as memorizing a phone book. However, memory is more than a special skill. It is the foundation of cognition. Ashcraft (1989) defined cognition as "the coordinated operation of active mental processes within a multicomponent memory system" (p. 39). Memory is simply retention of information. It is retention long enough that a stimulus can be perceived and long enough that the information can be used again. "A memory" lasts a few milliseconds or a lifetime. The multiple dimensions of memory indicate that it would be misleading to speak of localization of memory or diagnosis of memory as a single entity.

Multistore Theories of Information Processing

Guides to memory research in the 1960s were multistore theories that specified flow of information among three storage components (Figure 3–1; Atkinson and Shiffrin, 1971). Each component was distinguished according to capacity, duration, and form of information in the component. *Sensory memory* (or "detection system") holds a vast array of sensations for less than a second in modality-specific form, such as an "echoic" repre-

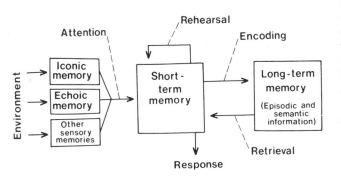

FIGURE 3–1 Three levels of memory have implications for language function. Processing for comprehension and production takes place within the capacity and time constraints of short-term memory, also called "working memory." The knowledge-base for communication is housed in long-term memory. (Reprinted by permission from Smith, A.D., and Fullerton, A.M., Age differences in episodic and semantic memory: Implications for language and cognition. In D.S. Beasley and G.A. Davis (Eds.), *Aging: Communication Processes and Disorders.* New York: Grune & Stratton, 1981)

sentation of sounds. Attended information proceeds to **short-term memory** (STM), which has a small capacity and can retain information for about 20 seconds. The contents of STM were thought to be encoded in acoustic or phonemic forms. These contents may be "transferred" to **long-term memory** (LTM), a vast storehouse of experiences and knowledge thought to have a "semantic" form. The multistore approach ran into many problems. Because different forms of representation are retained for varying durations, some researchers began to view memory with respect to "levels-of-processing." Accordingly, duration of retention is determined by elaborateness or depth of processing (Craik and Lockhart, 1972). The idea of a continuum exposed weaknesses in the idea of memory as distinct storage bins.

A distinction between a "psychology of the present" and a "psychology of the past" seems to be valid (Eysenck and Keane, 1990). These dimensions of memory have been recognized by many disciplines but have been defined and labeled differently. In cognitive psychology, STM was also known as primary memory; LTM, as secondary memory. Literature from neuroscience and the clinic divides memory differently and refers to STM as memories lasting a few hours, such as remembering what happened earlier in the day.

Clinical specialists have evaluated immediate, delayed, and remote memories. In this scheme, immediate recall refers to memory span associated with the STM in multistore models. Delayed memory is defined as recalling what happened earlier in the day (e.g., Tanridag, Kirshner, and Casey, 1987). According to the multistore approach, however, delayed memory is explained as recall from LTM based on acquisition of information a few hours earlier. This text follows the apparently prevailing orientation in cognitive psychology, which is based on the notion of an active or working memory.

An Active Memory

Language comprehension and formulation involve a psychology of the present. It is mental activity similar to *what is happening inside your head at this moment as you read this sentence.* The processing of this moment occurs under constraints of duration and capacity known as **working memory** (WM) (Baddeley, 1986). Working memory is the limited operating "space" for the activity of cognition. It is more than the STM of digit span or immediate memory span. The need for a distinction between working memory and STM was indicated in studies of patient KF, who had a digit span of only two items (e.g.,

Warrington and Shallice, 1969). The patient had an intact LTM, and so dissociation of STM supported making a distinction between LTM and a transient memory. Yet, KF also understood sentences quite well, indicating that a healthy immediate memory span is not essential for comprehension. Despite a small STM, enough work space was available for the processes of comprehension to operate properly (see also Waters, Caplan, and Hildebrandt, 1991). Working memory encompasses a capacity for processes as well as for transient information. A process is also transient, and we can only do so much at one time. WM and LTM are the features of memory that support processing and knowledge, respectively.

One longstanding question pertains to the **representation** or *encoding* of information either in a transient active state in WM or in a permanent passive state for the long haul in LTM. The meaning of "encoding" here differs from its sense in classical communication theory (e.g., Figure 1–3). Here it refers to a process of representing environmental input in the cognitive system so that the system can make further decisions about a stimulus. A representation of a stimulus is called a **percept,** which mimics the form of the stimulus. Representations exist for active encoding of LTM, so a reference to problems of "representation" is a bit vague. Paivio (1986) proposed two forms of representation with his **dual coding** hypothesis. He argued that the mind uses a verbal (i.e., symbolic) format or a nonverbal format (i.e., "quasi-pictorial" imagery). Many questions remain about forms of mental representation, including whether verbal and nonverbal forms are used in both WM and LTM.

While performing a task, working memory contains active information and previously encountered information held briefly, so active information can be related to the previous input (i.e., a few words ago). In Baddeley's theory, this brief retention device is called a **buffer.** When reading a story, "part of the short-term memory system is set aside as a buffer which contains propositions from earlier in the text" (Fletcher, 1981, p. 565). As indicated by this quote, some writers have used STM in the same sense as WM. No matter what things are called, the processor contains information in a presently active state and in a "short-term" buffer. The clinical memory span may involve retrieving buffered information. Baddeley (1986) identified different buffers according to format of representation. One buffer is a *visuospatial sketch-pad* holding onto images, like drawing on a note pad while solving a puzzle. The verbal buffer may be an *articulatory buffer* (or "articulatory loop") in a speech-based form or a *phonological buffer* in a sound-based form. In process models of reading and writing, a *graphemic buffer* provides "a temporary storage system for the internal representation of a word" (Hillis and Caramazza, 1989, p. 228).

Processing in Working Memory

WM can be said to house mental activity, and introducing WM naturally leads to a discussion of basic features of cognitive processing. Figure 3–1 is still helpful in showing the dual direction of information flow in the cognitive system. Processes are said to be **bottom-up** (or *data-driven*) to the extent that they are directed by the environment. Processes may be dictated by loudness, color, or sentence length. Processing is also said to be **top-down** (or *concept-driven*) to the extent that it is directed by what we know in LTM. For example, when comprehending a command like "Jump," we fill in the agent of the action from our knowledge of language. The agent is not in the stimulus. A theory may emphasize one direction, but comprehensive accounts of a function such as language comprehension usually address the influences of bottom-up and top-down processing.

As suggested in Chapter 1, processing occurs at different levels of awareness. Automatic processes are **obligatory,** because they happen no matter what. They happen when we hear or see a word. They occur so quickly that they escape conscious awareness, and they are studied with "fast tasks" in which response latency is measured in fractions of a second (Eysenck and Keane, 1990). Strategic processing is **optional** (controlled, intentional), and it is studied with "slow tasks" that permit conscious planning. These processes clog the system, whereas obligatory processes take up little or no room in WM. Processing for everyday linguistic communication is automatic and obligatory. When we hear an utterance, some comprehension happens whether we want it to or not.

The constraints of the work space present a problem for the **allocation of resources** in complex tasks. Studies of memory and attention converge on resource allocation. The problem is known as dividing attention so that we can do two things at once. Divided attention and WM capacity are studied with a *dual task* or *concurrent task* paradigm in which someone does two tasks at once (Eysenck and Keane, 1990). Dissimilar tasks, such as writing and listening to music, are easier than similar tasks, such as writing and listening to a speech. Practice may make it easier to do similar tasks at once, indicating that processes become more automatic and take up less room. One part of Baddeley's (1986) theory and theories of attention is a **central executive** (or *executive control system*) that manages the amount of work to be done at one time. Like a good executive, it does not do real work; it just deals with distractions so that work gets done. It distributes work according to schemas and plans stored in LTM. Ashcraft (1989) wrote that it "orchestrates" processes toward a goal, keeping track of what has happened and what should come next. He was also suspicious of the control system and wondered if it represents a desperate attempt to explain thinking with "a little thinking person" inside a thinking person.

Knowledge in Long-Term Memory

At an elemental level, language functions depend on knowledge of words and meanings. Philosophers and linguists figure out what people should know about words and meanings, and cognitive psychologists determine what people actually know and how they know it. Distinction between words and

meanings forms a basis for differential diagnosis, and diagnosis may entail making finer differentiations than this. This segment on LTM emphasizes storage of these types of information in the mind of the language user.

Framework for the Study of LTM. LTM is similar to a library system that acquires books, stores them, and has procedures for access. Two of these features are processes in working memory. *Acquisition* is the process of putting information into LTM and, in diagrams such as Figure 3–1, is the arrow going to LTM. Some disorders identified with LTM may be understood better as disorders of acquisition. Clinicians question whether treatment of aphasia should be aimed at acquisition (or "reacquisition"). *Access* is the process of locating information in LTM. As if the brain were a metaphor for cognition, access is said to occur as **activation** of stored information. It is essential for comprehension (i.e., accessing meaning) and expression (i.e., accessing words). In Figure 3–1, the idea of retrieval is shown with the arrow leaving LTM and is difficult to separate from the idea of access. Many speech-language pathologists believe that treatment of aphasia should be directed to improving access rather than acquisition.

Storage pertains to the inactive contents of LTM. Unlike a library, the mental store cannot be examined directly. As one watches people enter and leave a library, experimenters infer the nature of storage with tasks of acquisition (e.g., word-list learning), recognition (e.g., reporting that a stimulus was seen before), and recall (e.g., reproducing a stimulus heard previously). When we assess storage, we are witnessing the result of access processes in relation to storage. Theory addresses the type, form, and organization of information. As in distinguishing fiction and nonfiction in a library, Tulving (1972) proposed that LTM stores episodic, semantic, and lexical types of information. Anderson (1983) took another approach by dividing LTM into declarative and procedural knowledge, corresponding to a philosophical distinction between "knowing that" and "knowing how." The idea of declarative memory includes episodic and semantic memories, so procedural memory (i.e., knowing how to do something) is another type of information thought to require a place in a theory of knowledge. Theories of typology are indicative of disagreements in cognitive psychology. Dual coding theory of verbal and imagistic representation specifies the main options for hypotheses about the form of knowledge. Finally, organization is necessary to account for the lightning speed of access.

Episodic Memory: Our Experiences. Episodic memory is a record of events or episodes that occurred at a particular place and time. Also known as **autobiographical memory,** it is considered to be unique to an individual. It would represent what someone had for breakfast the previous day or what happened at a soccer match years before. We might interview a patient to assess episodic memory on a temporal gradient from what happened yesterday (i.e., "recent memory") or 20 years ago (i.e., "remote memory"). In the laboratory, investigators have examined memory for names and faces from high school graduating classes (Bahrick, Bahrick, and Wittlinger, 1975) and memory for significant events such as the John F. Kennedy assassination (Brown, Rips, and Shevell, 1985). We may think of episodes as being stored as images or movies waiting to be played back in the working memory of recollecting or dreaming. However, the form of our "memories" is debatable, because we could store our experiences as a file of statements (e.g., Eysenck and Keane, 1990; Solso, 1991). If this argument were about libraries, then the debate might be whether nonfiction is represented in printed or photographic form.

Semantic Memory: Our Conceptual Knowledge. Semantic memory is also known as *world knowledge* as well as conceptual knowledge. It is the storage of information about places, plants, animals, foods, actions, space, time, and so on. The core of semantic memory is considered to be universal, except for variations among cultures and levels of expertise. Basic theories tend to address a restricted domain: namely, our knowledge of objects. LTM might contain a description or photograph of every tree, chair, and bird that we have encountered. However, this idea does not enable us to recognize new or strange trees, chairs, and birds. It is more likely that LTM takes a more economical approach by representing concepts instead of specific objects. A **concept,** the basic unit of semantic memory, is the mental representation of a class of objects or actions (Smith, 1988). Although we speak of concepts by using words, we must recognize the difference between concepts and the lexicon. The concept [tree] may be a universal element of semantic memory, but the word for it varies from language to language. For this text, a concept is represented in brackets.

To encompass a class of objects such as fire engines, a concept has been considered to be an abstraction of some kind. Called the defining-feature or set-theoretic theory, an early depiction was to think of a class of objects such as [fire engine] as defined according to shared attributes. A concept was described as a list of categorical features (e.g., vehicle) and attributes (e.g., has ladders, used for fires). Thus, [fire engine] is coded as "vehicle," "has ladders," "used for fires," and so on. This theory was modified by correcting for the rigidity of fixed features. A notion of *characteristic attributes* (e.g., red) was added for features that we think are typical, considering that some fire engines are yellow (Smith, Shoben, and Rips, 1974). Also, access is related to form. Accessing concepts was thought to entail scanning and comparing lists of features. While the feature-comparison model failed to predict the outcome of several experiments, Ashcraft (1989) suggested that "the feature list approach to semantic memory died of inattention, rather than of some fatal empirical blow" (p. 297).

A significant change in depicting the form of concepts led to **semantic networks.** Categorical and attributive features are concepts, too. Instead of copying them over and over in lists, a more economical system is to store a concept according to its connections with other concepts. That is, [red] need be recorded once and can be linked to all concepts that are red. In a network, categories and attributes are represented as "nodes" connected to each other. A streamlined version is shown in Figure 3–2. Networks were conceived first as being hierarchical and then the principles of organization expanded as if networks are three-dimensional (Collins and Loftus, 1975). This theory seemed to be especially suited for depicting variations of relatedness among concepts, and relatedness was translated into a distance metaphor. Accessing a concept in the network was portrayed as an automatic **spreading activation** from one node to another. One procedure for testing semantic distances has been the *concept comparison task*, in which a neurologically intact subject is asked to verify sentences such as the following:

(1a) A fire engine is a vehicle.
(1b) A fire engine is a truck.

A common finding was that (1a) took longer to verify than (1b), indicating that [truck] is closer than [vehicle] to [fire engine] (Figure 3–2).

Theory was bolstered with the notion of "natural concepts" in order to depict knowledge in the human mind rather than a logical organization of concepts. For example, we might think of [bird] as an animal that flies, but not all birds fly. People establish connections such as "all busboys are short," which we call beliefs. A theory should accommodate concepts like [feminism], for which there may be little agreement as to defining features. Thus, natural concepts may consist solely of characteristic connections. Also, categorical relations have "fuzzy boundaries." Some in-

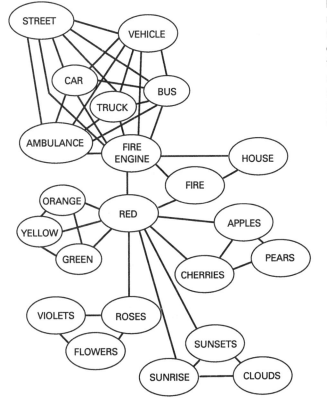

FIGURE 3–2 A simple semantic network suggestive of semantic relatedness or "distance" between concepts. (Reprinted by permission from Collins, A.M., & Loftus, E.F., A spreading-activation theory of semantic processing. *Psychological Bulletin*, 82, 1975, p. 412. American Psychological Association, publisher.)

stances of a category are more typical than others. The notion of **prototypicality** has been useful in portraying natural conceptual organization (Rosch and Mervis, 1975). Both robins and ostriches are birds; but, at the core of a category, we think of robins more often as birds. Unusual examples are peripheral and exist at the fuzzy boundary of a category.

So far in this discussion, the long-term representation of knowledge seems to be simply an arrangement of concepts. A richer world knowledge is constructed by representing **complex concepts** or conceptual combinations formed by the varied types of relationships between concepts (Smith, 1988). Combinations include modification, such as [large man], intensification, such as [very large], and instantiation, such as [man eats lasagna]. Types of relationships between concepts have also been presented by labeling the connections between concepts in a semantic network (e.g., Figure 3–3). That is, the connections in a network can be labeled as categorical relations (i.e., *isa*), such as [Bob *isa* person]. Complex concepts are also established with respect to how objects relate to actions, which have been a focus of linguistic and cognitive investigation. Linguists refer to **thematic relations** or **theta-roles** when referring to language (Cowper, 1992). The thematic relation of **agent** is the "doer" of an action. The **theme** (or patient) is the recipient of an action. Also, objects can be a **goal** or **location** of an action. In *The girl gives flowers to the teacher, flowers* is the theme and *teacher* is the goal. These concepts are often depicted as **propositions** or a predicate-argument structure, such as [give, girl, flowers, teacher]. Agent and theme are arguments around the verb. In a network, propositions are connections among concept nodes for actions and objects. More elaborate knowledge, such as going to a restaurant, is considered to exist within the network structure (Abbott, Black, and Smith, 1985).

In cognitive neuropsychology, single cases are examined with respect to process models that put access and/or storage in a box called the "semantic system." Corresponding to theory of semantic memory, the semantic system is formed and organized on its own terms, independent of modalities (Figure 3–4a). Stimulus processing begins with a modality-formed percept of an object or a word. The percept points to a concept in the semantic system. Yet, in dealing with a few cases with apparent semantic deficits in one modality, a few neuropsychologists suggested that we possess modality-specific semantic systems (Riddoch, Humphreys, Coltheart, and Funnell, 1988; Shallice, 1988). One version of this idea specifies a "verbal" semantic system and a "visual" semantic system (Figure 3–4b). This could be the way neuropsychologists differentiate categorical features and physical features, or these semantic systems may relate to arguments in cognitive psychology over the extent to which knowledge is represented as imagery. Other cognitive neuropsychologists believe that the special dysfunctions can be explained with one semantic system (e.g., Hillis, Rapp, Romani, and Caramazza, 1990).

Lexical Memory: Our Words. Research has indicated that words are stored separately from concepts (Collins and Loftus, 1975). Logical evidence includes different words with the same meaning (i.e., synonyms) and similar-sounding words with different meanings (i.e., homonyms). Lexical memory or the **mental lexicon** contains *what we know about words*, which includes the form of words (such as what they sound like, what they look like, and relationships between phonology and orthography). Such knowledge seems real when we think of the words we use but do not know how to spell. One notion was that the lexicon contains a single abstract form for a word, called a "logogen" (Morton, 1970). The lexicon also contains information about how a word can function in a sentence. This lexical-grammatical information was called the "lemma" by Levelt (1989).

Another question is the representation of **morphological structure** in the mental lexicon. Complex words consist of stems (i.e., base morphemes) and affixes (e.g., writing). One issue is whether stems and affixes are stored together "as words" or separately "as

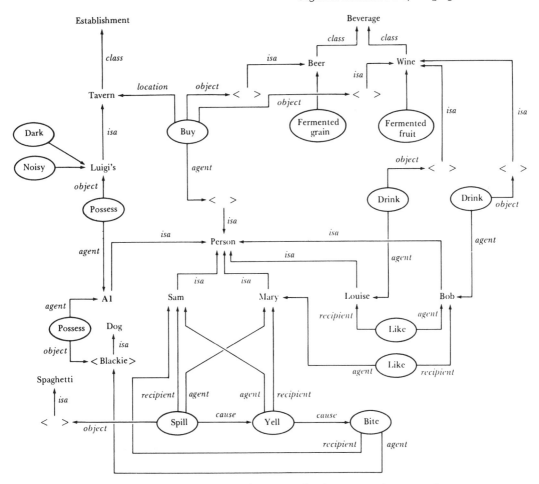

FIGURE 3–3 This depiction of a network of concepts in semantic memory is indicative of the complexity of semantic organization. Connections between concepts are defined by a few types of relationships. A person may search through a network like this to retrieve a word. (Reprinted by permission from Lindsay, P.H. and Norman, D.A., *Human information processing*, 2nd ed. New York: Academic Press, 1977)

morphemes" so that a complex word must be composed each time it is accessed or produced. Most research deals with orthography (e.g., Lima and Pollatsek, 1983), but some of it addresses phonemic form (e.g., Emmorey, 1989). Some evidence supports the idea that stems are stored by themselves (Taft, 1979). Other evidence supports the idea that each word has a place in LTM, although compound words may be more decomposed (An-

drews, 1986). The study of aphasia indicates that paraphasias can be formulated as a composition of normally unrelated parts, as in producing *walkness* (Badecker and Caramazza, 1991). Also, **open class** or content words (e.g., nouns, verbs, adverbs) might be stored differently from **closed class** or function words (e.g., articles, auxiliaries) (Matthei and Kean, 1989; Taft, 1990). Agrammatic aphasia has been a source of data addressing

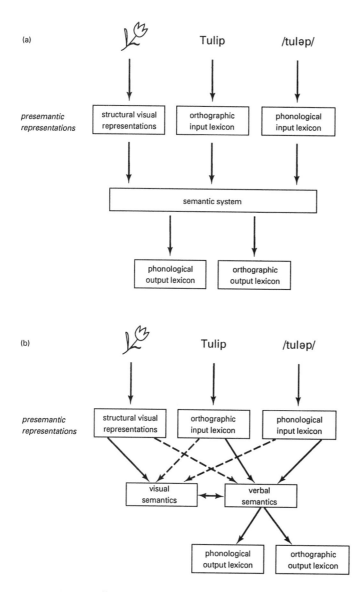

FIGURE 3–4 Relationships among lexical, visual, and semantic representations often proposed in cognitive neuropsychology. Two hypotheses have been debated: (a) semantic memory is independent of lexical and visual-object representations; (b) semantic memory is divided into visual and verbal forms. (Reprinted by permission from Hillis, A.E., Rapp, B.C., Romani, C., & Caramazza, A., Selective impairment of semantics in lexical processing. *Cognitive Neuropsychology, 7,* 1990, pp. 194, 223. Lawrence Erlbaum, publisher.)

- - - - - - routes proposed by some, but not all, proponents of the representational account this question, and observations may have more to do with access strategies than with storage (Chapter 5).

In rounding out a picture of lexical memory, let us consider the entry *bank*. We know its sound and spelling. We know that it can be a noun and a verb. Also, the lexicon contains **subcategorization rules** that specify how a word can relate to other words. As a noun, *bank* can be preceded by *a* or *the*. Verb subcategorization specifies how a verb might enter into relations with objects. As a verb, *bank* can be transitive, meaning that it can be followed by an object-theme, as in "to bank money." Grammatical information points to what *bank* means. Knowledge of what a word can mean is slightly different from concepts in semantic memory per se. That is, we know of [slopes on a river's edge] and [buildings that protect money]. We may know [tilting an airplane]. Yet, it is additional information to know that *bank* refers to these concepts. Many of us have knowledge of [row of oars on a boat] but may not know that *bank* is used to refer to this concept. Thus, knowledge of what words mean is a connection between words in lexical memory and concepts in semantic memory. Possible connections may not exist in the mind of a language user. Interface between a lexicon and semantic memory is knowledge specific to a language, which may be what some researchers refer to when speaking of *lexical-semantics*. The "mental dictionary" does not contain everything found in a real dictionary (Aitchison, 1987).

The Neurological Bases of Memory

The brain cannot be understood by only localizing functions, and theory of the brain's role in behavior depends on utilizing theory of cognition (Chapter 2). The multiple dimensions of memory should make it evident that looking for a "location of memory" is overly simplistic, just as diagnosing "impairment of memory" is an obscuring generalization. The neural bases for memory have been studied on several fronts. Neurobiologists have been examining neural tissue at the microscopic level. Neuropsychologists have related memory impairments to brain injuries (Chapter 6). Effects of drugs and electroshock therapy have been exploited. Little is known for certain, and many conclusions are based on logical relationships between cognitive theory and what is known so far about how the brain works.

Reading the literature on memory and the brain requires caution with respect to the various definitions of terms. For example, Rose (1989), a biochemist, defined STM as retention "for half an hour or so," so STM was thought to be the early stage of consolidating a permanent memory trace. In his *Memory and Brain*, Squire (1987) declared that "recent formulations of the working-memory hypothesis provide a bridge to biological considerations of memory stages and STM" (p. 137). Because working memory is a feature of cognitive processing in general, its place in the brain is distributed and is intrinsic to each of the areas active while we perform a task. An early account of transient retention was the reverberating circuit (Hebb, 1949), which was a circular arrangement of neurons permitting ongoing excitation. However, such circuits have not been observed, and single neurons can change temporarily to account for brief retention. Still, Squire (1987) concluded that holding neural coding for a few seconds starts a "sequence of synaptic changes leading to permanent memory storage" (p. 149).

A great deal of neurobiological research is a search for the "engram" or the neural encoding of a memory (Thompson and Donegan, 1986). Beginning in the 1960s, the approach "was to take over the models for studying animal learning which the psychologists had developed . . . and to ask what types of biological change took place during such learning" (Rose, 1989, p. 243). Neurobiologists have said that "learning can be broadly defined as any lasting change in behavior resulting from previous experience" (Cotman and Lynch, 1989, p. 201). This is the observable manifestation of the cognitive view of learning as the acquisition of a long-lasting or permanent representation of information.

Neurobiological paradigms have included studying sea mollusks' response to stimuli and looking for chemical changes in the brains of young chicks during and after imprinting (Rose, 1989). Featured in Johnson's (1991) entertaining book on the study of memory, Gary Lynch electrically stimulated artificially stored slices of the hippocampus (i.e., a nucleus within the temporal lobe). He was looking for a mechanism underlying changes caused by stimulation called *long-term potentiation*. He focused on the synapse and found the creation of new synapses. "The formation of long-term memory depends ultimately on changes in synaptic connectivity" (Squire, 1987, p. 145). Forming a long-term memory is called *consolidation*, which is "the process by which memory gradually becomes resistant to disruption by an amnestic agent" (p. 206).

While scientists seem to be zeroing in on the synapse for the mechanism of storage, another question pertains to the location of stored information. One view is that a memory is *localized* in a particular place, and this view is represented by the functional localizationists, discussed in Chapter 2, and Penfield's experiments with cortical mapping. The other view is that an engram is *distributed* throughout a wide area of cortex. In the 1940s, a proponent of this theory was Lashley, who failed to find a specific region in a rat's brain that was responsible for learning to find food in a maze (Squire, 1987). A similar idea is being examined in the field of artificial intelligence with computer modeling based on principles similar to neural structure and the excitation or inhibition of neural connections. This approach is known as **parallel distributed processing** (PDP), *connectionist models,* or *neural networks* developed by McClelland and Rumelhart (1985) and others. The idea is that "information about a person, object, or event is stored in several inter-connected units rather than in a single place" so that "the system can function reasonably well even if a unit is damaged or imperfect information is supplied to it" (Eysenck and Keane, 1990, p. 169). Seidenberg and McClelland (1989) proposed a network model for storage

of the lexicon. Individual words are not represented. Instead, information about word form is distributed over phonological and orthographic units. This theory is compatible with localization if an engram is distributed over a microscopic region specialized for a type of memory. After all, a pinhead of cortex contains millions of synapses.

WORD RECOGNITION AND COMPREHENSION

Word recognition involves indicating that we have heard or seen a word before. It happens when the percept of a stimulus is matched to a stored representation of the word in lexical memory. Recognize "penumbra"? Activating a word in the mental lexicon need not lead to comprehension, but things happen during the spreading activation of a lexical network. This section introduces the investigative strategies of psycholinguistics, especially for discovering the automatic obligatory processes that happen beneath our awareness. Occasionally we may wrestle with paradoxes between common sense and theory of processes inaccessible to reason. Yet, theory of automatic processes has to make sense only as an explanation of data.

Lexical Access

Two tasks have been employed widely for studying lexical access, which is the activation of a word in lexical memory. In a **lexical decision task** (LDT), a word or a nonword is usually presented as a letter-string on a computer screen (e.g., CAT or ANK). A subject must quickly decide if the string is a word and then press a response-choice button that stops a timer. Nonwords are "possible words" because they conform to rules of spelling in the language being used. It is assumed that the decision depends on finding a match between the percept of the stimulus and a representation in lexical memory. **Word-naming** (also, *pronunciation task*) often does not include the presentation of nonwords. These tasks are frequently used together, because their differences can be revealing. The most basic issue is whether lexical access occurs in these tasks. Other issues pertain to two processing phases that can occur when performing the tasks. The **pre-lexical phase** is what happens up to the instant of recognition. A **post-lexical phase** can occur because lexical activation may not avoid stirring up other information in a network, especially if the lexicon also contains grammatical information and pointers to meanings. When a stimulus-word activates meaning, we refer to the result as comprehension. Recognize "umbrella"?

While it makes sense that lexical access is required for an LDT, we can be skeptical about word-naming. After all, we can pronounce "ANK," which is not represented in the mental lexicon. One question is whether word-naming entails lexical access before pronunciation or bypasses the lexicon before pronunciation. Assuming that word frequency affects lexical access, Forster and Chambers (1973) found that high-frequency words are recognized faster in LDTs and naming tasks. There was also a correlation between decision and naming latencies for words but no correlation between LDT latency and naming nonwords. In this way, experiments supported an assumption that is hard to grasp with common sense, but the necessity for lexical access in word-naming is still debated (McRae, Jared, and Seidenberg, 1990; Seidenberg and McClelland, 1989). Although word-naming may be assumed to include lexical access, researchers approach this task cautiously; "one cannot assume that a variable affects lexical access simply because it affects pronunciation latency" (Balotta and Chumbley, 1985, p. 90).

Do these recognition tasks include post-lexical activation? Various experiments have supported an estimate that lexical access is completed in 100 to 300 milliseconds (msec) from stimulus presentation (McRae, et al., 1990). For common words, word-naming takes around 500 msec to response, and most of this time is consumed by articulatory programming. Lexical decision for single words takes around 600 msec (Forster and Cham-

bers, 1973). It is suspected that the longer time in LDTs is taken by a decision phase that follows lexical access.

Auditory word recognition has been investigated by Marslen-Wilson and Tyler (1980). Their **cohort theory** assumes that obligatory processes act with maximum efficiency and access the lexicon as quickly as possible. Word recognition is a continuous process of mapping a percept to lexical representations. The process starts when the first sound or syllable activates possibilities called a cohort; that is, all the possibilities for "in-". Word candidates are eliminated rapidly as more of the stimulus is heard (e.g., "infan-"). The point at which one candidate remains is the *recognition point* (e.g., "infantile"). This seemingly cumbersome process makes sense for a system operating without thinking; it is not a strategy. With LDTs and word-naming tasks in experiments, a *gating* procedure presents parts of a word increasing in length in order to discover the recognition points. In one study, recognition points for prefixed words occurred as soon as possible rather than a little later with respect to the word stem (Tyler, Marslen-Wilson, Rentoul, and Hanney, 1988).

Visual word recognition presents its own variations on lexical access (Figure 3–5). The process begins with analysis of a letter-string leading to mental representation of the stimulus (i.e., iconic percept). From this point, two routes to the lexicon are known as the **dual coding hypothesis.** One is *direct* mapping of the percept onto a stored representation. The *indirect* route inserts a **recoding** operation, which converts the orthographic percept into a sound-based representation. This phonological representation is mapped onto a stored representation for recognition. Word pronunciation has demonstrated recoding with the **regularity effect,** in which spellings pronounced irregularly (e.g., *move, cove, love*) take longer to name than spellings pronounced regularly (e.g., *hope, cope, nope*). This effect may be restricted to uncommon words (Seidenberg, Waters, Barnes, and Tanenhaus, 1984). Many researchers believe that the indirect route is most likely taken when

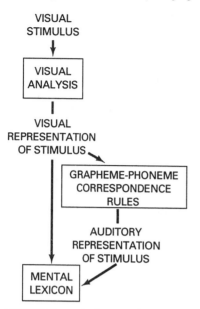

VISUAL
STIMULUS

VISUAL
ANALYSIS

VISUAL
REPRESENTATION
OF STIMULUS

GRAPHEME-PHONEME
CORRESPONDENCE
RULES

AUDITORY
REPRESENTATION
OF STIMULUS

MENTAL
LEXICON

FIGURE 3–5 A theory of printed word recognition in which a representation of a stimulus is related to a representation of the lexical item in the mental lexicon. Sometimes the graphemic representation is first automatically recoded into a phonemic code. (Reprinted by permission from Garnham, A., *Psycholinguistics: Central topics.* London: Methuen, 1985, p. 60.)

someone is learning to read or when reading material is difficult.

Study of word recognition expanded with use of a **priming task.** In this paradigm, a **prime** (e.g., JUICE) is presented before the recognition test word or nonword called the **target** (e.g., MOOSE) (Chiarello, 1985). Subjects respond only to the target. The *interstimulus interval* (ISI) or *stimulus onset asynchrony* (SOA) is usually a small fraction of a second (Table 3–1). The presence of a related word is thought to reduce the activation threshold of nearby words in a network. To test this hypothesis, related primes are compared with unrelated primes presented prior to the target. The wink of time in an SOA is enough for a related prime to increase speed of response over the presence of an unrelated prime. Word-form priming is ex-

plained on the basis of relationships in the lexical network. This task has indicated that phonological activation is inevitable during reading (Perfetti, Bell, and Delaney, 1988).

Post-Lexical Access: Comprehension

Seeing or hearing a word automatically stirs up meaning, and simple comprehension phenomena are studied with semantic priming. A word such as DOCTOR is shown as a prime before showing a target for recognition response (e.g., NURSE) (Meyer and Schvaneveldt, 1971). A **semantic priming effect** is indicated with a response that is faster than when an unrelated prime (e.g., TABLE) is presented. The greatest implication of this phenomenon is what it says about the prime or, namely, what it says about mental events upon just seeing or hearing a word. The prime activates conceptual information, and this activation spreads from the prime's concept node to related regions of semantic memory, decreasing their activation thresholds (Collins and Loftus, 1975). Looking back at Figure 3–2, it is as if seeing CAR sensitizes nearby areas so that [TRUCK] would be momentarily easier to access. **Facilitation** is the effect when a related prime produces faster recognition than a neutral prime (e.g., XXXX). Facilitation can vary from 17 to 56 msec, depending on length of SOA from 300 to 2,000 msec (Neely, 1976). An unrelated prime slows recognition relative to the neutral prime (i.e., inhibition), as if a prime such as PEARS steers the spread of activation away from [TRUCK].

What if the prime is a polysemous word such as BANK? Like thoughtless activation of recognition cohorts, does BANK activate all known meanings? This **multiple access hypothesis** is examined with targets that represent the different meanings (e.g., MONEY or RIVER). Facilitation of one target would indicate activation of only one meaning; but studies show that facilitation occurs for both meanings, supporting the theory of multiple access. We may think that the relative familiarity or **dominance of meanings** for BANK might influence multiple access. *River* is asso-

TABLE 3–1 Basic features of the primed lexical decision task (LDT) in which time is measured for deciding if a TARGET letter-string is a word. Context-effects are studied by presenting a PRIME prior to the target (Chiarello, 1985; Neely, 1976). Stimulus onset asynchrony (SOA) is the interval between prime and target. Facilitation and inhibition are determined in comparison to a neutral prime.

Relationship	Prime	SOA	Target	Effect of Prime
Phonological	JUICE		MOOSE	
Orthographic	BEAK		BEAR	
Semantic	DOCTOR		NURSE	Facilitation of 30 msec
Neutral	XXXXX		NURSE	Inhibition of 16 msec
Unrelated	TABLE		NURSE	

ciated less frequently with *bank* than is *money*. Simpson and Burgess (1985) compared dominant and subordinate meanings of primes with SOAs from 16 to 750 msec. Dominant targets such as MONEY were facilitated at all SOAs. For subordinate targets such as RIVER, priming increased from nothing at 16 msecs to facilitation equaling dominant targets at 300 msec. After 300 msec, dominant facilitation was maintained, but subordinate facilitation gradually declined. It seemed that before 300 msec, meanings are accessed sequentially in order of familiarity; after 300 msec, controlled allocation of resources inhibits less familiar meanings. Thus, an ambiguous word stimulates **ordered** access to multiple meanings.

Word Recognition in the Brain

When considering functional asymmetry of the cerebral hemispheres, a few more twists on recognition paradigms can be encountered. Usually word-naming is employed, and the word is shown to the right or the left hemifield. Studies are trained on the **imageability** of words in order to provoke the right hemisphere into responding. Concrete words such as "tree" are assumed to evoke more imagery than abstract words such as "hope." Several studies showed a greater right field (LH) preference for low-imagery words than high-imagery words, indicating that the RH becomes more involved with high-imagery words (e.g., Ellis and Shepherd, 1974; Hines, 1977). This is known as the *RH imageability hypothesis*, which added that the lexicon is specially stored in the RH along with associated imagery. Conflicting results surfaced, and skepticism arose because of failures to control for difficulties inherent to the hemifield paradigm (Schwartz, Montagner, and Kirsner, 1987). Also, word frequency was not controlled in early comparisons of concrete and abstract words. An LDT, which is more likely than naming to produce post-lexical phenomena, produced no support for RH or bilateral storage of high-imagery words (McMullen and Bryden, 1987). Concrete words may be activated in the LH; and with impulses crossing the commissures, imagery might then be activated in the RH.

To examine priming with the hemifield paradigm, the recognition target is presented to the right (LH) or the left (RH); and the preceding prime is presented to the center or to the same field as the target. Priming allows for comparisons of automatic/obligatory and strategic/controlled processing. Increasing the SOA increases the opportunity for controlled processing. Additional semantic or imagistic processing is likely to occur when the SOA is longer than 400 msec (Neely, 1977). Semantic facilitation also increases as the proportion of related pairs in a stimulus-list increases; density of relatedness in a block of trials may promote strategic use of expectations. Varying the density of related pairs, Chiarello (1985) studied three primes at an SOA of 500 msec. He found orthographic priming (e.g., BEAK-BEAR) in the LVF (RH). Phonological priming (e.g., JUICE-MOOSE) occurred in the RVF (LH). Semantic priming (e.g., INCH-YARD) was much greater than form priming and occurred in both visual fields. Then, Chiarello compared semantic primes that were abstract (e.g., MIND-BRAIN) or concrete (e.g., HEAD-BRAIN) (Chiarello, Senehi, and Nuding, 1987). The RH was involved at least equally with the LH in automatic semantic and concrete word priming. The LH assumed a greater role over the RH for controlled post-lexical semantic and abstract word priming. The RH appears to have a larger role in lexical access than had been originally expected (Burgess and Simpson, 1988).

Caplan (1984) called for a physiology of language. A neural response to a sensory stimulus is called an **evoked potential** (EP). A response evoked by an auditory stimulus is called an AEP; visual stimuli evoke a VEP. EPs are hidden in the complex EEG, and a specific response is teased from an EEG by a computer that averages waveforms and eliminates irrelevant background. These signals can be contaminated from the environment, requiring a copper-shielded soundproof room for experiments. Subjects are supposed to be

still, and trials containing obvious artifact are rejected for an analysis. Campbell and his colleagues (1986) "assume that any evoked potential is due to artifact unless proven otherwise" (p. 28). Another problem is that an EP recorded at one region probably arises from the cumulative interaction of cortical and subcortical regions. Despite their artifactual complexity, EPs "remain the only technique for millisecond-by-millisecond analysis of language physiology" (Picton and Stuss, 1984, p. 306). Can an EP be indicative of the brain's secretion of a cognitive event?

EPs appear as peaks and valleys measured in amplitude and latency. The "spikes" are responses in different levels of the nervous system. *Principal component analysis* (PCA) exposes these levels of neural activity. A summated waveform is divided into early, middle, and late phases and into fast and slow components (Table 3–2). Early fast components are indicative of sensory and perceptual levels of processing. Identifiable responses are P (positive) or N (negative). When labeled by position in a series of responses, an N1 is the first negative component. Latency may also be used for identification, such as a P300. However, it is position (i.e., P3) that is related to a cognitive process; P3s of 275 msec and 875 msec are considered to be "functionally identical" (Campbell, et al., 1986).

There have been several studies of EPs to words with lexical decision tasks. A posterior

TABLE 3–2   Phases or components of the neurological response to a stimulus, measured in the evoked response potential (ERP). Most cognitive processes of language functions are associated with late positive components (LPCs) or late negative components (LNCs).

Phases/components		msec	Location	Function
Early	Fast	0–10	Eye or ear to brain stem	Sensation
Middle		10–60	Thalamus to primary cortex	Sensation to perception
	Slow	60–300	Posterior association areas	N150 word recognition "attentional priming"
Late		300 and longer		P3 N400 semantic processes

N150 was evoked for recognizing printed words following varied contexts, and it was interpreted as an "early attentional priming" of the LH (Neville, Kutas, Chesney, and Schmidt, 1986). Auditory stimuli have been avoided because of difficulty in time-locking the EEG to a temporal stimulus, but Woodward, Owens, and Thompson (1990) used the gating paradigm and asked subjects to listen to parts of a word, considering its meaning. The investigators identified an N2-P3 complex that covaried with word duration and recognition point. On average, N2 occurred after 480 msec and around 200 msec after recognition points, and P3 happened later at 830 msec and around 500 msec after recognition points. Figure 3–6 shows examples of these EPs separated from their EEGs. The whole latencies varied widely among words. Considering speeds that have been measured for lexical access, it was decided that the neg-

ative-positive complex includes post-lexical semantic processes, which would be likely because of the task instructions. An N400 may also occur after lexical access. Holcomb and Neville (1990) utilized a priming task for auditory and visual related and unrelated stimuli (e.g., DOG-CAT, CAR-PEN). Modalities differed in distribution of response over the scalp, and EPs had N400 components that were larger to unrelated words. The N400 response appeared to be tied to language processing.

SENTENCE COMPREHENSION

For studying disorders, Tyler (1988) suggested that "researchers have, on the whole, been primarily interested in whether a patient (or group of patients) has difficulty with particular types of linguistic information, but

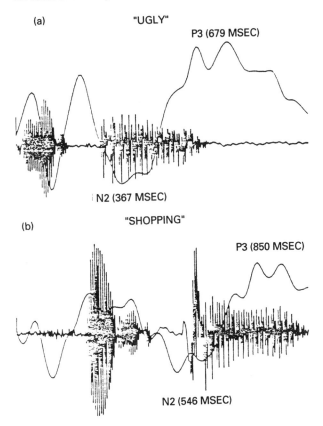

(a) "UGLY"

P3 (679 MSEC)

N2 (367 MSEC)

(b) "SHOPPING"

P3 (850 MSEC)

N2 (546 MSEC)

FIGURE 3–6 Neurophysiological response to *ugly* and *shopping*, recorded at the left parietal lobe and averaged for a group of subjects. The N2 and P3 components occur at different latencies for different words and may correspond to cognitive events "activated" by words. (Reprinted by permission from Woodward, S.H., Owens, J., & Thompson, L.W., Word-to-word variation in ERP component latencies: Spoken words. *Brain and Language,* 38, 1990, p. 495. Academic Press, publisher.)

they rarely attempt to locate the source of the difficulty in a particular aspect of the comprehension process" (p. 376). This section surveys the study of sentence comprehension processes in psycholinguistic laboratories. Only part of the story is told here. Lines of investigation are merely introduced so that we can have a sense for comprehension.

A Framework for the Study of Comprehension

Like word comprehension, sentence comprehension happens with automatic and obligatory **core processes.** According to Tyler (1987), core processes operate on a *principle of optimal efficiency* by assigning "an analysis to the speech input at the theoretically earliest point at which the type of analysis in question can be assigned" (p. 146). Also, they operate on a *principle of bottom-up priority,* because access to knowledge is initially determined by stimulus cues. Core processes are supplemented with capacity-consuming con-

trolled processes, and researchers try to distinguish automatic and strategic components of the time to make a response in a comprehension task.

Comprehension is initially assumed to rely on three subsystems: a lexical processor, a syntactic processor, and a semantic or interpretive processor (Figure 3–7; Cairns, 1984; Garnham, 1985). Research begins with the question of whether these processors exist as modular subsystems. The arrows suggest that a module depends on being informed by representations computed by another module. One issue was whether these modules operate serially (Figure 3–7a) or in an interactive/parallel fashion (Figure 3–7b). Now, interactive processing seems unavoidable for explaining research, and contemporary questions pertain to the manner in which interactive processing occurs. The main task for the **language system** (LS) is to utilize cues in an utterance to activate complex concepts. This task includes **thematic role assignment,** or figuring out *who is doing what to whom.*

FIGURE 3–7 The major subsystems of sentence comprehension arranged according to serial theory and the preferred interactive-parallel theory. Lexical access, for example, is elaborated in Figure 3–5.

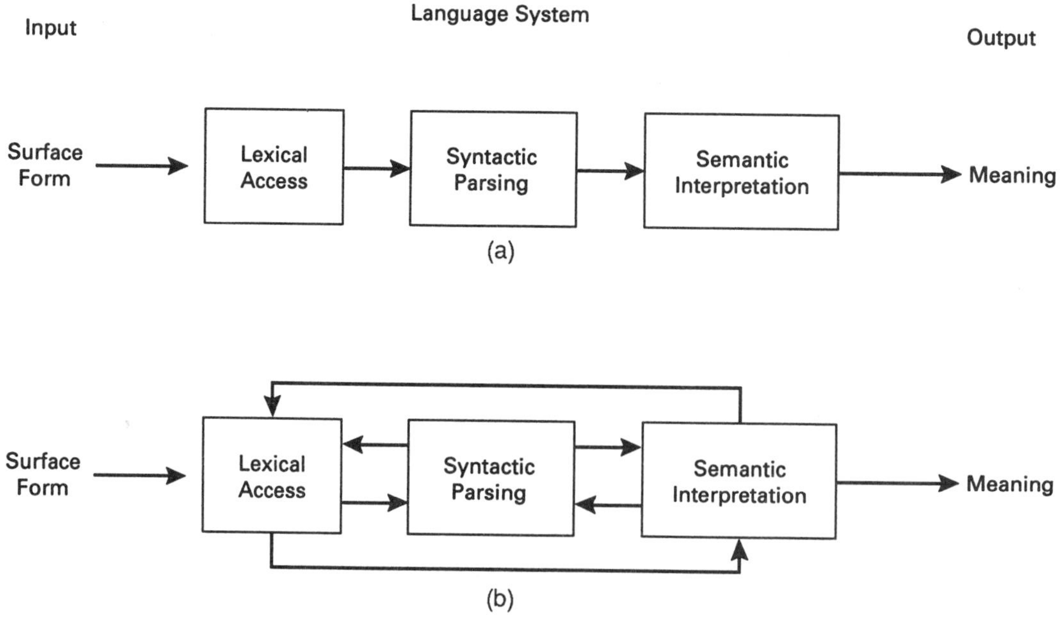

Speech-language pathologists' customary approach to assessment may interfere with recognizing a dominant approach in psycholinguistic research. Most clinical tests of comprehension are **off-line tasks,** in which a sentence is presented completely before a response. The response is generated from cumulative processing while the sentence was heard or read. In picture-choice or question-answering procedures, response is additionally a result of processes that occur after a sentence has been comprehended and that can be unrelated to comprehension. The post-comprehension period may consist of infiltrating strategic processing and response-making factors such as having to choose from among four complex drawings.

Many psycholinguists prefer **on-line tasks,** in which response can be tied to a point within an utterance and measurements can be influenced mainly by core comprehension processes. For example, eye movement can be detected as someone is quietly reading. This movement actually consists of alternating fixations and shifts called *saccadic movement.* Duration of eye fixation is indicative of cognitive effort at the fixation point, especially for a critical word or phrase in a sentence (Rayner and Pollatsek, 1989; Rayner, Sereno, Morris, Schmauder, and Clifton, 1989). Theories are tested by designing conditions that may induce variation of processing load across a sentence. When eye movement is observed, a subject does not have to make an overt response that might add decisions to comprehension. When overt responses, such as pressing a button, are obtained, they are often incidental to comprehension. In some studies, subjects press a button when they hear a sound or word in an utterance. To induce subjects to comprehend anyway, subjects are promised that they will be tested later. In these ways, researchers try to get as close as possible to the "click of comprehension" (Foss and Hakes, 1978).

Lexical Access in Sentences

According to Marslen-Wilson and Tyler (1980), auditory comprehension starts with the first word of an utterance. Recognition points occur quite early in a word when there is disambiguating context, thus keeping sentence comprehension moving along at a brisk pace; "after only about half a word has been heard (within an average of 250 msec from speech onset), the input has not only begun to be mapped onto the mental lexicon, but has also begun to be syntactically and semantically interpreted" (Tyler, 1987, p. 146). The word-familiarity effect on lexical access was detected by Foss (1969), who measured response latency for identifying a sound that followed a word, called the *phoneme-monitoring task:*

(2a) The traveling bassoon player found himself without funds.

(2b) The itinerant bassoon player found himself without funds.

Pressing a button when hearing /b/ took longer following less frequent words (2b), indicative of the different activation thresholds for words in lexical memory. Also, eye fixation was longer for uncommon nouns and adjectives (Rayner, et al., 1989).

What about the automatic post-lexical access of meaning, especially the activation of multiple meanings with polysemous words such as BANK? Using the phoneme-monitoring task, Foss (1970) found that response time after an ambiguous word (3a) is slower than after an unambiguous word (3b).

(3a) The men started to drill before they were ordered to do so.

(3b) The men started to march before they were ordered to do so.

This **ambiguity effect** is explained as an automatic activation of multiple meanings. However, the context before these words is bland, and we might wonder if a biasing context (4b) would limit the activation of meanings for a polysemous word such as *bugs* (Swinney and Hakes, 1976).

(4a) Rumor had it that, for years, the government building had been plagued with problems.

The man was not surprised when he found several bugs in the corner of his room.

(4b) Rumor had it that, for years, the government building had been plagued with problems. The man was not surprised when he found several spiders, roaches, and other bugs in the corner of his room.

In a comparison of these contexts with *bugs* (insects or a spying device) and *insects* using phoneme-monitoring for /c/, an ambiguity effect of 42 msec occurred for neutral context. There was no ambiguity effect for the biasing context. *Bugs* had the same processing load as *insects*, indicating that a **context effect** eliminated multiple access for a polysemous word. Is this context effect a penetration of autonomous activation? The answer is not clear. Contrary to Foss' presentation of /b/ immediately after an ambiguous word, /c/ was presented two syllables later.

Swinney (1979) recognized this problem and designed another study with the same stimuli but with a different task so that a response could be taken from a point immediately after the ambiguous word. He replaced phoneme monitoring with an LDT and called the task **cross-modal priming.** Wearing headphones for hearing the sentences, a subject sits in front of a computer for viewing a word or nonword at a point while sentences are being heard. Subjects are promised that comprehension will be tested later, and lexical decision time is the measure of processing load. In Swinney's study, the prime was *bugs* in the sentences *(4a, 4b),* and a visual target (i.e., ANT, SPY, or SEW) was presented right after the prime. This time, ambiguous primes facilitated recognition of each related target in each context, even when context biased interpretation to one meaning (i.e., ANT). In a subsequent experiment, the context effect occurred with targets presented four syllables after primes. Combined with Swinney's earlier study, these results indicated that the ambiguity effect (i.e., multiple access) occurs immediately, whereas the context effect with selected access occurs later.

In sentences, words can automatically acti-

vate multiple meanings. Thus, lexical access can be an autonomous module unaffected by information from other modules. Subsequent context effects can be attributed to the semantic interpreter. However, contextual information can penetrate lexical access. When the gating procedure was applied to complex words such as CORRESPONDING (5), the recognition point occurred before the word was completed when there was a syntactic bias in a context without semantic assistance (Tyler and Marslen-Wilson, 1986).

(5) Dinners and pineapples were old bracelets. For many brushes they had been regularly CORRESPON--- with each other.

Also, if semantic context is strong enough, selected access to the biased meaning can happen very soon after a polysemous word; ordered access of meanings can occur as well (Simpson, 1984). With a weak context for a polysemous word, especially for a subordinate meaning, further work by the semantic interpreter becomes necessary for selecting the intended concept. Besides activating meanings, lexical access informs the parser by activating grammatical categories and subcategorization restrictions stored in the mental lexicon.

Syntactic Processing: Parsing

The parser assigns grammatical categories and computes structural relations among words and phrases. Lexical activation informs the parser that a word can be a noun or a verb, and the parser assigns one category. The challenge of assigning structure is shown with structurally ambiguous sentences such as 6 and 7.

(6a) They fed (her dog) biscuits.
(6b) They fed her (dog biscuits).
(7a) They (are fighting) dogs.
(7b) They are (fighting dogs).

These strings of words can be parsed differently, and the parse is related to assignment of grammatical function to *dog* in 6 and *fight-*

ing in 7 (i.e., verb or adjective). In conversation, these ambiguities are resolved with cues such as pausing and stress. Researchers strip away these cues, leaving the parser on its own. Then, sources of resolution are added to a stimulus in order to determine how the parser works. One issue is whether parsing can take place without semantic cues; "the distinction between parsing and interpretation is far from clear-cut" (Altman, 1989, p. 1).

Modern psycholinguistics began in the 1960s by drawing upon linguistic theory to determine the influence of syntactic complexity on cognition. Types of structure were compared, and linguistic devices were identified as mental processes (Fodor, Bever, and Garrett, 1974). Researchers also wondered if embedding a subordinate clause within a main clause would burden the system. In the 1980s, researchers became interested in inducing parsing mistakes by presenting ambiguous strings of words at the beginning of sentences.

(8) The steel ships are transporting *is expensive.*

This sentence would be easier to comprehend if *that* were included in what turns out to be an embedded relative clause. The reduced relative clause in 8 creates a **garden-path sentence,** because it is possible that a reader is led astray initially by assigning a noun phrase to *the steel ships* rather than making *steel* a noun. The error cannot be recognized until reading the phrase *is expensive.* The parser's making mistakes and then correcting them give us some clues as to how the parser might work.

Frazier's theory of parsing has been the soul of many studies of garden-path phenomena (Frazier and Rayner, 1982). Her idea is familiar. Consistent with the principle of optimal efficiency, the parser assigns a complete structure at the earliest opportunity. The parser also assigns the simplest structure, a notion with linguistic refinements known as "minimal attachment" and which is somewhat controversial (Kennedy, Murray, Jennings, and Reid, 1989). Finally, according to a "revision as last resort principle," a listener or reader revises the assignment if it turns out to be ungrammatical. Automaticity and autonomy lead a parser into making a lot of mistakes and corrections.

Garden-path sentences become an ideal examination of whether structure is applied judiciously to a whole sentence or, instead, is slapped on with the first available parse. Let us become familiar with basic features of studies employing garden-path sentences such as 8. Many of these studies rely on duration of eye fixation as the measure of relative processing load. The crucial comparison is between the garden-path sentence and its unreduced disambiguated counterpart, such as *The steel that ships are transporting is expensive.* The **critical element** for measurement is the point at which an error can be recognized in the reduced sentence (i.e., *is expensive*). A **garden-path effect** occurs when the critical fixation is longer for reduced than for unreduced relatives. More time as well as regressive eye movements indicate that a subject was "garden-pathed" into an erroneous **initial parse** and had to revise in order to assign the **ultimate parse.** Thinking of other modules of comprehension, Ferreira and Clifton (1986) stated that "it is important to distinguish between *initial* and *eventual* use of nonsyntactic information" (p. 348). They added that "if the syntactic processor (or parser) is modular, it should initially construct a syntactic representation without consulting nonsyntactic information sources, such as semantic or pragmatic information or discourse structure" (p. 348).

What information does the parser use to assign a structure? Verbs are a strong source of lexical **subcategorization** rules. Some verbs take a direct object, and others cannot take a direct object (Mitchell, 1989).

(9a) After the private had *saluted* the sergeant he requested permission to end the exercise.
(9b) After the private had *fainted* the sergeant he requested permission to end the exercise.

For 9a, we would readily assign *the sergeant* to the initial clause; but for 9b, our parser would shift and begin another clause with *the ser-*

geant. Another cue is **number agreement,** which, in *10,* determines the attachment of [things that were stolen] (Mitchell, 1989).

(10) The police recovered the photographs of the painting which (was/were) stolen.

Also, it is reasonable to suspect that world knowledge from the interpreter can influence an initial parse. Rayner, Carlson, and Frazier (1983) studied **plausibility** of the beginning of a sentence to determine if subjects apply a quick initial parse based on knowledge of likely scenarios.

(12a) The florist sent the flowers *was very* pleased.
(12b) The performer sent the flowers *was very* pleased.

A comparison of *12* to unreduced versions showed that subjects were garden-pathed into parsing the beginning as someone sending flowers. Eye fixation on *was very* did not distinguish *12a* and *12b,* indicating that information about who usually sends or receives flowers did not bias the initial parse. Thus, initial parsing can be impervious to world knowledge.

Semantic Processing: Interpretation

The semantic interpreter is the center for integration. It resolves ambiguities and assigns thematic roles to the information it receives from lexical access and initial parsing. World knowledge is especially useful to the semantic subsystem. This section deals with more modest goals, beginning with the activation of regions of semantic memory. We hear statements like *13* and *14* all the time (e.g., "Fred is a jerk").

(13a) A canary is a bird.
(13b) A canary is an animal.
(14a) A robin is a bird.
(14b) A chicken is a bird.

In the concept-comparison tasks mentioned previously, time to verify these straightforward assertions was measured (Collins and

Loftus, 1975). Understanding these sentences involves a comparison of concepts, and *13b* takes longer than *13a* because [bird] is closer than [animal] to [canary]. Prototypicality contributes to *14a* being verified faster than *14b.* Speed of verification (if not comprehension) has something to do with the basic structure and spreading activation of semantic memory.

When an utterance has lexical and structural ambiguity, the automatic autonomy of lexical access and initial parsing deposit irrelevant meanings and incorrect structures into working memory. Experimental context effects indicate that these meanings are inhibited and initial parses are revised. The ambiguity effect is often eliminated two syllables or words after the ambiguous word (e.g., Swinney, 1979). In a version of cross-modal priming, an ambiguous prime was presented at the end of a sentence; and target words were presented at SOAs of 0, 200, and 600 msec (Tanenhaus, Leiman, and Seidenberg, 1979). The ambiguity effect occurred at 0 msec but not at 200 msec. In an on-line cross-modal priming study (see *15*), targets were shown immediately (position-1) or two syllables after ambiguous primes like *port* (Seidenberg, Tanenhaus, Leiman, and Bienkowski, 1982).

(15) The waiter poured the port into the glasses.

1   2
WINE
SHIP

Presenting targets at either of these positions was similar to manipulating the SOA in a basic LDT. Both targets were facilitated in position-1. Only the appropriate target was facilitated at position-2. We can also be garden-pathed into an interpretation of an ambiguous word that turns out to be incorrect and must be revised, as with *16* (Conrad and Rips, 1986).

(16) The old man's glasses were filled with sherry.

Interaction of bottom-up and top-down processing allows context to modify interpretations continually as we listen to sentences.

This introduction to psycholinguistics is restricted to considering the goal of determining *who is doing what to whom*. As indicated earlier, the distinction between the parser and interpreter in meeting this goal "is far from clear-cut" (Altman, 1989). Our interpreter is often said to engage in a **mapping** of thematic roles onto representations generated by lexical access and the parser. This operation may also occur in the reverse order, and in many instances it may be difficult to tease a parsing assignment of phrase structure apart from the assignment of who is the agent or recipient of an action (e.g., *12a, 12b*). An eye-movement study examined the role of animacy in parsing the initial word-string of *17* (Ferreira and Clifton, 1986).

(17a) The defendant examined *by the lawyer* turned out to be unreliable.
(17b) The evidence examined *by the lawyer* turned out to be unreliable.

Fixation on the critical phrase *by the lawyer* was longer for *17a* than for *17b*. This was a garden-path effect in that the additional time was needed for revising an initial parse of *The defendant examined*. The grammatical subject can be an agent for a verb that takes only animate agents. This initial parse assigns thematic roles, which a garden-pathed person has to revise upon discovering that the lawyer did the examining.

MacWhinney and Bates compared cues that we use for assigning thematic roles and developed what they call a *competition model* to explain processing differences across languages (Bates, et al., 1991; MacWhinney, Bates, and Kliegl, 1984). Let us just increase our familiarity with the cues by trying to decide who is doing what in *18*.

(18) The ball grab the cats.

English speakers lean heavily on **word order** and might initially assign the role of agent to *ball*, because noun-verb-noun (N-V-N) structures are usually agent-action structures thematically. Italian speakers are likely to assign agency to *the cats* because of a reliance on **inflectional agreements** between nouns and verbs. German speakers are likely to prefer *cats* for a different reason: namely, **animacy** agreement with the action. Thus, across languages, types of cues differ in information value. Word order is less important than other cues in Italian and German, and word order is more important in English. In another investigation, English speakers maintained a preference for word order as a basis for assigning agents, whereas Dutch speakers relied more on case inflection (McDonald, 1987).

LANGUAGE PRODUCTION

Verbal production has not been studied nearly as much as comprehension. Theories of language formulation processes have had the appearance of taking a theory of comprehension and reversing it or turning it upside-down. Any theory specifies three major phases of the expressive function (Figure 3–8). We start with an idea or meaning to convey, called a "pre-linguistic" phase. Meaning, which is presumably an activation of semantic memory, is converted into our language. Then, linguistic form tells the motor system what to do. Danks' (1977) version of this framework shows an interactive relationship among these phases that is monitored by the executive control system. Yet, it does not tell us much about each phase or how these major subsystems map onto each other. Regarding research, the information-processing paradigm has been applied to the study of word-retrieval (e.g., Loftus and Loftus, 1974), and priming has been used to influence sentences elicited by pictures (Bock, 1987). Mainly theories are tested with respect to their predictions of normal speech errors (e.g., Dell, 1988; Stemberger, 1984).

A few clinical investigators such as Schwartz (1987) interpret patterns of expressive disorder with respect to Garrett's (1984) theory of sentence production. The outline in Figure 3–9 packages processing sub-

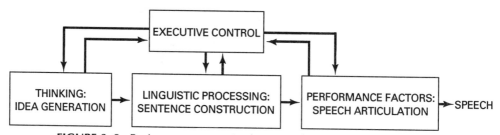

FIGURE 3–8 Basic components in theories of sentence production. (Reprinted by permission from Danks, J.H., Producing ideas and sentences. In S. Rosenberg (Ed.), *Sentence production: Developments in research and theory.* Hillsdale, NJ: Lawrence Erlbaum, 1977, p. 230.

systems in boxes that compute successive levels of mental representation. Formulation begins with conceptualization and ends in two motor stages: "regular processes" for speech programming and "coding processes" for execution of movement. Two levels of linguistic processes make up the middle of this mainly serial model. The **message-level representation** is said to drive subsequent processes. Garrett (1984) wrote that "language production is the development, under message-level control, of sentence-level representations that are sufficient to determine an appropriate control structure for articulation" (p. 173). The message level is especially important for pragmatic and discourse-level features of verbal behavior (Ch. 8).

This model is more subtle than one that would have semantics, syntax, and the lexicon ordered in a row. It suggests that components of language are formulated interactively at two levels, and these linguistic levels are specified to a degree of detail that is not presented here (Garrett, 1984). One level of syntax is close to semantics in a sense that is comparable to generating a deep structure. Another level is close to the lexicon in a way that is comparable to generating a surface structure. The **functional level** representation is generated by *logical and syntactic processes.* It contains conceptually specified slots for content words and specification of thematic roles of agent, recipient, and so on. Then, *syntactic and phonological processes* develop a **positional level** representation. This representation contains a syntactic frame

(i.e., grammatical morphemes and intonation cues) and the phonological form of words inserted into the frame.

Garrett argued that normal errors or slips of the tongue are explained by the existence of these levels. The process level generating **exchanges** was thought to be indicated by the linguistic relationship between exchanged units and the distance between units. A greater distance between exchanged units reflects a deeper source of error. Let us consider Garrett's samples.

(19) "I have a pinched *neck* in my *nerve.*"
(20) "She was a real *rack pat.*"

A mistake at the functional level is indicated in *19.* Appropriate lexical items are selected but are inserted incorrectly into thematic slots. Most exchanges across the phrase boundary involve whole words within a grammatical class (e.g., nouns). Contrary to *19,* phonologic similarity seemed rarely to be a factor in this type of exchange. In *20,* the speaker got through the functional level without mishap. Sound exchanges are generated at the stage of word form specification. Garrett's observations indicate that morphemic and phonemic exchanges tend to occur within a phrase. Phrasal constituents have been formulated. Also, open class words and grammatical morphemes may be generated at different stages. Exchanges occur mostly between open class words (i.e., nouns, verbs). However, **shifts** of position occur mostly with function words and inflectional endings (e.g.,

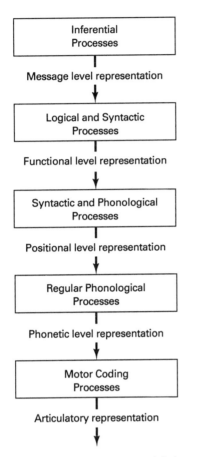

FIGURE 3-9 Garrett's serial theory of sentence formulation, an elaboration of Figure 3–8. A convention of such diagrams is that the boxes designate processing subsystems which compute mental representations outside the boxes. (Derived by permission from Garrett, M.F., The organization of processing structure for language production: Applications to aphasic speech. In D. Caplan, A.R. Lecours, & A. Smith (Eds.), *Biological perspectives on language*. Cambridge, MA: MIT Press, 1984, p. 174.)

"It certainly run outs fast"). Garrett (1982) concluded that "closed class vocabulary seems to be recruited at the point where the detailed surface form of sentences is being integrated, whereas the open class vocabulary is retrieved at an earlier stage when the

functional roles of words and phrases are being determined" (p. 218).

Advances in theory are often presented as modifications of Garrett's precedent or of a simpler idea that semantics precedes syntax which precedes phonology. Theories are evolving in the same direction in which theories of comprehension shifted from serial to parallel-interactive autonomy. There is evidence for a phonological input to formation of basic syntactic form. When faced with retrieving a phonologically difficult word for one syntactic frame, speakers sometimes shift to another syntactic frame (Bock, 1987). Phonological similarities between exchanged words, as in 19, may be more common than Garrett thought (Dell and Reich, 1981). Exchanges of similar-sounding words across phrases indicates that the positional level sometimes feeds back to the deeper syntactic processes of the functional level. PDP or connectionist theory has also contributed to predicting probabilities for the occurrence of normal speech errors (Dell, 1988) and explaining the tip-of-the-tongue state (Burke, MacKay, Worthley, and Wade, 1991).

SUMMARY AND IMPLICATIONS

The phenomena of "language" disorder are the phenomena of language comprehension and formulation. Theory of comprehension and formulation is a problem for the psycholinguistic branch of cognitive psychology. Research is devoted to discovering attributes of knowledge and processes that explain the results of experiments. Based on the thinking expressed by Caramazza's transparency assumption, we should be interested in how these discoveries help us explain the symptoms of language impairments. One of the basic diagnostic questions is whether a disorder can be an erasure of information stored in long-term memory or a disruption of processes in working memory. It we become concerned about a patient's memory, then we must investigate whether symptoms are caused by impaired acquisition, storage, or access; and we may search for a problem specific to episodic, semantic, or lexical stores. Another basic question is whether it is possible for brain injury to damage the general features of cognition, such as attention or executive control, that provide a hospitable environment for linguistic and other large modular systems to do their specific jobs.

Early in this chapter, Howard and Patterson were quoted regarding the diagnosis of an aphasic person's disorder. Especially for the patient with a focal lesion in the perisylvian region, they had stated that we need to identify component(s) of the language system that are impaired and those that are relatively spared. Chapter 2 referred to the long-held belief that a patient's behavior arises from interacting abnormal and normal processes. Interactive cognitive theory is an initial foundation with which researchers can predict deficit patterns and clinicians can identify treatment goals based on observing these patterns. For example, basic research may identify an impairment of the parser. If we were to mark this box in Figure 3–7b, we could see that evidence for this impairment would also have to be compatible with retention of lexical access and interpretive mechanisms and with the effect of parsing disorder on the operation of these mechanisms (Chapter 5). This thinking indicates that aphasia might

offer evidence for interdependencies among comprehension subsystems. It is also the manner in which theory of normal cognition shapes our ideas about the nature of language disorders.

Because aphasia may be conceptualized according to cognitive theories, it would be natural to believe that language disorders can be studied and assessed simply by applying the methods of modern psycholinguistics. Yet, differences between neurologically intact and brain-damaged subjects create problems with respect to the basic assumptions underlying psycholinguistic research. Some methods employ response modes that are disrupted in aphasia, forcing clinical researchers to modify psycholinguistic procedures. To study recognition, word-naming cannot be used with aphasic persons because of their problems with word production. A greater challenge may be the reliance on latencies of accurate responses in order to identify processes used by normal subjects. Brain damage impairs systems and causes errors so that response times would have a quite different meaning. Many aphasiologists ignore response latency and rely on comparing task-oriented capacities and analyzing patterns of errors on a task.

CHAPTER

4

INVESTIGATION OF APHASIA

This chapter focuses on what aphasic people tend to have in common. Information comes from studies of groups defined as having aphasia without further differentiation. It also comes from the broadly defined fluent and nonfluent aphasias caused by posterior and anterior lesions. The chapter emphasizes auditory comprehension deficit as a general feature of aphasia. For expression, it focuses on basic attributes of word-finding. Grammatical features are usually examined with respect to syndromes (Chapter 5).

EXPERIMENTAL FRAMEWORKS

Probably the most basic clinical question pertains to determination of disorder. Impairment is identified with reference to a norm. In research, a **mean score** by a brain-injured

group is compared with a mean from a "normal" or neurologically intact group. Another approach is to determine the number of experimental subjects who are **beneath a cut-off score** or on the low end of a range for a normal group. These approaches to group comparisons can lead to different generalizations about the brain-damaged group. A statistically significant difference from a normal average may portray the experimental group as deficient. With a cut-off score, we may find that a large portion of the same group is not measurably impaired. Moreover, a particular performance may or may not be interpreted as a deficit. Let us think about an aphasic group that scores 16 of 20, while normal controls score 19.5. If 16 differs significantly from 19.5 and is beneath a cut-off score, we may point out the deficit it reveals (e.g., Young and De Haan, 1988). If the deficient score is significantly **above chance performance,** we may emphasize that a function has been retained (e.g., Coslett and Saffran, 1989). We may see the glass as half empty or half full. This nuance applies to hunts for dissociations or specific impairments, and it points to making distinctions between loss of function and reduced efficiency of a retained function.

For differentiating among types of disorder, basic research employs **between-group designs** in the form of comparing groups defined according to site of lesion or type of neuropathology. Left-hemisphere damage (LHD) is compared with right-hemisphere damage (RHD). Stroke (CVA) is compared with closed head injury (CHI). To determine whether performance is deficient, we would add a neurologically intact control group. When subjects are assumed to have aphasia caused by perisylvian damage, aphasic LHDs may be compared with presumably nonaphasic LHDs. When the principle of double dissociation is considered (Chapter 2), the investigator may determine whether a deficit or capability relates to a particular LHD, any LHD, or any focal brain damage. Yet, with differing definitions of aphasia, this research can be murky. An "aphasic" group may be restricted to persons with single, unilateral lesions (e.g., Brookshire and Nicholas, 1984) or may contain a mix of persons with CVAs and head injuries (e.g., Clark and Flowers, 1987). Finding characteristics specific to a group addresses the issue of "when is aphasia aphasia" (Chapter 1).

What are the effects of rate, length, concreteness, and complexity on comprehension? What kind of errors are made on a naming task? A **within-group design** is employed for learning as much as we can about aphasia, which characterizes a great deal of the research reported in this chapter. One risk applies to between-group studies as well. Finding enough subjects is not easy, especially when we want to study a group that we can assume is homogeneous with respect to selection criteria (e.g., focal lesion, normal hearing, fluent aphasia). Brain-damaged experimental groups vary widely in size as well as

composition. Studies of five, ten, or 12 aphasic subjects are common. Investigators are often careful about drawing conclusions from results that suggest a characterization of a larger population.

THE NATURE OF APHASIA

After working with hundreds of cases, Schuell and her colleagues (1964) concluded that all cases of aphasia have deficits of comprehension, memory span, and word retrieval. An aphasia should be revealed in all modalities. This section introduces issues that even address the manner in which aphasia may be defined. Does aphasia extend to nonverbal areas of "intelligence"? Does the disorder consume a wider domain of symbolic function? The third question underlies many studies of specific abilities. That is, is aphasia a loss of knowledge or a disruption of processes? Or, might it involve both?

Language Disorder and Intelligence

A patient's wife is likely to say that "he doesn't talk but his mind is OK." As noted before, Darley (1982) defined aphasia as a language disorder that is "disproportionate to impairment of other intellective functions." Early in the twentieth century, Pierre Marie seemed to go against the grain of syndrome diagnosis such as "expressive aphasia." He noticed that all cases had some degree of comprehension deficit. He went further by arguing that aphasic people have some sort of "intellectual" deficit. It is difficult to ascertain what Marie meant. Discovery of intellectual deficit may have been Marie's way of dealing with comprehension deficit. However, patients with apparently more than a language problem propelled researchers into examining many functions besides language. Prior to the birth of cognitive sciences, varied higher cortical functions were embraced collectively beneath the umbrella of intelligence.

When assessing the range of a patient's cognitive capacities, clinical neuropsychologists initially relied on the **Wechsler Adult**

Intelligence Scale (WAIS) (Wechsler, 1981). It is divided into verbal and performance scales that seemed to correspond to the verbal-nonverbal dichotomy that has been so prevalent in differentiating dysfunctions (Table 4–1). Aphasic people usually score much worse on the verbal subtests than on the nonverbal subtests (McFie, 1975), a within-group pattern consistent with the notion of language-specific disorder. In the first use of standardized IQ tests with aphasic patients, Weisenburg and McBride (1935) compared results against the norm. The results indicated that aphasic people frequently have nonverbal deficits. With a German version of the WAIS, Orgass and Poeck (1969) found a mean performance IQ of 80 in 30 subjects, which was below the norm of 100 and significantly lower than the performance IQ of nonaphasic persons with LHD and RHD. In France, Alajouanine and Lhermitte (1964) reported similar results. Thus, aphasia is observed as disproportionate impairment of language skills, because performance on nonverbal tasks can be impaired, too.

The overall score from tests like the WAIS was thought to measure general intelligence, especially a mystic factor called *g* weaving through all mental functions. Because of their language deficits, the performance score was viewed as the fairest measure of *g* for aphasic persons. If we can believe this assumption, then deficient performance scores are suggestive of a deficient *g*. Often administered by speech-language pathologists, Raven's **Coloured Progressive Matrices** (RCPM) was thought to be predictive of *g* (Raven, Court, and Raven, 1976). It relies on presentation of geometric designs. In each set of items, 12 items increase in difficulty, from completing simple figures to reasoning with a less than apparent pattern of figures. In a study of 111 aphasic subjects, those with severe comprehension deficit were well below nonaphasic brain-damaged groups; moderate to mild aphasias were comparable to RHD subjects (Kertesz and McCabe, 1975). In another study, small aphasic and RHD groups were also similar in that both had the most difficulty with items requiring reasoning by analogy, and most errors involved "repetition of a pattern" (Horner and Nailling, 1980). If visuospatial tests measure *g*, then we may be tempted to conclude that aphasia pulls general intelligence along with it, casting doubt on whether aphasia should be considered to be a language-specific disorder.

Aphasic persons also have difficulty with visuospatial problem-solving tasks. The "Tower of Hanoi" puzzle was given to 18 subjects (Prescott, Loverso, and Selinger, 1984). It looks simple enough, with three disks of varied sizes stacked on one of three pegs. The disks must be transferred, one at a time, from the first peg to the third peg, with no disk placed on a smaller one. Aphasic subjects required twice the number of moves as normal subjects to solve the problem. Some were successful within the cut-off score of 11 moves; but seven gave up, and a few others took 50 moves to a solution. Later, aphasic LHDs did not differ from subjects with RHD, and the investigators mused, "One might ask what these nonverbal tests measure" (Prescott, Gruber, Olson, and Fuller, 1987, p. 255). Prescott's question is appropriate as investigators move toward considering the cognitive bases of tasks.

TABLE 4–1 Subtests in the Wechsler Adult Intelligence Scale. Vocabulary is sometimes omitted (Lezak, 1983).

Verbal	*Performance*
Information (general knowledge)	Digit symbol (timed matching)
Comprehension (judgment, reasoning)	Picture completion
Arithmetic	Block design (manual reproduction)
Similarities (word pairs, concepts)	Picture arrangement (stories)
Digit span (forward and backward)	Object assembly (e.g., puzzles)
Vocabulary (definitions)	

Deficits outside the realm of language were found to be associated with severity of aphasia. Difficulty with Raven's matrices was mostly confined to the aphasias with severe comprehension deficits (Kertesz and Mc-Cabe, 1975). Zangwill (1964) found deficits with the RCPM in aphasic persons with constructional apraxia, a motor disorder involving the ability to produce spatial designs (Chapter 7). Assessed with replication of block designs, the presence of constructional apraxia is related to severity of comprehension deficit (Benton, Hamsher, Varney, and Spreen, 1983). Severe comprehension deficit occurs with lesions including the inferior parietal lobe, which has a role in visuospatial abilities on both sides of the brain. Deficits beyond the perisylvian area may also be due to the chronic remote effects of stroke (Chapter 2). Moreover, heightened caution goes into intepreting classical tests of intelligence. The WAIS's verbal scale goes beyond the automatic processing of everyday language use. It tests conceptualization, judgment, and reasoning. The performance scale requires dexterity, and clinical neuropsychologists prefer to supplement this section with tests in which input functions (e.g., spatial perception) can be evaluated with minimal response requirement. Therefore, remote effects of lesions and confounds in testing permit the conclusion that difficulties co-occurring with language disorder are not necessarily a component of a single disorder. Aphasic people may simply have disorders in addition to their aphasia.

The vague notion of *g* was replaced with the idea that we possess multiple cognitive skills or "intelligences." *Crystallized* intelligence was thought to rely on previously acquired knowledge and was measured with tests in the verbal section of the WAIS. *Fluid* intelligence supposedly acquires information and solves novel problems. It was identified to a lesser extent with the performance section. The crystallized form seemed to remain stable as fluid intelligence declines with aging (Horn and Donaldson, 1976). Gardner (1983) argued that there are six specialized "frames of mind," consisting of linguistic, logical-

mathematical, musical, spatial, bodily-kinesthetic, and personal capacities. Sternberg (1985) proposed three intellectual capacities: contextual (i.e., adapting to the environment and common sense), experiential (i.e., using knowledge for solving novel problems and solving familiar problems quickly), and internal (i.e., planning and evaluating). At a conference on aphasia and intelligence, someone concluded that "it is doubtful whether the notion of intelligence as a unitary capacity is helpful in analyzing the psychological changes brought about by cerebral damage" (Lebrun and Hoops, 1974, p. 45). Theory of intelligence has become consistent with the notion of modularity of large functional systems that often work together in the performance of the many tasks used in clinical assessment.

Pantomimic Asymbolia

Symbols can take many forms. In his classic introduction to speech pathology, Van Riper maintained that aphasia is a deficit of "symbolization" (Van Riper and Emerick, 1990), or the mental processes of comprehending and retrieving symbols. In 1870, Finkelnburg described cases in which verbal and nonverbal symbol use were impaired (cited in Duffy and Liles, 1979). A pious Catholic woman could not initiate the sign of the cross. A violinist was able to play by ear but could not read musical notation. We may wonder if it is in the nature of aphasia for patients to have problems with symbols beyond the use of their verbal language, leading to the notion that aphasia should actually be called "asymbolia."

Aphasia in deaf users of ASL seems to address this question, but actually it may only skirt the edges. "Despite the important differences in form, signed and spoken languages clearly share underlying structural principles. Like spoken language, sign language exhibits formal structuring at the lexical and grammatical levels, similar kind and degree of morphological patterning, and a complex, highly rule-governed grammatical and syntactic patterning" (Poizner, et al., 1987, p. 21). Aphasia in ASL indicates that the cognitive bases of linguistic performance should be generalizable to ASL. It does not provide evidence for the question of asymbolia. Similarly, after a stroke, the composer Ravel recognized musical patterns but had difficulties reading musical notation, naming notes, and finding their location on the keyboard of his piano (Alajouanine, 1948). He was having trouble with a specialized language system. Aphasia in ASL is a regular aphasia, and the question here is whether aphasia is a more consuming disorder that would be more evident in hearing persons. The clinical implication is whether highly symbolic augmentative modes of communication would be weakened as part of aphasia or, instead, can be an easy extension of unimpaired capacities.

So, what is this implied nonlinguistic symbolic capacity? Nonverbal symbolization has been studied primarily with respect to manual gesturing, in contrast to pictographic systems such as Blissymbols (Silverman, 1989). Gesturing is a multidimensional behavior. A gesture may be intentional, or it may be an unintentional extension of emotional reaction. Intentional gestures vary in their "iconicity." *Iconic* gestures are near replicas of their referents (e.g., pantomime). Others, such as saluting, are arbitrary conventions shared by a community and may be considered to be more symbolic than pantomime. Two gestural systems have been employed in the study of aphasia. One is ASL, and the other is a set of modified American Indian signs called Amer-Ind (Skelly, 1979). ASL contains many arbitrary symbols, but Amer-Ind is loaded with pantomimic representations of referents. The iconicity of these systems has been examined according to their **transparency:** namely, the extent to which someone unfamiliar with the code can guess a gesture's meaning. Amer-Ind was 54 percent guessable, and ASL was 10 to 30 percent guessable (Daniloff, Lloyd, and Fristoe, 1983). Automatic reactions, single arbitrary conventions, and pantomimic gesture may reside outside the circle of features that are inherent to language.

Another consideration is that motor impairments of hemiparesis or limb apraxia can obscure a view of symbolic behavior, just as dysarthria can mask language behavior. In the study of aphasia, the influence of paralysis can be avoided by having everyone use the unimpaired limb. Limb apraxia is tricky, because it does not usually occur in spontaneous behavior but occurs when someone is asked to perform a movement upon instruction or imitation (DeRenzi, Motti, and Nichelli, 1980). In a sense, it is only a problem in the clinic. Limb apraxia has been controlled for by testing for its presence and then figuring test results into the experimental analysis (Duffy and Duffy, 1981) or by selecting subjects without this disorder (Daniloff, Fritelli, Buckingham, Hoffman, and Daniloff, 1986).

A dissociation of propositional from subpropositional gesturing is often seen in aphasic patients (Duffy and Buck, 1979). Facial expression and vocal reactions to humor are retained (Buck and Duffy, 1980; Gardner, Ling, Flamm, and Silverman, 1975). In a study of pantomime, Duffy and Duffy (1981) found that aphasic subjects' mean performance was significantly worse than that of normal adults. Gesturing the use of common objects was correlated with a measure of overall verbal ability, indicating that language and pantomime deficits could be related. The correlation with language, however, did not separate apraxia from asymbolia as factors. With more statistical analysis, Duffy and Duffy concluded that apraxia contributed little to pantomime performance. Screened for apraxia, aphasic subjects were impaired at imitating Amer-Ind and ASL; and they had more difficulty with a matched group of ASL signs (Daniloff, et al., 1986). Because of the possibility of the motor confound, many investigators decided to focus on gesture recognition for the purpose of addressing the theoretical question of a pantomimic asymbolia.

Pantomime recognition provides an opportunity to determine, as with verbal deficits in aphasia, whether a central disorder can be inferred from coexisting receptive and expressive deficit. To assess recognition, a researcher produces a gesture, and a subject must identify the referent in a set of pictures. Evidence of asymbolia came from group mean deficit (Duffy, Duffy, and Pearson, 1975), correlation with a measure of overall language ability (Duffy and Duffy, 1981), and correlation with receptive language ability (Ferro, Santos, Castro-Caldas, and Mariano, 1980). Aphasic persons also had more difficulty recognizing pantomime than facial emotion (Walker-Batson, Barton, Wendt, and Reynolds, 1987). Yet, when the number of aphasic subjects scoring below a cut-off score was computed, the proportion of subjects with recognition deficits varied from 41 to 74 percent (Gainotti and Lemmo, 1976; Seron, Van Der Kaa, Remitz, and Van Der Linden, 1979; Varney, 1982). Range of aphasic scores in Duffy and Duffy's study overlapped considerably with the normal range. Some studies showed no relationship between pantomime recognition deficit and severity of aphasia (Daniloff, Noll, Fristoe, and Lloyd, 1982; Feyereisen and Seron, 1982). Thus, many aphasic persons do not have pantomime recognition deficit, and it is usually mild if they do have it.

Most investigations of the asymbolia question have relied on pantomime to represent symbols. The issue of whether aphasia is a sweeping asymbolia is not resolved by this research, and figuring out what the issue is depends on what should be called a symbol. There are anecdotal indications that aphasia includes or spreads to arbitrary conventional gestures. A speech-language pathologist is concerned about the communicative avenues available to persons with symbolic disorder; for many aphasic persons, pantomime is one of them.

Disorder of Knowledge or Processing

This section deals with a basic question about the language-specific disorder itself. Schuell (1969) pondered whether aphasia is a deficit of linguistic competence, performance, or both. This question has been contemplated since the earliest study of aphasia (e.g., Jackson, 1879). Is it a *loss* of words from a vocabulary, or is it an *interference* with the

use of words that are not erased? The answer was indicated in clinical observations that sentences are understood at some times but not others. An object is not named one moment, but is named later without assistance (Head, 1920). Thus, Lenneberg (1967) concluded that "neither discrete words nor discrete grammatical rules are neatly eliminated" (p. 207). Schuell and her colleagues (1964) decided that "the language storage system is at least relatively intact" (p. 336) because of the nature of recovery or "the aphasic's spontaneous application of the rules of his language as his available vocabulary increases, and his utterances increase in length and fluency" (Schuell, 1969, p. 119). The issue of competence or performance deficit continues to lie at the heart of many investigations of specific functions. One adjustment in contemporary research is that the issue is restated with respect to the status of knowledge and processing.

Schnitzer (1978) described a common strategy for determining the status of knowledge. No one task or type of task can address knowledge. All types of activities that utilize knowledge are examined, such as metalinguistic tasks along with comprehension and production tasks. Metalinguistic tasks include choosing the correct sentence from a pair (Gardner, Denes, and Zurif, 1975) and arranging phrases into a sentence (von Stockert and Bader, 1976). Grammaticality judgment involves asking a subject to decide whether a sentence is "good" (under a smiling face) or "bad" (under a frowning face) (Shankweiler, Crain, Gorrell, and Tuller, 1989; Wulfeck, 1988). Because metalinguistic tasks are strategic, a deficit on such tasks may mean that problems exist in conscious processing. Yet, "a deficiency which affected all of the linguistic abilities," wrote Schnitzer, "would have to be either a remarkable coincidence or (more likely) a deficiency in the linguistic competence underlying all modalities" (p. 347). Caplan (1985) added that "disturbances found only in one language task have been considered to be disturbances in performances, sparing competence, while disturbances found in all language-related tasks reflect a disturbance of the central set of representations, that is, of competence" (p. 133). Success with just one language task indicates that knowledge is retained to some degree.

AUDITORY COMPREHENSION

The clinical impression is that comprehension deficit exists in all cases of aphasia (Basso, et al., 1978; Schuell and Jenkins, 1961b; Smith, 1971), but there is some uncertainty as to whether this is so (Boller, Kim, and Mack, 1977). Comprehension is a private event, and we infer its status from behavior. A patient responds with a quizzical look, does not follow instructions, or gives an odd answer to a question. Mild deficit is difficult to detect in conversation. Some aphasic persons have such serious problems that they appear not to be paying attention. Others mask severe deficit with nods and easy phrases such as, "Oh yes, I think so" or "That's good," even to a question like "Where do you live?" By presenting language stimuli without natural context and by asking for simple responses, we try to avoid the overestimates or underestimates of ability that can occur from observing conversation.

Aphasia and Auditory Agnosia

An impaired ability to recognize sounds despite adequate hearing is called **auditory agnosia.** Some patients have trouble only with environmental sounds, such as water pouring or a door squeaking. This is called **auditory sound agnosia** (or nonverbal auditory agnosia) (Bauer and Rubens, 1985). Others do not recognize speech sounds; this is called **auditory verbal agnosia** or word deafness. "Pure word deafness" can occur without significant impairment of reading and expression. These agnosias are usually caused by *bilateral infarcts* in the temporal lobe.

Persons with the most severe aphasias may have normal nonverbal sound recognition or may have a severe agnosia along with the language comprehension deficit (Faglioni, Spinnler, and Vignolo, 1969; Varney, 1980). If aphasic subjects make semantically related errors when pointing to pictures of sound sources, we might suspect that sound agnosia and aphasia have a common basis. However, studies of this question produced mixed results (Spinnler and Vignolo, 1966; Strohner, Cohen, Kelter, and Woll, 1978). When aphasic people do not recognize environmental sounds, some impaired verbal mediation may be slipping into a recognition task. This was indicated when 13 subjects, impaired on word comprehension, were normal in recognizing sounds that would be difficult for the average person to label (i.e., bird calls) (Riege, Metter, and Hanson, 1980). Auditory sound agnosia does not seem to be connected to language dysfunction. When it occurs in aphasic persons, it is a distinct disorder that is an "accident of location" of lesion.

Speech Perception

Speech perception is assessed with a **discrimination** task, in which subjects hear CV-syllable pairs (e.g., /pa/, /ba/) or nonsense word pairs (e.g., *ursit, ursat*) and then make same-different judgments (Benton, Hamsher, Varney, and Spreen, 1983). Natural speech is presented with live voice or recordings, but acoustic variables are manipulated more precisely with synthetic speech (Riedel and Studdert-Kennedy, 1985). Another method is **identification** or "labeling"; a subject points to a letter designating the phoneme. Some aphasiologists believed that nearly all aphasic people have a problem with speech perception (e.g., Blumstein, 1981). However, in one study, only 14 of 80 aphasic subjects were beneath the normal range for discrimination (Varney, 1984). Of those with impairment, most improved to normal perception within four months after onset. Of nine fluent aphasic subjects at least one year after onset, six were normal for discrimination (Franklin, 1989). Here are some key findings:

1. The task matters. Discrimination is easier than identification (Blumstein, Tartter, Nigro, and

Statlender, 1984; Riedel and Studdert-Kennedy, 1985). Considering that discrimination can be normal when identification is impaired, Riedel and Studdert-Kennedy concluded that signs of speech perception deficit need not be blamed on auditory processing and could be part of language deficit. That is, impairment is seen more often with labeling than with the "prelinguistic" discrimination task.

2. The difference between sounds matters. More discrimination errors occur with sounds differing by one phonemic feature than by multiple features (Blumstein, Baker, and Goodglass, 1977; Miceli, Caltagirone, Gainotti, and Payer-Rigo, 1978).

3. Place contrasts are more difficult to discriminate than voicing contrasts (Miceli, et al., 1978; Blumstein, et al., 1984).

4. Voice onset time is a problem for some patients (Gandour and Dardarananda, 1982; Itoh, Tatsumi, Sasanuma, and Fukusako, 1986).

5. Aphasic people may have a more basic difficulty with temporal cues (Carpenter and Rutherford, 1973). Perception improved when formant transitions were extended (Tallal and Newcombe, 1978). However, in subsequent studies, extending the transitions did not help. Formant transitions may be irrelevant to perceiving place, and difficulty with place "lies in ... the first 30-odd msec of the stimulus" (Blumstein, et al., 1984, pp. 148–49). Riedel and Studdert-Kennedy (1985) found no difference between long and short CV-pair intervals, contradicting others (e.g., Tallal and Newcombe, 1978).

6. These deficits occur across syndromes (Basso, Casati, and Vignolo, 1977; Miceli, Gainotti, Caltagirone, and Masullo, 1980; Varney and Benton, 1979).

Word Comprehension

Many patients do not have problems with single words when pointing to pictures. When sentences are difficult to understand, a deficit with words indicates severe receptive disorder. In one study, 43 percent of aphasic subjects made no errors (Schuell and Jenkins, 1961b); in another study, 45 percent were within normal range (Varney, 1984). Common words are easier than rare words (Schuell, Jenkins, and Landis, 1961). One is-

sue is whether aphasia produces **category-specific deficits.** Syntactic categories were studied by comparing nouns and verbs. Some patients were equally impaired for nouns and verbs, some were impaired for verbs but not nouns, and others had the opposite pattern (Miceli, Silveri, Nocentini, and Caramazza, 1988). Semantic categories have been explored with single cases, contributing to theories of "knowledge systems." Two cases of global aphasia had islands of good comprehension with respect to foods and living things (Warrington and McCarthy, 1983, 1987). In a group dominated by Wernicke's aphasia, body part names were harder to comprehend than clothing and object names, but each impairment was slight (Gentilini, Faglioni, and DeRenzi, 1988).

Sentence Comprehension

Sentence comprehension is assessed with respect to choosing a picture, following instructions, answering yes-no questions, and verifying that a sentence is true. Experiments may be constructed with standard tests or tasks uniquely created for answering a question. A common device is the *Token Test* and its derivatives (Chapter 10): subjects follow instructions of increasing length and complexity by pointing to or manipulating "tokens" of various shape, size, and color. A challenge to any method is whether conclusions can be generalized to other conditions. Aphasic people can show no deficit in sentence verification but have poor performance on the Token Test (Elmore-Nicholas and Brookshire, 1981). Caplan (1987) has argued that many forms of assessment, such as picture-choice and the Token Test, do not permit study of syntactic and semantic features that are important for comprehension. He preferred presenting sentences and having subjects manipulate toy animals so that they could show whether they are deriving thematic roles (i.e., "who is doing what to whom") from surface forms (Chapter 10). Sometimes deficits are hard to find. When accuracy is normal, deficit may be seen in slowness of response (e.g., Brookshire and Nicholas, 1980; Schulte, 1986). Also, most clinical procedures are off-line, meaning that a response is based on strategic processing added to the core processes of sentence comprehension.

Length and Complexity. Sentences challenge a weakened comprehension mechanism with their length and complexity (Lasky, Weidner, and Johnson, 1976; Shewan and Canter, 1971; Weidner and Lasky, 1976). However, longer sentences can be easier, which happened for 12 subjects when information was added from *Which one is the knife?* to *Which one is the knife that cuts?* (Clark and Flowers, 1987; also, Pierce, 1982). The key factor may lie in whether an addition is an **informational redundancy** or adds another computation to the decisions of the language system. The following introduces the notion that there is much for us to think about when assessing a patient's sentence comprehension.

It is difficult to increase complexity without adding words. Clinical researchers tried to pry length and complexity apart to evaluate each, as if length indicates something about short-term memory and complexity is more of a "language" factor. At first, syntactic complexity was specified according to number of transformations from active declarative sentences. Shewan (1979) compared *1a* and *1b* to assess complexity and used much longer sentences to assess length with a picture-pointing task.

(1a) The people arrived by train.
(1b) The milk was not drunk by her.

Trouble with comprehension may not show up until sentences are long and complex. On the Token Test, designed to be sensitive to mild deficit, 91 percent of aphasic persons were impaired, 93 percent on a short version (DeRenzi, 1979; Hartje, Kerschensteiner, Poeck, and Orgass, 1973). In one study, some adjustments were made to Token Test commands in order to examine syntactic complexity while controlling for length (i.e., *b* is

more complex than *a*) (Curtiss, Jackson, Kempler, Hanson, and Metter, 1986):

(2a) Touch the red circle.
(2b) Touch each yellow circle.
(3a) Touch the small blue circle and the small red circle.
(3b) Before you touch the green square, touch the white circle.

Complexity had an effect only for short sentences, but *2b* also required more visual scanning of tokens besides being more complex according to syntactic theory. Similarly, *3a* has a more complex response than *3b*, indicating that complexity need not, by itself, determine difficulty of comprehension. What someone must do with the sentence may be the final determiner of difficulty. *3b* may also be difficult because of the difference between order of events in the surface structure and their order of occurrence in response. To study this question, Ansell and Flowers (1982a) used adverbials *before* than *after* with similar commands.

(4a) After touching the white square, touch the red circle.
(4b) Touch the red square, after touching the green circle.

The adverbial was the only factor affecting aphasic subjects (N = 12) with mild to moderate comprehension deficit. There were fewer order errors with *before* and *after*. Event order made no difference, and it did not matter whether the main clause came first (*4b*) or second (*4a*). One reason for doing research is that logical complexity does not always correspond to empirical (or cognitive) complexity.

Syntactic Factors. Aphasic persons may comprehend sentences of the same length differently because of structural differences. Researchers have addressed an assortment of linguistic features, such as agent-object order, negation, verb tense, and lots of prepositions (Lesser, 1974; Parisi and Pizzamiglio, 1970). Aphasia differs from normal in number of errors and response speed but tends not to differ in order of difficulty (Parisi and Pizzamiglio, 1970; Shewan and Canter, 1971). Syntactic forms are compared to determine if some forms are more impaired than others. Deficit isolated on one form may provide a clue to a processing disruption.

One syntactic factor is the use of **word order** to signify thematic role. *Canonical order* is the most common order in which logical subject (S) and object (O) are expressed in a language. To assess comprehension based on word order, we have someone choose between pictured agent-theme arrangements or manipulate toys to display an action. In a test of object manipulation for large groups of aphasic subjects (N = 37 to N = 56), sentences preserving the canonical subject-verb-object (SVO) order of English (5b) were easier than deviations from canonical order (5a) (Caplan, Baker, and Dehaut, 1985).

(5a) S-O relative: The elephant that the monkey hit hugged the rabbit.

(5b) O-S relative: The elephant hit the monkey that hugged the rabbit.

(6a) Clefted S: It was the woman that shot the man.

(6b) Clefted O: It was the farmer that the painter kicked.

In *5a*, the object of *hit* appears before the subject. In a study of mild aphasia (N = 8), canonical structures (6a) were understood almost without error; deficit was located in noncanonical forms (6b) (Ansell and Flowers, 1982b). Deviation from canonical order poses a problem for aphasic persons.

Another syntactic flashpoint in aphasia is **center-embedding,** which is one aspect of the problem Caplan's subjects had with *5a*. Despite the fact that 7b is longer than 7a, 7b was easier to understand than 7a (Goodglass, Blumstein, Gleason, Hyde, Green, and Statlender, 1979).

(7a) The man greeted by his wife was smoking a pipe.

(7b) The man was greeted by his wife, and he was smoking his pipe.

(8) The frog hit the monkey and patted the elephant.

Other sentences with compound verb phrases (VPs) (8) were easier than sentences with relative clauses of the embedded or branching type (5a, 5b) (Butler-Hinz, Caplan, and Waters, 1990). Conjoining the ideas expressed with embedding (e.g., 7b) seems to help an aphasic person get the message.

Pronouns, reflexives, and empty noun phrases (NPs) address a structural factor called **coreferencing** of referentially dependent NPs. In Government-Binding theory of syntax (see Cowper, 1992), linking a pronoun or reflexive with an antecedent (i.e., *coindexing*) is determined by the hierarchical structure of the sentence. Butler-Hinz, Caplan, and Waters (1990) had subjects manipulate dolls upon listening to 11 types of sentences, including the following:

(9a) Pronoun: The old man tickled him.

(9b) Reflexive: The father tickled himself.

(9c) Empty NP (object-control): The boy convinced the old man to wash.

(9d) Empty NP (subject-control): The boy promised the old man to wash.

Reflexives (9b), their antecedents close in tree structure, were easier than pronouns and empty NPs (9a, 9c, 9d), their antecedents being more distant. Also, object-control coreferencing (9c) was easier than subject-control (9d), perhaps related to subcategorization of *convince* and *promise*. The difference between these two sentences is also expressed in terms of **filler-gap dependencies.** The "gap" represents the absence of an explicit agent for *wash*, much like the absence of "you" in a command. The job of the language processor is to fill the gap with an understanding of who is washing. In 9d the agent is the boy, which is farther from *wash* than the old man who is to be washing in 9c. The greater distance may make 9d more difficult for aphasic patients.

Semantic Factors. The **reversibility** of subject and object is said to manipulate semantic constraints on thematic role, because reversibility is determined by the kind of agents that can perform actions.

(10a) The *nurse* kissed the *girl*.
(10b) The *girl* drank the *milk*.
(10c) It was the *plants* that the *boy* watered.

A reversible sentence (*10a*) minimizes semantic constraints, because either NP could be the agent or object; and a listener relies on NP order to figure out who is doing what to whom. Semantic constraints are enhanced with nonreversible NPs (*10b*). Reversible sentences were harder across a range of aphasias (Heeschen, 1980), but Ansell and Flowers (1982b) found that this difficulty does not have to be part of mild comprehension deficit. Clefted sentences, however, allowed reversibility to become a factor. Reversible sentences (*6a, 6b*) were more difficult than nonreversible sentences (*10c*). Aphasic people are aided by the semantic restrictions on switching subjects and objects relative to verb meaning. In another study, aphasic subjects (N = 18) were able to use surface cues to make comprehension easier (Pierce, 1982). For reversible sentences, assigning thematic roles was improved with the additions in *11*.

(11a) The boy is *being* hit by the girl.
(11b) The man takes the boy *over* to the girl.

Plausibility is related to reversibility and refers to a statement's relationship to conceptual or world knowledge. Implausible situations may be improbable or absurdly impossible. Aphasic people find comprehension easier when sentences correspond to their world (*12a*) than when sentences represent unlikely events (*12b*) (Caramazza and Zurif, 1976; Deloche and Seron, 1981; Heilman and Scholes, 1976; Heeschen, 1980; Kudo, 1984).

(12a) The patient calls the nurse.
(12b) The thief arrests the policeman.
(13) The woman greeting her husband was smoking a pipe.

However, plausibility did not matter when sentences such as *7a* were made less probable as in *13*, which may not conflict with the familiar for some people (Goodglass, Blumstein, et al., 1979). Aphasic subjects responded accurately and quickly to absurdities in a verification task (e.g., *The clothes are washing the woman*) (Brookshire and Nicholas, 1980). Congruence between a statement and one's world knowledge makes comprehension easier in contrast to possible but implausible events.

Negation has been thought of as a semantic factor representing denial of an affirmative sense. Comprehension is usually tested when a negative marker conveys negative intent, and negated statements cause problems in aphasia (Davis and Hess, 1986; Elmore-Nicholas and Brookshire, 1981; Just, Davis, and Carpenter, 1977). However, negative intent does not require a negative surface marker. In natural context, the affirmative *Must you bite the pen?* implies that a person should not bite the pen. Aphasic subjects (N = 18) had problems with such utterances, while having little difficulty comprehending negative markers with affirmative intent (e.g., *Won't you close the door?*) (Wilcox, Davis, and Leonard, 1978).

Explaining Comprehension Disorder

Clinical aphasiologists have contemplated different functional causes of comprehension disorders in aphasia. Focusing on auditory comprehension, some speculation has been aimed at peculiarities of the auditory modality. However, the apparent centrality of aphasia should direct us to factors that would be common to reading as well. In any case, the theories surveyed here have tended not to discriminate among syndromes and have been addressed to aphasia in general.

Auditory Processing. Distortion of the acoustic signal in the mind of an aphasic person could be the impairment causing comprehension disability. One possibility pertains to the speed of speech. That is, "the basic impairment underlying speech comprehension deficits in aphasia is a failure to analyze rapidly changing acoustic events"

(Riedel and Studdert-Kennedy, 1985, p. 229). Aphasic subjects could perceive the order of two sounds when there was enough time between them, so normal intervals may be too brief for a patient to use intact perceptual capacity (Swisher and Hirsch, 1972). Tallal and Newcombe (1978) argued that the main deficit in aphasia is a problem with perception of rapid verbal and nonverbal sequences. Later, Riedel and Studdert-Kennedy (1985) found no support for this theory.

If impairment of speech perception is responsible for comprehension problems, then research should demonstrate a relationship. Varney (1984) found that all 14 aphasic subjects with impaired perception had deficient word comprehension, but eight of 12 with the worst word comprehension had normal perception. In another study, some subjects with impaired perception passed a sentence comprehension test, whereas others with good perception had poor comprehension (Carpenter and Rutherford, 1973). Relationships were minimal in other studies (e.g., Baker, Blumstein, and Goodglass, 1981; Gandour and Dardarananda, 1982; Miceli, et al., 1980). Also, increasing vowel length did not improve sentence comprehension (Blumstein, Katz, Goodglass, Shrier, and Dworetsky, 1985). In Varney's study, most patients with impaired speech perception progressed to normal within four months in perception and word comprehension. Riedel and Studdert-Kennedy (1985) were critical of methods and said that "both the perceptual tests and the Token Test are extremely artificial and require consistent levels of attention over relatively long periods of time" (p. 231). Regarding aphasic comprehension, Shewan (1982) concluded that "explanations of these problems on the basis of auditory perceptual disturbances are no longer widely accepted" (p. 61).

Rate has also been evaluated with respect to linguistic units larger than sounds or syllables. This level involves temporal phenomena that can be controlled more easily by a speaker, leading to a suggestion that a speaker should slow down to help a patient comprehend. This common advice to friends of clients is most workable when the comprehension mechanism is in pretty good shape and can function if given enough time. This hunch was supported when rate of word presentation was reduced (Lasky, et al., 1976); Poeck and Pietron, 1981; Weidner and Lasky, 1976). Pausing between major syntactic constituents helped in other studies (Blumstein, et al., 1985; Liles and Brookshire, 1975). However, aphasic subjects were not aided by two- or five-second pauses in complex commands (Hageman and Lewis, 1983; Liles and Brookshire, 1975), and pauses between words did not help for a picture-pointing task (Blumstein, et al., 1985). Brookshire and Nicholas (1984) found inconsistencies with reduced rate and four-second pauses in Token Test commands and recommended that "previous reports of the effects of pauses and slow rate upon aphasic listeners' comprehension should be interpreted with caution" (p. 327).

STM or Working Memory. Perhaps, the language system just does not have enough room to operate. Baffling data are sometimes explained in terms of a **trade-off effect,** indicating that some things are more difficult than others because of constraints on processing resources (e.g., Pierce, et al., 1990). Frazier and Friederici (1991) contemplated aspects of language comprehension that would suffer from reduced computational capacity of the processor. Little is known about working memory capacity in aphasia. Most research addresses STM. The previous chapter noted that perhaps memory span relates to one feature of processing capacity—the short-term buffer, which does not seem to be necessary for single sentence comprehension (Vallar and Baddeley, 1984). Patients have difficulty repeating digits, letters, or words (e.g., Albert, 1976; Black and Strub, 1978; Tanridag, et al., 1987). Many score poorly on tests of memory span, but either receptive or expressive elements in the task could be the root of the problem. Comparisons of memory span and comprehension in aphasia indicate that semantic processing (i.e., number of content words in Token Test commands) may lean on STM, but syntactic processing of complex sentences does not relate to measures of STM (Martin, 1987; Martin and Feher, 1990).

Taking more time to respond to an utterance may allow more time for comprehension to occur, perhaps on a more consciously controlled basis. An imposed delay has been a basic feature of immediate memory research, partly to examine rehearsal that could occur during the interval. Enforced delay of response did not improve short-term recall for nonfluent subjects but did help fluent subjects, indicating that the "articulatory loop" of the short-term buffer suffered from non-fluency (Rothi and Hutchinson, 1981). Delays were no help for following Token Test commands (DeRenzi, Faglioni, and Previdi, 1978; Toppin and Brookshire, 1978) and were detrimental in one study (Brookshire, 1978b). Yorkston, Marshall, and Butler (1977) concluded that a delay inhibits impulsive initiation of response before the stimulus is presented completely (called "anticipatory errors"). Persons with mild aphasia may function better when a speaker gives them more time to respond, but this time may be needed to contemplate the meaning of what was said or to formulate a satisfying response. There was no group effect of waiting in Schulte's (1986) study of following Revised Token Test commands, but single subjects showed the varied results of previous studies. In general, temporal factors may be considered on an individual basis, and very little is known regarding conditions other than following commands with tokens.

Brookshire (1978a) speculated that a variety of perceptual and memory-related deficits could cause problems with sentence comprehension. McNeil has also contemplated various problems of attention and resource allocation to account for aphasic comprehension (McNeil and Hageman, 1979; McNeil and Kimelman, 1986). Brookshire proposed that aphasia could involve slow rise time, abnormal noise buildup, retention deficit, and information capacity deficit; and he made these notions explicit by relating them to location of errors in Token Test commands.

With a version of this test and a similar test with objects, investigators have been unable to discover these patterns (Hageman and Folkestad, 1986; LaPointe, Holtzapple, and Graham, 1986).

An Impaired Language System. In the context of extensive study of the auditory system, it seemed daring to think that aphasic comprehension could be a language disorder instead of an auditory processing disorder. Word comprehension tests expose central language disorder with type of error in pointing to pictures. One foil is phonemically related to the stimulus, and another is semantically related. A third, unrelated foil may expose random responding. Among their few errors, aphasic patients make substantially more semantic than phonemic and random errors, indicating that difficulty with word comprehension tends to be an interpretive problem with perceived lexical forms (Gainotti, Caltagirone, and Ibba, 1975; Schuell and Jenkins, 1961b). When foils are varied according to semantic relatedness, errors tend to be in the picture most related to the correct meaning (Pizzamiglio and Appiciafuoco, 1971). The conceptual relatedness of errors indicates that access to semantic memory can be merely imprecise. An activated lexical representation points to the correct area of meaning in semantic memory but not the correct concept (Butterworth, et al., 1984; Pierce, et al., 1990). The few cases of apparent category-specific deficit indicate that some regions of semantic memory can be more accessible than others.

Early attempts to explain sentence comprehension deficit addressed what was called quantitative and qualitative differences from normal performance. Investigators compared syntactic forms and looked for order of difficulty, which was presumed to reflect the manner in which language is processed (e.g., Parisi and Pizzamiglio, 1970; Shewan and Canter, 1971). The type of difference from normal subjects might provide some direction for subsequent research by telling us whether aphasic comprehension is an inefficient normal mechanism or consists of processing anomalies that do not exist in the normal language system. The studies showed that aphasia differed from normal in number of errors and speed of response but did not differ in order of difficulty, leading to a vague characterization of aphasic comprehension as a quantitative but not qualitative difference from normal.

In the cross-linguistic search for universal features of aphasia, the use of word order cues to meaning has been examined. Evidence presented previously indicated that English speakers have difficulty with atypical expressions of agent-verb relations (e.g., passive sentences). However, from their study of English-speaking subjects, Caplan and Hildebrandt (1988) concluded that aphasic people can use word order to comprehend thematic roles, except for the most severely impaired. In some languages, canonical order differs from the Indo-European SVO. Canonical order in Japanese is SOV. Using the object manipulation task, Hagiwara and Caplan (1990) studied 30 Japanese aphasic individuals. Sentences with SOV order were understood with less difficulty than those deviating from canonical order, indicating that the structure producing difficulty is not fixed but is specific to the language being spoken. The more universal characterization of the problem is that it is related to deviations from canonical form. This description of the problem indicates that top-down processing brings an expectation of canonical order to comprehension, and an aphasic person brings intact knowledge of basic order to this task.

WORD-FINDING

All aphasic people have some kind of difficulty with word-finding, which can be observed in conversation. Object-naming places word-finding under a microscope.

Object-Naming

Word-finding impairment is most often researched, assessed, and treated with object-naming or *confrontation naming*. In an influential paper on the varieties of naming errors, Geschwind (1967) wrote that "we are speaking of naming in the narrower sense and not of word-finding in the flow of speech" (p. 97). "Naming" is naming things. It is a convenient tool for diagnosing the presence of a disorder, because the norm is not to make mistakes in naming pictures of common objects. Objects can be presented through different modalities by their sound, feel, or smell. The central impairment in aphasia causes the same word-finding problem, no matter which modality is used (Goodglass, Barton, and Kaplan, 1968).

Stimulus Variables. Investigation may focus on the stimulus presented for confrontation naming. Researchers wondered if **visual clarity** of an object matters for aphasic persons trying to name it. Bisiach (1966) compared realistic pictures, line drawings, and drawings obscured by lines. The obscured objects reduced naming scores, in spite of an ability to perceive the obscured objects. What if we heighten **object realism,** especially if we think that a realistic context matters? In one study, real objects were easier to name than line drawings, but clinical importance of the small statistical difference was questioned (Benton, Smith, and Lang, 1972). Realism made no difference for Corlew and Nation (1975). Similarly, Hatfield and others (1977) compared objects, photographs, and line drawings and concluded that realism has little effect on naming accuracy.

Instead of an object being presented, it may be described in a task called **naming to description** or to definition. A stimulus might be, "It is good for telling time and can be worn on your wrist." The stimulus should lead someone to think of an object. Aphasic subjects made more errors, especially more "no response" errors, when naming to description than when naming pictured objects (Barton, Maruszewski, and Urrea, 1969; Goodglass and Stuss, 1979). Comprehension problems may confound interpretation of performance as a deficit of formulation. However, for a visually impaired person, naming to a verbal stimulus is an alternative to objects for assessing naming ability.

Sentence completion, such as "You tell time with a — — —," is intended to elicit a name and is often regarded to be a naming task. However, there need be no object to name. The sentential context along with automaticity of elicitation makes it seem like a controlled model of extended expression. The carrier phrase elicits more accurate word-finding than naming (Barton, et al., 1969) and is often used as a cue to improve naming. However, scores for a test of aphasia show that an object and a carrier phrase (e.g., "You write and erase with a — — —") can be comparable in eliciting the same word (Porch, 1981). Pettit, McNeil, and Keith (1989) presented a picture and carrier phrase to elicit inflectional variations of nouns and verbs (e.g., "Here's a dog. Here are two— — —."). The next chapter examines elicitation of grammatical forms.

Lexical Variables. The other observable feature of confrontation naming is the lexical response. A common variable is the **familiarity of words,** determined by norms of frequency of word usage. Common words are easier than rare words for an aphasic person to retrieve (e.g., Gardner, 1973; Rochford and Williams, 1965). **Elaboration** of correct naming may be observed in mildly impaired fluent patients (Marshall, Neuburger, and Starch, 1985). They would provide more details from the stimulus, such as "farmer with a pitchfork" or would try to be more specific, such as "pie, two-layer chocolate." In the search for **category-specific impairment,** a problem with naming fruits and vegetables was uncovered (Hart, Berndt, and Caramazza, 1985), but semantic-specificity has not yet been shown to be a widespread feature of aphasia. In assessing syntactic category, objects elicit nouns; actions elicit verbs. In one study, verbs were more difficult to retrieve (Williams and Canter, 1987), but other investigators found no difference

(Basso, Razzano, Faglioni, and Zanobio, 1990).

Attention is also given to the type of deficient naming response. An aphasic person may be unusually slow to name objects or may fail to produce names. Schuell and Jenkins (1961b) observed errors corresponding to the paraphasias defined in Chapter 1. Group means showed that 29 percent of the errors were semantic associations, 19 percent were sound approximations, and 52 percent were irrelevant names or omissions. However, this pattern did not characterize many individuals. For severely impaired patients, errors were 72 percent irrelevant and omitted responses, but for mildly impaired patients, errors were 75 percent semantic associations. Nonfluent patients were more accurate than fluent groups (Goodglass and Stuss, 1979). Nonfluent patients' errors tended to be semantically related (Gardner, 1973).

Divergence and Word Fluency

Confrontation naming converges on one idea and one response. Divergent cognition generates a quantity and variety of responses, such as thinking of things that can be done with an object (Chapey, Rigrodsky, and Morrison, 1977). Divergent word-finding entails generating numerous words to a single stimulus or idea. A series of words is elicited in **word fluency tasks.** Someone would be asked to produce words starting with a letter or belonging to a category such as vegetables or countries. The latter task has been called "category naming" (Grossman, 1981), "word-naming" (Joanette, Goulet, and Le Dorze, 1988), or a "controlled-association task" (Cappa, Papagno, and Vallar, 1990). Hough (1989), who called it "category generation," separated "natural object concepts" (e.g., sports, fruit) from "ad hoc categories," such as things for a garage sale or for holding a door open. In assessment, there is usually a limit of around 60 seconds for producing as many words as possible. Speed maximizes the number of words produced, but still the task can be highly strategic in the mind of the speaker.

Borkowski, Benton, and Spreen (1967) obtained data on production of "as many words as you can in 60 seconds" that begin with a letter. Six letters were difficult for normal adults: *J* elicited only 4.83 associations. Moderate difficulty was observed with *N* (8.23). Easy letters went into the **FAS test,** with these three letters eliciting 10.22 to 11.50 words from persons without brain damage. The FAS test became a common test and part of one aphasia battery (Spreen and Benton, 1977). Damage to the left or right hemisphere caused a large drop in production. Persons with LHD did worse than those with RHD, but only for difficult letters. Persons with LHD, RHD, and bilateral damage were impaired in another study; and a discriminant analysis showed that only 48 percent of patients could be classified as to side of lesion using this method (Wertz, Dronkers, and Shubitowski, 1986). At around seven words per letter, the task did not clearly distinguish nonfluent and fluent groups studied by Collins, McNeil, Lentz, Shubitowski, and Rosenbek (1984). Fluent aphasias produced more words in another study (Bayles, Boone, Tomoeda, Slauson, and Kaszniak, 1989).

In a **categorical word fluency** task, a patient is asked to produce as many members of a category as possible in 60 seconds. Grossman (1981) used 10 categories such as sports, birds, furniture, tools, clothes, and weapons. A small group of normal adults produced 14.66 words per category. Persons with RHD were impaired with 11.48 words. Aphasia entailed a precipitous drop. Nonfluent patients produced 5.29 words, and fluent patients produced 6.71. These levels are fairly consistent. In a study of five categories, including tools and crimes, normal adults averaged 13.51 words, but mildly impaired fluent aphasic persons produced 6.76 (Adams, Reich, and Flowers, 1989). Word fluency contains factors that may not be specific to aphasia or to the language system. It seems to detect cerebral dysfunction in general. Morever, the skill assessed is a fluctuating one, as normal adults average 22.5 animal names in a one-minute period but display a range of nine to 41 words

(Borod, Goodglass, and Kaplan, 1980; Goodglass and Kaplan, 1983).

Word-Finding in Discourse

More natural conditions, such as conversation, involve an extended flow of interrelated words. A common clinical condition is **picture description,** in which an object is shown in the context of an action to elicit words in sentences. Naming and description were equally successful in eliciting nouns for nonfluent and fluent subjects (Basso, et al., 1990). When action-naming was compared to description for eliciting verbs, scores were again comparable for most types of aphasia; however, anomic cases did better with descriptions, leading to the conclusion that "performance on a single word confrontation-naming task may not be highly predictive of performance in connected speech" (Williams and Canter, 1987, p. 132). Goodglass, Hyde, and Blumstein (1969) figured that naming tends to elicit "picturable" words, such as *bird,* and that conversation would contain more nonpicturable words, such as *animal, time, year, wife.* Aphasic subjects used more nonpicturable than picturable nouns in spontaneous speech.

Marshall (1976) studied word-retrieval behaviors during conversation as "a situation whereby the aphasic, unprompted by the clinician, illustrates that he is unable to retrieve a word and initiates some effort to do so without assistance from the clinician" (p. 445). These efforts included semantic and phonemic paraphasia, circumlocution, indefinite terms (e.g., "the one," "stuff"), and taking or requesting more time. Patients often took an uncomfortable amount of time before retrieving an intended word. Also, a patient may try to correct an error. Unassisted **self-correction** was studied for a variety of word-finding tasks, such as confrontation naming, answering questions, and sentence completion (Marshall and Tompkins, 1982). Types of self-correction were *cued-corrections* when a patient produced a related response prior to the target response, *effortful corrections* when a patient produced a series of partial responses leading to the target response, and *immediate corrections* when a patient quickly provided the target response. Subjects classified as low-verbal engaged in as much self-correction as high-verbal subjects, but the more severely impaired were less successful. These groups did not differ as to type of self-correction, except that the less-impaired subjects had more immediate self-corrections.

Speaking rate differentiates nonfluent from fluent aphasias and is one measure that can be sensitive to deficit in mild aphasias. Normal rate in *words per minute* (wpm) has been considered to be 100 to 175 wpm (Howes, 1964; Kerschensteiner, Poeck, and Brunner, 1972). Kerschensteiner used the following categories to characterize variation among aphasic patients:

very slow	—	0 to 50 wpm
slow	—	51 to 90 wpm
normal	—	above 90 wpm

Of 47 aphasic subjects, 17 were very slow, 13 were slow, and 17 were normal. In research on communicative efficiency, *syllables per minute* discriminated normal from aphasic groups (Yorkston and Beukelman, 1980). Normal elderly adults produced 193 syllables per minute. Mildly aphasic patients produced 121 syllables per minute.

Content analysis is exploited widely for measuring the informational efficiency of expression. Clinicians usually examine descriptive discourse, which is usually elicited with complex drawings such as the "Cookie Theft," a kitchen scene of children reaching for cookies and a woman washing dishes (Goodglass and Kaplan, 1983). Yorkston and Beukelman (1980) divided a sample into units the size of a word or short phrase. A content unit was defined "as a grouping of information that was always expressed as a unit by normal speakers" (p. 30). Examples included *cookies, from the jar, mother,* and *in the kitchen.* Content units tended to be specific concepts rather than clausal units. Two measures were **number of content units,** re-flecting amount of information conveyed, and **content units per minute,** or efficiency of communication. Number of units did not distinguish subject groups, but efficiency was discriminating. Normal elderly subjects produced 33.7 units per minute. Mildly aphasic subjects produced a normal amount of information but at a slower pace of only 18.7 units per minute.

Explaining Word-Finding Disorder

Should we believe that all word-finding deficits are aphasia because all aphasias include word-finding deficit? Logic does not lead to this conclusion. In the restricted arena of object-naming, errors may signify a disorder but do not necessarily signify aphasia. Geschwind (1967) wrote of **nonaphasic misnaming** and **aphasic misnaming,** implying that misnaming may be caused by an impaired language system or another disorder. Hypotheses about other causes of naming problems can be developed from a process-model for the naming task. This model may help us to locate areas of cognition that are pertinent to word-finding in discourse.

Naming engages processes from vision to muscle contraction. Along the way, lexical access must take place; but, unlike word recognition (Chapter 3), activation of meaning precedes lexical activation when naming something accurately. The stimulus is an object, not a word. The model of naming in Figure 4–1 begins with recognition of the object, a subprocess that depends on perception (see Chapter 7). Recognition activates a representation of the object-class that is stored in LTM. The "recognition unit," as some call it (Ellis and Young, 1988), then activates a concept in semantic memory (or the "semantic system"). Then the concept points to a word in lexical memory, called the "phonological output lexicon" in Figure 4–1. This phonological form then guides speech production. With respect to this task-analysis, we can imagine points of potential difficulty leading to a poor response, beginning with blindness and ending with muscle paralysis.

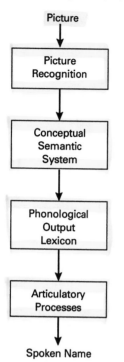

Picture

↓

Picture
Recognition

↓

Conceptual
Semantic
System

↓

Phonological
Output
Lexicon

↓

Articulatory
Processes

↓

Spoken Name

FIGURE 4–1 A typical model of object naming. Components are represented similarly elsewhere (e.g., Figures 3–4, 7–1). As suggested with Figure 2–9, diagnosis entails determining the impaired component that is responsible for misnaming. (Reprinted by permission from Bruce, C. & Howard, D., Why don't Broca's aphasics cue themselves? An investigation of phonemic cueing and tip of the tongue information. *Neuropsychologia*, 26, 1988, p. 261. Pergamon Press, publisher.)

One researcher put it this way: (a) "The first step is the identification of the object as a member of a category whose stored representation provides a good match with the stimulus object" (b) "Once a category representation has been activated, then the corresponding label is retrieved" (Brownell, Bihrle, and Michelow, 1986, p. 50). The question: Where is the "functional lesion" responsible for aphasic misnaming?

Clinicians have long differentiated object recognition disorder from language disorder by employing a strategy of **task-comparison** rather than depending on one task for the diagnosis. Similar to the analysis of drawing on command (Chapter 2), our guide is a model for the task that exposed the impairment (i.e., misnaming). We do our best to examine one component at a time. For assessing recognition, a patient may be asked to manipulate objects. If performance leads us to suspect visual agnosia, then we present objects to each modality independently to see if misnaming occurs only for vision. A patient may arrange pictures of objects into categories, which also touches upon conceptualization in semantic memory. With these tests, the patient does not have to access the mental lexicon or articulate words. If these tasks are performed normally, then the locus of the problem is later in the naming function. Motor evaluation may rule out an articulatory disorder. If we eliminate problems of recognition and speech, then we can begin to suspect that misnaming is caused by impaired processes related to language functions. Aphasic and agnosic misnaming are used to support the modular theory of independent recognition and lexical processes (Brownell, et al., 1986).

Now, let us consider the formidable problem of distinguishing between two central components of object-naming: the conceptual or semantic system and the lexical system. Distinguishing deficient semantic knowledge from deficient lexical knowledge is akin to distinguishing between misnaming an object because we do not know what it is and misnaming an object because we do not know its name. With respect to processes, disturbed access to concepts may exist apart from impaired access to the lexicon, while knowledge of both remains intact. All of these possibilities are rarely contemplated in studies of misnaming and other word-finding problems. Researchers may adopt the glossy notion of **lexical-semantic disorder,** because connections between systems make it hard to pry them apart with our tests. Presenting words activates the mental lexicon, which automatically activates concepts (Chapter 3); similarly, presenting objects activates semantic memory, which may activate related lexicon.

Goldstein (1948) suggested that aphasic word-finding problems come from deficient "categorical behavior" or "abstract attitude." In modern jargon, problems might be identified with the semantic system. Assessment involves matching and sorting objects according to various common features. Aphasic groups exhibited impairment on such tasks and did worse than persons with RH damage (Cohen, Kelter, and Woll, 1980; Gainotti, Carlomagno, Craca, and Silveri, 1986; Grossman and Wilson, 1987). In another study, pictures and words were presented in two tasks of matching items according to category (e.g., dogs) or function (e.g., for cutting). The two tasks were pooled in data analysis, which revealed deficit concentrated in posterior-fluent aphasia (McCleary and Hirst, 1986). The greatest problem for this group was with functional relations. While fluent subjects were much more impaired in naming than the anterior-nonfluent group, there was no relationship between naming scores and feature-matching scores. Other subjects were like normal controls when sorting objects into semantic categories (Milton, Wertz, Katz, and Prutting, 1981). Yet, results with posterior-fluent aphasias reinforced a common impression that semantic disorder dominates in these patients.

When words are explicitly introduced in a sorting or matching task, a subject must access the mental lexicon. Such tests tap into knowledge of what words mean or connections between lexical and semantic stores, and most evidence for lexical-semantic deficit in posterior-fluent aphasias comes from such tasks (e.g., Grober, Perecman, Keller, and Brown, 1980). Nonfluent and fluent subjects exhibited knowledge of categorical and functional organization when asked to put words into requested categories. Persons with fluent aphasias had particular problems when sorting on their own (McCleary, 1988). In order to compare conceptual knowledge to naming, Goodglass and Baker (1976) utilized a word comprehension task to assess lexical-semantic sensibility. Subjects were asked if a word goes with a picture (e.g., an orange). Besides being the object name, words were

categorical associates (*apple*), attributes (*juicy*), and so on. High-comprehending subjects understood associated meanings similarly to normals. Low-comprehending patients were dissimilar to normals, indicating to these investigators that these patients had a constricted lexical-semantic system. Naming scores were related to scores on the word comprehension test, which may have simply indicated that low-comprehending aphasic persons also have the most severe naming problems.

In another study, a hospital staff was asked to judge the typicality of objects so that the investigators could compare the naming of high-typical examples of a category (e.g., kitchen chair) and the naming of low-typical examples (e.g., beach chair) (Brownell, et al., 1986). Object familiarity varied, while the **basic name** could be the same (e.g., *chair*). Normally, a basic name is elicited by highly typical examples. A **subordinate label** (e.g., *kitchen chair*) and **superordinate label** (e.g., *furniture*) may also be produced. Low-typical examples tend to elicit more subordinate labels than basic names. With subjects who had fluent or nonfluent aphasia, typical objects elicited many more basic names than atypical objects. Both groups had difficulty producing subordinate names but conveyed the concepts with compensatory strategies. Instead of saying "racing car," a nonfluent patient might say "car, goes fast"; fluent patients might give the attribute without the basic name. Because aphasic subjects exhibited more than one way to convey an idea, Brownell concluded that the functional lesion is clearly outside the conceptual/semantic system per se.

In terms of Garrett's formulation model (Figure 3–9), Brownell and his colleagues (1986) located damage for most aphasic subjects in the positional level, where lexical forms are activated in relation to their positions in a sentence (also Le Dorze and Nespoulous, 1989). This focus on impaired lexical assess in aphasia has been reinforced with some attention given to the "tip-of-the-tongue" state, in which properties of the correct word can be conveyed instead of the word itself. Barton (1971) instructed aphasic subjects to point, upon naming failure, to the target word's first letter, number of syllables, and "big" or "small" for indicating size of the target word. Subjects guessed these properties accurately over 60 percent of the time, in spite of being unable to say the word. It was as if an object activated the concept and parts of lexical form. In another study, some aphasic subjects were less successful in reporting features of unspoken words, and a few others could not do it at all (Goodglass, Kaplan, Weintraub, and Ackerman, 1976).

Finally, the word-fluency task provides an opportunity for a different kind of qualitative analysis of word-retrieval based on lexical-semantic connections. Letter-fluency tasks induce generation of words from a lexical base by having patients fish for commonalities of form. The categorical-fluency task induces generation of words from a semantic base. Grossman (1981) examined the succession of words produced to a category such as *birds*. Responses were given scores identified with prototypicality bands extending from the most typical members of a category to the least typical members. Bands were defined according to ratings of typicality. Ideal members of a category were assigned a 1.00 (e.g., "robin"), whereas the most peripheral instances or items not belonging to a semantic field were assigned a 7.00 (e.g., "fish"). Normal adults and persons with RH damage produced most of their responses from three bands between 1.00 and 2.99 (Grossman, 1981). Nonfluent aphasic subjects produced prototypical examples as the normals did. In contrast, patients with Wernicke's aphasia were likely to produce words in the most distant bands, especially words that did not belong in the category. They started with examples of high typicality and progressed to examples of low typicality. They "often cross the borders around a referential field" (p. 327). Attention keeps turning to posteriorly damaged patients for the possibility that the guiding forces of semantic memory somehow cannot keep lexical-retrieval from going astray.

SENTENCE PRODUCTION

Sentence production exposes differences among aphasic patients, which is the dominant theme of the next chapter. Yet, sentence-specific features of aphasia have been addressed with respect to the categories of nonfluent and fluent aphasias. Caramazza and Berndt (1978) proposed that syntactic and semantic abilities can be dissociated, and the dissociation is related to anterior and posterior lesions in the left hemisphere (Table 2–1). Anterior aphasias tend to be agrammatic while preserving lexical-semantic abilities, whereas posterior aphasias preserve syntax despite lexical-semantic difficulties. Despite the intense search for dissociations, some aspects of sentence formulation may be shared by all cases of aphasia.

Clinical researchers have been interested in whether the **condition for eliciting discourse** makes a difference in lexical and grammatical features of sentences. The concern is whether standardized test conditions reveal the way an aphasic person talks in natural circumstances. Roberts and Wertz 1989) compared a test of describing object functions to conversation with 20 subjects. Utterances and clauses were longer and word-finding was more accurate in conversation, but syntactic structures were formed better in the object-function test. The results indicated that formal assessment may not be indicative of sentences produced naturally. When within-sentence factors (e.g., syntax) are compared with parameters of discourse (e.g., cohesion), aphasic subjects are often intact with respect to discourse in the midst of sentence-level reductions such as number of words, content efficiency, and syntactic complexity (e.g., Brenneise-Sarchad, Nicholas, and Brookshire, 1991; Ernest-Baron, Brookshire, and Nicholas, 1987).

Cross-linguistic studies addressed the status of **word order** in picture descriptions (Bates, Friederici, Wulfeck, and Juarez, 1988). Grammatical order errors would be possible at the word level if someone were to utter *ing-walk* and at the phrase level if someone were to say *man the*. Such errors did not occur in English, Italian, and German. The preservation of comprehension for canonical order has also been observed for production. Three-element productions were examined. Canonical SVO order was used 81 percent of the time across syndromes and the three languages. Also, order around a locative preposition was correct across syndromes and languages around 70 percent of the time. These results were well above chance, and aphasic subjects did not differ from normals. There was also an indication that the canonical order of SOV is preserved in Turkish speakers (Bates and Wulfeck, 1989). Resilience of canonical word order appears to be a general feature of aphasia. In production, canonical order may even be overused as a "safe harbor," especially for speakers of Italian and German.

APHASIA IN BILINGUAL PERSONS

A speech-language pathologist in the United States might be evaluating the following individual: an 80-year-old male whose native language is German, who learned French as a second language, and who then learned English after settling in America at the age of 18 (Perecman, 1984). Does aphasia occur equally in these languages? This question was examined with problematic retrospectives, and estimates of equal impairment varied from 20 to 90 percent (Chapter 1). For a group of ten aphasic bilinguals, accuracy and latency of object-naming in English and Spanish did not differ (Vogel and Costello, 1986). There was no significant difference between English and Spanish on verbal subtests of an aphasia battery (Porch and de Berkeley-Wykes, 1985). How aphasia appears in bilinguals should depend on site of lesion in relation to the manner in which multiple languages are organized in the brain. Investigators have become skeptical about the notion that the right hemisphere makes room for using multiple languages, and evidence has indicated that

bilinguals rely on the LH for both languages (Chapter 2).

Bilingualism is hard to study. Bilinguals vary in (a) proficiency in the second language, (b) age of learning the second language, (c) manner of learning the second language (e.g., naturally or formally), (d) context of learning the second language (e.g., where it is predominant), (e) affective factors (i.e., cultural attitudes toward a language), and (f) linguistic relationship between languages used (i.e., similarity between languages) (Obler, Zatorre, Galloway, and Vaid, 1982). Cross-linguistic investigations illuminate the importance of similarity between languages. Differences in use of grammatical inflection can make grammatical problems seem to be different in two languages. Also, uncertainty arises from the interdisciplinary study of bilingual people with head injuries as well as stroke. Is the disorder really aphasia? Studies with only language tests may not demonstrate dissociation of language from other cognitive functions (e.g., Paradis and Goldblum, 1989).

Contemplation of aphasia in bilinguals began long ago with Ribot and Pitres, who were curious about patients who were more severely impaired in one language than the other. They wondered if differences have something to do with which language is the native tongue or which language is the most familiar at the time of brain damage (Paradis, 1977). The *rule of Ribot* ("primacy rule") stated that the native or first-learned language is usually less impaired. The *rule of Pitres* was associated with "habit strength" and stated that the most frequently used language is less impaired. Comparison of languages on this basis has run into difficulty, largely on the basis of how to define familiarity. Of two languages used in everyday life, one may be first learned and currently used at home, whereas both are used extensively at work (e.g., Junque, Vendrell, Vendrell-Brucet, and Tobena, 1989). Research has been unable to support one rule or the other as a broad generalization, when languages are impaired differently. An unusual pattern is

alternating aphasia, in which expression with one language is impaired one day, the other language is impaired the next day, and so on (Paradis, Goldblum, and Abidi, 1982). Comprehension and expression can be dissociated. Good comprehension can be retained in two languages, whereas verbal expression is severely impaired in one language. The implication for rehabilitation is that we should not anticipate a pattern of impairment for each client.

Modern understanding of bilingualism indicates that aphasia should be clearly distinguished from normal bilingual behavior occurring in aphasic individuals (Grosjean, 1989). Bilingual behavior may be seen as abnormal to a monolingual clinician who is not familiar with bilingual behavior. One feature of bilingual behavior is **language mixing,** which occurs mainly in a bilingual mode (Chapter 1). Mixing is "any case in which elements from one language are used in the context of another language" (Perecman, 1984). The concept of "interference" appears in the literature, but linguists prefer the broader notion of mixing, which can be quite intentional. The language chosen for conversation between bilinguals is the *base language*. Once the base language is chosen, another language is mixed in by *code-switching* (i.e., reverting completely to the other language for a word, phrase, or sentence) or by *borrowing* a word from the other language and integrating it with the base language, such as a French speaker using "weekend" or "brunch" including attachment of French inflection.

Perecman (1984) estimated that language mixing occurs in less than 10 percent of multilingual aphasias, and more often in Wernicke's aphasia than other syndromes. She tried to differentiate aphasic language mixing from nonaphasic mixing. "Lexical-level mixing," such as word borrowing, occurs in normal and aphasic bilinguals. In an object-naming task, some patients occasionally name in the unsolicited language (Vogel and Costello, 1986). Perecman claimed that "utterance-level mixing" is a phenomenon of aphasia as opposed to normal language use; patients respond in a language different from the one in which they are addressed. Another capacity of bilingual persons is **translation,** and Perecman (1984) was curious about spontaneous translation, or an immediate unsolicited translation of one's own or someone else's utterance into another language. In reviewing literature, she found few reports of spontaneous translation. One aphasic woman who repeated sentences in another language could not translate on request. Another study compared languages for word-level tasks of comprehension, naming, and translation. Initial severity of deficit differed between languages for word comprehension and translation, favoring the native language used with family (Junque, et al., 1989).

Grosjean (1985, 1989) was concerned about analyses like Perecman's, especially regarding the notion that utterance-level mixing is necessarily a sign of disorder. Responding in another language may normally occur in conversation, depending on the pragmatic application of code-switching rules when the bilingual mode is appropriate. Grosjean suspected that impairments might occur in the management of languages with respect to linguistic status of a communicative partner, such as (a) using the wrong base language with a monolingual interlocutor, (b) extensive code-switching with a monolingual, (c) language mixing while reading a monolingual text, and (d) failing to switch or translate upon request. Therefore, utterance-level mixing is a pragmatic violation when a monolingual clinician is speaking to a bilingual client but may be quite natural when a clinician is bilingual. Data does not appear to be available on the extent to which these behaviors occur in a group of aphasic persons in comparison with matched controls when speaking to monolingual and bilingual clinicians.

SUMMARY AND IMPLICATIONS

In giving us an idea of what aphasia is, basic investigation has given us some ideas about directing observation for diagnosing and assessing this disorder. Of course, assessment leads to treatment objectives. We know, for example, that treatment will emphasize language more than other areas of function. In general, aphasia is a difficulty with words, not concepts. However, we need to check on nonverbal symbolic behavior if we think that gesture might compensate for verbal deficits. For most cases of aphasia, we probably do not have to restore an erased knowledge of language as if a patient had to learn language all over again. Instead, our treatment of deficit will be aimed at processes used for comprehension and formulation.

For a long time, aphasiologists employed few guidelines for identifying disorder in the language system. For language comprehension, early attempts to diagnose disorder were related to a length-complexity distinction. Then, researchers tried to uncover specific comprehension problems by manipulating linguistic components of stimuli, such as syntactic or semantic features. Caplan (1987) suggested that "syntactic comprehension impairments are often independent primary disorders of sentence processing" (p. 323), rather than a result of some peripheral or general feature of cognition such as short-term memory. He also concluded that the syntactic processor is not impaired in an "all-or-none" fashion but rather is impaired partially. The same syntactic problems occur with reading sentences as well, indicating that the disorder has to be identified with something that is applied to both forms of input (Samuels and Benson, 1979). Once diagnosis of comprehension began to be directed at specific kinds of impairment, studies of the language system were usually related to the study of syndromes.

CHAPTER

5

THE SYNDROMES OF APHASIA

Stroke causes aphasias. This chapter is oriented around deficits that distinguish one aphasic person from another. Distinctions are often made in terms of prototypical syndromes summarized in Chapter 1. Broca's aphasia is by far the most thoroughly scrutinized type. It is "the flagship of the neuropsychology of language" (Grodzinsky, 1991). Through the study of this syndrome, aphasiology has taken on characteristics of contemporary psycholinguistics.

CLASSIFICATION CONTROVERSIES

A *clinical syndrome* is "a group of findings, signs and/or symptoms which occur together in a given disease process with sufficient frequency to suggest the presence of that disease process" (Benson, 1979a, p. 57). The clin-ical syndromes of aphasia may be related to differences in prognosis and strategies of treatment. The notion of *theoretical syndromes* pertains to what a pattern of behaviors can tell us about cognition and its relation to the brain. Much research is motivated to determine if a clinical syndrome is caused by a particular cognitive impairment, but theoretically sound syndromes may turn out to be somewhat different from clinical syndromes.

Clinical Classification

For the first century of serious interest in aphasia, keeping track of syndrome classifications was an imposing task. It began with modality-based theoretical syndromes proposed by nineteenth-century diagrammakers. Later, Head (1920) suggested a revolutionary classification based on the linguistic features of impairment (e.g., nominal aphasia, syntactic aphasia). Simpler dichotomies appeared, such as syntagmatic and paradigmatic forms (Jakobson, 1971) and Type A and Type B aphasias (Howes, 1967). More elaborate systems were introduced (Luria, 1966; Wepman and Jones, 1964). Students had to learn these systems as part of the history of clinical aphasiology. We could not figure out which was best or correct. The Boston system has emerged as a worldwide clinical classification (Table 1–2).

Speech-language pathologists got into an argument over whether aphasia should be subdivided at all. Darley (1982) thought it wise to classify the two sides of the debate as "the splitters" and "the lumpers." Wertz (1983) declared that classification "was born in Boston and slain by Darley and Schuell." Before the influence of modern psycholinguistics, Schuell decided that "we cannot really separate the *semantic* from the *structural* aspects of language" (in Sies, 1974, p. 75). She said that "both kinds of impairment are found in the same patients and both are related to the overall severity of the existing language deficit" (p. 76); "the dichotomy assumed in categorizing aphasia as amnesic versus syntactical . . . is artificial" (Schuell, et al., 1964, p. 101). This view became known as the **unidimensional theory**, stating that aphasia varies only along a dimension of severity in a single disorder and, thus, there are no qualitative differences of disorder. Schuell and Wepman debated this point with respect to statistical analyses applied to their aphasia tests (Jones and Wepman, 1961; Schuell and Jenkins, 1961a; Schuell, Jenkins, and Carroll, 1962).

In a book dedicated to Schuell, Darley (1982) wrote disdainfully about "adjectivists." Darley argued that "little clinical purpose is served by proliferating adjectives, which are presumed to designate different 'types' of aphasia. . . . They are based on different, at times incomplete or biased, observations; they reflect what people look for and believe in" (p. 42). He supported his opinion by reviewing studies that showed similarities between fluent and nonfluent categories and among more specific syndromes. He said that any observed differences are mere "idiosyncracies" (Darley, 1983). He claimed that syndromes are "useless"; "little is to be gained clinically by splitting aphasia into subgroups; much is to be gained by lumping together patients who share a common core of disability that justifies the adoption of a unified rationale of treatment" (Darley, 1982, p. 42). "I *don't* do something different on the basis of the adjective that they or anyone else supplies" (Darley, 1983, p. 281). At a conference, Holland (1983) debated Darley by saying that syndromes are revealed with "a higher power microscope through which to view aphasic patients" and that there is clinical merit in precision of description "if the goal is to fit the patient correctly with what might help" (p. 289).

Early in aphasiology, syndromes were defined according to the general status of language ability in each modality. Schuell supported a unitary view by displaying severity of deficit across modalities and did not compare results to site of lesion. Her conclusion about variation of aphasia is correct with respect to what she looked for. Schuell helped to establish the notion that aphasias are multimodality disorders. Modern classification was built on information that was not sought in Schuell's examination method. The Boston system depended on linguistic variation in the verbal modality, with comprehension still diagnosed along a severity continuum. Patterns of deficit were linked to lesion site with the emerging technology of localization. Thus, both points of view were related to approaches to observation, leading to the possibility that a point of view can motivate observational strategy and vice versa. Darley saw observational bias in syndrome research, but others might see this research as consisting of paradigms that are appropriate for testing a hypothesis. As Chapter 1 indicated, the "fallacy of objectivity" implies that there will always be a bias, and the task of science is to minimize bias and interpret results with re-

spect to an honest recognition of biasing influences. In the feud over syndromes, bias
lives on both sides of the fence.

A few clinicians thought that syndromes
are supposed to characterize 100 percent of a
caseload. Yet, syndromes are not intended to
bear this burden and should reflect the outcome of certain focal lesions (Chapter 2).
Benson (1979a) concluded that "only about
half of the cases of aphasia seen routinely in a
clinical practice can clearly be placed into
one or another of the syndromes and even
this figure is dependent on some degree of
diagnostic flexibility" (p. 136). Data on the
prevalence of syndromes is sometimes divided into cases with unequivocal diagnoses
and those with equivocal diagnoses. The low
yield of unequivocal diagnoses stems from
the fact that many aphasias are caused by
large lesions or lesions overlapping functional
regions. "In view of the many potential complicating factors . . . it is not at all surprising
that pure examples of the aphasic syndromes
are not common, and in fact it is remarkable
that the recognizable syndromes shine
through as often as they do" (Benson, 1979a,
p. 137).

Theoretical Syndromes

In the worldwide study of aphasia, there is
now little argument that the clinical syndromes are valid descriptions of variation
among forms of aphasia. However, debate
has not ceased. Now, there is plenty of argument over the theoretical usefulness of the
clinical syndromes. In contrast to Schuell's
and Darley's unitary theory of aphasia, the
syndromes are offered as support for a **multidimensional theory,** stating that the aphasias
reflect functional lesions in distinct components of the language system. Broca's and
Wernicke's aphasias seem to represent a double dissociation between the syntactic and
semantic systems. Associated sites of lesion
are suggestive of relationships between cognitive subsystems and brain function, an ex-
citing prospect for going beyond hemispheric

asymmetry in specifying functional organization of the brain.

Schwartz (1984) advised "that much of the
disharmony in contemporary aphasiology
stems from the misguided attempt to utilize a
single classificatory scheme to achieve a variety of noncomplementary ends" (p. 4). These
noncomplementary ends can be divided
roughly into the purposes of clinical classification and theoretical classification. In clinical syndromes, deficits co-occur with a reliable regularity and are related to lesions at
the level of gross neuroanatomy. Schwartz
suggested that "these are not inconsequential
facts; they are simply off-target as far as the
neurolinguistic enterprise is concerned" (p.
4). This enterprise seeks evidence in language
disorders for the modularity of processes like
the syntactic parser. In Broca's aphasia,
agrammatism co-occurs with comprehension
deficit, but this observation by itself does not
identify a process that accounts for both deficits. Caramazza (1984) has sought "psycho-
logically strong" syndromes representing a set
of symptoms that "*cooccurs necessarily*" because of damage to a component of
cognition.

Caramazza (1986) wrote that the transparency assumption (Chapter 3) "must be accepted if we are to use the performance of
brain-damaged patients to inform and constrain theories of normal cognitive processing" (p. 52). He put forth a framework for
cognitive neuropsychology with a *fractionation assumption*, stating that "brain damage
will, on occasion, result in the total and selective disruption of processing components or
modules; that is, brain damage can fractio-
nate the cognitive system along psycho-
linguistically significant lines" (Caramazza
and Berndt, 1985, p. 29). "Fractionations" are
like dissociations. An objective is "to explain
patients' impairments in terms of some hypothesized damage to the normal cognitive
system" (Caramazza and Badecker, 1991, p.
211). Caramazza went further by taking on
group research. He insisted that rigorous case
study is the only methodology that can live

with the assumptions of cognitive neuropsychology. He sparked a series of defenses from many who are doing group research (e.g., Caplan, 1988; Zurif, Gardner, and Brownell, 1989).

Debates are the fire in the belly of any discipline, and the "Caramazza Wars" have been especially thought-provoking. The following offers a brief characterization of what has transpired:

Caramazza's argument: The mean score for a normal group is likely to be representative, because the group can be assumed to be homogeneous. Such homogeneity cannot be assumed for brain-damaged subjects. The lesion is a natural manipulation that introduces variation as if an experimental task were done differently for each subject. The mean cannot be representative of any member of the group. Extreme scores, in particular, indicate that a group is made up of different specific cognitive disorders. Grouping subjects into loosely defined clinical syndromes does not enhance homogeneity because lesions are unspecified or quite variable (Chapter 2). Such grouping is "useless" if not "harmful" for making inferences about normal cognition (Caramazza, 1986). Behavioral support for this contention includes the wide variability in the use of grammatical morphemes among 20 patients diagnosed as having agrammatic aphasia (Miceli, Silveri, Romani, and Caramazza, 1989). Thus, "valid inferences about the structure of normal cognitive systems from patterns of impaired performance are only possible for single-patient studies" (Caramazza and McCloskey, 1988, p. 519). A patient's disorder is too specific to be hidden in a group mean.

The cases against Caramazza's position: Using a symptom pattern to infer location of a functional lesion seems to ignore compensatory processes that may contribute to performance (Caplan, 1991). Moreover, group research is an established approach in cognitive psychology, and statistics contain mechanisms that account for variability. Grodzinsky (1991) claimed that Miceli's study does not support Caramazza, because much of the variability was in quantity of omissions and errors rather than type of difficulty. Agrammatism is defined by type of omission and error, and quantitative variation merely reflects the severity of agrammatism. Case studies have limited generalizability,

and the "problem of extreme scores can apply equally to scores collected from a single patient" (Zurif, et al., 1989, p. 242). The best approach may be to combine single case and group designs in one research program utilizing procedures that permit comparison between individual and group data (Bates, McDonald, MacWhinney, and Appelbaum, 1991).

Caramazza's replies: Caramazza sensed that objections to his position did not take into account the specific purpose for which he recommended case studies and rejected the use of syndromes. "Generalize to what?" (Caramazza, 1986). The goal is to figure out the cognitive system, not to characterize a group. "This is not to say that one cannot approach syndromes scientifically; but it does follow that, in syndrome-based studies, one can only derive information about the consequences of the clinical categorization" (Caramazza and Badecker, 1991, p. 216). That is, we can learn interesting things about Wernicke's aphasia, but it is too general a level of observation for developing cognitive theory.

Darley (1982) and Caramazza (1986) both claimed that aphasic syndromes are useless. Darley argued that clinical syndromes do not exist; if we assume that they do exist, then they would be useless as a basis for planning language treatment. Caramazza has allowed that clinical syndromes exist and serve useful purposes for clinical management and investigation. For him, it is useless to infer the nature of cognition for a group defined according to clinical classification. When four subjects in a group of five perform one way on a task, advocates of group studies emphasize the performance of the four, whereas advocates of single-case research are especially curious about what the fifth subject was doing.

AGRAMMATISM

Agrammatism, the symptom, is the definitive feature of Broca's aphasia, the syndrome. In contemporary research, subjects are often defined as being agrammatic, possibly in an attempt to focus on a specific symptom. These subjects may not have Broca's aphasia according to classical criteria (Kolk and van Grunsven, 1985). Some investigators use "agrammatism" instead of "Broca's aphasia" to refer to a syndrome of comprehension and production deficits (e.g., Caplan, 1985). For Heeschen (1985), agrammatic and Broca's aphasia are the same. A writer may use "agrammatism" to refer to all types of grammatical deficit or may distinguish it from paragrammatism. Also, the case against group research was carried mainly by a "case against agrammatism" (Badecker and Caramazza, 1985).

Linguistic Description

Linguistic description of agrammatism has been important, because, as Lapointe (1985) put it, "the psycholinguistic account to be given later depends crucially on properties of the linguistic elements that are manipulated by the impaired, agrammatic speech production system" (p. 112).

Grammatical Morphemes. Traditionally, agrammatism has been identified as omissions of grammatical morphemes. These morphemes include function words (or closed-class words) and inflectional endings marking subject-verb agreement, verb tense, and conjugational forms in languages other than English. The prominence of omissions causes sentences to be shorter than normal. Omission of function words is a typical phenomenon in English-speaking persons with Broca's aphasia. It is heard in descriptions of the *Boston Diagnostic Aphasia Examination's* Cookie Theft picture, which showed a woman washing dishes while water overflows from the sink (Goodglass and Kaplan, 1983). In the following sentences, *1* is an example of moderate impairment (Caramazza and Hillis, 1989). Sentence 2 is a milder agrammatism, elicited with a picture of a girl giving flowers to a teacher (Saffran, Schwartz, and Marin, 1980; Schwartz, 1987):

(1) "Mother washing sink . . . water flowing floor. . . ."

(2) "Girl is handing flowers to teacher."

Harold Goodglass and colleagues in Boston pioneered investigation of this disorder. Their early research indicated that stress and position in the sentence have something to do with likelihood of omission. An unstressed initial functor such as *the* is more likely to be dropped than a stressed initial functor such as *can't* (Goodglass, Fodor, and Schulhoff, 1967).

Do grammatical morphemes differ in difficulty, so that we can rank stimuli for eliciting these forms in treatment? To answer this question, Goodglass and Berko (1960) constructed a sentence-completion task to elicit inflections. DeVilliers (1974) ranked the appearance of eight grammatical morphemes in obligatory contexts. Berko-Gleason and Goodglass developed a story-completion task to elicit 14 syntactic forms (Gleason, Goodglass, Green, Ackerman, and Hyde, 1975). Pluralized nouns and progressive verbs were among the easiest forms to produce, whereas it was very difficult to add *-s* for subject-verb agreement and produce the future auxiliary.

One of the significant discoveries of cross-linguistic studies is that agrammatism is not just a problem of omission. Articles are omitted more often in English than in other languages. Inflections and functors are substituted in German (Bates, Friederici, and Wulfeck, 1987b), Hungarian (MacWhinney and Osman-Sagi, 1991), Italian (Miceli, et al., 1989), French (Nespoulous, Dordain, Perron, Ska, Bub, Caplan, Mehler, and Lecours, 1988), and Hebrew (Grodzinsky, 1984). Expanding our idea of agrammatism may include different types of agrammatism. Two Italian cases indicated that morphological and syntactic dimensions of grammar can be dissociated (Miceli, Mazzucchi, Menn, and Goodglass, 1983). In Miceli's view, deficits in morphology concentrate on whole words such as functors, whereas syntactic deficits are problems with inflectional attachments and clausal structure. One feature of the variability in Miceli's 20 subjects was the absence of consistent co-occurrence of impaired functors and inflections (Miceli, et al., 1989). Studies of Italian speakers led to defining agrammatism as "the omission of freestanding grammatical morphemes *with or without* the substitution of bound grammatical morphemes" (Miceli, et al., 1989, p. 450). Another distinction was seen in a Polish patient with pronounced structural simplification but mild morphological deficit for all grammatical morphemes (Jarema and Kadzielawa, 1987). Similarly, Berndt (1987) distinguished omissions from structural simplification.

Main Verbs. Of the open-class content words produced, noun phrases appear more often than verb phrases (Myerson and Goodglass, 1972). Action-naming is more difficult than object-naming, which may be discussed as a dissociation of verbs from nouns (McCarthy and Warrington, 1985; Miceli, Silveri, Villa, and Caramazza, 1984; Williams and Canter, 1987; Zingeser and Berndt, 1990). In Chinese, verbs do not have the complexity of conjugation. With this factor out of the way, Chinese persons with agrammatism still had more difficulty retrieving verbs (Bates, Chen, Tzeng, Li, and Opie, 1991). The verb-finding problem was observed in descriptions of the girl giving flowers to her teacher.

(3) The young . . . the girl . . . the little girl is . . . the flower."
(4) "The girl is flower the woman."

Saffran and others (1980) concluded that the main verb's place was marked with the auxiliary *is*. However, Badecker and Caramazza (1985) used this data as an opportunity to note that agrammatic utterance can be ambiguous regarding the intended construction. They suggested that 3 could be an inappropriate use of the *be* form. Saffran's data also included examples of using nouns as verbs, as in 5.

(5) "The girl is rosing the teacher."

The *-ing* verb form is used more often than other verb inflections (Goodglass and Geschwind, 1976), and some suggest that agrammatic patients are often nominalizing a verb; that is, turning it into a noun. Thus, example 1 may be just a series of nouns to someone with agrammatism. Lapointe's (1985) idea

was that reliance on V + *ing* in English is an example of a broader deficit involving simplification of verbs, because agrammatic Italians produce the simpler past participle more than the present participle.

Word Order. Subjects with Broca's aphasia were asked to describe simple actions and object locations (Saffran, et al., 1980). They reversed NPs 40 percent of the time when the NPs were alike in animacy (e.g., "The sink is in the pencil"). This has been called the **animacy effect.** However, three-element utterances were nearly always in NVN order; errors such as NNV were not observed. Cross-linguistic studies indicated that morphemic order is resilient across syndromes (Bates, et al., 1988). The only sign of incorrect word order was the use of noncanonical OV forms 20 percent of the time in two-element utterances (e.g., "banana . . . eat"); error was related to verb subcategorization in relation to animacy of agents and recipients. Researchers hesitated in attributing such errors to a syntactic disorder, because severe cases appeared to abandon attempts to produce a sentence and resorted to labeling elements in a picture. It was noted previously that canonical order, such as SVO in English, seems to be overused as a "safe harbor." In situations focused on a recipient of an action (e.g., *ball was kicked*), patients with Broca's aphasia might say "kicked ball."

Simplification. Myerson and Goodglass (1972) examined a patient who conveyed negation by tagging "no" onto the beginning or end of a phrase instead of embedding it between a NP and VP. Patients often produce utterances in a simplified form. In the story-completion task, simple imperatives (e.g., *Sit down*) and noun phrases (e.g., *twelve cups, funny story*) were among the easiest structures to produce (Gleason, et al., 1975). Subjects found it difficult to construct noun phrases with two adjectives (e.g., *small red car*). Subjects in this study concatenated information, such as saying "a large house, a white house" instead of *a large white house*, or saying "girl tall and boy short" instead of *the girl is taller than the boy* (Gleason, et al.,

1975). In a study of naming, subjects elaborated by saying "the man and the man is old" instead of *the old man* (Brownell, et al., 1986). The same agrammatic behavior occurs in repetition, such as repeating *The old woman is washing the window* as "The woman is old and washing the window" (Ostrin and Schwartz, 1986). Embedding information, even to put adjectives into an NP, is hard for someone with agrammatism.

Explaining Expressive Agrammatism

Several twists and turns have developed in linguistic classification of symptoms. Main verbs and word order are being associated with syntax, whereas functors and inflections are being associated with morphology (e.g., Heeschen, 1985; Miceli, et al., 1983). One implication of research is that we should not be satisfied with "agrammatism" for describing a deficit. The patient may have a more specific deficit leading to more focused and, maybe, more efficient treatment. Schwartz, Linebarger, and Saffran (1985) warned that "it is one thing to describe agrammatism in syntactic terms and quite another to locate the responsible deficit in a mechanism that constructs syntactic representations" (p. 86).

Impaired "Syntax"? Initially, researchers attributed symptoms to an isolated problem with syntax. A "no-syntax hypothesis" was an easy target for accusations of vagueness (Kolk and van Grunsven, 1985). The ambiguity is partly a failure to specify whether syntactic knowledge or processing is impaired. Some essayists suggested that a "syntactic processor" is damaged, mainly indicating that the disorder is "modular" or affects one component of the language system (Caramazza and Berndt, 1978). Full consideration of the issues must deal with comprehension, but this section focuses on ideas about the impairment of formulation processes.

One class of hypotheses has been put forth by linguists claiming that agrammatic patients formulate sentences with an "underspecified syntactic representation" (Grodzinsky, Swinney, and Zurif, 1985) or

an "impoverished syntactic representation" (Caplan, 1985). Both ideas seem to pertain to the generation of representations during the formulation process as opposed to the representation of syntactic knowledge in LTM. Both ideas characterize a limitation on generation of a phrase structure or "syntactic tree" during sentence formulation. Grodzinsky proposed that a complete tree is formed but some terminal nodes are missing. Caplan proposed that patients do not construct a hierarchical tree. Instead, they activate a linear NVN form in the spirit of Bates' safe harbor notion. According to each view, agrammatic productions are not likely to be just a series of names. A patient is more likely to have activated a partial structural frame during formulation.

Another class of explanation refers to theory of language formulation (e.g., Figure 3–9). Agrammatism might even shed some light on such theory. The varied patterns of agrammatism prompted Goodglass and Menn (1985) to say that "it seems dubious that the term syntax can translate into a single process" (p. 21). Agrammatism has become a moving target, making it difficult to pose one theory. Garrett (1984) concentrated on omission of function words as a *closed-class theory* of agrammatism. His idea was that symptoms are caused by a **damaged positional level** mechanism, because this is where function words are selected. Ostrin and Schwartz (1986) thought that phrase simplification also originates in a damaged positional level. Retained canonical word order is indicative of a spared functional level. When someone has order errors and problems with grammatical morphemes, one or two mechanisms could be damaged (Caramazza and Berndt, 1985).

One challenge for the positional level explanation is the agrammatic patient's problem with retrieving main verbs (Lapointe, 1985). How does this fit into a theory of sentence formulation? Access to verbs should facilitate framing a sentence because of the subcategorization rules that specify types of nouns that can accompany a verb. Zingeser and Berndt (1990) proposed that a **verb-finding deficit** is causally linked to sentence formulation difficulties. After all, people with anomic aphasia retrieve verbs and produce good sentences (Miceli, et al., 1984). With respect to Garrett's theory of formulation, subcategorization is part of the lexical entry for a verb, and lexical entries are retrieved at the positional level. In operations at this level, the verb determines positioning of nouns in the sentence frame that is generated adequately at the functional level. Thus, verb-finding deficit may contribute to a fuller understanding of positional level impairment.

Debate rages as to whether agrammatism is a legitimate entity. Miceli and others (1989) said that their data "can no longer be ignored just for the obstinate protection of a fictional category of dubious theoretical value" (p. 475). Support for rethinking our way of looking at grammatical features of language comes from the substitutions and verb-finding problems in so-called agrammatic patients (Badecker and Caramazza, 1985) and the overlap of symptoms between patients who are supposed to be different with respect to the agrammatism-paragrammatism distinction (Bates, et al., 1991; Heeschen and Kolk, 1988). Moreover, a telegraphic utterance can be analyzed linguistically in a number of ways (Badecker and Caramazza, 1985). The other side of the debate has been presented mainly by Caplan (1986, 1987a), who suggested that verb-finding deficit is another disorder that an agrammatic patient can have, and by Grodzinsky (1991), who argued for refocusing on the similarities among patients. Caplan (1991) suggested that variability of functors and inflections in Broca's aphasia is indicative of the complexity of sentence formulation. In his opinion, agrammatism is an appropriate classification, and we just have much more to learn about the intricacies of grammatical processes.

Effort and Adaptation. Goodglass (1976) entertained the possibility that effort of production, especially with the burden of apraxia of speech, results in the elimination of less salient words such as functors. Thus, telegraphic utterance is an adaptive "econ-omy of effort." If patients did not have motor problems, they would produce complete sentences. However, patients with little apraxia omit grammatical morphemes. Economy of effort does not account for substitution errors.

Bates, Wulfeck, and MacWhinney (1991) contemplated cognitive effort in the access of grammatical forms. They used the **competition model** (Chapter 3) as a basis for an alternative to closed-class theory. Competition is between **cue validity** (i.e., information value of a linguistic form) and **cue cost** (i.e., amount and type of processing involved in using a linguistic form). Bates predicted that elements with high cue cost will be impaired across all syndromes, and elements with high cue validity will tend to be retained. Cue validity appears to be variable across languages. Articles carry more information value in German than English and are omitted much less in German. Sparing canonical word order may reflect automaticity of activation of basic phrase structure.

One of Goldstein's (1948) main contributions to thinking about aphasia was his view that symptoms are the product of impairment and the organism's adaptive response to the impairment. When we identify a functional lesion in a component of a cognitive model, we should notice that other components are left untouched. Spared components should be adaptive. Kolk and Heeschen (1990) differentiated **impairment symptoms,** attributable to a damaged processor (i.e., negative symptoms), from **adaptation symptoms,** attributable to compensatory adjustments by the cognitive system (i.e., positive symptoms). These investigators claimed that omissions are symptoms of adaptation and substitutions are symptoms of impairment. The idea that omissions are a normal adjustment was supported by referring to the common use of elliptical expressions by neurologically intact persons (e.g., "more milk," "too late"). Kolk and Heeschen referred to experiments presenting stimuli that reduced information value of elliptical expression, and agrammatic omissions decreased significantly. They also decided that structural simplification points to impairment. Their theory, called **synchrony reduction,** was that agrammatic patients are slow to activate structural representations; this slowness reduces the synchrony required to combine elements of a sentence and, thus, makes complex structures difficult to produce.

BROCA'S APHASIA

Broca's aphasia is the co-occurrence of agrammatism and a moderate-to-mild comprehension deficit. While comprehension deficit is consistent with the notion that aphasia is a multimodality impairment, the impression of "expressive aphasia" lingers from the depths of aphasiology's history. Whether an agrammatic patient must have deficient comprehension is somewhat controversial. Broca's aphasia is still a swaggering flagship in a contentious sea. Study of comprehension addresses overlapping questions of whether aphasia is impaired knowledge or processes and whether one disorder can be so central that it disrupts both expression and comprehension.

Comprehension Ability

Comprehension has been said to be "good" or "relatively preserved" in Broca's aphasia (Zurif, et al., 1976; Wulfeck, 1988). However, terms like "good" are relative; in the clinic, this syndrome is diagnosed with a range of deficiency. When diagnosing with the Boston Diagnostic Aphasia Examination (Goodglass and Kaplan, 1983), the profile for Broca's aphasia allows a range from the 50th to the 90th percentile for auditory comprehension. According to the Western Aphasia Battery (Kertesz, 1982), the patient can be in a range of 4 to 10 points for this function. In development of Shewan's (1979) test of sentence comprehension (Chapter 10), three major syndromes were compared. Of 21 total points, the syndromes ranked as follows: anomic aphasia, 14.8; Broca's aphasia, 12.5; Wernicke's aphasia, 9.73.

The study that made comprehension deficit interesting was Caramazza and Zurif's (1976) comparison between reversible (6*a*) and nonreversible (6*b*) statements with patients diagnosed as having Broca's and conduction aphasia.

(6a) The *girl* that the *boy* is chasing is tall.

(6b) The *apple* that the *boy* is eating is red.

Subjects chose interpretations from two pictures, and the foil had either a different element for the situation or a reversal of agent and theme. The subjects with Broca's aphasia had significant difficulty with reversible statements (6*a*). They also made more order errors than lexical errors, indicating that lexical items were identified but their thematic roles were sometimes difficult to determine. Caramazza and Zurif concluded that people with Broca's aphasia can use semantic constraints to comprehend thematic roles (e.g., apples do not eat) but have difficulty when they must rely on the syntactic feature of word order. In addition to center-embedded clauses, passive sentence structure in English also proved to be difficult (Samuels and Benson, 1979; Schwartz, Saffran, and Marin, 1980).

Caramazza and Zurif (1976) thought that available data was "contrary to the view that Broca's aphasics have retained a normal tacit knowledge of their language" (p. 581). Later it was decided that "disruption of the syntactic processing mechanism undermines the Broca patient's ability to utilize syntactic information in all language performances that require syntactic analysis" (Berndt and Caramazza, 1980, pp. 272–73). Despite this wavering over knowledge and processes, the basic conclusion was that Broca's aphasia is a central syntactic disorder with an agrammatic comprehension that parallels linguistic expression. In particular, people with Broca's aphasia acquired a reputation for having difficulty with word order when it is the main cue to thematic roles. Some researchers put subjects into the Broca category according to an "inability to interpret other than simple active structures or semantically constrained sentences" (Rosenberg, Zurif, Brownell, Garrett, and Bradley, 1985, p. 292; also, Shapiro and Levine, 1990). If Broca's aphasia is indeed distinctive because of focal damage to a module of language comprehension, other aphasias should not have the same problem. However, Caramazza and Zurif's subjects with conduction aphasia had the same performance pattern, leading Darley (1982) to declare that syndromes are a figment of the Boston imagination. Thus, several issues remained following the early studies of Broca's aphasia.

Problematic Features of Sentences

Just as grammatical morphemes drop out of speech, patients with Broca's aphasia are suspected to process sentences as if these morphemes are absent. Studies had subjects comprehend sentences in which **functors** matter for interpretation. Heilman and Scholes (1976) presented sentences like 7 in a picture-choice task with word-order and lexical foils.

(7a) She showed her baby the pictures.
(7b) She showed her the baby pictures.

In these sentences, *the* cues the structuring and thematic roles of other words. Again, subjects with Broca's and conduction aphasias had difficulty making word-order decisions. Then, investigators arranged stimuli so that subjects could respond to the indefiniteness of *a* and the definiteness of *the* (Goodenough, Zurif, Weintraub, and von Stockert, 1977). Subjects with Broca's aphasia failed to distinguish the articles, contrary to those with anomic aphasia. Broca subjects were also impaired in the use of stress and juncture which, like functors, resolve syntactic ambiguities, as in *They fed her dog biscuits* (Baum, Daniloff, Daniloff, and Lewis, 1982). People with Broca's aphasia developed a reputation for being insensitive to functors, although they responded appropriately to sentences like *Bill walking the dog* and *Bill the walking dog* (Caplan, Matthei, and Gigley, 1981).

Inflectional cues to thematic roles were examined in cross-linguistic research. In highly inflected languages, case inflection tags the thematic roles of nouns. In studies of Serbo-Croatian, agrammatic subjects were deficient in using case inflection for showing actions between toy animals (Smith and Bates, 1987). They had no impairment in the use of semantic information. Case and gender cues were compared to animacy cues for showing agent-object relations between toy animals and objects. Subjects with anomic aphasia were also impaired for inflections, although Broca's aphasia presented much greater impairment. Convergent combinations of case and gender cues enhanced performance significantly for agrammatic subjects. In a similar study of Turkish and Hungarian, subjects across three syndromes were impaired in using case markings (MacWhinney, Osman-Sagi, and Slobin, 1991). Subjects with Wernicke's aphasia had the greatest difficulty. In other cross-linguistic study, the use of morphology was impaired in all aphasic groups (Bates, Friederici, and Wulfeck, 1987a).

Following Caramazza and Zurif (1976), it was suspected that agrammatic aphasia includes a deficit in dealing with **word order** when making thematic decisions about NPs in a sentence. Schwartz and others (1980) presented statements like *The square is on top of the circle* and *The cow kicks the horse*, and subjects made more reversal errors than lexical-semantic errors. Chance performance with reversible passives indicated that these sentences were not understood. In Caramazza and Zurif's study, the finding that nonreversible sentences are easier than reversibles indicated that semantic cues can be used to interpret thematic roles. However, their subjects may have benefited from picture-foils like an apple eating a boy (*6a*) and relied on world knowledge to comprehend nonreversibles. When manipulating **plausibility** in reversible sentences without creating bizarre impossibility, researchers showed that plausible reversibles can be understood better than implausible but possible reversibles with Broca's and Wernicke's aphasia (Deloche and Seron, 1981; Heeschen, 1980). Thus, thematic roles appeared to be hard to detect when relying mainly on word order (i.e., reversibles), and deviation from canonical order exacerbates this problem (i.e., passive reversibles). Thematic decisions are easier with semantic cues (i.e., nonreversibles) and are complicated by implausibility in conditions created for research.

Sherman and Schweickert (1989) tried to deal with problems in Caramazza and Zurif's (1976) design so that more complete observations could be made concerning syntactic complexity, semantic reversibility, and plausibility of events. The investigators also wanted to address theoretical reservations about Caramazza and Zurif's conclusions (e.g., Grodzinsky, 1986). Sherman and Schweickert looked for deficits by comparing five agrammatic aphasic subjects to normal controls. As in the earlier study, the foil in picture-pairs forced a decision about thematic roles of NPs in sentences such as 8, which is only a sample of the several conditions presented.

(8a) The dog is pulling the clown.
(8b) The tree is climbing the girl.
(8c) The cowboy is carried by the Indian.
(8d) The cowboy that the boot is polishing is clean.

Relative to the 1976 study, conditions were expanded to include reversible actives (8a), reversible passives (8c), and implausible versions of each type of sentence (8b, 8d). Aphasic subjects could interpret most actives (96.3 percent correct) and passives (81.3 percent). Comprehension of reversible passives was generally impaired but was also at above-chance levels. Pronounced deficiency occurred with center-embedding. Results reinforced Caramazza and Zurif's conclusions. For plausible events, reversible sentences led to more errors than nonreversibles. Plausibility was easier than implausibility, an effect that was pronounced for center-embedded sentences. Thus, people with Broca's aphasia seem to process semantic constraints to overcome limitations with word order.

Sherman and Schweickert (1989) were impressed with syntactic capacities displayed by their agrammatic subjects, especially in comprehension of active and passive sentences. Reversible sentences need not be difficult (Gallaher and Canter, 1982), or agrammatic persons can comprehend them at above-chance levels (Wulfeck, 1988). Dutch subjects made few errors for active reversible statements, and those with Broca's aphasia did better than Wernicke subjects on passives (Friederici and Graetz, 1987). In comparison of English, German, and Italian, use of **canonical order** with the toy animal manipulation task did not decline in any syndrome (Bates, et al., 1987a). When order is the main cue to thematic roles, it is a problem when sentences are in a noncanonical sequence. However, passive sentences may present less difficulty than was thought originally, and deviation from canonicity may be more problematic in sentences complicated by relative clauses.

Relative difficulty of inflection, word order, and semantic information differs across languages due to variation of cue validity among languages. Inflectional morphology is more important in Italian than English, whereas the reverse is the case for word order. German and Italian patients relied on word order cues in an apparent compensation for morphological deficit (Bates, et al., 1987a). In many studies, sentences were constructed so that subjects had to rely on either inflection or word order. Yet, to ensure communication, we often combine cues, creating **cue redundancy** (Bates, et al., 1991). For Serbo-Croatian, combination of order, case, and gender cues enabled subjects with Broca's aphasia to comprehend almost normally (Smith and Bates, 1987). Canonical word order was used successfully for Turkish and Hungarian, and switches of order did not pose a problem when case markings were available (MacWhinney, et al., 1991).

Explanation: Locating a Functional Lesion

Limited short-term memory may have little to do with grammatical comprehension deficits (Martin, 1987). Just as a pattern of deficit in expression is suggestive of damage to a particular subprocess of language formulation, a pattern of difficulty might point to a weak subprocess of comprehension. We may be inclined to consider the syntactic subsystem to be the location of disorder, but we should assess whether knowledge or processing is impaired. Also, impairments of a process may be considered with respect to the major subsystems of sentence comprehension (Figure 3–7).

Linguistic Knowledge. Lost knowledge would be a deep central deficit, because the same knowledge is applied to expression and comprehension. As indicated in Chapter 4, theory of lost knowledge (or competence) should be supported by impairment across any task in which the knowledge is required. A deficit isolated in syntactic knowledge should be supported by showing that semantic knowledge is intact. Metalinguistic tasks have been employed extensively, partly because they involve "shallow processing" (Linebarger, Schwartz, and Saffran, 1983) or may circumvent processes of comprehension and expression tasks (Baum, 1989).

As Caramazza and Zurif (1976) suggested, initial studies indicated that knowledge of syntax (i.e., word order) is erased in Broca's aphasia. When arranging words into sentences, subjects had difficulty marking NPs with articles and tended to group content words together (von Stockert and Bader, 1976; Zurif, Caramazza, and Myerson, 1972; Zurif, Green, Caramazza, and Goodenough, 1976). A conceptual dissociation was demonstrated by Semenza, Denes, Lucchese, and Bisiacchi (1980), who compared seven Broca's and seven Wernicke's aphasias. Subjects with Broca's aphasia were unimpaired in detecting class relations between a target picture (e.g., fisherman) and two choices (e.g., sailor, diver). They were impaired when the task involved picking out a thematically related idea (e.g., fisherman: fish, river). Subjects with Wernicke's aphasia had the opposite pattern of performance. While Semenza's results were suggestive of a deep impairment pertaining to conceptual relationships expressed

in syntactic form, the other studies of word-sorting were suspect because they involve processes used in language formulation (Caramazza and Hillis, 1989).

Word-sorting was replaced by **grammaticality judgment,** in which subjects just indicated whether a sentence is good or bad. Agrammatic subjects were good at detecting violations of agreement (Grossman and Haberman, 1982), use of prepositions (Friederici, 1982; Branchereau and Nespoulous, 1989), verb subcategorization and noun inflection for Serbo-Croatian (Lukatela, Crain, and Shankweiler, 1988), and other violations including errors of word order (Linebarger, et al., 1983; Wulfeck, 1988). In one study, subjects made on-line responses to spoken sentences by pressing the "bad" button at the point when they heard an error (Shankweiler, Crain, Gorrell, and Tuller, 1989). Location of inflection and functor errors was manipulated, and subjects with Broca's aphasia displayed a response pattern similar to normal controls. In another study, subjects pressed a button after the whole sentence was heard (Wulfeck, Bates, and Capasso, 1991). Groups of Italian and English speakers were successful enough to display knowledge of syntax. Errors of morphology were harder to deal with than errors of word order for English speakers. As expected from the cue validity of inflection, Italian subjects found it easier to detect inflectional errors.

Grammatical judgments support the view that people with Broca's aphasia retain the representation of phrase structure and grammatical morphology in long-term memory. A study of word-sorting also exhibited retained knowledge of articles and SVO order (Gallaher, 1981). From cross-linguistic studies, Bates, Wulfeck, and MacWhinney (1991) concluded that linguistic competence remains intact for Broca's and Wernicke's aphasias. Thus, we should not say things such as "the patient has lost his language" or "she does not know language." We should turn to processing to explain comprehension deficit and its parallels with agrammatic expression.

Lexical Access. In the exploration of whether Broca's aphasia is a valid theoretical syndrome, researchers develop hypotheses with respect to whether damage to one subsystem of comprehension accounts for comprehension problems exhibited by these patients. A corollary is that other subsystems remain intact. The attention given to syntax should lead us to believe that lexical access is one of these intact subsystems. In one study, a lexical decision task (LDT) was used for comparing access to open- and closed-class words (Bradley, Garrett, and Zurif, 1980). Diagnosis of deficit hinged on normal subjects, who had a frequency effect for open-class words but not for closed-class functors. Subjects with Broca's aphasia did not exhibit this difference. Bradley proposed a **lexical hypothesis,** which stated that agrammatic comprehension is an impairment in accessing functors, an idea that fits nicely with the earlier indications of insensitivity to functors and the closed-class theory of agrammatism. However, several investigators could not replicate the frequency effect with normal adults, thereby weakening the basis for claiming that aphasic patients are different (e.g., Kolk and Blomert, 1985; Taft, 1990); and Gordon and Caramazza (1983) could not replicate the findings for aphasic subjects.

Claims of intact semantic processing in Broca's aphasia may be shown in the obligatory activation that occurs with lexical access. When primes preceded lexical targets in LDTs, recognition was facilitated by semantic relatedness across several syndromes; but subjects were impaired in judging the relatedness of the same words (Blumstein, Milberg, and Shrier, 1982; Milberg and Blumstein, 1981). Then, priming pairs were presented in such a way as to bias an ambiguous prime (e.g., BANK) for a target (e.g., RIVER) (Milberg, Blumstein, and Dworetzky, 1987). That is, SHORE-BANK should speed response to RIVER, and MONEY-BANK should steer the system to a conceptual region far from [rivers]. Subjects with Broca's aphasia surprisingly had no priming effects relative to unrelated primes. However, Milberg's research design suffered some criticism (e.g.,

Chertkow, Bub, and Seidenberg, 1989; Hagoort, 1989; Milberg and Blumstein, 1989). Katz (1988) simplified the task by presenting one-word primes (e.g., BANK) for targets such as MONEY or RIVER. This time, agrammatic subjects displayed semantic priming for both meanings of BANK. Even with severe comprehension deficit, aphasic patients appear to be able to activate regions of semantic memory. Lexical-semantic impairments are more evident in slow tasks permitting consciously controlled processing.

Despite evidence for lexical access capacity and the large shadow over Bradley's closed-class lexical hypothesis, Swinney, Zurif, and Nicol (1989) saw possibilities for the view that comprehension in Broca's aphasia is diminished by a disruption of lexical access. With a cross-modal priming task, Swinney examined the multiple access of meanings for ambiguous words (e.g., *plant*) in spoken sentences such as 9.

(9) The gardener was responsible for watering every plant * on the enormous estate.

While listening to this sentence, four Broca's and four Wernicke's aphasic subjects made a recognition decision about letter-strings (e.g., TREE, FACTORY, PAGE, FUNERAL) shown immediately after the ambiguous prime (*). Wernicke subjects exhibited normal immediate access of multiple meanings, but Broca subjects were primed only for dominant meanings (i.e., TREE). The investigators concluded that Broca's aphasia includes an impaired automatic exhaustive access of meanings and speculated that agrammatic patients may merely be slow to access secondary meanings. Moreover, performance with Wernicke's aphasia supported the notion of modularity of impairment in an "encapsulated" mechanism. Swinney's conclusions were attacked by Caramazza and Badecker (1991) in the continuing effort to discredit the use of groups to infer the status of cognition. Caramazza suggested that a later prime should have been used to see if exhaustive access is indeed just slow.

The central role of verbs in predicate-argument structure and problems with verb-finding in agrammatism led Shapiro and Levine (1990) to study verb access in a cross-modal priming task. Judiciously placed word recognition was the means of measuring processing complexity for verbs. One difference of complexity is illustrated with *10*. The verb *put* is simpler, because it must take a theme (*new suit*) and location (*on the shelf*). In *10b*, *donated* should be more complex, because location (i.e., *to the charity*) is optional.

(10a) The happy officer put * the new suit on * the shelf.

(10b) The sad girl donated * the new suit to * the charity.

Subjects with Broca's aphasia performed like normal controls. Process time was longer after verbs allowing multiple argument structures (e.g., *10b*), an effect that dissipated downstream after the preposition. Fluent aphasic subjects were not sensitive to argument structure, indicating that they are impaired in the access of lexical subcategorization. The expressive problem with verbs in Broca's aphasia does not appear to extend to core processing in sentence comprehension. The mixed conclusions in the cross-modal priming experiments may enhance our appetite for more psycholinguistic investigation of lexical access with aphasia.

The Syntactic Parser. Thinking of comprehension as the interactive operation of encapsulated subprocessors, we may believe for now that lexical access generates fairly adequate information for other modules in Broca's aphasia. However, theorists started to worry about ambiguity of the idea of a damaged syntactic processor. Goodglass and Menn (1985) declared that the idea "is quite fuzzy." Many aphasiologists have referred to a computational device called the parser and yet have made scant reference to theories in psycholinguistics such as Frazier's simplest parse and paradigms like those employing garden-path sentences. Promoting his "case against agrammatism," Caramazza complained that "without some indication of how

the hypothesized parsing component can be made sense of computationally, the proposal goes no further than positing an underspecified linguistic faculty for the sake of collecting several intuitively related phenomena under a single generalization" (Badecker and Caramazza, 1985, p. 120).

One class of theory of syntactic impairment is based on linguistics and arises from speculation about "syntactic representations" that we may try to relate to the cognitive notion of the parse. Linguists tend to argue that aphasia includes a modular disorder of syntax in contrast to unidimensional theories and lexical-semantic hypotheses. They were concerned about word-order factors in off-line experiments with sentences of varied complexity (e.g., Hildebrandt, Caplan, and Evans, 1987; Chapter 4). They also focused on the now disputed chance-level performance observed in 1980 with reversible passive sentences. Caplan and Futter (1986) studied an agrammatic patient's manipulation of toy animals in response to passives and other constructions. Finding chance response to reversible passives, they concluded that the subject failed to assign a hierarchical phrase structure. Their **linearity hypothesis** stated that the subject used a linear SVO assignment of thematic roles to understand NVN sentences, consistent with the idea that canonical order is easy to comprehend across languages (Bates, et al., 1987a).

Linguistic aphasiology contains its disagreements. Grodzinsky (1986) claimed that patients generate hierarchical representations and that impairment is an incomplete structural representation (also Grodzinsky and Marek, 1988). For example, in Government-Binding theory of passives, a "trace" that designates thematic role is said to be left in the wake of movement of NPs from their canonical position (Cowper, 1992). Grodzinsky's **trace-deletion hypothesis** states that agrammatic patients delete traces from structural representations and end up assigning thematic roles randomly. Caplan (1987a) disagreed, and Sherman and Schweickert (1989) claimed that they failed to support explicit predictions by Caplan and Grodzinsky.

Grodzinsky (1989) turned to a study of relative clauses to support his theory but also claimed that "the present account is an abstraction, and . . . does not make claims about 'traces' being deleted from the patients' heads" (p. 485). In Chapter 1, it is emphasized that dysfunction exists in internal phenomena. A linguist may back off from an appearance of speculating about cognition, but this is the domain of disorder. Linguistic approaches tend to ignore issues such as whether impairment lies in automatic or controlled parses. Yet, in talk about "structural representations," linguistic theories are suggestive of the nature of activated representations used for parsing.

Another class of theories is more psycholinguistic in terminology and appears to give more attention to difficulties with grammatical morphemes. Friederici (1988) has been a leading proponent of an **impaired parsing hypothesis.** This theory was intended initially to counter any suggestion that syntactic knowledge is lost. Sensitivity to grammatical morphemes in off-line and metalinguistic tasks is indicative of intact knowledge. These tasks also allow time to compensate for difficulty with core processing. In on-line tasks of word-monitoring, agrammatic subjects responded slower to functors than to content words, in contrast to normal controls (Friederici, 1983; Swinney, Zurif, and Cutler, 1980; Tyler and Cobb, 1987). This finding may be compatible with the lexical hypothesis, but Friederici (1988) claimed that grammatical morphemes are recognized and disorder is "a computational failure involving the structural information carried by closed-class elements" (p. 281). The patient does not activate syntactic representations fast enough for integration with semantic information. Agrammatic deficit is a "computational mismatch."

Syntactic priming in LDTs is studied to see if disorder can be located in the core activation of syntactic representations. Baum (1988) wanted to determine if grammatical primes (e.g., *It's true that the boys*) facilitate response to a target (e.g., *play*) relative to an ungrammatical prime (e.g., *It's true that the boy*). With 500 msec between stimuli, syntactic priming did not occur for Broca subjects as it did for normal controls. Haarmann and Kolk (1991) varied SOA and presented primes like *We can* and targets like TALK or NOSE. Broca subjects were facilitated at 1,100-msec intervals but not at 300 or 700 msec. Like Friederici, Haarmann and Kolk suggested that people with Broca's aphasia are slow to activate syntactic representations. In another study, two types of prime-target pairs were presented auditorily (Blumstein, Milberg, Dworetzky, Rosen, and Gershberg, 1991). One type was a single phrase (e.g., *is-going*), and another crossed phrase boundaries (e.g., *he-goes*). Target recognition was compared against a baseline (e.g., *pru-goes*). Unlike normals, Broca subjects were not facilitated within a phrase. Broca subjects had a normal lack of facilitation across phrase boundaries. With erroneous pairs (e.g., *could-going, they-goes*), these aphasic subjects also displayed normal inhibition or slowed recognition relative to baseline. Failed facilitation was attributed to impaired automatic activation. Normal inhibitory priming was attributed to retention of controlled processing.

There has been no shortage of ideas about what could go wrong in the realm of syntax, especially in Broca's aphasia. While retaining storage of inflectional lexicon, a patient may be slow to use these cues when activating an initial parse. Given time in off-line tasks, a capacity for slowly activating syntactic representations may be exhibited. In either case, syntactic analysis may be rigidly linear or incomplete. Linguistic and psycholinguistic theories point to a rejection of all-or-none notions of a demolished syntactic device and acceptance of theory expressing some form of partial impairment. Moreover, clinical reliance on off-line comprehension tasks may be insufficient for diagnosing the cognitive disorder.

Semantic Interpretation. So far, the comprehension deficit in Broca's aphasia is attributed to impaired obligatory processes leading to delayed and/or incomplete parsing, especially of noncanonical and complex sentences. Semantic processing can be weakened by receiving faulty information from other components of the system. Yet, the **semantic constraint hypothesis** states that intact semantic processes are a source of controlled adaptation to these limitations. In many comprehension situations presented clinically, "all that is required is knowledge of the lexical items and how they can be sensibly combined, based on knowledge of the world" (Sherman and Schweickert, 1989, p. 434). Even if there are insensitivities to grammatical morphemes or word order, people with Broca's aphasia comprehend, and their deficits are too subtle to be exposed in many picture-decision tasks. When pictured events are absurd, "the analysis required is even further removed from the sentence; the subject simply needs to be able to distinguish depictions of probable and improbable real-world occurrences" (Sherman and Schweickert, 1989, p. 435).

Another possibility, suggested first by Schwartz and others (1980), is based on an assumption that lexical and syntactic processes are functional in Broca's aphasia. These aphasiologists challenged the notion of syntactic deficit because of patients' success with grammatical judgment and problems with comprehension (Linebarger, et al., 1983). Instead, they proposed an **impaired mapping hypothesis,** which states that patients fail to assign thematic roles to realized syntactic representations. Zurif and Grodzinsky (1983) disagreed by saying, in part, that off-line judgments are not good indicators of processing ability. Schwartz and her colleagues reinforced their position with a study of plausibility judgments. Agrammatic patients were sensitive to some thematic oddities (e.g., *The worm swallowed the bird*) but had difficulty when NPs were moved away from canonical positions (e.g., *We saw the bird that the worm swallowed*) (Schwartz, Linebarger, Saffran, and Pate, 1987; Saffran and Schwartz, 1988). Grodzinsky (1989) thought that the basis for the mapping hypothesis is a syntactic difference between sentences and that his trace-deletion hypothesis makes the same predictions. Others believe that people with Broca's aphasia are able to assign thematic roles within limits of syntactic capacity (Caplan, 1985; Kolk and van Grunsven, 1985).

Centrality of Broca's Aphasia

Co-occurrence of similar deficits in expression and comprehension led to the proposition that a single, deep, central disorder is responsible for both problems in Broca's aphasia. Loss of knowledge could account for both impairments, but this explanation has been discounted. Among theories of processing, the lexical access hypothesis could account for both problems. However, Shapiro and Levine indicated that verb access is not as impaired as verb retrieval for production. Theories of expressive and receptive deficit have some similarities. Friederici's idea that a slow parser cannot keep up with other subsystems is similar to Kolk and Heeschen's theory of synchrony reduction for formulation. Caplan's linearity hypothesis is reminiscent of Bates' "safe harbor" of canonical structure in expression. Without explicit identity of receptive and formulative dysfunction, a production-specific disorder may be compatible with a comprehension problem based merely on the slowing of core processes, which tend to be lexical and syntactic.

We may wonder if a relationship between expression and comprehension has been proved, especially as a cohesive feature of Broca's aphasia (Kolk, van Grunsven, and Keyser, 1985). In most studies, either comprehension or production has been examined. Production has rarely been compared directly to subtle receptive skills. Conclusions from one study have been examined with respect to impressions of previous work on the other function. A deep central disorder may not be necessary to produce expressive agrammatism. Researchers have described patients with agrammatism but without an apparent comprehension deficit (Caramazza and Hillis, 1989; Miceli, et al., 1983; Nespoulous, et al., 1988).

WERNICKE'S APHASIA AND JARGON

Wernicke's aphasia is the most severely impaired fluent syndrome. It is caused by a focal lesion in the posterior superior region of the temporal lobe and is characterized by jargon and severe comprehension deficit. Also, because of poor recognition of expressive deficit, patients are not at all self-conscious about their neologisms and other paraphasias. As with the tendency to identify agrammatic aphasia instead of Broca's aphasia, the term **jargonaphasia** is seen frequently in a presumed reference to patients with Wernicke's aphasia. This aphasia, associated with semantically anomalous sentence production, is often thought to arise from a disorder in the semantic realm that is a double dissociative contrast to agrammatic aphasia.

One curious finding in surveys of aphasic populations is a consistent tendency for people with Wernicke's aphasia to be older (i.e., in their 60s) than people with Broca's aphasia (i.e., in their 50s). Coppens (1991) reviewed these studies and the many explanations inspired by this finding. One of the more reasonable explanations is a selection bias in the studies, attributable to a tendency for fluent aphasias to survive longer because lesions are smaller than in nonfluent aphasias and a tendency for Wernicke's aphasia in the acute stage to have the same pattern of deficit through the chronic stage. The age difference is not pronounced at one month post onset. Cognitive changes in normal aging could be another factor, although evidence is inconclusive.

Comprehension Deficit

An outstanding feature of this aphasia is severe comprehension deficit. When syndromes are compared, this group usually makes the most errors, except when global aphasia is included. In the Boston Diagnostic Aphasia Examination's criteria for diagnosis, the upper end of the range for this function is the 45th percentile, or below average (Goodglass and Kaplan, 1983). Someone with Wernicke's aphasia may be in a room with a group

of people and act as if he or she does not even hear the conversations. Proximity of the lesion to the primary auditory area in the temporal lobe, as well as severity of deficit, led some investigators to suspect that the processing of linguistic stimuli does not go beyond speech perception. The deficit appears as "pure word deafness," but the syndrome suggests a difference because of the jargon that is unique to Wernicke's aphasia (Kirshner, Webb, and Duncan, 1981). Speech perception deficits are not specific to this syndrome (Basso, et al., 1977; Blumstein, et al., 1977; Miceli, et al., 1980) and are often not sufficient to reduce language comprehension substantially (Carpenter and Rutherford, 1973; Shewan, 1982). Nevertheless, variation of lesion size and location may create an "auditory-predominant" subgroup in which auditory processing is substantially below reading (Heilman, Rothi, Campanella, and Wolfson, 1979; Kirshner, Casey, Henson, and Heinrich, 1989). Damage in the auditory region can add a modality-specific component to an aphasia with clear impact on other modalities.

Wernicke's aphasia has been swept up with Broca's aphasia in efforts to determine if aphasias include a broad double dissociation of semantic and syntactic functions, contrary to Schuell's opinion that these aspects of language use are inseparable. Wernicke's aphasia might be a problem in the semantic domain, whereas syntactic capacities remain intact. Many of the studies mentioned before are not helpful because Broca's aphasia was often compared with mixed groups of posterior or fluent aphasias. We can get an idea of how it went with Wernicke's aphasia from Caramazza and Zurif's (1976) pivotal study of reversibility in sentences along with lexical and ordering foils in picture choices (e.g., 6a, 6b, p. 108). They were "perplexed" about the performance pattern of five Wernicke subjects. These subjects were above chance on the task, indicating comprehension capacity. Wernicke subjects had equal difficulty with syntactic and semantic factors, including the basis for errors, so Caramazza and Zurif could not point to a modular impairment.

They wrote frankly about an issue that may pertain to other studies: "The good level of performance in the Wernicke's patients may have been due simply to a bias in the selection of patients; since patients had to have enough comprehension skills to be able to understand our instructions and perform the experimental task, we likely included only very mildly impaired, atypical Wernicke's aphasics" (p. 579).

How well does the impaired language system in Wernicke's aphasia deal with lexical access? Kohn and Friedman (1986) decided that a case with mild Wernicke's aphasia had a post-access disorder two months post onset. The diagnosis of a patient called "HN" was not reported with respect to test criteria; however, scores on the Boston Diagnostic Aphasia Examination were given. HN was said to have semantic and phonemic paraphasias. His 8 of 15 points in following commands pushes the upper limit for comprehension, but his 102 of 105 in naming is unusual for Wernicke's aphasia. He could repeat words, indicative of lexical access or activation of a lexical representation. He had occasional difficulty with word comprehension in picture-pointing tasks, which was called a "phonological-semantic dissociation." Kohn and Friedman were intrigued by the fact that when he could not comprehend a word, HN spelled it aloud and did not figure out its meaning until he wrote it and read it aloud. It was as if an orthographic-to-phonological route to meaning was working more efficiently. This phenomenon is also seen in patients with anomic aphasia. Moreover, patients with more typical Wernicke's aphasia do not repeat words very well, which does not necessarily mean that patients are unable to access the lexicon for recognition.

Four Wernicke subjects showed a normal priming effect in an on-line study of sentence comprehension using the cross-modal lexical priming procedure (Swinney, et al., 1989). These subjects, who had to be able to perform the task, seemed to access multiple meanings automatically after ambiguous words (example 9, p. 112). Milberg and Blumstein (1981) were surprised to find se-

mantic priming effects for Wernicke's aphasia in simple LDTs, especially effects that did not occur for Broca's aphasia (also, Blumstein, et al., 1982; Milberg, et al., 1987). Yet, Wernicke subjects also had many more errors making lexical decisions, and they performed much worse than Broca subjects in making judgments about the semantic relatedness of word-pairs. In total, these studies indicate that Wernicke's aphasia maintains automatic access to semantic memory through the lexicon, but controlled decisions on the lexical-semantic dimension can be difficult. Like Kohn and Friedman, Swinney and his colleagues decided that comprehension disorder may exist in another component of sentence processing.

As indicated before, early studies of varied syntactic forms showed that Wernicke's aphasia, while characteristic of more severe impairment generally, does not differ from other syndromes in the relative difficulty of these forms (e.g., Parisi and Pizzamiglio, 1970; Shewan and Canter, 1971). The syntactic component of sentence comprehension has been evaluated with respect to the processing of grammatical morphemes and word order in making decisions about thematic roles of nouns. In cross-linguistic research, the use of subject-verb agreement cues was impaired for Wernicke's aphasia as well as Broca's aphasia (Bates, et al., 1987a). In the study of Turkish and Hungarian, the subjects with Wernicke's aphasia had more difficulty than Broca and anomic subjects in dealing with case markings. Also, Wernicke's aphasia has been included in the basic finding that processing canonical order is preserved. In earlier research, these patients could order phrases into sentences (von Stockert and Bader, 1976). This syndrome also possesses the same deficit with noncanonical order in passive sentences (Heeschen, 1980).

Unique syntactic problems in Wernicke's aphasia were indicated in two studies. Word order had an impact that was not observed for Broca's aphasia with respect to the Dutch language. Wernicke subjects had more difficulty for a particular agent-object order that can occur in active and passive sentences

(Friederici and Graetz, 1987). Another hint of unique disorder occurred in Blumstein's study of syntactic priming. Wernicke's aphasia did not exhibit inhibitory priming, which was considered to be a disturbance in controlled processing of syntactically erroneous word-pairs. Broca's aphasia exhibited impaired automatic processing (Blumstein, et al., 1991). This contrast is consistent with the earlier conclusion regarding controlled processing for semantic relatedness judgments.

The ability to deal with semantic and pragmatic features of sentences has been mixed. Nonreversible sentences were easier than reversibles, which is a sensitivity to verb-restrictions on possible NP-arguments (Heeschen, 1980). Plausible situations were easier in one study (Heeschen, 1980) but not in another study (Deloche and Seron, 1981), indicating that Wernicke patients may or may not be influenced by their world knowledge.

Semantic and Neologistic Jargon

Jargon consists of fluent, extended verbalization that contains semantic and unrelated paraphasias and neologisms. We were introduced to this form of aphasia with Gardner's (1974) sample, presented early in the first chapter. It has complete sentences with lots of functors and inflections that seem to be in the right places. Yet, the sample is hard to interpret, containing one neologism (i.e., "repuceration") and words like "barbers" that have no obvious connection to context. Because of its minimal neologisms, we would refer to this sample as *semantic jargon.* Another example is seen in the conversation between patient "RH" and an experimenter ("E") (Tyler, 1988, pp. 380–81; reprinted by permission of the publisher, Lawrence Erlbaum):

(11)   E: Do you do much reading?

       RH: No I don't no its all gone I don't.

       E: That must be frustrating.

       RH: I'd to I . . . I . . . like to me that's very good . . . I'd have something here a long time and have this but now . . . I suppose all I can do the . . . box.

       E: Television? What do you like to watch?

       RH: Well . . . no anything I want really because I can't the others at all . . . I can't this going . . . er . . . there's nothing for me to go or sometimes the . . . erm . . . phew . . . wait a minute . . . er.

This speech is loaded with indefinite terms such as "something," "anything," and "nothing." In describing a picture, Wernicke subjects generated as many words as normal subjects but fewer substantive words than normals and subjects with Broca's aphasia (Gleason, Goodglass, Obler, Green, Hyde, and Weintraub, 1980). Wernicke subjects used many more verbs than nouns, opposite the pattern indicative of verb-finding difficulty in Broca's aphasia. Wernicke subjects used more indefinite "pointing" words (e.g., *this, here*) than did normals and Broca subjects.

Buckingham and Kertesz (1976) gave us several examples of neologistic jargon:

(12) "I appreciate that *farshethe,* because they have *protocertive*" (p. 66).

(13) "I would say that the *mik daysis nosis* or *chpicters*" (p. 70).

From many examples provided by Buckingham (1981b), one patient described a picture of a woman washing dishes; Schwartz (1987) translated a transcription of the neologisms:

(14) "Anything [?] I mean, she is a beautiful girl. And this is the same with her. And now it's coming there and [?] Now what about here or anything like that . . . what any." [Examiner: "Anything else?"] Nothing the *kee-ser-eez* the, these are *day-ver-eez* and these and this one and these are living. This one's right in and these are . . . uh . . . and that's nothing . . . I can see things like this. You know, this type of thing. I can *dru-bit,* but so what" (p. 54; reprinted by permission of the publisher, Academic Press).

Neologisms tend to contain only phonological sequences that are permissible in the patient's language, with rare exceptions such as "chpicters" in *12.* When repeating sentences, people with Wernicke's aphasia produce the same types of errors, which is thought to result in part from the comprehension problem (Li and Williams, 1990).

Expression dominated either by semantic paraphasia or by neologism has been thought to be indicative of variability of Wernicke's aphasia along a severity continuum (Kertesz and Benson, 1970). Moreover, a study of spontaneous recovery showed that some patients with this diagnosis in the acute stage recover spontaneously to a pattern like anomic aphasia, whereas other patients progress slowly and continue to have a Wernicke's aphasia through the chronic period (Kertesz and McCabe, 1977). Progression proceeds from a neologistic jargon to a semantic jargon. If we can assume that comprehension varies accordingly, then some studies of this syndrome may be restricted to those with semantic jargon and enough comprehension and self-awareness to follow instructions and possess the so-called therapeutic set mentioned in the first chapter.

We may wonder what someone with these expressive symptoms does in the clinic when asked to name objects. When errors were counted, success levels differed among syndromes (Table 5–1). Most errors were made with Wernicke's aphasia. Unlike those with Broca's aphasia, Wernicke patients retrieved nouns more easily in picture description than confrontation naming (Williams and Canter, 1982). As with Broca's aphasia, actions were harder to name than objects in picture description and confrontation naming (Williams

and Canter, 1987). Patients with Wernicke's aphasia also benefited less than the others from phonemic cueing (Kohn and Goodglass, 1985; Pease and Goodglass, 1978) and were less likely to exhibit the tip-of-the-tongue state (Goodglass, et al., 1976). Naming to description and object-naming were equal in eliciting words for persons with anomic aphasia in contrast to Broca's and Wernicke's aphasias, in which naming to description was harder (Goodglass and Stuss, 1979). While naming was extremely difficult for patients with Wernicke's aphasia, syndromes did not differ in the production of semantic errors, contrary to impressions of extended spontaneous verbal expression (Kohn and Goodglass, 1985). Broca's, Wernicke's, and conduction aphasias did not differ in the production of errors labeled as phonemic paraphasias, whereas few of these errors occur with anomic aphasia. Object-naming may constrict expressive lexical processes such that syndrome differences are not exposed.

"Where Do Neologisms Come From?"

Buckingham (1981b) asked this question and suggested conditions for proving four hypotheses. This discussion focuses on the two main ideas that have been tossed around. First, neologisms might arise from defective realization of lexical form, an extreme version of the disorder producing phonemic paraphasias (see section on conduction aphasia; Lecours, 1982). This was called the **conduction theory** (Kertesz and Benson, 1970). For a

TABLE 5–1 Two studies of object-naming with major syndromes of aphasia, both showing greatest number of errors with Wernicke's aphasia.

	Williams and Canter (1982) High-frequency Words	Low-frequency Words	Kohn and Goodglass (1985)
Maximum score	20.0	20.0	85.0
Wernicke's	7.8	6.1	39.1
Anomic, anterior	12.1	10.9	54.5
Anomic, posterior			42.9
Conduction	10.0	6.8	59.4
Broca's	11.7	12.5	50.4

neologism to be extreme phonemic para-phasia, a patient should be producing pho-nemic paraphasias, neologisms, and ambig-uous transformations. Also, the patient "should *not* be simultaneously producing ver-bal paraphasia at other points in his speech output, or we could never, in principle, rule them out as possible inputs to the phonemic transformations" (Buckingham, 1981b, p. 50). The conduction theory was ruled out, be-cause subjects exhibited no "middle ground" between frank neologisms and obvious pho-nemic paraphasias (Buckingham and Kertesz, 1976). Then, Buckingham (1987) decided that he "will not rule out the possibility that some bizarre lexical productions could stem from severe phonemic paraphasia" (p. 383).

Second, a few **two-stage theories** state that a patient has an anomia but fills empty lexical slots with neologisms. Damage is deeper into the system than that proposed in conduction theory. Unlike those with Broca's aphasia, persons with Wernicke's aphasia ex-hibited little tip-of-the-tongue information about a word upon word-finding failure (Goodglass, et al., 1976). A case study of a patient called RD led to one view of the word-finding problem (Ellis, Miller, and Sin, 1983; Miller and Ellis, 1987). RD produced paraphasias in naming, spontaneous speech, and reading aloud. There was a strong effect of word frequency, with low-frequency words having a high error rate. Also, errors tended to have a phonological similarity to targets, especially with respect to number of syllables. A *lexical activation hypothesis* stated that flow of activation is reduced between semantic and phonological systems, locating disorder between Garrett's functional level and proc-esses generating positional level representa-tions. Buckingham's (1981a) first idea about the next stage was a *masking theory*. When there is a word-finding block or failed lexical activation, neologisms become "strings of well-formed phonemes or syllables that fill in the gaps and compensate for words not re-trievable from the lexicon" (p. 198). These gap fillers may be generated by perseveration from a previous word or neologism in the manner of alliteration (the same initial sound), assonance (rhyming), or stereotypic repetition of an affix.

Later, Buckingham (1987) borrowed two devices from a couple of sources and tinkered with Garrett's formulation model. The mech-anisms are a random generator, which is an abnormal process (Butterworth, 1979), and a scan-copier (Shattuck-Hufnagel, 1979). Buck-ingham put both mechanisms into the syn-tactic and lexical system that computes posi-tional level representations (Figure 3–9). Both devices pertain to forming the phonological shape of a lexical item. Butterworth observed brief hesitations before neologisms that did not occur before verbal and phonemic para-phasias. Thus, there may be something unique about the origin of neologisms. But-terworth and Buckingham proposed that a *random generator* of syllabic segments is re-sponsible for neologisms, despite the fact that these forms tend to follow phonological rules of the language used. As with the masking theory, the random generator is assumed to fill gaps left by an underlying anomia. The random generator is a special idea: it is one of the few hypotheses in which brain damage creates an abnormal process instead of dam-aging a normal one. An impaired scan-copier was considered to be responsible for pho-nemic paraphasias.

The Notion of Paragrammatism

Theory of expressive disorder in Wer-nicke's aphasia has so far focused on open-class, content words. The structural frame-work of sentences has been ignored, as if the disorder affects only lexical slot-filling. Schwartz (1987) admired *12* and *13* (p. 118) for their complex coordination and subor-dination, suggesting that the syntactic as-pects of language formulation are relatively spared and thus separated from lexical as-pects. The extensive study of grammar in Broca's aphasia is evidence for the impression that "unless the patient's speech was agram-matic, it has been assumed that the patient did not have a syntactic deficit" (Martin and Blossom-Stach, 1986, p. 229).

Nevertheless, jargonaphasia has had a reputation for containing errors of grammar called *paragrammatism*. Errors would mainly be substitutions of functors and inflections. According to Goodglass and Kaplan (1983), "*most* inflections and small grammatical words fall smoothly into place, but with unsystematic substitutions or omissions of both grammatical morphemes and lexical words (i.e., nouns, verbs, adjectives), and tangled grammatical organization" (p. 7). However, there are relatively few linguistic studies of syntax in jargon. It is a tough corpus, because it can be hard to tell a syntactic error from a semantic one in these strange utterances. Compounding interpretation problems is the inexquisite syntax spoken by average neurologically intact persons. Picking over grammar in jargon leaves us wondering what can be called a deficit. In the study of descriptive discourse by Gleason and others (1980), Wernicke subjects used fewer and simpler structures than normal controls. Aphasic subjects tended to sequence phrases instead of embedding them. Thus, we may add simplification to the lengthening list of characteristics of paragrammatism that are also reported as agrammatism.

Cross-linguistic comparisons of Broca's and Wernicke's aphasias included a comparison of omissions and substitutions. Consistent with the classical agrammatism-paragrammatism distinction, grammatical morphemes were omitted much more frequently in Broca's aphasia in German (Bates, et al., 1987b). The classical dichotomy was in trouble with the extent to which grammatical substitutions were observed in Broca's aphasia. Substitution errors, which are difficult to detect in English, occurred with similar frequency in both syndromes, especially in richly inflected languages. In studies of German and Dutch aphasias, Heeschen and Kolk (1988) detected differences between the syndromes in spontaneous speech, in which Broca's aphasia has a higher proportion of omissions than substitutions, whereas Wernicke's aphasia has a mixture or a predominance of substitutions. Moreover, sparing of canonical word order was observed in both syndromes (Bates, Friederici, et al., 1988).

"We conclude that the contrast between agrammatism (attributed to Broca's aphasia) and paragrammatism (attributed to Wernicke's aphasia) has been greatly exaggerated" (Bates, et al., 1991, p. 137).

Because of similarities in grammatical mistakes in Wernicke's and Broca's aphasias, others argued that there is no difference in syntactic disorder (Heeschen, 1985), or that the traditional distinction needs "conceptual realignment" (Goodglass and Menn, 1985). Thus, it has been recommended that the distinction between agrammatism and paragrammatism be discarded. Kolk and Heeschen (1990) attributed the different manifestations of language formulation to different adaptive capabilities. Particularly because of their lack of awareness of their jargon, people with Wernicke's aphasia do not employ adaptive strategies. This idea was related to differences in sentence repetition. Patients with agrammatism have more of a mixture of omissions and substitutions than in spontaneous speech, whereas those with jargon have no task effect (Heeschen and Kolk, 1988). Kolk and Heeschen admitted that equivalence of disorder was not proved. Much more comparative research needs to be done. Moreover, theoretical proposals should be more explicitly related to observations so that studies can be derived from well-thought-out predictions. A failure to adapt does not seem to go far in explaining why people with jargonaphasia talk the way they do.

Paragrammatism on the Bubble

Martin and Blossom-Stach (1986) explored paragrammatism with case WS. He had a lesion in the temporal-parietal region, was diagnosed at one month post onset as having Wernicke's aphasia, but then had pronounced improvement of comprehension by the time of study two months later. WS was like the group with rapid spontaneous recovery observed by Kertesz and McCabe (1977). Lexical errors were mainly phonemic paraphasias, and comprehension was well above the ceiling for Wernicke's aphasia. Moreover, the corpus for analysis was the patient's writing in homework assignments and a personal journal he started about one month post onset. WS was classified as having a fluent aphasia with syntactic problems. He may have had a pattern of conduction aphasia on his way to anomic aphasia. Categories of error that most interested the investigators were full word exchanges (*15*) and partial word or phrase exchanges (*16*) (Martin and Blossom-Stach, 1986, pp. 231, 232). The examples are from the journal and homework, including writing a sentence when given a word.

(15a) "I do think I *need* anything I *have*."

(15b) "*It* [Memorial Day] is almost here when *June* comes."

(15c) "Carol has shown my speech therapy has improved much when *I* showed *her* my tests."

(15d) "*She* was given an Oscar by *Meryl Streep*." [homework, *given*]

(15e) "The *pupil* gave *her* an A+." [homework, *pupil*]

(16a) "Bob talked about Dr. Adam's living in Toronto." (Bob talked to Dr. Adams about living in Toronto.)

(16b) "The Astros listened to the radio tonight." (I listened to the Astros on the radio tonight.)

(16c) "My railroad train bought a new switch." [homework, *switch*]

(16d) "The batter was out when the ball missed." [homework, *out*]

Other input to the analysis was a word-arrangement task in the homework, which has not been clearly related to theory of spontaneous formulation.

Like the investigators, we might analyze these exchanges in the manner in which Garrett related normal errors to levels of his formulation model (see *19*, *20*, Chapter 3). Two features of the exchanges are that they occur across phrase boundaries, and they occur within a grammatical category (e.g., verbs in *15a*, prepositions in *16a*). These are supposedly indicative of functional level dys-

function (Garrett, 1984). Another thing to consider is whether pronouns and grammatical morphemes, presumed to be chosen at the positional level, are consistent with the correct or incorrect sentence. For example, "she" in *15d* and "her" in *15e* agree with the switched version. Different pronouns would have been selected for the correct version. Similarly, the "-s" in *16a* and the preposition in *16b* are appropriate for the incorrect sentence. The thought was that errors occurred in meaning formation prior to selection of elements appropriate for positional structure. It was concluded that "both the full and partial exchange errors occurred during construction of a deep level of representation, or, in Garrett's model, at the functional level of representation" (Martin and Blossom-Stach, 1986, p. 216).

We may also notice that some of these switches create thematic role-assignment problems that are possible in the world (*15d*), implausible (*15e*), or impossible (*16c*). Some of these sentences are like those presented in a study of reversibility and plausibility in comprehension. Patient WS was given a comprehension test that exposed a deficit in making word-order decisions about active and passive reversible sentences. The researchers suggested that the functional level problem includes a central "difficulty in mapping semantic relationships onto grammatical roles" (Martin and Blossom-Stach, 1986, p. 216), or a mapping problem akin to the one Schwartz used to explain agrammatic comprehension. These researchers entertained many possibilities, perhaps partly as a function of ambiguity in interpretation of WS's intent.

WS's paragrammatism lies on a bubble between syndromes and between deficit and normalcy. Without normal controls, how did Martin and Blossom-Stach (1986) decide that errors were deficits? At first, they said that "these errors are pathological in that they occurred in writing rather than speech" (p. 211). Yet, it is rare that we see error-free writing before it is edited. Then, they compared rate of errors to normal linguistic errors in Garrett's research. Frequency of errors in

WS's writing was much greater. Garrett had suggested that we should expect one error per week in normal conversation. Nevertheless, speech errors do not tell us what to expect in unedited writing and tasks in which patients are given a word or words.

Semantic Disorganization?

Most of the disorders hypothesized so far for Wernicke's aphasia have been associated with either comprehension or formulation processes. The possibility of deep central disorder is usually considered with respect to semantic memory. A loss or disorganization of conceptual knowledge might produce paraphasias and reduce comprehension. For example, number of semantic paraphasias was correlated strongly with number of semantic errors on a word-comprehension test (Gainotti, 1976). As indicated in Chapter 4, Grossman (1981) addressed the categorical word fluency of Wernicke subjects in his fluent group. They were more likely than others to produce atypical members of a category, crossing the borders of a referential field. The dissociation of semantic deficit from syntactic deficit was suggested mainly in association with broad comparisons between posterior-fluent aphasia and anterior-nonfluent aphasia. Thinking of generalities, we should again be aware of the difficult distinction between semantic and lexical storage, or the difference between not knowing an object and not knowing its name, as a basis for word-finding block in Wernicke's aphasia.

In one study employing pictures of objects and mentioned earlier for Broca's aphasia, a double dissociation was indicated when Wernicke subjects identified thematic relations between objects more easily than categorical relations. This pattern was opposite the one demonstrated by Broca subjects (Semenza, et al., 1980). In another study, Wernicke subjects were impaired in relating objects according to action, function, and physical attributes (Cohen, et al., 1980). More recently, 13 persons with Wernicke's aphasia were compared with groups having anomic, Broca's, and global aphasia (Koemeda-Lutz, Cohen, and Meier, 1987). Subjects were shown three objects (e.g., apple, banana, pear) and, when ready, were then shown a series of objects one at a time (e.g., peach, chair). Subjects had to press a button indicating "yes" or "no" as to whether each object belonged to the class of objects presented initially. Some decisions were based on category; others were based on property (e.g., yellow, light). For half the items, the classification name was shown beneath the initial objects. Showing the label helped aphasic subjects. However, Wernicke's aphasia did not exhibit a unique problem. Results indicated that semantic content and structure are preserved in aphasia and that access processes are impaired instead.

As discussed in Chapter 4, use of words in matching and sorting tasks turns them into the so-called lexical-semantic test of the knowledge of what words mean. Buckingham (1981a) had suggested that "brain damage will often loosen up the organization of the mental dictionary and thereby disrupt the system of verbal concepts" (p. 199). Fluent aphasias have more frequently exhibited organizational difficulties when words are involved, such as in categorical word fluency. In Goodglass and Baker's (1976) word recognition study, low-comprehending subjects had a pattern of associate recognition that differed from normal controls. These patients were thought to have a constricted semantic structure. Another approach resulted in a different conclusion, when Rinnert and Whitaker (1973) inventoried relationships between semantic paraphasias and targets and compared them to normal word associations. Sixty percent of error-targets corresponded to association norms for the error or the target. It was concluded that "semantic confusions are more *like* than *unlike* normal word associations" (p. 66). Buckingham and Rekart (1979) studied word retrieval errors for one subject with Wernicke's aphasia and concluded that the errors were similar to the "slips" of normal speakers. We can go back to studies of semantic priming, which indicate a fairly stable lexical-semantic knowledge and a capacity for automatic access but problems in controlled access to this knowledge.

CONDUCTION APHASIA AND PHONEMIC PARAPHASIA

Conduction aphasia has seemed to be a two-headed disorder. Researchers have been curious about either the demonstrative repetition deficit or the phonemic paraphasias in spontaneous speech. The former concern was related to short-term memory deficit, and the latter spawned studies of the end-stages of language and speech production. For a while, repetition deficit was the definitive disorder, and neurological explanation put conduction aphasia into the category of **disconnection syndrome** (Geschwind, 1965). Good comprehension and fluent sentence production indicated that auditory and speech centers are intact (Chapter 2). The auditory center just could not send impulses to the speech center. However, disconnection did not account for other features of the syndrome such as phonemic paraphasias and sentence comprehension deficits exposed in comparisons with Broca's aphasia.

Working Memory and Sentence Comprehension

The unique deficit of repetition was purported initially to demonstrate the distinctiveness of memory stores through a "selective impairment of short-term memory" (Saffran and Marin, 1975; Shallice and Warrington, 1977; Warrington and Shallice, 1969). When memory span was viewed to be a gross indicator of processing capacity, researchers wondered about the impact of deficient STM on a logically dependent function such as auditory language comprehension. Studies suggested that there is more to processing capacity than what is measured by memory span, because patients with compressed STMs had pretty good sentence comprehension (Chapters 3, 4). The theoretical basis for the lack of relationship between STM and comprehension is that memory

span reflects transient buffer capacity and ignores processing capacity of working memory. Another reason is that automatic cognitive processes, including core obligatory comprehension processes, are thought to take up little room in the processing system.

Isolated deficient memory span signified **impaired phonological encoding** and, in particular, was considered to be evidence for "fractionation" of a phonological buffer from an articulatory buffer in working memory (Vallar and Baddeley, 1984a). More information is needed to diagnose this disorder, and two cases demonstrate the relevant evidence. Case PV, a 31-year-old woman who had suffered a stroke, perceived speech normally in discrimination and rhyme judgment. She repeated single words but could not repeat digit and word sequences longer than three items (Vallar and Baddeley, 1984a). Thus, her system for analyzing stimuli was spared, but her ability to hold onto a mental representation was impaired. Case AE, a 48-year-old woman who had suffered a posterior CVA, had an auditory digit span of 1.5 (Friedrich, Glenn, and Marin, 1984). A deficit of phonological encoding was indicated when she did not exhibit a normal phonological similarity effect, in which phonologically similar letters are harder to retain than phonologically dissimilar letters. Unlike normal adults, PV and AE had longer spans for visual stimuli. PV exhibited reduced duration for subspan material, and AE had no recency effect for supraspan lists.

The investigators also explored comprehension abilities in these cases. PV could comprehend short sentences (around six words long) and long sentences of around 16 words. Impairment became apparent only when verification of long sentences was made more difficult (Vallar and Baddeley, 1984b). Later, PV displayed a variety of syntactic comprehension and judgment abilities, except when syntactic anomalies occurred between widely separated elements in short stories (Vallar and Baddeley, 1987). Friedrich, Martin, and Kemper (1985) presented AE with active, passive, and locative reversible sentences, some of which were borrowed from the study of Broca's aphasia by Schwartz and others (1980). Unlike the agrammatic patients in Schwartz's study, AE identified thematic roles in active reversibles but had difficulty with thematic roles in passives and locatives. Contrary to the typical pattern between modalities in aphasia, performance improved from auditory stimuli to reading. Friedrich concluded that AE could map SVO relations onto basic NVN structure but had a syntactic deficit with the passive exception to canonical order. This deficit is one example of the growing interest in comprehension deficit in conduction aphasia.

Suspicion of **syntactic comprehension deficit** began with studies showing groups with conduction aphasia performing like those with Broca's aphasia (Caramazza and Zurif, 1976; Goodglass, et al., 1979; Heilman and Scholes, 1976). Patient MC was deficient in comprehending passives and center-embedded relative clauses, which was described as a syntactic disorder (Caramazza, Basili, Koller, and Berndt, 1981). Caplan (1987b) disagreed by noting that most errors occurred with lexical foils and not with the role-reversal foils that would be indicative of syntactic deficit. Peach, Canter, and Gallaher (1988) compared ten subjects with conduction aphasia and ten with anomic aphasia, and they used stimulus materials prepared for an earlier study of Broca's aphasia (Gallaher and Canter, 1982). Both groups scored well on a clinical test of comprehension and would be judged as having a very mild comprehension deficit. Only active sentences were presented, and analysis focused on nature of errors. Both groups were accurate around 70 percent of the time. As did those with Broca's aphasia, the two groups of mild fluent aphasia made significantly more subject-object order errors than lexical errors. AE's order errors came with passive sentences (Friedrich, et al., 1985). Peach concluded that the three syndromes demonstrate a syntactic comprehension deficit, although only one of these syndromes has agrammatic expression.

The dilemma, expressed by Peach and others (1988), is to explain how three clinical syndromes can have a syntactic comprehension deficit. One way out of this dilemma is to recall the impressive body of literature on agrammatic aphasia and realize that identity of disorders cannot be claimed until the same experiments have been done with each syndrome. Syntactic processing is complex (and/or elusive), and syntactic comprehension deficit is a "fuzzy" description of the area in which a few tests expose problems. There may be different reasons for the similar outcomes on comprehension tests. Can the subtle deficits with conduction aphasia be attributed to a partial malfunction of the syntactic parser, as in Broca's aphasia, or can another problem affect the comprehension system similarly? Peach did not examine the short-term buffer status of his subjects, but PV, AE, and MC were diagnosed as having a deficit of auditory STM or phonological encoding. Caramazza and his colleagues (1981) attributed comprehension deficit to this disorder. Friedrich and others (1985) speculated that the processing of grammatical morphemes is particularly dependent on phonological buffering. The dilemma is not resolved, and we may be interested in more comparisons of syndromes when on-line studies of comprehension are devised.

Phonological Output

Now let us switch to expressive deficit in repetition tasks as well as spontaneous verbalization. While the expressive deficit in Broca's aphasia led to wondering if agrammatic expression is caused by a central disorder underlying comprehension deficit as well, discovery of apparent syntactic comprehension deficit led Friedrich and others (1985) to wonder if a deep central deficit contributes to language production in conduction aphasia. Clinical experience suggests that syntactic problems are absent (Goodglass and Kaplan, 1983), enhancing the mystery of comprehension deficit (Peach, et al., 1988). People with conduction aphasia can be quite fluent conversationalists. In a variety of tasks, including repetition of complex sentences, AE exhibited little difficulty in producing grammatical forms, including relative clauses (Friedrich, et al., 1985).

The main clinical impression of conduction aphasia is the appearance of phonemic paraphasias, which are also heard in Wernicke's aphasia. We cannot escape controversy, because the notion of phonological impairment turns out to be as fuzzy as other disorders identified only with respect to major linguistic components. Intense study was motivated by Blumstein (1973), who examined the conversational speech of patients with conduction, Broca's, and Wernicke's aphasias. Subjects with Broca's aphasia made more speech-sound errors that the others, but groups were identical in the kind of phonemic errors produced. The study left the impression that these aphasias have the same phonological disorder. "Phonemic paraphasia" might label any sound-level error in any case of aphasia. A more profound implication is that all cases with "phonemic paraphasias" would be treated with the same strategy. On the other hand, the awkward speech with Broca's aphasia and fluency of conduction aphasia indicate that similar categories of phonological error could be generated from different disorders.

Level of observation can make a difference in detecting disorder (Canter, Trost, and Burns, 1985). The usual clinical strategy is conducting *perceptual analysis,* or listening to speech and classifying behaviors (e.g., Blumstein, 1973). A modern approach, called phonological process analysis, exposes regularities in varied errors by examining the linguistic context of errors (Parsons, Lambier, and Miller, 1988). *Acoustic analysis* records speech output with devices such as a spectrograph. Parameters include sound duration (Williams and Seaver, 1986) and voice onset time (VOT) (Blumstein, Cooper, Goodglass, Statlender, and Gottlieb, 1980). *Physiologic analyses* measure events within the speech mechanism, such as muscle contraction or velar movement (Itoh, Sasanuma, Hirose, Yoshioka, and Sawashima, 1983). It is thought that, as observation gets further

from the actual events of production, the likelihood of erroneous diagnosis increases. The opportunity for error is greatest in perceptual analysis, which is susceptible to variation among researchers in classification of phonological phenomena. Investigators believed Blumstein's perceptually based results but did not believe her interpretation.

If the brain is organized into functionally distinct regions, then the different sites of lesion for conduction aphasia and apraxia of speech (AOS) lead us to believe that phonological disorders differ. A broad distinction has been drawn between phonemic and phonetic levels of speech production (Lecours and Nespoulous, 1988). Garrett's theory points to three levels of phonological production that bring the end-stage of motor execution into this discussion. Various attempts to specify functional levels have been employed in generating hypotheses for studying phonological disorders (Table 5–2). Conduction aphasia is suspected of being a language disorder, where phonemic shapes are formed. Apraxia of speech is portrayed as disruption of programming the motor system for speaking, once phonemic shapes have been activated. Dysarthrias are impairments in the neurological execution of muscle contractions required for speech. Because AOS tends to occur with Broca's aphasia, the most controversial distinction has been between apraxic and aphasic phenomena. Some researchers just want to see if groups differ in a parameter of speech (e.g., Williams and Seaver, 1986). Others make assumptions about what their observations indicate about the status of underlying functional systems (e.g., Canter, et al., 1985; Kohn, 1984).

When we listen to the speech of Broca's and fluent aphasias, we hear sound substitutions and additions. Researchers in Japan and the United States listened carefully and detected differences in naming and word repetition (Canter, et al., 1985; Monoi, Fukusako, Itoh, and Sasanuma, 1983). Canter studied ten Broca's, five Wernicke's, and five conduction aphasias. Monoi examined three subjects with Broca's aphasia and three with conduction aphasia. Sound and syllable sequence errors were more common in fluent aphasia. Conduction aphasia possessed more transpositions; that is, a substitution from elsewhere in the same word. Buckingham (1989) called them "linear ordering derailments," which can be anticipatory (e.g., "papple") or perseverative (e.g., "gingerged"). Speech with Broca's aphasia contained more transitional disruptions from one sound or syllable to the next and distortions that were not observed in fluent aphasias. Both studies indicated that errors increased as a function of motoric complexity in Broca's speech but not in fluent aphasias. All groups usually made one-feature errors (namely, an incorrect sound close to the target); but three-feature errors were more likely in fluent aphasia. Broca's speech contained more errors in the word-initial position; fluent aphasias had more errors in the final position (Table 5–1). Kohn (1989; Kohn and Smith, 1990) conducted an extensive analysis of patient CM, who had conduction aphasia. Many errors were like normal speech errors, including word-interactions in which a segment of one word was "copied" into another word. Unlike with normal errors, a few word-interactions occurred across several words in an utterance.

By examining many features of speech production, researchers indicated that clinical symptoms are indicative of different phonological disorders in anterior and posterior aphasias (Canter, 1988). Acoustic analysis has been used to remove observation from listener perception. Spectrographic measures indicated that sound duration was longer in subjects with Broca's aphasia than in those with conduction, Wernicke's, and anomic aphasias (Williams and Seaver, 1986). Thus, we may be right in thinking that we hear slower speech in nonfluent aphasia. Synergy in VOT was found with fluent aphasias but was lacking in Broca's aphasia or patients with apraxia of speech (Blumstein, et al., 1980; Itoh, Sasanuma, Tatsumi, Murakami, Fukusako, and Suzuki, 1982). Itoh and others (1983) found asynchronous velar movement in anterior aphasia, whereas timing was normal in fluent aphasias. The results together were indicative of impaired temporal pro-

TABLE 5–2 Differential diagnosis of phonological disorders, including the terminology used to designate functional levels. (Garrett's terminology (Figure 3–9) is represented in boldface.)

Disorder	CNS Location	Functional Location	Speech Symptoms
Conduction aphasia	Posterior cortex	**Phonological process (positional level)** Pre-motor stage Scan-copier device	Fluency More errors in final position Sequence errors Transpositions anticipatory perseverative No distortions
Apraxia of speech	Anterior, pre-motor cortex	**Regular phonological processes (phonetic)** Pre-articulatory or motor programming Sub-phonemic	Laborious More errors in initial position Transition errors Distortions and substitutions
Dysarthria	Motor cortex and below	**Motor coding process (articulatory)** Execution	Varied distortion and substitution Respiratory and phonatory deficit Impairment at all functional levels

gramming of laryngeal and oropharyngeal movement in AOS but not in fluent aphasia. Thus, phonemic paraphasia in conduction aphasia has been diagnosed as a disorder at a "pre-articulatory" phonemic level, whereas apraxia of speech has been diagnosed as a motoric, phonetic impairment that is imposed on a patient's agrammatic aphasia. The person with apraxia of speech produces an accurate lexical representation with difficulty; the person with conduction aphasia produces an inaccurate lexical representation smoothly.

Explaining Repetition and Phonological Impairments

The repetition deficit in conduction aphasia seems to emerge from the disorder causing phonemic paraphasias (Kohn, 1984). Phonemic paraphasias occur when repeating words, phrases, or sentences (Li and Williams, 1990). This connection has not been obvious, because as sentences become longer and less familiar, repetition elicits a deterioration of verbalization that is not observed in spontaneous or conversational speaking. The impairment of phonological encoding may be a link between the major symptoms. Kohn and Smith (1990) suggested that the similarity of many phonemic paraphasias to normal speech errors is indicative of an impaired mental representation of a phonological string; distant word-interactions, a few separated by several words, were suggestive of an "inability to clear a phonemic output buffer." That is, pieces of lexical items activated for previous production remain stuck in a temporary holding region of working memory.

Buckingham (1987) worked from Garrett's theory in identifying a cognitive location of the disorder producing phonemic paraphasias. In his view, this problem arises from a computational breakdown in generating the phonological shape of content (or open-class) words during positional level operations. According to Garrett (1984), positional level disorders should be revealed in errors across word boundaries, such as normal sound exchanges between words (e.g., 20, Chapter 3).

Evidence for such errors in conduction aphasia has been sparse, because researchers focused on one-word productions (Pate, Saffran, and Martin, 1987). Such errors occurred in Kohn and Smith's (1990) study but not in Pate's study of one case. In any case, Buckingham used the notion of a *scan-copier* as the positional level mechanism where damage occurs. His account is complex, but it appears that the copier operates on lexical items already activated into a buffer (i.e., "phonological output buffer"). It scans these forms and turns them into a production-ready state. The distinction between a buffer and a scan-copier corresponds to the intuition that lexical access is accomplished because of the similarity of errors to targets, and impairment occurs in some additional operation on the lexical item.

ANOMIC APHASIA

Sometimes called amnesic aphasia, this syndrome is the mildest form of language-specific disorder. Comprehension seems unimpaired until we test for complex levels and reading. Fluent speech differs from Wernicke's and conduction aphasias because of its lack of paraphasias. The patient fills word-finding gaps with vague terms and circumlocutions. Anomic aphasia is usually associated with a posterior lesion sparing Wernicke's area; however, the same general characteristics can be observed after frontal lesions that do not cause agrammatic aphasia, so frontal anomic aphasia may be studied in comparison to posterior anomic aphasia (e.g., Kohn and Goodglass, 1985). Anomic aphasia may be the end-stage of recovery in some persons who have Wernicke's aphasia soon after onset. These circumstances in the diagnosis of anomic aphasia illustrate a difference between clinical and theoretical syndromes. Common symptom patterns tend to be identified as clinical syndromes, but theoretical syndromes are presumed to be linked to a site of lesion causing a particular cognitive dysfunction.

Language Comprehension

People with anomic aphasia comprehend better than those with other kinds of aphasia, but they still have a deficit. The mean score for anomic aphasia on Shewan's (1979) auditory sentence comprehension test is 14.8 of 21 maximum points. According to the Boston Diagnostic Aphasia Examination, the range for this syndrome is the 60th to 90th percentile (Goodglass and Kaplan, 1983). As with Broca's aphasia, this range is above Wernicke's aphasia, which has a 50th percentile ceiling. The difference from Broca's aphasia is that anomic aphasia has a higher floor for the range. The Western Aphasia Battery is similar in that the range for anomic aphasia is 7 to 10 points, with a maximum score of 10, and the range for Broca's aphasia is 4 to 10 (Kertesz, 1982).

Perhaps because of the lexical focus of expressive impairment, the comprehension disorder has been suspected of being a semantic dissociation from syntax, like the semantic problems attributed to Wernicke's aphasia. Yet, few comparisons to Broca's aphasia have included a group defined explicitly as having anomic aphasia. Cross-linguistic research has little to say about anomic aphasia, except for what we might be willing to generalize from the commonalities of Broca's and Wernicke's aphasias. Anomic aphasia gets lost in groups defined as having "high-comprehension" along with Broca's and conduction aphasias, even in studies of semantic processes (e.g., Chenery, Ingram, and Murdoch, 1990). Lexical decision research is appropriate for anomic aphasia, but Blumstein and her colleagues (1982) studied every major syndrome except anomic aphasia and later focused on Broca's and Wernicke's aphasias (Milberg, et al., 1987). We may associate anomic aphasia with features of mild fluent aphasia mentioned sporadically in Chapter 4. In a study with an anomic group, these subjects exhibited a normal sensitivity to articles, whereas the subjects with Broca's aphasia did not (Goodenough, et al., 1977). However, in highly inflected Serbo-Croatian, people with anomic aphasia had a deficit in comprehending inflections (Smith and Bates, 1987). In the lexical-semantic domain, subtle problems with words were detected, in that anomic subjects had a greater deficit in detecting connotative meaning than did Broca and conduction subjects (Gardner and Denes, 1973).

Word-Finding Disorder

The magnet for our attention regarding anomic aphasia is the special deficit for retrieving words. When naming objects, the patient illustrated near the end of Chapter 1 would name some quickly, take several seconds to name others, and would use circumlocutions to designate others. In general, accuracy scores for naming are equivalent to Broca's aphasia, except when posterior and anterior anomic aphasias are separated (Table 5–1). Posterior anomic aphasia includes a serious naming deficit. In the research, groups did not differ in frequency of semantic paraphasias. Anomic aphasia was distinctive in the use of circumlocutions instead of targeted words (Kohn and Goodglass, 1985). Only the comparison between frontal anomic aphasia and conduction aphasia produced a significant difference in phonemic paraphasias, with fewer phonemic paraphasias in the frontal group. With respect to stimuli in naming tasks, naming descriptions and naming objects were equal for persons with anomic aphasia, as opposed to Broca's and Wernicke's aphasias, in which naming to description was more difficult (Goodglass and Stuss, 1979).

People with anomic aphasia do better than persons with other aphasias in retrieving verbs (Miceli, et al., 1984; Williams and Canter, 1987). In Williams and Canter's study, action-naming was more impaired than object-naming for all syndromes. However, persons with anomic aphasia had nearly twice the correct action-naming responses (51 percent) relative to Broca's aphasia (26 percent), although these groups were nearly equal in object-naming scores. Also, noun retrieval did not differ between tasks of naming and description; the difference for verb-finding, favoring picture description, was greatest for the anomic group but was not statistically significant.

One question is whether word-finding problems can be related to storage of lexical-semantic information. This problem is possible, considering results for fluent aphasias in object and word sorting and matching tasks. A semantic priming task was employed to see if the difference between high- and low-comprehending aphasias found by Goodglass and Baker (1976) would be observed again (Chenery, et al., 1990). This time, most high-comprehending subjects had anomic aphasia, and semantic activation in lexical decision was compared to controlled naming and semantic judgment tasks. Related primes had various relationships to target words. High- and low-comprehending groups showed semantic priming effects, indicative of subconscious access to semantic knowledge. Unlike low-comprehending subjects, high-comprehending subjects retained the ability to make semantic judgments. Thus, automatic and controlled access as well as storage are well preserved in aphasic people with good comprehension.

The patient EST had a temporal meningioma removed from his left lateral ventricle, and an aphasia test indicated that he had anomic aphasia (Ellis and Young, 1988). Scores on naming tests were in the range of 20 to 40 percent correct. A case study was designed to determine the locus of word-finding deficit in the cognitive system used for this function. Nearly errorless performance on object sorting and matching according to semantic categories indicated that EST could "comprehend objects," or that conceptual knowledge was intact. In general, the conceptual accuracy of circumlocution tells us that world knowledge and recognition are spared. This capacity corresponds to Chenery's conclusions for high-comprehending subjects and a semantic priming task. EST got all items correct in a word comprehension task in which four pictured choices were semantically related, indicative of intact lexical-semantic access. He recognized famous faces but had trouble naming them (Flude, Ellis, and Kay, 1989).

EST's disorder was put squarely in "activating entries for words within the speech output lexicon" (Ellis and Young, 1988, p. 121). High-frequency words were easier than low-frequency words in spontaneous production, which was indicative of normally varying activation thresholds in lexical-semantic storage. Final diagnosis was identified as a reduction of "the *amount* of activation reaching the (intact) speech output lexicon from the (intact) semantic system" (Ellis and Young, 1988, p. 122). This proposal is similar to the lexical activation hypothesis for explaining paraphasias in patient RD's Wernicke's aphasia (Miller and Ellis, 1987). As discussed in the section on Wernicke's aphasia, two-stage theories indicate that a difference between disorders may exist in what the impaired cognitive system does to fill the gaps left by inadequate lexical activation. The theory is that someone with many neologisms has a random segmental generator to fill the gaps. For anomic aphasia and EST in particular, retained storage of meanings and the lexicon begins to account for the ability to use circumlocutions to fill the gaps. There is no random generator. The scan-copier seems to be fine. Let us ask our friends in cognitive neuropsychology to explain the rest.

SUMMARY AND IMPLICATIONS

One contribution of psycholinguistic theory to aphasiology is to show why general functions such as auditory comprehension have not been easily related to the brain. It may be more appropriate, if not easier, to relate subsystems like lexical access or syntactic parsing to the brain. Clinical syndromes were thought to contribute to this endeavor by exposing specific cognitive impairments in relation to consistent sites of lesion. Yet we can be impressed with Schuell's sense that semantics and syntax are inseparable. Syntactic and semantic impairments have been somewhat difficult to tease apart in comparisons of Broca's and fluent aphasias. The agrammatism-paragrammatism dichotomy may not be valid in its traditional form. There is an increasing dissatisfaction with diagnosis in terms of "fuzzy" categories.

Cognitive neuropsychologists have been arguing that clinical language behavior should be interpreted with respect to a psycholinguistic theory of normal function. To say that someone has Broca's aphasia or agrammatism or that something is like Broca's aphasia does not explain anything. It is only a description of a pattern of behavior. Group differences or unique problems can be exposed when assessment is set up to distinguish knowledge and process, semantic and lexical information, and automatic and controlled processes, rather than being set up to distinguish clinical syndromes. We are recognizing differences between metalinguistic and comprehension tasks and between off-line and on-line tasks. We can not only distinguish central and peripheral disorders, we can also distinguish among central disorders.

Psycholinguistic aphasiology can be said to have clinical value because we believe that a better understanding of language function and dysfunction helps us to do therapy better. This rhetoric has to be supported with clear relationships between observable phenomena and inferred disorders. Howard and Patterson (1989) recommended that diagnosis determine the impaired and spared components of a patient's language system. Some of the possibilities are shown in Figures 3–7 and 3–9. Treatment goals would be based partly on a desire to repair damaged cognitive subsystems so that they will operate better. Objectives might include the following:

For Broca's Aphasia:

(1a) Increase speed of lexical access in order to improve comprehension.

(1b) Improve the parsing mechanism in order to improve comprehension.

(1c) Improve semantic mapping in order to improve comprehension.

(2a) Improve computation of positional level representations in order to improve use of grammatical morphemes in expression.

(2b) Increase speed of activation of structural representations in order to improve use of grammatical morphemes in expression.

For Wernicke's Aphasia:

(1) Improve conceptual organization around the edges of typicality in order to improve comprehension and expression.

(2a) Dismantle the random generator that is causing neologisms.

(2b) Increase flow of activation from the semantic system to the mental lexicon in order to improve word-finding.

This is the sound of cognitive objectives. Such goals may frighten a behaviorally oriented clinician, and they must be translated into relevant behaviors or tasks in order to be useful. We should be concerned, however, about the number of disorders proposed to explain some deficits and the less than obvious explicitness of other disorders. Different theories indicate that we should assess someone with Broca's or Wernicke's aphasia further to determine a specific disorder within each category, and they indicate that more basic research is needed to compare and clarify theories of disorder.

6

MULTIFOCAL NEUROPATHOLOGIES AND DISORDERS

Traumatic brain injury (TBI) and progressive neuropathologies are quite different conditions. With sudden impact, TBI tends to happen to teenagers and young adults. We know the cause, and it is avoidable. Alzheimer's disease sneaks up on the thoughts and memories of the elderly. Its cause has been an agonizing mystery. Nevertheless, both conditions usually disrupt language behavior. Both have been at the center of controversy over when a language disorder is aphasia. Primary impairments have been associated with attention, memory, and executive control. By the end of the 1970s, head trauma and progressive disease had turned heads in the health care system, generating funds for research and rehabilitation centers with encouragement from newly formed family support groups. Speech-language pathologists became team members for coordinating assessment, treatment, and counseling services for multiply-impaired individuals and their families. This chapter introduces pathological conditions and cognitive impairments, and it addresses the nature of language difficulties found with these conditions.

NEUROPSYCHOLOGICAL ASSESSMENT

Clinical neuropsychologists conduct comprehensive assessment of patients' cognition, personality, and capacity for reentering the community (Lezak, 1983). Methodology was based initially on tests already available for evaluating intelligence and personality in education, industry, and the military. The **Wechsler Adult Intelligence Scale** (WAIS) is introduced in Chapter 4, and clinical aphasiologists are familiar with other batteries and specific procedures.

The **Halstead-Reitan Neuropsychological Test Battery** is packaged at the Reitan Neuropsychology Laboratory in Arizona (Reitan and Wolfson, 1985). The package for adults contains the WAIS; tests of attention, rhythm, and thinking; and the *Minnesota Multiphasic Personality Inventory* (MMPI). The collection includes an aphasia screening test in use since 1935 (Halstead and Wepman, 1949; Wheeler and Reitan, 1962). Reitan's company provides a computer program called the *Neuropsychological Deficit Scale*, which facilitates interpretation of raw scores. A software package is also available that transforms scores into an image of the probable site of lesion.

The **Woodcock-Johnson Psycho-Educational Battery** (Woodcock and Johnson, 1989) contains two major batteries. *Tests of Cognitive Ability* sample visual perception, verbal memory, and other skills. *Tests of Achievement* examine reading, writing, and arithmetic, as well as world knowledge. Both sections have a short standard component and a supplemental component for more thorough testing. The standard portion of the cognitive tests produces a score of broad cognitive ability; supplemental testing yields summary scores related to seven factors, such as short-term memory, processing speed, visual processing, fluid reasoning, and knowledge.

Standardized administration and scoring for Luria's (1966) flexible methodology were adapted as the **Luria-Nebraska Neuropsychological Battery** (LNNB) (Golden, Hammeke, and Purisch, 1980; Golden, 1984). It contains 11 subtests for varied skills, and three scales summarize performance (e.g., left- and right-hemisphere scales). The LNNB has been controversial. Its emphasis on reliable measurement collides with a "process approach" emphasizing flexible administration and analysis of response strategies (Kaplan, 1988). Spiers (1981) asked, "Have they come to praise Luria or to bury him?" and decided that the test is not as comprehensive as claimed.

Attention is assessed with the digit-symbol test of the WAIS or a similar visual search and scanning test called the **Symbol Digit Modalities Test** (Smith, 1973), in which numbers are matched to a series of abstract symbols as quickly as possible. The **Trail Making Test** in the Halstead-Reitan battery examines attention and concentration by having a patient draw lines to connect numbered or lettered circles in sequence (Reitan and Tarshes, 1959). The popular **Wechsler Memory Scale** contains questions about current information and surroundings, a digit span test, paragraphs for retelling, word-pair recall, and geometric figures to draw from memory (Wechsler, 1945). The test yields a score called the Memory Quotient (MQ).

Besides object matching, tests of visual perception include judging line orientation and discriminating between forms. Integration entails recognizing the whole or pattern in an array of parts or details. A patient tries to identify the missing part of an incomplete figure (e.g., the WAIS, Raven's matrices) or name a fragmented object, as in the **Hooper Visual Organization Test** (Hooper, 1958). Constructional ability, which is skilled movement based on visual stimuli, is tested by replicating geometric designs and by drawing. A **draw-a-person test** is relatively culture-free, and the **complex figure test** involves copying a geometric design. Drawing tasks may have copying and memory components (i.e., stimulus present or absent).

TRAUMATIC BRAIN INJURY (TBI)

It was kind of a freak accident. I was on a motorcycle and I didn't have my helmet buckled. I just put it on, you know, and didn't buckle it. I was comin' down the road, and there's like an island in the road, you know, there was an island with two telephone poles in the middle, and I bounced off both those poles. Bounced off and flew 40 feet through the air and lost my helmet in the meantime. And my brains were leaking out on the ground, and then I got to the hospital, and I was in a coma for four months. I was supposed to croak but I didn't. I fooled them all.

Gary was 18 when he rode his cycle off the road. Head injury is the most common cause of death under age 38 in the United States.

The highest incidence is between ages 10 and 29. The most typical head-injured person is male, single, of lower socioeconomic status, and high school–educated or less (Anderson and McLaurin, 1980; Cooper, 1982). About 500,000 persons suffer head trauma each year, and more than half are caused by traffic accidents. Falls are the next major cause. Most injuries occur in the summer and fall, and the most common contributing factor is alcohol use. In a study in Virginia, 12 percent of head injuries were precipitated by interpersonal violence, with 80 percent of these being self-inflicted or stemming from domestic problems (Rimel and Jane, 1983).

Mechanics of Brain Injury

With Luria's (1970b) distinction between penetrating and nonpenetrating projectiles, head injuries have been broadly classified according to whether the skull is displaced, meninges are torn, or cortex is violated. A common classification is *open* (i.e., penetrating) and *closed* (i.e., nonpenetrating) head injuries. Mechanisms of injury are quite variable. Some researchers prefer to describe the damage to their subjects instead of classifying in a way that overly simplifies. War produced large samples of penetrating lesions, which taught us a great deal about cerebral dysfunction. Small-caliber weapons provided Luria (1970b) with "cleanly punched out" lesions to study. Investigations followed World War I (Goldstein, 1942), World War II (Luria, 1966; Newcombe, 1969; Russell and Espir, 1961), and the Vietnam War (Mohr, Weiss, Caveness, Dillon, Kistler, Meirowsky, and Rish, 1980).

An active civilian population is susceptible to blunt, nonpenetrating trauma or **closed head injury** (CHI). A moving object strikes a blow when the head is stationary, or the head is moving and strikes a stationary object, such as in motor vehicle accidents and falls. Bone fragments may lacerate cortex. However, without laceration, violence to the cerebrum distinguishes the injury (Figure 6–1). Primary damage at the moment of impact causes contusion (i.e., bruising) that is superficial or ex-

tends into cortex and white matter. Violent movement of the brain and the bony configuration of the skull result in *multifocal contusion*, usually of **anterior frontal lobes** (i.e., prefrontal areas 9, 10, 11, 12) and **temporal lobes** (i.e., area 38). *Diffuse axonal injury* (DAI) stems from swirling motions and pressure waves caused by rapid acceleration-deceleration. This stretching (or "shearing") of white fiber tracts within the cerebrum and brain stem occurs more with high-speed traffic accidents than with blows or falls. *Secondary effects* include swelling, hemorrhage, and pulmonary complications. Surgery may be performed to evacuate subdural hematomas. Widespread embolism can occur within hours. Sometimes secondary effects are dominant, as in a person who is conscious for a while before lapsing into a coma.

CHI: Cognitive Impairments

The remaining discussion focuses on closed head injury because of its uniquely multidimensional deficits. Levels of functioning are summarized in Table 6–1, a popular means of depicting experimental subjects' severity of dysfunction. Consciousness and orientation are reduced in the acute period after injury, but an aroused patient may experience rapid progress. Hagen (1981) described a clinician's dilemma: "If the traditional language assessment instruments are applied, one may obtain a diagnosis and embark on a course of treatment only to find that all aspects of patient management are inappropriate the following day or week. However, if one waits until the patient 'stabilizes,' not only will 2–3 months of valuable treatment time be lost, but the patient may develop coping strategies that interfere with the effectiveness of treatment" (p. 73).

Coma. In an emergency room, a patient may be classified as a "talker" or a "nontalker." Consciousness is quickly analyzed with respect to state of **arousal** (i.e., primitive wakefulness) or, if the patient is aroused, degree of **awareness** or understanding of surroundings. Rimel and Jane (1983) found 25 percent of

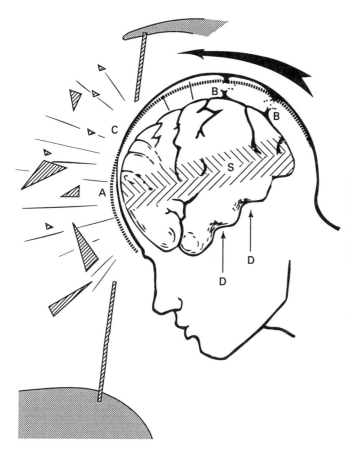

FIGURE 6–1 Mechanisms of closed head injury: (A) pre-injury contour of the skull; (C) contour after impact with inbending at A and outbending at the vertex; (B) torn subdural veins upon rotation of the brain; (S) shearing of intracerebral tracts; and (D) direct trauma to anterior frontal and temporal lobes. (Reprinted by permission from Grubb, R.L. & Coxe, W.S., Central nervous system trauma: Cranial. In S.G. Eliasson, A.L. Prensky, & W.B. Hardin (Eds.), *Neurological pathophysiology* (Second Edition). New York: Oxford University Press, 1978, p. 330.)

TABLE 6–1 General status and progress are often portrayed with this scale, developed at Rancho Los Amigos Hospital (Hagen, 1981, 1984). Only a few dimensions of each level are shown here, which is insufficient for intended use.

Levels of Cognitive Functioning

I   *No response.*

II   *Generalized response:* inconsistent, nonpurposeful, or gross response to stimuli.

III   *Localized response:* inconsistent, but responses related to stimuli.

IV   *Confused-agitated:* bizarre and indiscriminant behavior, incoherent utterance, short attention span, uncooperative.

V   *Confused, inappropriate, non-agitated:* follows simple commands, better attention span, distractible, unable to learn new things.

VI   *Confused-appropriate:* some goal-direction, remote memory returning, recent memory still deficient, increased appropriateness.

VII   *Automatic-appropriate:* oriented in familiar situations and routines, improved but shallow recall of activities, judgment still impaired.

VIII   *Purposeful and appropriate:* aware, appropriate, retains remote and recent information.

---

head-injured people to be nontalkers at hospital admission. Nontalkers can be difficult to arouse, and loss of consciousness is known as *coma*. Depth of coma is usually evaluated in four components. *Pupils* are checked for size and reaction to light. Pressing the thumb by the eyebrow might elicit a *motor response*. There might be abnormal *respiration*, such as hyperventilation. Finally, does *eye gaze* respond to commands? The **Glasgow Coma Scale** is a well-known version of this assessment (Jennett and Teasdale, 1981). It involves observation of eye opening, motor response, and verbal performance. Each category is rated, and a "coma score" is computed. Depth and duration of coma may be an early guide to severity of damage but are not necessarily related to severity of language disturbance (Brooks, Aughton, Bond, Jones, and Rizvi, 1980). The duration of coma is usually reported in descriptions of experimental subjects. Damage is often classified as severe if coma lasts more than 24 hours.

Attention. Arousal and awareness are base states of attention. They may be known in cognitive psychology as "consciousness" or the awareness of environmental events and one's own thoughts and memories (Solso, 1991). The relationship between attention and the nervous system is considered with respect to multiple levels and features of attention (see Chapter 7). Arousal of cortex to environmental stimuli of any type depends on intactness of the reticular activating system in the brain stem (Trexler and Zappala, 1988). Awareness exists from stupor (or "obtundation") to alertness. An alert patient can be distractible, and bilateral damage to diffuse projections to frontal and temporal cortex may be responsible for distractibility (Table 7–1).

Selective attention is the ability to focus on a part of an external environment of competing stimuli and on a part of the internal environment of competing thoughts and memories. Study of phenomena like the "cocktail party effect" involved presenting different messages to each ear and having a subject shadow one of the messages by repeating it (Eysenck and Keane, 1990; Solso, 1991). Bottom-up selectivity responds to color, loudness, and other salient features of a stimulus. Motivation and expectation provide top-down influences. Selective attention may be managed by a *thalamofrontal gating system* of thalamic connections with prefrontal cortex and the limbic system (Trexler and Zappala, 1988). This system is commonly damaged in CHI, and patients may have a hard time concentrating on a task long enough to complete it. They may be easily distracted by irrelevant stimuli. Focused attention is required for the effective operation of any functional system.

Perception and Recognition. CHIs may perform poorly on visuospatial tasks in a test battery (e.g., Luzzatti, Willmes, Taricco, Colombo, and Chiesa, 1989). The clinical neuropsychologist tries to figure out the role of attention, memory, and motor processes in performance of such tasks. The analysis of perception and recognition are main topics of the next chapter but cannot be avoided with CHI. Perception is the internal representation of a stimulus. Recognition depends on adequate perception; and recognizing a word, object, or person also involves access to previously acquired memories. Impairment of these processes is caused by damage to posterior sensory regions, and it usually takes bilateral damage to produce an agnosia (Bauer and Rubens, 1985). Patient JB was involved in a traffic accident that caused mainly left parieto-occipital damage and was able to perceive and recognize objects (Humphreys, Riddoch, and Quinlan, 1988). Young and De Haan (1988) presented patient PH who, years after his accident, remained unable to copy complex shapes or recognize familiar people. A person with *prosopagnosia* does not recognize faces but does recognize people by their voices or clothing (Chapter 7). The patient knows who people are, indicative of intact semantic memory. The instructive thing about PH was that he could not identify people when asked to judge explicitly whether faces were familiar, but he exhibited *covert recognition* by matching familiar faces faster than unfamiliar faces.

Memory. Another common consequence of CHI is **post-traumatic amnesia** (PTA), a vacillating period of diminished awareness in which a patient cannot remember events occurring before and after the accident. PTA is observed with many talkers and after non-talkers regain consciousness. It is temporary but usually lasts much longer than the duration of coma. A brief assessment is the *Galveston Orientation and Amnesia Test* (GOAT) (Levin, O'Donnell, and Grossman, 1979). A patient is asked about location, time, and date and about recollections of what happened after and before injury. A complete neuropsychological evaluation can be done during this period, but the examiner expects random changes in pattern of deficit.

The multidimensionality of memory raises a few questions about amnesia, and it turns out that amnesia has been revealing about the nature of memory. For example, clinicians wonder if the "memory loss" is actually a problem of acquisition or retrieval rather than an erasure from storage. Two distinct types of impairment are instructive. **Retrograde amnesia** involves forgetting events occurring before injury, and persons with CHI usually do not recall the 30-minute period prior to injury. Severe deficit extends further into the past (i.e., "remote memory"), and the GOAT has a clinician record the date of the first retrograde event reported. Recovery includes a shrinkage of this amnesic period. Also, a patient forgets ongoing events after the injury, or "recent memory." This **anterograde amnesia** is the more prominent component of PTA, which ends when a patient "remembers today what happened yesterday and does not begin each day with a blank mind" (Jennett and Teasdale, 1981, p. 89). The patient begins to recognize the speech-language pathologist. Figure 6–2 charts recall from periods of one patient's life before and after trauma at five, eight, and 16 months post onset (Barbizet, 1970). The retrograde period decreased from two years to two weeks prior to injury, and the anterograde period of PTA lasted three months after arousal from coma. At 16 months, the residual "lacuna" (i.e., memory gap) covered about six months of this patient's life. The remaining pre-traumatic memory gap is usually long-lasting.

Amnesia has varied causes, such as Korsakoff's syndrome, due to chronic alcoholism, and an infection called herpes simplex encephalitis. Most research is done with Korsakoff's syndrome. Because of the problem with autobiographical memories, amnesias seemed to support theory of two types of information storage. Amnesia could be a deficit of episodic memory, leaving the semantic memory system intact (Shallice, 1988). Patient KC, five years after a severe injury, could not remember episodes of his life. Yet, he could remember facts such as the floor plan of his childhood home and names of friends and schools attended. He could discuss the nature of his work prior to injury but could not recall events that had occurred while on the job (Tulving, Schacter, McLachlan, and Moscovitch, 1988). Cohen and Squire (1980; Squire, 1987) felt that amnesias might be content-specific but in terms of the distinction between declarative and procedural storage (Chapter 3). Patients have difficulty with episodic and semantic information (i.e., declarative memory), especially in anterograde amnesia, and they retain knowledge of skill performance (i.e., procedural memory).

Amnesia may be a problem with processes rather than a loss of storage. Assuming that pre-traumatic memories were acquired normally, then retrograde amnesia can be either a destruction of stored memories or a retrieval problem. A damaged retrieval mechanism is suggested by the gradual spontaneous return of remote memories; however, this does not account for the retrieval of memories of the distant past better than memories of the more recent past (Squire, 1987). Anterograde amnesia could be an impairment of acquisition. New declarative memories may

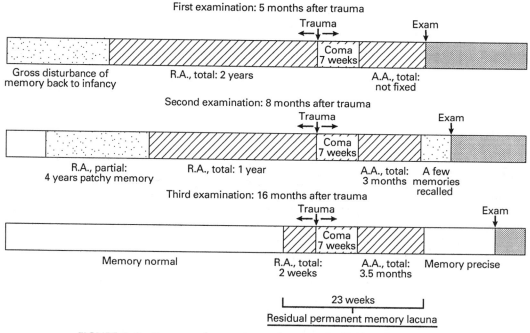

FIGURE 6–2 Recovery from retrograde amnesia (R.A) and anterograde amnesia (A.A.) by a patient assessed 5, 8, and 16 months after trauma. The period of retrograde amnesia decreased toward the moment of trauma. (Reprinted by permission from Barbizet, J., *Human memory and its pathology.* New York: W.H. Freeman, 1970, p. 126.)

be difficult to acquire because of deficient semantic encoding of stimuli (Freedman and Cermak, 1986). Graf and Schacter (1985; Schacter, 1987) indicated that a problem with retrieval of newly acquired information can be discerned when we distinguish automatic and controlled, effortful processing. They proposed that **implicit memory** (i.e., recall without awareness) is intact and that **explicit memory** (i.e., conscious recollection) is impaired. Explicit recall is tested with free-recall and other tasks in which someone is trying to remember; implicit recall is tested by having someone do something other than a memory task (i.e., word completion), and the experimenter checks to see if performance is influenced by retention. This notion was supported subsequently by a study of mild CHI in which consciousness had been lost for 20 minutes or less (Mutter, Howard, Howard, and Wiggs, 1990).

"Frontal Lobe Syndrome" and Executive Control. The pre-frontal damage in CHI, far forward of the motor regions, is associated with the so-called "frontal lobe syndrome" (Mattson and Levin, 1990). The pre-frontal area is a vast region of cortex (Figure 1–2). Deficits occur in intellectual skill, executive function, and personality (Benson and Stuss, 1986). Further differentiation is made with respect to the most forward region or *frontal poles*, the *orbitofrontal* region above the eyes, and a *dorsolateral* region posteriorly and laterally. Damage to the most forward regions is not often associated with cognitive deficit but does change personality. Impaired frontal poles and medial frontal lobes cause **arousal disorder,** characterized by apathy and a lack of initiative giving an impression of depression. Orbitofrontal damage releases inhibitions, permitting outrageous displays known as **behavior disorder.** Behavior disorder includes sexual inappropriateness and attempts to escape the hospital called "elopement."

Dysexecutive syndrome is observed as a disorganization of behavior sequences. Patients have difficulty shifting response sets and evaluating their performance. According to Duncan's (1986) theory, executive function starts with *goal lists,* such as taking a shower, getting dressed, and eating breakfast before going to work. An *action-list* is the mental operations and overt actions engaged in meeting these goals. Self-monitoring or *means-ends analysis* compares current states and goal states, ensuring that goals are being met. Executive control applies to any information-processing domain, and "disorganization should manifest itself in the widest possible variety of tasks" (Duncan, 1986, p. 279). Dysexecutive syndrome can be exposed in complex problem-solving tasks such as the "Tower of Hanoi" puzzle (Chapter 4). Simpler tasks include arranging pictures in a logical sequence or telling a story. We should watch for approaches to solving problems. A patient may be systematic or engage in trial and error (Hagen, 1981). The patient may leave pictures in the initial random order, seemingly satisfied that this is a good solution. Arousal problems appear when a patient stops in the middle of a task and needs repeated instructions or prodding to keep going.

One pertinent task in the neuropsychological battery is the **Wisconsin Card Sorting Test** (WCST) (Grant and Berg, 1948). It contains 64 cards depicting one to four colored shapes. Patients must determine a sorting strategy according to a criterion that an examiner has in mind (e.g., color or shape) and that is deduced from the examiner's feedback (i.e., "right" or "wrong"). Once a patient uses one criterion consistently, the examiner changes the criterion. The test is used to assess concentration and attention-shifting, and Shallice (1988) thought of the WCST as a test of executive control or what he called the "supervisory system." Another procedure is

the **Twenty Questions Task,** in which a patient must guess the pictured object that the examiner is thinking of from a random array of objects (Goldstein and Levin, 1991). The patient must use a strategy of asking "yes" and "no" questions. Impairment is indicated in taking more trials than normal controls to guess the target item. Persons with CHI tend to ask questions about specific objects rather than categorical questions, despite having knowledge of the categories and ability to remember previous questions.

Language Deficits with CHI

Traumatic brain injury can cause severe sensory and motor disorders that mask language capacities. Mild trauma is followed by a rapid recovery to seemingly normal language function. This section deals with deficits that have been clearly exposed through traditional clinical tests. Studies have differed broadly in subject characteristics and assessment strategy. Functions were investigated in one study that were not investigated in the others. The following summarizes some of these studies:

— Levin, Grossman, and Kelly (1976) published one of the first studies of formal language assessment. Fifty persons with CHI of varied severity were given several tests from a battery originally designed for stroke-related aphasia. Proportion of subjects who were deficient was reported, such as 12 percent in reading comprehension of words and phrases, 40 percent in object-naming, 4 percent in sentence repetition, and 10 percent in writing sentences to dictation. Impairments were most severe and widespread across language functions with 14 subjects in a coma for more than 24 hours.

— Sarno, Buonaguro, and Levita (1987) examined 25 CHIs averaging 38 years of age and nearly four months after injury. Four tasks from a standard aphasia battery consisted of naming, sentence repetition, word fluency, and the Token Test of sentence comprehension. CHIs were impaired in all tasks to levels found in stroke-related aphasia.

— Fifteen persons with traumatic brain injury were given a standardized language battery. At a mean age of 28 and at one month to over four years post onset, these subjects had deficits in all areas of language function (Bernstein-Ellis, Wertz, Dronkers, and Milton, 1985). However, in comparison to LH stroke-related disorder, TBIs were better in writing and, indicative of perceptual deficits, were much worse in two tasks of object-matching.

— Thirty severe CHIs (i.e., coma more than 24 hours) received an Italian translation of a German test for aphasia plus some more naming tasks and tests of other cognitive functions (Luzzatti, et al., 1989). On the aphasia test, CHIs averaged in the range for mild language deficit but with wide variation among subjects. Subjects were also impaired on Raven's test of shape perception and pattern integration.

While only 40 percent of Levin and others' (1976) patients had object-naming deficits, "anomia is the primary linguistic deficit reported after CHI" (Hartley and Levin, 1990, p. 356). When there is a deficit, it is most pronounced in word fluency. Several investigators employed a letter-fluency task (Adamovich and Henderson, 1984; Gruen, Frankle, and Schwartz, 1990; Wertz, et al., 1986), and words produced per letter varied as to cognitive level (VI, 5.0; VII, 8.3; VII, 11.6) (Lohman, Ziggas, and Pierce, 1989). Lohman and others (1989) explored categorical fluency in 11 CHIs in Levels V to VII. They found substantial reductions relative to normal controls in words produced for nine categories, such as clothes (9.1 vs. 16.9), furniture (8.0 vs. 12.6), and birds (6.4 vs. 12.7). Typicality of words differed from normals only for vehicles and weapons, which was indicative of fairly good semantic organization. The lexical-semantic system was evaluated with a task in which subjects made judgments about the categorical relatedness of word-pairs (Haut, Petros, Frank, and Haut, 1991). Results suggested that CHI preserves lexical-semantic memory but slows access to this knowledge both before and after one year post onset.

Word-finding difficulties may appear in the information efficiency of extended utterance. Ehrlich (1988) elicited picture descriptions from 10 severe CHIs at various times post onset and conducted a content

analysis. There was no significant difference from normal controls in syllables per minute and number of content units produced. However, CHIs produced fewer content units per minute. Glosser and Deser (1991) studied interviews with nine patients at Levels V to VII and a mean age of 24.3. CHIs exhibited paraphasias but did not produce more indefinite words than normal controls. CHIs also exhibited syntactic errors and grammatical omissions but spoke at a normal level of syntactic complexity.

Discussion so far has avoided diagnosing these impairments as aphasia. Despite the mechanical complications of a severe blow to the head, many patients can still have relatively focal lesions. In the study by Luzzatti and others (1989), 16 of 30 subjects had unilateral lesions according to CT scan. Thus, it is likely that some CHIs exhibit classical aphasic symptoms. Sarno (1980) had concluded that 32 percent of a large group had aphasia but others had a "subclinical aphasia," with no apparent deficit in conversation but still an impairment in word fluency. Regarding their study of 25 CHIs, Sarno and others (1987) decided that they had found "parallel aphasias which characterized both CHI and CVA aphasic patients" (p. 336). "CHI and CVA aphasic patients revealed many more similarities than differences in linguistic performance and overall communicative effectiveness" (p. 335). Furthermore, Sarno concluded that "the traditional language rehabilitation approaches implemented with CVA aphasic patients are appropriate for the management of aphasia in CHI patients as well" (p. 336).

In characterizing CHIs as a group, there has been some debate over the extent to which deficits in aphasia tests must be diagnosed as aphasia. Holland (1982b) said that CHI patients "will not be terribly responsive to the traditional methods by which we have come to treat aphasia" (p. 345). The other side of the issue began with a study by Heilman, Safran, and Geschwind (1971), who administered an unspecified aphasia examination to 750 patients with CHI and decided that only 2 percent had aphasia (also, Schwartz-Cowley and Stepanik, 1989). Heilman focused on naming and made Geschwind's (1967) distinction between types of misnaming. The few CHIs diagnosed as aphasic made errors with all types of material in all situations. Also, they did not display the "nonaphasic misnaming" observed from head-injured persons who had normal spontaneous speech. In discussing misnaming, Holland (1982b) argued that impaired language behavior need not be indicative of aphasia. Errors with CHI may be perceptually based or confabulatory. Persons with stroke and CHI exhibit anomia, the symptom, but those with CHI may not necessarily exhibit anomic aphasia, the syndrome.

Another depiction of language deficit is to compare it to syndromes of aphasia, especially when a language test has interpretation devices that place patterns of performance into aphasia classifications. Heilman and his colleagues (1971) classified 13 of the 2 percent who had aphasia and found that nine had anomic aphasia and four had Wernicke's aphasia. Subsequent investigators have supported this observation, indicating further that CHIs tend to be similar to these fluent aphasias (e.g., Thomsen, 1975). Hartley and Levin (1990) said that acute or severe CHIs may be like Wernicke's aphasia, which is usually a transient state accompanied by disorientation and resolves to anomic aphasia as orientation improves. An exception occurred in the analysis by Luzzatti and others (1989). Of the 18 CHIs classified as aphasic, 11 were diagnosed as having Broca's aphasia. However, six were classified this way because of dysarthria. These diagnoses were tied to performance on a test for aphasia. Deficits on Luzzatti's other cognitive tests were not figured into this diagnostic equation. If aphasia is a system-specific dysfunction, then language tests alone do not permit a diagnosis of such a disorder. The influence of dysarthria shows that pattern of test scores may be one thing, whereas diagnosis of disorder is something else.

Aphasia tests tend to tap into only particular types of information for comprehension and expression. Patients are not pressed for knowledge that might be education-dependent or from episodic memory. For example, asking, "Is grass green?" is different from asking, "Was last night's dinner good?" These sentences are similar linguistically but access different types of content in LTM. One of these questions may circumvent language problems based in anterograde amnesia. This thought should bring us to the difference between **primary disorder,** which is the cognitive system(s) impaired by brain injury, and **secondary symptoms,** which are the manifestations of the primary disorder in behavior. This distinction is particularly useful when the type of behavior impaired does not readily correspond to the cognitive system that is impaired. For example, as Holland (1982b) suggested, a naming error may be a secondary symptom of object recognition impairment. We should consider manifestations of inattention, amnesia, or executive dysfunction in language behavior, as well as manifestations of an impaired language system. Wertz (1985) diagnosed **language of confusion** instead of aphasia. We return to the idea in Chapter 1 that diagnosis is an interpretation of behavior with respect to what it tells us about the status of cognitive functions.

Holland (1982b) did not mince words: "If the language problems seen in closed head injured patients don't look like aphasia, sound like aphasia, act like aphasia, feel, smell or taste like aphasia, then they aren't aphasia" (p. 345). Studies indicate that when patients with CHI are tested beyond language function alone, they display disorders that are uncommon in aphasia caused by stroke. Holland (1982b) asserted that "it is in the area of language pragmatics that aphasia and head injured language most vividly contrast" (p. 347). Gobble and others (1987) reported that patients recover "the ability to put sentences together grammatically" but still have problems comprehending complex language and expressing ideas in an organized way (see Chapter 8). After 18 years of examining 2,500 head-injured cases, Hagen (1981) decided that CHI produces three groups: (a) those with *disorganized language* secondary to conceptual impairment; (b) those with predominant *specific language disorder,* or aphasia, with minimal other cognitive deficits; and (c) those with *residual cognitive impairment* without language dysfunction.

PROGRESSIVE DEMENTIA

Because we are living longer, illnesses of old age will strain families and health care systems into the twenty-first century. About 15 percent of persons over age 85 suffer some form of dementia arising from various causes. About 65 percent of these are likely to have **dementia of Alzheimer's type** (DAT), also known as senile dementia of Alzheimer's type (SDAT). The nightly news reports possible discoveries of the cause or early diagnostic signs of this terrible disease, the main topic in this section on dementia. Speech-language pathologists may evaluate language abilities and, especially in a nursing home setting, may recommend adjustments in the communicative environment to make life easier for someone with dementia. Moreover, because many neurologists refer to language problems as "aphasia," the study of dementia is embroiled in debates over when aphasia is aphasia.

Neuropathologies

Alzheimer's disease is one of several progressive neuropathologies with a gradual onset and relentless deterioration of function. One characteristic change is a presence of *neurofibrillary tangles,* which are unusual triangular and looped fibers in the cytoplasm of nerve cells. A microscope also picks up granular deposits and remains of degenerated nerve fibers called *neuritic plaques.* These phenomena signify a gradual disruption of patterns of neural connection (Damasio, Van Hoesen, and Hyman, 1990). Alzheimer's disease should no longer be thought to be a condition of "diffuse" brain damage. It has a definite multifocal pattern of pathology. Neurofibrillary tangles are pronounced in granular layers II and IV of the **inferior temporal lobe,** which has connections with the

hippocampus. Tangles also accumulate in **posterior association regions** of cerebral cortex, and the magnitude of pathology is greater with increasing distance from primary sensory regions. Area 22 of the temporal lobe, which contains Wernicke's area, is much more damaged than auditory areas 41 and 42. Most damage occurs in pyramidal layers III and V of the parieto-temporal junction (e.g., area 39), confirmed in PET studies of cerebral metabolism (Chawluk, Grossman, Calcano-Perez, Alavi, Hurtig, and Reivich, 1990). In an individual, hemispheres may differ in the density of tangles. Thus, impairment can be selective, and there is a heightened awareness of individual variability of deficit patterns.

Subcortical pathologies are distinguished from cortical diseases by the prominence of motor disorders with the former. **Parkinson's disease** arises from cell loss in the substantia nigra of the midbrain. This reduces the transmission of an inhibitory neurotransmitter called dopamine to the corpus striatum within the cerebrum. Around 40 percent of these patients have an apparent dementia along with the tremors and rigidity of motor function (Ross, Cummings, and Benson, 1990). In **Huntington's disease,** the basic defect is an inherited atrophy of the caudate nucleus in the striatum (Figure 2–3). Remote hypometabolism in cerebral cortex has been seen with parkinsonism and Huntington's disease (Metter, 1987).

Other neuropathological conditions are responsible for broad changes in cognitive function. Multiple cerebrovascular accidents are the second most common cause of dementia in the elderly (Ross, et al., 1990). We are likely to see diagnoses such as **multi-infarct dementia** (MID) or stroke-related dementia (SRD). **Viral encephalitis** is an inflammation of cerebral tissue. When **human immunodeficiency virus** (HIV) infiltrates the CNS, it reduces concentration, increases forgetfulness, and produces apathy. Speech becomes effortful as the body loses strength. Distinct language impairment is not evident until the terminal stage (Navia, Jordan, and Price, 1986).

Diagnosis and General Characteristics

His wife forgets that water is running in the tub, and he decides it is time to see a doctor when she gets lost while driving the car. He says he feels her withdrawing from him. Now, she tries to brush her teeth with her comb. Before long, she will not know who he is. One frustration about the frightening suspicion that someone has Alzheimer's disease is the difficulty in confirming diagnosis at the beginning. "The confirmation of the diagnostic hypothesis is a matter of histologic study of the post-mortem brain specimen" (Damasio, et al., 1990, p. 91).

Diagnosis is termed "probable dementia of Alzheimer's type" according to criteria developed at the National Institutes of Health in Washington, D.C. (McKhann, Drachman, Folstein, Katzman, Price, and Stadlan, 1984). It is identified clinically in two or more declining cognitive areas, namely language (e.g., mistaken names), memory (e.g., forgetting appointments), visuospatial orientation (e.g., getting lost in familiar surroundings), and judgment (e.g., not wearing a coat in freezing weather). DAT is seriously considered in the absence of other explanations such as depression, multiple infarcts, alcoholism, malnutrition, or other diseases. Diagnosis may be confirmed with a biopsy of tissue containing tangles and plaques exceeding age-related expectations (Damasio, et al., 1990). Neuropsychological tests uncover patterns of deficits; but only a few tests, such as the similarities and block design subtests of the WAIS, may be sensitive to the incipient phase of disease. Screening tests are used extensively to diagnose severity of deficit. A common test is the **Mini-Mental State Examination** (Folstein, Folstein, and McHugh, 1975). Others include the **Mattis Dementia Rating Scale** (Mattis, 1976) and the **Short Portable Mental Status Questionnaire** (Pfeiffer, 1975).

The course of Alzheimer's disease is a gradual continuum of changes, portrayed as three phases encompassing six to 12 years (Cummings and Benson, 1983). Changes in language behavior have been identified with these stages (Obler and Albert, 1981). Experimental subjects are often classified according to stage or severity of deficit, and severity simply corresponds to progression after onset (Table 6–2). The individual in *Stage I* conducts household chores carelessly but can still follow well-established routines. Conversation contains word-finding errors. The next stage is sensed with an increasing burden on family members. Roles reverse, and a spouse becomes a parenting caregiver. In *Stage II*, memory impairments are more obvious and disruptive. The individual puts on shoes before socks. There is frequent pacing and then staring into space. Sensory and motor deficits arise after the early and middle stages. In terminal *Stage III*, neuromuscular disability appears as limb rigidity or flexed posture. The individual is now sitting motionless in a corner of a room and becomes totally dependent on others for basic tasks of daily living.

The Memory System

The first sign of progressive dementia is forgetfulness. Memory has been investigated to determine whether deficit is a degraded long-term store or impaired acquisition or retrieval processes. Modular deficits would be indicated in difficulties with retaining a specific type of information such as words or objects. Problems surrounding LTM would be anticipated knowing that neurofibrillary tangles disrupt connections with the hippocampus in the temporal lobe. In one study, subjects with DAT showed deficient recall of well-known events and people from each decade between 1930 and 1970 (Wilson, Kaszniak, and Fox, 1981), contrasting with Korsakoff subjects, who recalled remote events better than recent ones (Albert, Butters, and Levin, 1979). Yet, families of persons with DAT become most distressed about failures to retain what was said a few minutes earlier.

In cognitive psychology, retention of specific events (i.e., episodic memory) has been studied with list-recall tasks. Free recall of lists of ten or more items permits study of immediate retrieval of information in working memory (e.g., a recency effect) and acqui-

TABLE 6–2 Stages in the progression of dementia of Alzheimer's type (DAT).

	Other Terms	Intelligence	Personality	Language
Stage I	Early Mild	Forgetful Disoriented Careless	Apathetic Anxious Irritable	Usually comprehends Vague words in talk Naming may be impaired Word fluency impaired Good repetition
Stage II	Middle Moderate	Recent events forgotten Math skills reduced	Restless	Comprehension reduced Paraphasias, jargon Irrelevant talk Naming becomes wordy Poor self-monitoring
Stage III	Late Severe	Recent events fade fast Remote memory impaired Family not recognized Incontinence		Becomes unresponsive Becomes mute

sition of less information from the middle of a list for LTM. Mild and moderate DATs have a reduction of recall across all list positions but maintain the normal serial position effect of higher recall of the last few and initial items (Martin, Brouwers, Cox, and Fedio, 1985). Recency can be resilient in dementia, indicating an accessibility of information in working memory (Spinnler, Della Salla, Bandera, and Baddeley, 1988). Learning to recall drawings of common objects, DATs were unable to retain these memories ten minutes later (Hart, Kwentus, Harkins, and Taylor, 1988). Acquisition of new information of any type seems to be the main source of memory problems in early DAT. Memory traces developed in initial learning may be weaker than normal or may decay faster than normal so that traces cannot be consolidated enough to achieve long-term retention.

Studies of working memory address buffer capacity with span tests, the encoding of stimuli with material-specific effects on immediate recall, and duration of representation with subspan recall. Memory span for digits is reduced. Morris (1987) found that auditory span (4.9 digits) is better than visual digit span (3.9). Both verbal and nonverbal visual memory span were reduced by 22 per-

cent in mild and moderate DATs, indicating that reduction of capacity is not necessarily material-specific (Spinnler, et al., 1988). Morris (1987) examined encoding in early DAT. Intact phonological encoding was indicated when acoustically similar letters were harder to recall than dissimilar letters, contrary to findings for conduction aphasia. Decreased recall as word length increased was indicative of an intact articulatory loop. Persons with DAT can repeat subspan material immediately. However, when recall of subspan lists is delayed for a few seconds and rehearsal is prohibited during this period, abnormally fast forgetting is found regularly (Dannenbaum, Parkinson, and Inman, 1988; Kopelman, 1985). In a study of mild DATs, Morris (1986) introduced distractors in the delay period that do not normally prohibit rehearsal; recall still declined. Morris thought of subvocal rehearsal (i.e., "recycling") or elaborative encoding (e.g., "chunking") as executive control functions. He decided that limited resources weaken an executive that is supposed to allow rehearsal to occur.

Language Deficit

Language behavior is one window through which families observe a loved one's mental capacities slowly decline. Through the 1980s, a research group at the University of Arizona generated many studies of language in dementia (Bayles, Boone, Tomoeda, Slauson, and Kaszniak, 1989; Bayles and Kaszniak, 1987). Murdoch and others (1987) recommended that "presence of language disorder be included in the mandatory diagnostic criteria" for Alzheimer's disease (p. 136). Ross, Cummings, and Benson (1990) wrote that "language impairment correlates with dementia severity, allowing linguistic changes to be used for clinical staging of DAT" (p. 341). For observing linguistic changes, neurologists and rehabilitation specialists have relied extensively on clinical procedures designed to assess language in aphasia (e.g., Appell, Kertesz, and Fisman, 1982; Cummings, Benson, Hill, and Read, 1985).

In a study of naming, Bayles and Tomoeda (1983) compared persons with DAT, Parkinson's disease, Huntington's disease, and multi-infarct dementia. Only moderate DATs had significant naming deficit, leading to a suggestion that naming deficit is absent in early DAT. Yet, deficit has been observed in mild DAT (Martin and Fedio, 1983; Flicker, Ferris, Crook, and Bartus, 1987), although impairment was slight for high-frequency words (Shuttleworth and Huber, 1988). Deficit was more apparent in categorical word fluency (Huff, Corkin, and Growdin, 1986) and was comparable between animal-name fluency and letter fluency (Shuttleworth and Huber, 1988). In a "supermarket verbal fluency test," which is part of the Mattis Dementia Rating Scale, subjects produced names of things in a grocery store. People with DAT produced fewer words and fewer categories of information (e.g., meats, vegetables), and organization of response was worse in moderate DAT than in mild DAT. Moderately severe DATs used fewer words per category produced. Word fluency was related to naming, indicative of a general word-retrieval deficiency (Martin and Fedio, 1983; Ober, Dronkers, Koss, Delis, and Friedland, 1986; Troster, Salmon, McCullough, and Butters, 1989).

Word-finding deficiency in discourse has been examined with measures of information efficiency in picture descriptions. One team of investigators came up with a *conciseness index*, which is a ratio of "central facts" with respect to total words produced, and an *anomia index*, which pertains to the use of pronouns relative to nouns (Hier, Hagenlocker, and Shindler, 1985). DATs' descriptions had reduced conciseness and increased anomia, and both were more pronounced in late DAT than early DAT. With greater severity of dementia, there were more empty words and more indefinite use of pronouns. Glosser and Deser (1991) also found more indefinite terms and an absence of paraphasias in interviews. Another study included Yorkston and Beukelman's (1980) efficiency analysis. A group of DATs used fewer content units per minute than healthy elderly controls (i.e., 10.3 vs. 31.7 units); however, there was no difference in conciseness and anomia indices (Smith, Chenery, and Murdoch, 1989). The impression of reduced informational efficiency is accompanied by inconsistent findings with respect to some of the measures.

A few investigators examined syntactic aspects of expression. Hier noticed that syntax was a greater problem in multi-infarct dementia than DAT and that DATs had more difficulty with the lexicon than with syntax (Hier, et al., 1985). Similarly, conversation and writing to dictation had more lexical errors than syntactic errors (Kempler, Curtiss, and Jackson, 1987). Smith's DATs were unimpaired in the number of clauses structuring utterances (Smith, et al., 1989). In interviews, nine DATs produced complete sentences and were comparable to controls in complexity and number of syntactic errors (Glosser and Deser, 1991). Alzheimer's dementia appears to leave syntactic components of formulation relatively unimpaired.

Language comprehension has been examined more than might be suspected from titles of articles, because comprehension tasks are disguised as tests of semantic memory. A researcher might be oriented to studying object recognition with "word-picture association" tasks (Flicker, et al., 1987). Early DAT diminished word comprehension slightly, and difficulty was more evident in sentence comprehension (Bayles and Kaszniak, 1987). In a test of word comprehension, mild and moderate DATs were more inconsistent than normal controls (Knotek, Bayles, and Kaszniak, 1990). In another study, ten DATs were selected because of minimal comprehension deficit on an aphasia battery. They comprehended words when pictures differed substantially, but were slightly deficient when choices were semantically similar. Also, semantic knowledge was probed with questions about words and objects, and a slight impairment of 84 percent correct was noted for questions about specific attributes such as, "Is it sharp or dull?" or "Do you cut things with it or lift with it?" (Chertkow, Bub, and Seidenberg, 1989).

Language processing skills are pressed in attempts to find tasks that might be sensitive to early, mild Alzheimer's dementia. Bayles and her research team (1989) have employed a sentence disambiguation task, in which subjects are presented with various types of linguistic ambiguities and are asked to provide two meanings by paraphrasing the statements or to choose the meanings from pictures. Lexical ambiguity is assessed with statements such as, *The fans were noisy that night.* Bayles also evaluates structural ambiguities (e.g., *She asked how old George was*) and logical ambiguities (e.g., *The corrupt police can't stop drinking*). Difficulties with this task are pronounced in mild DAT. Sentence disambiguation is the most obvious example of extensive use of off-line and metalinguistic tasks in determining language capacities with dementia. Through the 1980s, researchers had not tried to garden-path DATs to examine core access and parsing processes.

Researchers have agreed that phonology and syntax are unimpaired in mild and moderate dementias. Bayles and Boone (1982) found that subjects could correct phonological and syntactic errors much more readily than semantic errors. Bayles (1986) has concluded that "semantic and pragmatic communicative functions emerge as having greater early vulnerability" (p. 464). The prominence

of word-finding problems has led to identifying the progression of linguistic deterioration vaguely in the area of "lexical-semantics." Many investigators have questioned whether language deficits result from a problem with the semantic system, which would have a more far-reaching impact than a problem centered on the mental lexicon.

Semantic Memory

Difficulty with naming tasks was thought to result from visual perceptual disorder rather than lexical retrieval disorder. Yet, perceptual difficulty was disputed. In Bayles and Tomoeda's (1983) study, most naming errors were semantically related to targets. A predominance of semantic errors has been found in other studies (e.g., Martin and Fedio, 1983). Perceptually based errors reappeared in another study (Shuttleworth and Huber, 1988). Object-matching ability declined as a function of severity of dementia. Persons with DAT seemed to vary in having a perceptual or lexical-semantic basis for misnaming. Another component in the naming task is object recognition (Figure 4–1), and contemplation of visual object agnosia is relatively rare in the literature on DAT. Some researchers weld perception and recognition together as one function (e.g., Shuttleworth and Huber, 1988). Agnosia is usually caused by bilateral damage and is seen at home when someone uses objects inappropriately. This disorder could be based on conceptual deficit, as suggested by Warrington's studies of single cases with cerebral atrophy or encephalitis (Warrington, 1975; Warrington and Shallice, 1984).

Again, let us try to conceive of the possibilities of impairment in the fuzzy category of lexical-semantic deficit. Vocabulary tests have been used to test conceptualization (e.g., Knotek, et al., 1990). Lexical memory is knowledge of words. Semantic memory is knowledge of concepts apart from words. Links between them are knowledge of what words mean. These networks could be erased or disorganized partially or totally. Proposing a deficit of storage is like proposing a deficit of linguistic competence, so that all tasks in which the knowledge is used should be impaired. It is thought that **category-specific deficits** can only be explained as a partial loss from semantic memory. Warrington and Shallice's (1984) cases of herpes simplex encephalitis identified and named inanimate objects much better than living things and foods, and these cases also manipulated objects much better than foods. On the other hand, a pattern of impaired and spared performances indicates damage to processes unique to impaired tasks. Automatic access of knowledge should be examined in addition to the more typical assessment of controlled processes with slow tasks.

Status of lexical-semantic knowledge is often inferred from performance on naming and other verbal tasks. Evidence for at least partial integrity of knowledge comes from production of superordinate categories in a word-fluency task (Troster, et al., 1989), ability to tell whether a picture or word is an example of a category (Huff, et al., 1986; Nebes, Boller, and Holland, 1986), and ability to match related words (Grober, Buschke, Kawas, and Fuld, 1985). Deficit has been indicated in reduction, constriction, and disorganization of categories in word-fluency tasks. In word association, persons with dementia tended to replace normally dominant paradigmatic or categorical responses with idiosyncratic thoughts, multiword responses, and perseverations (Gewirth, Shindler, and Hier, 1984; Santo Pietro and Goldfarb, 1985). Loss of knowledge was inferred when subjects made semantic errors with the same content items in word recognition and object-naming (Huff, et al., 1986). Variability of naming success, an attribute of aphasia, has been thought to be an indication of access impairment, whereas a consistent problem with the same items is indicative of lexical-semantic loss. For subjects with DAT given a naming test six months apart, 80 percent of errors were consistent (Henderson, Mack, Freed, Kempler, and Andersen, 1990). Dealing with semantic information about words is pervasive across many tasks (Abeysinghe, Bayles, and Trosset, 1990; Flicker, et al., 1987; Huff, Mack, Mahlmann, and Greenberg, 1988).

Tasks with object-stimuli may not require accessing lexical knowledge and, thus, provide a clearer window to semantic memory. Subjects with DAT correctly sorted animals, foods, and tools into these categories; but, when asked questions about categories and attributes of these objects, they had difficulty with questions about attributes of objects (Martin, 1987). A mixed dementia group was deficient when it was asked to rank attributes of objects according to importance (Grober, et al., 1985). Investigators have concluded that categorical information is more available to persons with DAT than information pertaining to attributes (Chertkow, et al., 1989; Flicker, et al., 1987; Martin, 1987). Misnaming was correlated with the difficulty in answering attribute-questions (Martin, 1987) and an insensitivity to semantically related pictures (Diesdfeldt, 1989).

When tasks tapped into automatic access, investigators became more impressed with the status of semantic memory. Nebes presented a continuous series of word-pairs, and subjects with DAT were timed in naming the second word of each pair (Nebes, 1985). Subjects performed better when the first word was semantically related than when the first word was unrelated. Nebes concluded that gross semantic structure and automatic processes are preserved in Alzheimer's disease. Persons with DAT actually have exhibited "hyperpriming" in LDTs; namely, a greater semantic facilitation than occurred for normal controls (Chertkow, et al., 1989). This surprising effect was found with some DATs but not others in another study (Albert and Milberg, 1989). Balota and Duchek (1991) felt that the word-naming recognition paradigm would reduce the possibility of controlled processing suspected to occur in LDTs. Because subjects had difficulty suppressing naming response to primes, they were asked to name each word in a dual-prime task (e.g., MUSIC-ORGAN-PIANO,

KIDNEY-ORGAN-PIANO, CEILING-OR-GAN-PIANO). First, response to the second prime was studied as if it were a target, and DATs again exhibited hyperpriming. Second, the triplets show that Balota and Duchek were interested in the influence of the first prime on biasing the ambiguous second prime. In measuring response to the third word, the researchers found no priming effects, indicative of some sort of subtle change in the automatic activation system.

Alzheimer's dementia appears to strike most forcefully at purposeful access and analysis rather than at subconscious automatic activation. The most consistent primary deficits associated with linguistic and other cognitive symptoms of Alzheimer's dementia are reduced maintenance of information in working memory and impaired deliberate use of semantic memory. Language deficits seem to center on the semantic component. Bayles (1986) concluded that "it is true that certain of the domains, notably the pragmatic and semantic, appear to have greater dependence on conscious thought and intellectual integrity than the phonologic and syntactic and are therefore more vulnerable to effects of dementing illness" (p. 466).

Is It Aphasia?

Some researchers speak of the language deficits in dementia as aphasia (e.g., Ross, et al., 1990). Bayles (1986) was quoted in the first chapter regarding speech-language pathologists' objections to identifying language in dementia as aphasia. Wertz (1985) recommended that the deficits be called **language of generalized intellectual impairment**. This disagreement is suggestive of a question as to whether focal left-hemisphere lesion and Alzheimer's disease cause the same language dysfunction. If we depend on etiology for answering this question, then we assume that dysfunction must differ in some way. If we depend solely on behavioral observation, the answer becomes debatable. Few studies have compared groups directly, especially with psycholinguistic methods in which hypothe-

sized cognitive differences can be tested with pertinent procedures.

Huff and others (1988) compared ten subjects with anomic aphasia resulting from stroke and ten with Alzheimer's disease (AD) on object-naming, naming to definitions, and other tests of knowledge of word meaning. Comparison with classical anomic aphasia makes sense because of broad similarities to mild DAT in level of comprehension and fluency. In naming tasks, the groups had the same number and pattern of errors. Most errors by far were omissions, and semantic errors outnumbered other types of errors. Error pattern was consistent in the first session, and it took a separation of a month between tests to expose more inconsistency in the CVA group. Groups did not differ in semantic judgments about word-pairs, which was sandwiched between two word-association tasks in order to determine task-priming effects. The only difference between groups in this study was that the stroke group had a much greater task-priming effect, displaying a greater benefit from previous exposure to items for word association. Huff concluded that stroke causes a greater deficit of lexical access and AD causes a greater loss of lexical-semantic knowledge, although it is unclear as to how task-priming provides the cutting edge in separating the disorders.

Two research teams examined picture description by persons with DAT and stroke-related anomic and Wernicke's aphasias (Hier, et al., 1985; Nicholas, Obler, Albert, and Helm-Estabrooks, 1985). The stroke groups did not differ from AD groups in quantity of words, comments on the task, empty phrases, value judgments, and conjunctions. Early DAT was like anomic aphasia, and late DAT was similar to Wernicke's aphasia. Distinction from Wernicke's aphasia was most evident, because DATs produced fewer phonemic and unrelated paraphasias and neologisms. Neologism was the most salient distinctive feature. Nicholas' study did little to settle arguments and was trotted out to support each side of the debate. Au, Albert, and Obler (1988) wrote that "linguistic measures on speech output of early to mid-stage patients with Alzheimer's disease have been compared to those of anomic aphasics and were not significantly different" (p. 167). Also citing Nicholas' study, Swindell, Boller, and Holland (1988) concluded that descriptive discourse is "sensitive in differentiating individuals with early Alzheimer's disease . . . from individuals with anomic and Wernicke's aphasias" (p. 413).

Appell, Kertesz, and Fisman (1982) examined DAT with a test that was designed to diagnose aphasia according to a cut-off score and syndrome according to pattern of scores. Among subjects with DAT, scores conformed mostly to anomic, Wernicke's, or global aphasia. The researchers concluded that DATs "were without exception aphasic to some degree" (p. 87). Later, they decided that "aphasic types in the present Alzheimer's sample appeared to be different from those found in a stroke and general aphasic sample. . . . The language impairment in Alzheimer's disease is part of a more pervasive cognitive disorganization. . . . At times aphasia is the presenting symptom" (p. 89). In figuring out why many investigators refer to language of dementia as aphasia, the key phrase is, "aphasia is the presenting symptom." Aphasia becomes a category of language behavior or descriptive label for deficient performance on a language test rather than a diagnosis of cognitive disorder. Furthermore, Appell wrote that observing aphasia "confirms the almost universal finding that language is disturbed" (p. 87). Any language disorder is called an aphasia, even though the disorder is sometimes "part of a more pervasive cognitive disorganization."

We have many concerns about approaches in traditional research. One pertains to the limited use of theory to specify the relevance of the chosen observation. Geschwind (1967) wrote of misnaming, such as referring to the hospital as a "hotel" and then calling doctors "bell boys." Such thematic errors have not been reported for aphasic misnaming. The broad category of "semantic error" may be insufficient for exposing such distinctions. A similar problem occurred in the study of phonological deficit in conduction and Broca's aphasias, where the mere level of observation influences answers to general questions. The semantic category may be too fuzzy for testing hypotheses about the distinctiveness of language disorders with closed head injury and Alzheimer's disease. It may be premature to define semantic errors as "aphasic errors" at the start of an investigation (Shuttleworth and Huber, 1988). As Bayles (1986) noted, some semantic phenomena may be related to general thought processes.

Another problem is a failure to consider varied verbal and nonverbal performances when it is possible that one disorder is language-specific and another lies in other aspects of cognition. When considering the entire landscape of verbal and nonverbal behavior, persons with Alzheimer's disease differ from those with focal CVA. That is, having administered a variety of tests, Bayles and others (1989) found that including tests of memory helped to differentiate stroke-related aphasias from those with DAT. Bayles (1986) has also suggested that DAT affects functional communicative phenomena that are spared in aphasia. When we evaluate this domain, the level of analysis again becomes important. A test of functional communication yielded the same score for moderate DAT and Wernicke's aphasia, but types of error made by the two groups differed. The DATs tended to be irrelevant, whereas aphasic subjects produced paraphasias (Fromm and Holland, 1989).

Most investigators agree that Alzheimer's disease and focal CVA cause different disorders. Disagreement originates in differing assumptions in the use of the term "aphasia." To many, aphasia stands for a primary impairment exclusively in the language system, and this "classical aphasia" is caused by focal lesion. Clinical researchers often say that behaviors of dementia are similar to an aphasia or are "aphasia-like." To others, "aphasia" is any deficit of language behavior caused by brain damage. The problem originates partly in a traditional dependence on clinical tests of language behavior as necessarily being tests of aphasia (Swindell, et al., 1988). At a conference on aphasia, some presenters decided that the Mini-Mental State Examination puts aphasic people at a disadvantage for measuring general cognitive functions because language is the primary medium of the test (Golper, Rau, Erksin, Langhans, and Houlihan, 1987). Someone in the audience commented that "I think you've presented empirical evidence that it's no more useful to give so-called 'intellectual' tests to an aphasic patient and call them demented than it is to give a language test to a demented patient and call them aphasic" (p. 134).

SUMMARY AND FURTHER IMPLICATIONS

As in the study of aphasia, study of behavior with traumatic brain injury and progressive multifocal pathologies has been aimed at determining the underlying cognitive or primary impairment. This ongoing endeavor is intended to determine what to look for in behavior that would be indicative of primary cognitive impairments. Especially with closed head injury, primary impairments involve generalized cognitive functions. Treatment objectives for CHI include the following:

1. To improve selective attention for stimuli pertinent to a task.
2. To extend concentration on a task.
3. To improve recognition of common objects.
4. To improve strategic encoding of new information.
5. To improve self-monitoring for a series of actions to meet a goal.

These do not tend to be objectives in the rehabilitation of aphasia caused by focal CVA. Goals for aphasias are considered for traumatically injured persons who have aphasia. With CHI, we may anticipate that goals focus on improving comprehension of complex levels of language and improving word-finding efficiency. Speech-language clinicians, in coordination with others on a rehabilitation team, are also likely to be dealing with manifestations of the listed cognitive impairments in language behavior. Problems of attention, memory, and executive function may be most evident in discourse (see Chapter 8).

This chapter forces students to consider the inconsistent labeling of neurologically impaired populations. The situation may have deep roots in the disparate orientations that disciplines bring to the study of language. To obtain information about this problem, a questionnaire was distributed to clinical aphasiologists. It began with a request to identify one's research population, and choices included "right hemisphere," "aphasia," "traumatic brain injury," and "dementia." The problem was confronted at the start of the questionnaire because of the inconsistent basis for identifying clinical groups. Some were identified by dysfunction; others, by a label for site of lesion; others, by a label for etiology. Some investigators might check aphasia and traumatic brain injury as two different groups. Others might check both as the same group. Thus, inconsistency begins by mixing terms for neural and cognitive phenomena. Because closed head injury has a multifocal component and Alzheimer's disease is also multifocal rather than diffuse, the variability of these pathologies may produce the neurological conditions for classical aphasia in some patients.

The viewpoint that any misnaming behavior is aphasia differs from Geschwind's (1967) recognition of nonaphasic misnaming. As indicated in Chapter 4, few neurologists as well as speech-language pathologists would deny that misnaming can be caused by disorders of object recognition. Thus, few would deny that nonaphasic misnaming is possible. Argument pertains to whether cognition is fractionated beyond the process for object recognition. Models of object-naming, however, do separate a conceptual system from a lexical system (e.g., Figures 4-1, 7-1). Many argue that Alzheimer's disease tends to diminish storage and access in the conceptual system, and word-finding ends up suffering because of it. Focal CVA is thought to disrupt access in the lexical system and spare the conceptual or semantic system. Wernicke's aphasia is suspected of including conceptual impairment, but its distinctive neologisms point to difficulties in lexical formulation. Some levels of observation do not distinguish language behavior with focal CVA and multifocal/diffuse lesion, but we cannot accept this finding as the only observation and ignore the difference in neuropathology. It is equally likely that the assessment is inadequate for exposing a difference in primary dysfunction of cognition. In statistics, this is known as a Type II error. When we ignore this possibility, we continue to diagnose as if behavior is the only domain to consider and as if the dysfunction does not exist inside the patient's head. The label (e.g, "aphasia") is not important per se. The important point is that if dysfunctions are different, then they should be given different names when recommending rehabilitative services.

CHAPTER

7

RIGHT-HEMISPHERE SYSTEMS AND DYSFUNCTIONS

We have associated the right hemisphere with visuospatial and musical skills, and clinical aphasiologists have thought of an intact RH as a source of compensatory strategy for aphasia due to LH damage (e.g., Fitch-West, 1983; Helm-Estabrooks, 1983). For a long time, people with right-hemisphere dysfunction (RHD) were not referred to speech-language clinics, because the patients do not display demonstrable word-finding and grammatical deficits. Neuropsychological evaluation exposes disorders of perception and orientation. These are not the domains of speech and language. Yet, some of the primary deficits might underlie language problems often occurring with RHD.

Two public figures exhibited quite different problems. Gardner (1982) described the conduct of Associate Justice William O. Douglas, who suffered a stroke with left hemiparesis in 1974. Justice Douglas seemed to recover rapidly and could talk and write. He checked himself out of rehabilitation, anxious to return to work. Denial of illness, called **anosognosia,** is common with RHD. Justice Douglas claimed that his weakened arm was injured in a fall. Returning to the bench, he insisted that he was the Chief Justice. In court, "he dozed, asked irrelevant questions, and sometimes rambled on." After being asked to resign, "he came back to his office, buzzed for his clerks . . . asked to participate in, draft, and even publish his own opinions separately; and he requested that a tenth seat be placed at the Justices' bench" (p. 310). In contrast, James Brady, an aide to President Reagan when both were wounded in 1981, worked courageously and diligently on his therapy and expended a great deal of energy encouraging others with brain injuries to do likewise. His speech was mildly slurred and monotonic, but in televised interviews his replies were relevant, coherent, and often buoyed with humor. While this chapter speaks of RHDs as one group, its intention is to present possibilities that may occur in different patterns in different people.

LEFT NEGLECT
AND SPATIAL ATTENTION

Sacks (1985) wrote of a woman who "appeared only half made-up, the left side of her face absurdly void of lipstick and rouge" (p. 74). Unilateral neglect of extrapersonal space is caused by damage in the parieto-temporal region. It is more frequent and/or obvious after RHD, so clinicians are more familiar with **left neglect**. Patients with posterior RHD bump into things on their left, leave food on the left side of the plate, put on clothes only on the right side, and draw only the right side of an object (Ellis and Young, 1988). Assessment includes a *crossing-out (or cancellation) test* of marking lines through circles scattered about a page. Someone with parietal RHD ignores the circles on the left. A *line-bisection test* entails asking a patient to mark the center of horizontal lines. Someone with left neglect marks to the right of midline (Heilman, Watson, and Valenstein, 1985; Lezak, 1983). This right displacement becomes greater as lines become longer, and displacement actually shifts leftward when lines are as short as one inch (Nichelli, Rinaldi, and Cubelli, 1989).

The mechanism underlying neglect is thought to be attention, and disorder is often called **hemi-inattention**. Experimental psychologists are especially interested in selective and divided attention (Table 7–1). Attention manages the processing of environmental stimuli and general processing load in working memory (Eysenck and Keane, 1990; Solso, 1991). Selective or focused attention is studied by presenting two (or more) inputs and asking a subject to respond to one (e.g., dichotic listening). The cocktail party was mentioned in the previous chapter to suggest a situation for focusing auditory attention. A common analogy for focused visual attention is that it is like a spotlight with an adjustable beam. Anything outside the spotlight's circle is processed minimally if at all. One neurotheory is that selective attention is handled

TABLE 7–1 Levels and functions of attention. The executive system is said to manage selective and divided attention.

	Other Terms	*CNS*	*Impairment*
Arousal	Primitive wakefulness	Brain stem	Coma
Awareness	Alertness Responsiveness Vigilance	Diffuse Cerebral	Obtundation drowsiness lethargy
Selective attention	Focused	Thalamo-frontal gating	Distractible Concentration impaired
	Auditory	Thalamo-temporal	Inattention
	Visuospatial	Thalamo-parietal/occipital	Unilateral neglect
Divided attention	Resource allocation	Intra- and interhemisphere processing capacity	

by a thalamic sorting system and the areas of cortex responsible for specific functions (Trexler and Zappala, 1988). Divided attention is also studied by presenting two (or more) inputs, but this time subjects are asked to respond to both. Issues pertain to allocation of cognitive resources in a limited-capacity operating system. Attentional devices operate automatically; that is, they can be unintentional, can happen without awareness, and consume little capacity. Attention can also be controlled, especially by the executive manager; then, it is volitional and consumes processing capacity.

Focusing attention seems to be managed by "special-purpose" attentional systems such as a spatial mechanism and an auditory mechanism. Left neglect is considered by many to be a defective "attention system specific to visuospatial processing" (Shallice, 1988, p. 320). The disorder is a "unilateral spatial neglect" or "hemispatial neglect." Posner and others conducted "the first study to link neglect empirically with the modern cognitive psychology of attention" (Shallice, 1988, pp. 316–17). *Covert attention,* or the cognitive spotlight, is impaired as opposed to overt shifts of eye movement (Posner, Walker, Friedrich, and Rafal, 1987). In Posner's theory, there are three stages in shifting covert attention: (1) disengagement from a current focus, (2) moving attention to a target, and (3) engagement of the target. Studies showed that a right parietal lesion prohibits disengagement from information coming from the ipsilateral field. Visual cues facilitate disengagement, permitting movement to information from the contralateral field and demonstrating that left neglect is not a deficit of perception.

Heilman added another system. Besides an impaired attentional system, an impaired *intentional system* for the RH may cause neglect (Heilman, et al., 1985; Verfaellie, Bowers, and Heilman, 1988). Intention in each hemisphere is associated more with response than with processing stimuli and pertains to a readiness to act and decisions going into determining action. In neglect, the left side is ignored because RHD reduces the in-clination to act upon visuospatial input. We may wonder if some theorists are emphasizing a bottom-up feature of selective attention and others are emphasizing a top-down feature. Mechanisms postulated for left neglect indicate that spatial attention is multifaceted: "one should view the distribution of attention over space as the result of a variety of neuronal subsystems that are called into action depending on the cognitive operation undertaken by the subject" (Cubelli, Nichelli, Bonito, De Tanti, and Inzaghi, 1991, p. 155). Like so many other impairments, neglect may occur for different reasons.

VISUOSPATIAL FUNCTIONS AND DYSFUNCTIONS

A broad double dissociation of linguistic and visuospatial systems has been portrayed eloquently by Gardner (1982) with respect to artistry. LH stroke impairs literary skills but "neurologists who had had the opportunity to work with aphasic painters claimed that not only did these painters retain their artistic capacity but in fact their works of art *improved* in quality following the loss of language" (p. 321). Conversely, RH stroke disrupts the work of the painter. Patients "neglect the left side of the canvas, typically drawing incomplete figures. . . . The overall contour of objects is disrupted" (p. 322). Each of us relies on the visuospatial system in our daily contact with the environment as well as for our own artistic proclivities. As noted in Chapter 2, both sides of the brain contribute to performing the tasks used to evaluate visuospatial skills.

Perception and Recognition: Objects and Faces

Since 1890, clinical neuropsychologists have identified two types of agnosia (Bauer and Rubens, 1985). *Apperceptive visual agnosia* is a perceptual deficit that causes recognition difficulty. *Associative visual agnosia* is a recognition problem without perceptual deficit. These diagnoses appropriately assume that we should distinguish between perception and recognition. Ellis and Young (1988) believed that "the issues raised by modern studies of agnosia demand a richer type of theory" (p. 33). That is, "it is rare to find an associative agnosic who does not show signs of piecemeal perception or who does not have to resort on occasion to a feature-by-feature analysis of visual stimuli. The interaction between these levels of impairment makes analysis of visual behavior extremely difficult and often confounds attempts at classification" (Bauer and Rubens, 1985, p. 202). Humphreys and Riddoch (1987) decided that there are five types of agnosia. Problems with object classification after LH infarcts and bilateral diseases were called a "semantic agnosia." Use of the term "agnosia," like that of "aphasia," may be overgeneralized to some extent.

Several researchers use object-naming for assessing object recognition, calling it an **identification task.** In the study of neurologically intact persons, naming does not pose the problem it does for clinicians who try to assess recognition by aphasic patients. The idea is that, if a person can name an object, then the person knows what it is. The model of object-naming in Figure 4–1 is expanded in Figure 7–1. Figure 4–1 omits perception, which is a prerequisite for recognition. Other processes leading to a naming response are nearly duplicated in Figures 4–1 and 7–1. The present figure indicates that perception is more complex than we might have thought. Stages were borrowed from Marr's (1982) influential theory of visual perception. Absence of boxes signifies representations that are computed by processes that operate on a stimulus and processes that draw from semantic and lexical stores in LTM.

As indicated in Chapter 3, the function of **perception** is to compute a mental representation or percept of a stimulus. The percept of an object may be a "structural description." According to Marr's theory, visual analysis yields an *initial representation,* or a two-dimensional "primal sketch" of an object according to the observer's vantage point. The *viewer-centered representation* fills out the per-

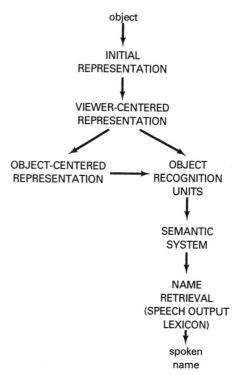

FIGURE 7–1 A model of object recognition when assessed with a naming task. Emphasis is on perception, a component omitted from the naming model in Figure 4–1. This model shows mental representations computed by implied processes. (Reprinted by permission from Ellis, A.W., & Young, A.W., *Human cognitive neuropsychology.* Hove, UK: Lawrence Erlbaum, 1988, p. 31.)

cept as a nearly three-dimensional or "2 ½-D" sketch. Perhaps because of its social or pragmatic importance, the ability to perceive faces is of particular interest to clinicians. A "facial percept" forms from parallel analyses of structural features, facial expression, and oral movement during speaking. One patient complained that faces look like flat white oval plates (Ellis and Young, 1988). This level of perception is assessed with the matching of duplicate pictures of an object or an unfamiliar face. *Object-centered representation,* a "3-D" percept, is independent of vantage point and, thus, is generalizable to seeing an object in any position. This level is tested with matching an object pictured at two different angles. One picture might show the object in a conventional position, and the other shows it at an unusual angle. This stage is conditional and may not be needed for objects in a conventional position relative to the viewer's vantage point.

When recognizing a word or object, we are indicating minimally that we have heard or seen it before. Cognitively, **recognition** is a mental match of a percept (e.g., viewer-centered representation) to a representation stored in LTM. Like lexical access, a percept is said to activate this representation. For common objects, a stored representation is not likely to be a "photograph" of a particular object, because it is unlikely that we remember every chair, tree, or car we have seen. Knowledge of what an object looks like is called an "imagen" (Paivio, 1986) or an *object recognition unit* (Ellis and Young, 1988). For face recognition, the facial percept activates a recognition unit of someone's appearance (e.g., "She's familiar"). The form of these units has been debated in cognitive psychology. Kosslyn's (1983) version was that LTM contains image files in a spatial medium (e.g., a crude "picture" of a bird) and propositional files of properties such as [birds have wings]. Kosslyn's propositional files are connected to image files and are what others say are conceptual nodes for physical attributes in semantic memory. Dual long-term representation also corresponds to the dual coding theory of encoding in working memory and is similar to the idea floated in cognitive neuropsychology that we have visual and verbal semantic systems (Figure 3-4b).

Someone with RHD can usually match objects in the same view. Disorder is revealed with objects presented in particular ways. Incomplete figures are presented to assess *closure*, and RHDs have more difficulty than those with LHD in finding a missing part or naming the figure (Benton, 1985). RHDs have difficulty naming *subjective contour illusions*, which are black-and-white contrasts that are suggestive of an object; depth perception might be impaired (Wasserstein, Zappulla, Rosen, Gerstman, and Rock, 1987).

Marr's theory of perception becomes pertinent when a patient has problems matching pictures showing an object in a typical and an unusual view (Layman and Greene, 1988). There seems to be a dissociation of object-centered perception from viewer-centered perception (Ellis and Young, 1988). Individuals with posterior RHD, usually in the parietal lobe, make errors of recognition and naming; but the errors are caused by a problem of object-centered perception when objects are distorted or in an unusual position. This disorder might have been called an apperceptive visual agnosia.

Other patients can have difficulty identifying objects visually without impaired visual perception. Disorder seems to occur at the stage in which a percept is related to an object recognition unit. A patient matches objects and names them when presented through tactile or auditory stimulation. This is classical associative or visual object agnosia as a recognition problem per se. It is discussed in Chapter 4 regarding diagnosis of naming impairments and in Chapter 6 as a problem occurring with closed head injury and dementia. Dissociations of recognition from perception tend to be caused by bilateral occipital lesions (Bauer and Rubens, 1985). They rarely occur with focal lesion in either hemisphere, but a few cases with left occipital damage have been reported. These patients might put ashes into a sugar bowl or become confused when setting a table (Shallice, 1987).

We can recognize an object without knowing what it is, which is tested in common paradigms in which a series of items is presented and a subject is asked if the item was seen or heard before. In an art museum, we may pass a bizarre contemporary sculpture for a second time, remembering it but still not relating it to known objects. Some clinical tests for object recognition require accessing knowledge about objects (i.e., the semantic system). This distinction between a shallow and deep recognition is included in a summary of receptive functions in Table 7-2. The semantic system is activated when matching or sorting objects according to

TABLE 7–2 Functional levels of cognitive response to stimuli. Terminology for impairment is omitted where distinctive disorder has not commonly been recognized.

	Cognitive Process; Subjective Experience	Terminology for Impairment
Sensation	"Initial detection of energy from the physical world" (Solso, 1991, p. 67)	Deafness Blindness Hemianopia
Simple perception	Viewer-centered representation of sensation as a percept; "I see it."	Agnosias: apperceptive post-sensory pre-categorical
Complex perception	Object-centered representation of sensation as a percept; "I see it."	
Shallow recognition	From percept, accessing a recognition unit stored in LTM; "I've seen it before."	
Deep recognition	From recognition unit, accessing a concept in semantic memory; "I know what it is."	Agnosias: associative categorical semantic
Word comprehension	From lexical unit, accessing a concept in semantic memory; "I know what it means."	Aphasia

functional relations (e.g., cup and spoon) or hierarchical relations (e.g., cup and glass). We should be familiar with these tests for the study of semantic organization (Chapters 4, 5, 6), but they also may be claimed to be an assessment of visual recognition (e.g., Warrington and Taylor, 1978). Object-naming assesses connections between a concept and the lexicon, as indicated in Figure 7–1. When we detect that a patient has trouble recognizing objects and people, we are merely scratching the surface. The problem may have causes in perception, access to recognition units, or access to conceptual information.

Difficulties with face recognition parallel problems with objects. RHDs' perceptual disorder manifests itself as an ability to recognize family and famous people and a deficit for the new faces of the neurologist or nurse. The problem is said to be confined to *unfamiliar faces*. Matching tests show that difficulty occurs when photographs display the same face in different angles and lighting conditions (Benton, Hamsher, Varney, and Spreen, 1983). Other patients have difficulty identifying family, friends, and famous people, and a deficit in familiar face recognition is called **prosopagnosia**. It usually occurs with visual object agnosia and bilateral occipitotemporal lesions (Benton, 1985; Bauer and Rubens, 1985). However, a few cases with posterior RHD have been reported (e.g., DeRenzi, 1986).

Patients with prosopagnosia can form a percept, indicated when matching unfamiliar faces even when a face is shown at different angles. When shown pictures of famous people, patients know they are looking at a face and can identify age, gender, and facial expression. They use voices and clothing to recognize acquaintances, so we could say they have not forgotten who people are. Semantic memory stores "person identity nodes" (e.g., vocation, beliefs, favorite foods) (Bruce and Young, 1986). A voice or name activates identity nodes. People with prosopagnosia just cannot access this knowledge through cues from the face. Many patients who do not exhibit explicit recognition by naming faces still possess implicit or **covert recognition** of familiar faces, which is detected with electrodermal response and other methods (for review, see Bruyer, 1991). A patient with herpes simplex encephalitis, on the other hand, failed to recognize familiar people from their faces, names, and voices (Hanley, Young, and Pearson, 1989). Further analysis indicated that he had deficient access to semantic memory rather than a prosopagnosia.

Posterior damage may cause an impairment of color perception called **achromatopsia.** Patients say that everything looks black and white or that colors have lost their brightness (Ellis and Young, 1988). Bilateral occipitotemporal lesions are responsible for this disorder, but a unilateral lesion in this region may produce hemiachromatopsia in the contralateral visual field (Benton, 1985). Deficits of color perception and recognition cannot be differentiated as neatly as they can with objects, bringing any thought of "color agnosia" into serious question. There are methodological problems in diagnosing a color agnosia, and "we know of no patient whose clinical data support this distinction" (Bauer and Rubens, 1985, p. 204). For example, color is a strictly visual phenomenon; it cannot be heard or touched, so recognition via naming cannot be assessed through other modalities as can be done with objects.

Neurologists have examined finger recognition (i.e., "Show me your ring finger") or finger localization (i.e., "Which finger am I touching?") because **finger agnosia** was thought to be a localizing sign to the parietal lobe. However, this idea has also been controversial over the years. Variations of the symptom motivate some studious testing (e.g., Benton, et al., 1983). Unilateral impairment of one hand indicates contralateral damage. Bilateral impairment with both hands involves one's own fingers and those of the examiner. The bilateral version is one of a combination of four symptoms called **Gerstmann's syndrome,** which also consists of right-left disorientation, writing disturbance,

and acalculia (Boller and Grafman, 1983). The syndrome has been linked to left parietal damage. One mystery is the cognitive factor that could draw these four deficits together.

Spatial Skills: Orientation and Construction

Dealing with spatial relationships between objects is a special skill. Holmes described a patient, wounded in World War I, who could recognize a spoon and a bowl but had difficulty locating a bowl with a spoon so that he could eat soup (cited in Ellis and Young, 1988). There can be a dissociation between visual (i.e., shape, hue) and spatial (i.e., location) perception or recognition, and an impairment with the latter is *spatial agnosia.* On the other hand, persons with visual object agnosia have difficulty recognizing objects but have no difficulty locating them. Motor operations in space can also be problematic for persons with RHD, such as a symptom known as *dressing apraxia* in which clothes are put on in a disorganized fashion.

Persons with RHD suddenly find it difficult to find their way around, especially in the maze of hospital corridors. By now, we should not be surprised that different types of disorientation may occur. One type is **topographical disorientation,** which occurs with neglect and frequently with prosopagnosia. A patient fails to orient to the immediate location and has difficulty reading maps, remembering familiar routes, and learning new ones (Myers, 1986). This disorder can be attributed to an inability to recognize landmarks, but it also occurs when object recognition is preserved (Ellis and Young, 1988). With **geographic disorientation** (also, "reduplicative paramnesia"), a patient relates to immediate surroundings such as the hospital but fails to conceive of general location, claiming to be in China or Africa when actually in Ohio (Fisher, 1982).

Constructional skills are manifested in motor tasks such as drawing or building something. Impairment is called **constructional apraxia.** Copying a Picasso-like abstract design, called the Rey-Osterrieth figure, exposes differences between right and left pari- etal damage. Parietal LHDs omit details in a coherent configuration. Parietal RHDs draw incoherent details. For the artist, "the result is a fragmented and disconnected drawing, whose parts, while often recognizable, do not flow or fit together into an organized whole" (Gardner, 1982, pp. 322–23). When drawing a person one month after hospital discharge, LHDs' drawings resembled a person and in- cluded detail of facial features, but RHDs' drawings were disorganized and were elabo- rated with extraneous detail (Swindell, Hol- land, Fromm, and Greenhouse, 1988). In an- other study, patients were asked to draw objects when given category names (e.g., fruits, tools) (Grossman, 1988). RHDs had a lower recognizability score than LHDs, al- though one fluent aphasic subject did draw "formless blobs." LHDs generally included necessary details, and groups did not differ statistically in incorporating extraneous de- tails. Coupled with impaired perception of fragmented objects, the disorganized ele- ments of drawing are often suggested to be indicative of a deficiency in **integration** capacity.

Mental Imagery

Object recognition, orientation in space, and construction depend on mental imagery. Images, which are "quasi-pictorial" mental representations, are percepts that can be re- tained for a brief time in a buffer. The object- centered feature of the perceptual problem with RHD points to a failure to execute **men- tal rotation** for stimulus encoding (Layman and Greene, 1988). This is thought to be a moving encoding process by which we can "turn objects around" (Finke, 1989). In a study of neurologically intact adults, Shepard and Metzler (1971) found that the time taken to match two identical shapes is a function of the degree of difference of orientation be- tween them. This has been a robust finding, but attempts to relate it to RH function with hemifield studies have been mixed. In one study, field asymmetry for mental rotation varied as a function of spatial ability; subjects

with low ability had an LVF (RH) preference, whereas those with high ability had an RVF (LH) preference (Voyer and Bryden, 1990). Nevertheless, impaired mental rotation so far has been associated with RHD. Layman and Greene (1988) were especially curious about someone with posterior RHD who did things in reverse, such as putting the wrong end of a spoon in a coffee cup and using his keys upside down. In Riddoch and Humphreys' (1986) terms, RHD impairs transformation of an unusual object representation onto a pro- totypical recognition unit.

Studies of geographic knowledge have been used to explore the notion that visu- ospatial imagery is a form of representation in LTM (Finke, 1989; Solso, 1991). Knowl- edge of the geography of a country may not be preserved as a "mental map." Instead, we may store propositions in the semantic net- work about locations and sizes of states and locations of cities (e.g., [Reno is east of Los Angeles]). This possibility is indicated in the distorted maps that people draw of the United States (e.g., Reno is actually west of Los Angeles). Subjects have been asked to estimate distances between cities on a map, indicating that we store spatial images of ge- ography. This procedure was applied to per- sons with focal RHD, and results indicated that these patients have a problem with ma- nipulating the internal representation of space. That is, it is a processing impairment rather than a loss of geographic knowledge (Morrow, et al., 1985).

When we ask someone to copy a picture just removed from view, the client must re- tain the percept in the visuospatial sketch pad. On the other hand, drawing on com- mand is guided by **image generation,** or the activation of physical information about an object stored in LTM (Figure 2–9). In eval- uating drawing on command, Grossman (1988) suspected that image-generation is de- ficient in RHDs and some LHDs. In the study of left neglect, some authors refer to a *representational theory* that differs from atten- tional theories. Bisiach and Luzzatti asked patients with RHD to imagine Milan's Piazza del Duomo, a square commanded by the 600-

year-old Milan cathedral. Asked to report buildings and streets on each side, patients could not report buildings on the left. Intact long-term storage of the neglected buildings was exhibited when the patients imagined the piazza in the opposite direction (Bisiach and Luzzatti, 1978). This phenomenon does not explain neglect of stimuli. It indicates that neglect is a comprehensive deficit in the active mental representation of visuospatial information from any source; or it is a manifestation of Posner's idea regarding disengagement of the spotlight, this time aimed covertly onto the internal environment.

The RH's reputation as well as impaired imagery in RHDs direct us to the conclusion that the RH is responsible for mental imagery. However, if we are to rely on lesion-deficit data, we should remember the need to demonstrate a double dissociation. Cases with LHD have also been reported to have image-generation deficit (Grossi, et al., 1986), including someone with apparent Broca's aphasia (Riddoch, 1990). Thus, the notion that the RH is the site of mental imagery can be challenged. A "principle of equivalence" states that similar parts of the visual system are activated when objects are perceived or imagined (Finke, 1989). Percepts are registered in right and left occipital lobes, and it usually takes bilateral lesions to impair object perception. Studies of LHD led to the revolutionary conclusion that image-generation is an LH capacity (Farah, 1988; Farah, Gazzaniga, Holtzman, and Kosslyn, 1985; Kosslyn, 1987). An LH role corresponds to cognitive theory, in which physical attributes of objects are said to be stored as propositions in semantic memory, so image-generation could be a constructive process rather than the mere activation of stored pictures.

Sergent (1990) surveyed the evidence used to support different views of the localization of image-generation. There were a few published studies of cerebral blood flow and metabolism, but only one by Roland and Friberg (cited in Sergent, 1990) examined cortical activation during image-generation without response to specific verbal stimuli. Subjects were asked to imagine a walk through their neighborhood, and 16 LH sites and 15 RH sites were especially active while subjects took this imaginary stroll. In an analysis of all types of investigation, Sergent found difficulties with paradigms and subsequent interpretations in support of this or that theory. For example, researchers employing physiologic measures did not use the control tasks of componential analysis to isolate the image-generation process. Sergent concluded that the evidence points to both hemispheres operating "simultaneously and conjointly" in the generation of visual imagery. Impaired imagery may contribute to the deficits with the Tower of Hanoi that puzzled Prescott with respect to what the task measures (Chapter 4). In aphasiology, we may question assumptions about the RH capacities that we can count on when believing that a treatment for aphasia draws upon these capacities.

AUDITORY DYSFUNCTIONS

RH specialization for processing pitch patterns and music has been shown with studies of RHD (Chapter 2). A patient may not be able to tolerate listening to the radio, a sign of **sensory** or **receptive amusia.** Sacks (1985) described an elderly woman who suffered an infarct in her right temporal lobe. In the early months after her stroke, she woke up to hearing familiar songs, but she was nearly deaf and no radio was turned on. She would ask, "Is the radio in my head?" Sacks called this a "musical epilepsy." What about other nonverbal sounds? RH-damaged subjects were generally normal in recognition of common sounds, although they made some errors based on sound similarity (Faglioni, Spinnler, and Vignolo, 1969; Spinnler and Vignolo, 1966). Like visual object agnosia, agnosia for environmental sounds usually occurs with bilateral temporal damage (Bauer and Rubens, 1985). What about voices? People with prosopagnosia, caused by bilateral occipitotemporal lesions, can recognize familiar people from their voices. However, some people with RHD are uniquely impaired for famous voices, whereas globally aphasic persons can recognize the sound of Johnny Carson or John F. Kennedy (Van Lancker and Krieman, 1986).

EMOTION

The RH has earned a reputation for having a role in emotion. Emotion is a feeling in the gut of limbic and autonomic nervous systems and is a message recognized in cognitive cortex. In dichotic listening, LEAs (RH) occurred for laughs and cries (King and Kimura, 1972) and for judging tonal sequences as positive or negative (Bryden, Ley, and Sugarman, 1982). In recognizing facial expressions, the usual LVF (RH) preference for neutral faces was enhanced (Ley and Bryden, 1979; Strauss and Moscovitch, 1981). An LVF (RH) preference for emotional words (e.g., *kill, love*) occurred for lexical decision (Graves, Landis, and Goodglass, 1981). Researchers have tried to induce an emotion and obtain an indication of concurrent hemisphere activity by looking for lateral eye movements or measuring EEG-alpha. Arousal was often not confirmed by autonomic measures, and asymmetries had to be interpreted gingerly with respect to stimuli used. Both hemispheres seemed to contribute to emotional qualities of behavior, but the RH was often dominant (Silberman and Weingartner, 1986). There was even leftward movement in the smiles of most normal right-handed adults (Moscovitch and Olds, 1982). The neurology of emotion has been shown to be a complex interaction of subsystems; and, with the lesion-deficit method, Cancelliere and Kertesz (1990) found that the basal ganglia has a central role in deficits with RHD.

Persons with RHD may display a flat affect or indifference that occurs with left neglect (Gainotti, 1972). Based on skin response, heart rate, and respiration, RHDs demonstrated **hypoarousal** to tactile stimulation (Heilman, Schwartz, and Watson, 1978) and emotional pictures (Morrow, Vrtunski, Kim, and Boller, 1981). Cognitively, RHDs had difficulty recognizing and remembering facial expressions and recognizing the emotional

significance of pictured situations (Cicone, Wapner, and Gardner, 1980; Dekosky, Heilman, Bowers, and Valenstein, 1980; Weddell, 1989). RHDs and LHDs had difficulty expressing emotions on request and recognizing emotions expressed by a clinician using facial and limb gesture, whereas RHDs were superior to LHDs in pantomime recognition and expression (Walker-Batson, Barton, Wendt, and Reynolds, 1987). Facial reactions of RHDs were inaccurate in response to pictures of familiar people, pleasant and unpleasant scenes, and unusual photographic effects (Buck and Duffy, 1980). A central disorder seemed unlikely, as impaired recognition was unrelated to production of facial emotion (Borod, Koff, Perlman-Lorch, and Nicholas, 1986). Separation of autonomic and cognitive systems was indicated when hypoarousal did not necessarily co-occur with deficient recognition of facial emotion (Zoccolotti, Scabini, and Violani, 1982).

RHD and LHD transform mood differently. The difference was described according to *valence of emotion*, in which the RH is assumed to be involved in negative emotion and the LH, in positive emotion. If this is true, we might be suspicious of those smiles (Borod, St. Clair, Koff, and Alpert, 1990). In a study of unilateral sodium amytal injection for surgical cases, the valence of emotional reactions was noted. Laughter or elation was elicited more often after RH injection or from the LH, whereas crying occurred more often with LH injection or from the RH (Lee, Loring, Meader, and Brooks, 1990). The results are consistent with clinical observations. RHDs joke and laugh excessively, a change in a "positive" direction and a presumed loss of the RH's negativity. Aphasic LHDs can be depressive and may cry excessively, a presumed loss of the LH's normal positive valence (Gainotti, 1972; Sackeim, Greenberg, Weiman, Gur, Hungerbuhler, and Geschwind, 1982). Depression seems greatest with anterior LHD. RHDs also vary. Some react to cartoons with excessive hilarity. Others are unresponsive (Gardner, Ling, Flamm, and Silverman, 1975). Posterior RHDs are more depressed than anterior RHDs, who are "unduly cheerful and apathetic" (Robinson, Kubos, Starr, Rao, and Price, 1984).

THE LANGUAGE SYSTEM AND RHD

People with RHD are thought to have relatively intact linguistic skills. With American Sign Language, "one RHD patient even correctly uses the left side of signing space to represent syntactic relations, despite her neglect of left hemispace in non-language tasks" (Klima, et al., 1988, p. 323). In this section, discussion of language behavior initially focuses on tasks assumed to examine the language system with minimal influence from other cognitive systems. Then, discussion turns to influences of visual attention, imagery, and emotion, not only in language with RHD but also in aphasic language.

Language-Specific Skills

Brownell (1988) stated that "RHD patients are most often non-aphasic in that they can normally process most words and sentences in isolation" (p. 248). This is the standard level of assessment in tests intended to identify language disorder or diagnose aphasias. For a long time, RHDs served in control groups in studies of aphasia, and their performance on some intriguing language tasks was relatively ignored except to the extent to which it pointed out deficits after LHD.

Comprehensive Testing. The *Porch Index of Communicative Ability,* a test of simple language skills, was given to two large groups with RHD (see Chapter 9). Above the 50th percentile for overall performance on this test, spoken language fell in the normal range (Porch and Palmer, 1986). With RHD, verbal expression came close to comprehension, differing from the aphasic pattern of verbal scores being more reduced than comprehension. A French battery, called the *Protocole d'Examen de la Fonction Linguistique* (PEFL) was given to 42 persons with RHD (Joanette, Lecours, Lepage, and Lamoureux, 1983). Some tasks were somewhat sophisticated,

such as verbal reasoning and producing sentences from certain nouns (e.g., *cleverness, competition*). The RHD group was deficient in 34 of 47 variables; 33 individuals exhibited deficits. Anterior lesions produced deficits differing in unspecified ways from posterior lesions, and results were related to educational background. Thus, RHD causes some problems with language tests, especially with more severe overall dysfunction and when the language system is pushed by demands on knowledge and reasoning.

Auditory Comprehension. RHDs displayed good word comprehension when given two picture choices but had trouble with four semantically similar alternatives (Coughlan and Warrington, 1978). Elsewhere, comprehension was statistically inferior to normal, but 50 RHDs averaged only 1.35 errors out of 20 items. Most errors were related to a word's meaning and to a diagnosis of general mental deficiency (Gainotti, Caltagirone, and Miceli, 1983). When controlling for neglect of the left side of picture displays, there was no difference from normal controls. Sentence comprehension was assessed with the Token Test, with its array of colored shapes. Persons with RHD displayed no deficit (Boller and Vignolo, 1966; DeRenzi, 1979; Lesser, 1976) or were deficient but did better than aphasic subjects (Brookshire, 1978b; DeRenzi and Faglioni, 1978; Hartje, Kerschensteiner, Poeck, and Orgass, 1973; Martino, Pizzamiglio, and Razzano, 1976; Swisher and Sarno, 1969). In a study of auditory digit and letter memory span, RHDs were not deficient, in stark contrast to aphasic LHDs (Tanridag, et al., 1987). In another study of verbal STM, posterior RHDs were close to normal but frontal patients were as deficient as aphasic subjects (Black and Strub, 1978). Problems with sentences may arise when determining thematic roles from agent-object order, especially in passive sentences (Heeschen, 1980; Hier and Kaplan, 1980).

Language Production. RHDs have named objects effectively (Boller, 1968; Porch and Palmer, 1986). The perceptual deficit with posterior RHD should not cause problems with simple drawings. When object-naming was used to assess recognition, RHDs had no difficulty with objects in conventional view; however, with objects presented in an unusual viewpoint, error rate was twice that of normals and substantially higher than LHDs (Layman and Greene, 1988). In another study, 12 RHDs were compared with mildly aphasic and normal subjects (Diggs and Basili, 1987). Statistical deficits were found in 20-item naming and object-description tasks (e.g., naming: normal, 18.4; RHD, 16.8; mild aphasia, 17.0).

Greater problems with word-finding arise with categorical and first-letter word fluency tests (Boller, 1968; Borkowski, et al., 1967; Wertz, et al., 1986). Only a "minority" of RHDs displayed minor deficit with naming tasks but not with either type of word fluency (Cappa, Papagno, and Vallar, 1990). In Diggs and Basili's study, RHDs were substantially impaired in producing animal names, things that roll, and functions of tin cans and bricks. RHDs had more difficulty with categorical fluency than with first-letter fluency (Joanette and Goulet, 1986). These patients did not produce bizarre words and differed from normals in number of words produced only after the first 30 seconds (Joanette, Goulet, and Le Dorze, 1988). More subtle features were examined in an earlier study of categorical fluency (e.g., birds, vehicles, sports). RHDs generated more clusters of related items than aphasic subjects, but the items in clusters were less central or typical than was found in nonfluent and fluent aphasic groups (e.g., "waterskiing, sailing, swimming" for sports) (Grossman, 1981).

Eisenson (1962) characterized extended verbal expression with RHD as "empty." From descriptions of a picture series called the Cowboy Story, propositions were counted as a measure of "information content" (Joanette, Goulet, Ska, and Nespoulous, 1986). Patients produced a normal number of words and clauses but a deficient number of propositions. Trupe and Hillis (1985) asked RH-damaged patients to describe a picture and tell what caused hospital admission. Again, content analysis revealed reduced in-

formativeness. Some patients were verbose, whereas others exhibited a paucity of utterance. Diggs and Basili (1987) obtained discourse from picture description and "What would happen if" situations, and subjects were deficient in number of "message units" for all tasks. Thus, Eisenson seems to have been correct.

Status of the Language System. In previous chapters, the language system was examined with regard to knowledge and processes that are specific to the use of language. Metalinguistic tasks supplement tasks of comprehension and formulation for studying knowledge in LTM. RHDs had difficulty arranging words into a sentence (Cavalli, DeRenzi, Faglioni, and Vitale, 1981), but subjects did much better than aphasic groups in detecting orally presented sentences violating agreement rules (Grossman and Haberman, 1982). RHDs made relatively few errors telling whether complex sentences were good or silly (Schwartz, et al., 1987). In another study (Schneiderman and Saddy, 1988), RHDs were asked to insert a word (e.g., *wool*) into a sentence that they read (e.g., *Susan brought the sweater that was mended*). Subjects displayed a variety of lexical and syntactic sensitivities in this condition. Yet, they had a deficit when the insertion shifted grammatical role in one part of the sentence, such as locating *daughter* in *Cindy saw her take his drink*, whereby the role of *her* changes. The investigators concluded that this "rigidity" of syntactic representation is "preliminary evidence for a linguistic deficit resulting from right-hemisphere damage" (p. 51).

Schneiderman and Saddy (1988) thought that their task examined the "core linguistic system." However, we should not associate this notion with automatic obligatory core comprehension processes (Chapter 3). Metalinguistic tasks involve conscious processing, and the investigators in question did not entertain a hypothesis about the processes required from stimulus to response so that all possible disorders could be considered. Their use of reading may have minimized demands on concentration and executive resource allocation, and it may be important to differentiate automatic processing in fast tasks from strategic processing in slow tasks when interpreting results with RHD (Tompkins, 1990). However, the linguistic specificity of difficulty is a challenging result having something to do with thematic roles. The result should find a more specific explanation in future research.

Scores on a language battery led Cappa and others (1990) to rule out phonological and syntactic disorders of comprehension. As has been done in the interpretation of problems with closed head injury and dementia, they pointed to *lexical-semantic deficits.* This ambiguously dual domain has been a hub of conjecture about language disorder with RHD, supported by preferences for semantic errors and Grossman's finding of less typicality in categorical divergent word-finding. Gainotti decided that a "semantic-lexical impairment" exists with accompanying mental deficiency. There has been little hint of deficient organization of semantic memory from grouping or matching objects according to properties and categories (Gainotti, et al., 1986; Koemeda-Lutz, et al., 1987). RHDs made good typicality judgments about fruits and vegetables (Grossman and Wilson, 1987). Reduced productivity in word-fluency only after 30 seconds indicates that problems may arise with processes that are "less automatic" than the core processes of everyday verbal expression (Joanette, et al., 1988). This lexical-semantic idea must be split, because the lexical system is contained in the language system, whereas semantic memory is a broad domain of knowledge that, as suggested earlier in this chapter, may even underlie the generation of imagery. Bayles' (1986) comment on the broad nature of semantics in the study of dementia applies to RHD as well.

When researchers propose that RHD can cause a "language disorder," they should be more explicit as to whether they are referring to an impairment of the language system or a secondary deficit of language behavior caused by a primary impairment of a system commonly associated with the RH. Studies of language should rule out the second possibility before deciding that the first possibility is correct. Proposing damage to the language system has dramatic implications for theory of the asymmetry of cerebral function. Opinions have differed. Diggs and Basili (1987) decided that perceptual and attentional deficits could not explain deficits of divergence. They said that RHDs had problems in "lexical-semantic abilities" and disorder lies in a "linguistic process" or "a larger linguistic-cognitive complex." Bryan (1988) reached a similar conclusion. Having compared RHDs to mildly aphasic patients, Joanette had another view: "It is not at all clear that the absence of superficial differences in the overall linguistic performances reflects a similar absence of qualitative differences in the cognitive mechanisms underlying these performances" (Joanette, et al., 1983, p. 242). Myers (1986) argued that language problems are explained by impairments of attention, perception, and organizational skills. Joanette's and Myers' view is dominant, as indicated in the following section.

Secondary Difficulties with Language

This section considers relationships between nonverbal capacities and the processing of language. RHDs exhibit problems in language behavior that can be readily explained as impairments of other cognitive systems. Language processing with aphasia is explored further with respect to information activated by language stimuli and the manner in which aphasic persons deal with prosodic features of utterances.

Visual Attention and Language. "A ROSE is a ROSE or a NOSE" (Patterson and Wilson, 1990). Some people with RHD make a few errors reading words aloud and, among the errors, tend to misread the beginning of words. They may also omit or misread words on the left side of a page. Either symptom is a form of **neglect dyslexia.** The deficit is not caused by homonymous hemianopia; errors occur even when words are in the intact field.

Patient VB made errors on 15 percent of words exposed for two seconds (Ellis, Flude, and Young, 1987). A good test is to present words that can still be words when the first letter is omitted or substituted (e.g., *blight*). VB understood erroneous targets according to the errors, so the impairment was in an early point in the process, such as perception or recognition. Of the errors, 66 percent were clear left-side errors, usually substitutions of the first one or two letters, irrespective of word length. To define neglect errors, Ellis identified a **neglect point** as the place in the target from which errors occur only to the left (e.g., "sl*ain*" for *train*, "pi*llow*" for *yellow*). The number of letters to the left of the neglect point usually was the same as the target, indicating that VB encoded letter slots but not the letters. Explanation centered on attentional theory of neglect in general; namely, an impairment in the control of attentional focus, with the spotlight engaged mainly to the right.

Another patient, SP, was presented to show that neglect dyslexia is more varied and more complex (Young, Newcombe, and Ellis, 1991). SP had left homonymous hemianopia and her symptoms of dyslexia were similar to VB's. SP also comprehended according errors. One exception was that, with unlimited reading time, SP made many more errors than VB. VB's errors had dropped to 8 percent in this condition. The investigators were interested in two features of SP's problem. One pertained to type of error as a function of position of a word on a page. Omissions tended to occur from the left side of a page, whereas initial-position errors occurred anywhere on the page. This led to the suspicion that different disorders underlie the general notion of neglect on the left side of a page. The second feature was initial-position deletions and substitutions and, especially, their dependence on the hemifield in which a word was seen. Deletion tended to occur when the left part of a word fell into the hemianopic field. Substitutions occurred when words were entirely in the intact right visual field. Young and Ellis retreated from

their original explanation of VB's deficit and concluded that different disorders contribute to the symptoms generally associated with neglect dyslexia.

Neglect dyslexia is quite varied. With right parietal lesion, neglect may occur much more often with nonword letter strings than with words. This difference led to a hypothesis that lexical access is intact and the problem with nonwords is attributable to a disorder of visuospatial attention (Brunn and Farah, 1991; Sieroff, Pollatsek, and Posner, 1988). Sieroff (1991) reached this conclusion after an examination of WC, who had had a stroke in the right parieto-occipital region. He was nearly perfect in reading words but displayed neglect dyslexia when letters of words were spaced apart. Regarding the two general symptoms of neglect dyslexia, VB and SP had neglect for words and side of the page (Ellis, et al., 1987; Young, et al., 1991), but JB had a deficit only for words (Riddoch, Humphreys, Cleton, and Ferry, 1990). Curiously, a patient with a left occipital lesion had a problem with the first letter when there could be many possible words with the letter changed (e.g., *-ose* as opposed to *-oap*) (Patterson and Wilson, 1990). Other rare cases of right neglect dyslexia with LH damage have been reported (e.g., Hillis and Caramazza, 1989; Warrington, 1991).

Imagery and Language. The possibility of dual coding in working memory has been considered for the representation of information prompted by words and sentences. **Concrete words** seem to evoke imagery as well as verbal coding, while abstract words may be coded solely within the verbal-symbolic system (Paivio, 1986). Sentences may arouse images as well. In a few studies, high-imagery/concrete sentences took longer to process than low-imagery/abstract sentences. Imagery was considered to account for the longer times. The opposite result has also occurred (Holmes and Langford, 1976), but some factors associated with imagery may not have been controlled. Eddy and Glass (1981) devised high- and low-imagery sentences comparable in concrete wording but differing as to whether imagery would be necessary to determine their truth value (e.g., *A Star of David has six points* vs. *The prince will some day be king*). High-imagery sentences took longer to verify. Imagery may be inherent to comprehension, or it may just happen incidentally. It may be part of off-line strategic processing for verification but not part of automatic comprehension (Glass, Millen, Beck, and Eddy, 1985). By activating "a wider range of stored information in semantic memory than a comparable verbal representation," it may facilitate inferential processing (Belmore, Yates, Bellack, Jones, and Rosenquist, 1982, p. 350).

Clinical investigation of this feature of language function is sparse. If imagery is an RH function, then RHD should disrupt the encoding of language likely to evoke imagery. RHDs without language disorder were given two-term series problems for a study of deductive reasoning (Caramazza, Gordon, Zurif, and Deluca, 1976). Subjects were presented questions such as, *John is taller than Bill; who is taller/shorter?* RHDs had a deficit when the two parts of the question were incongruent. Solving incongruent problems has been thought to require more imagery. Three-term series problems include two premises, as in those used by Read (1981) in studying patients with temporal lobectomies: *A is fatter than B; B is fatter than C; which is the fattest?* Incongruent problems were harder, but RHDs dealt with all problems normally. While there were some differences between the groups in these studies, the difference in outcome was difficult to explain. Goldenberg and Artner (1991) compared RHDs and LHDs who had ischemic strokes in the posterior cerebral artery. None of the LHDs had aphasia. Subjects were presented with high- and low-imagery sentence-pairs and were asked to decide which was correct. The only deficit occurred for LHDs on high-imagery sentences, but the magnitude of the difference from normal controls was very slight. RHDs' only deficit was on perceptual tasks.

Conversely, if imagery is associated with the RH, then aphasia should not include difficulty with imagery. Sentence comprehension might even be easier when imagery is likely to be evoked. The tendency to assess comprehension with picture-pointing tasks eliminates an area of comprehension dealing with nonpicturable meanings. Elmore-Nicholas and Brookshire (1981) wondered if this matters. They compared comprehension of sentences that can be verified with respect to common knowledge, such as, *A tree is taller than a flower* (picturable) and *A balloon is lighter than a book* (nonpicturable). Subjects found picturable, or imageable, relationships to be easier to verify than nonpicturable ones. High-imagery sentences (e.g., *The edge of a quarter is rough*) assert a physical attribute of an object, and low-imagery sentences (e.g., *A quarter is worth one-fourth of a dollar*) assert a categorical fact about an object. In a verification study, this factor did not matter to ten aphasic subjects who could comprehend simple sentences (Davis and Hess, 1986).

Emotion and Language. Thinking about effects of nonlinguistic processes on comprehending and producing utterances, we may wonder about talking with feeling. Does the problem of recognizing emotion in faces generalize to recognizing emotion in speech? Is muted emotion heard in the speech of RHD patients? A disorder called **aprosodia** has been diagnosed in RHDs, and Ross (1981) proposed that there are receptive and expressive forms of this deficit. Interpretation of intonation behavior is complicated by the fact that prosody also includes the suprasegmental components of tonal languages and the stress and juncture markers of meaning and structure in other languages such as English. A main question has been whether **affective** and **linguistic prosody** are dissociated due to RHD and/or LHD.

RHD subjects were deficient in identifying emotional tone in mundane sentences, detected in pointing to a happy, sad, or angry face (Heilman, Bowers, Speedie, and Coslett, 1984; Schlanger, Schlanger, and Gerstman, 1976). The disorder may be called *auditory affective agnosia* (Bauer and Rubens, 1985). Expression could have a flat intonational contour (Ross and Mesulam, 1979). Severely aphasic LHDs also had difficulty recognizing prosodic emotion (Schlanger, et al., 1976), and aphasic subjects had a similar deficit with emotional content (e.g., *My little cat is dead*) (Seron, Van Der Kaa, Van Der Linden, Remits, and Feyereisen, 1982). Tompkins and Flowers (1985) examined tasks used to infer impaired processing of emotion. They presented three tasks graded in difficulty from perception to recognition. They also examined access to knowledge of emotion. RHDs were more impaired than LHDs for all tasks, and LHDs were impaired only for the more demanding recognition task. Both groups exhibited knowledge of emotional concepts.

Cancelliere and Kertesz (1990) pursued the notion that there are clinical syndromes of aprosodia, especially determined by site of lesion. They gave a test of receptive and expressive emotional prosody to 46 patients with left or right lesions. Modeled after criteria for aphasic syndromes, the battery included a subtest of repetition. A classification was concocted based on ranges of test scores. It included a Broca's aprosodia (i.e., expression more impaired than comprehension), a Wernicke's aprosodia (i.e., severe deficit of comprehension), and conduction aprosodia (i.e., repetition more impaired than expression). The researchers found transcortical sensory aprosodias as well as Wernicke's and Broca's aprosodias with RHD. Contrary to Ross' (1981) idea that deficits are distinguished according to anterior and posterior RHD, the patterns of deficit were unrelated to site of lesion. The so-called Wernicke subjects could not be associated with a lesion in the temporal lobe opposite Wernicke's area in the LH. The aphasia model was a device to depict patterns and was not pursued seriously in the authors' discussion of results.

RHD may spare linguistic prosody in receptive and expressive tasks. One Thai RHD subject could recognize linguistic tones normally, consistent with expectations (Gandour and Dardarananda, 1983). English-speaking RHDs comprehended lexical stress normally (e.g., *black*board, black *board*), and most had no problem producing lexical stress (Behrens, 1988; Emmorey, 1987). They produced contrastive stress when answering "Who did what" questions (Behrens, 1988). Others could read aloud declarative sentence contours (Cooper, Soares, Nicol, Michelow, and Goloski, 1984). Shapiro and Danly (1985) compared sentence contours and affective prosody in a reading task and concluded that RHDs had deficits for both features of prosody. Other subjects had difficulty with contrastive stress answers to *Wh*-questions (Weintraub, Mesulam, and Kramer, 1981). Bryan (1989) found that RHDs, especially those with parietal lesions, were impaired comprehending and producing lexical stress (e.g., *convict*, and con*vict*) and discriminating and recognizing sentence contours.

Shapiro and Danly's study stirred debate and closer scrutiny (e.g., Ryalls, 1986). One controversy focused on the method used for detecting two production disorders with RHD: *aprosody* (restricted variability of pitch) and *hypermelodicity* (abnormally high variability of pitch). Colsher and others (1987) showed that when mean fundamental frequency is figured in variability, Shapiro and Danly's conclusions about anterior and posterior RHD must be reversed to say that aprosody results from posterior lesion and hypermelodicity results from anterior damage. Mean pitch and variability are normally related, but they were not correlated in Colsher's RHDs. The perception of hypermelodicity is based on a co-occurrence of high mean pitch and low pitch variability. Thinking about Shapiro and Danly, Behrens (1989) studied a wider variety of sentence contours with a different task (i.e., story completion). Her eight RHDs were deficient for producing declaratives and yes-no questions but had no problem with imperatives and *Wh*-questions. Behrens concluded that deficit for syntactic contours is only partial.

The unfolding issues with RHD have concentrated on whether aprosodia includes an impaired language system. This possibility seems to be odd initially, because syntactic functions, in particular, have not usually been associated with the RH. Yet, Bryan and Shapiro and Danly claimed to have discovered an exception because of deficits in recognizing lexical stress and producing declarative contours. However, Behrens did not find problems with linguistic stress and decided that the language system is spared. She thought that the selective contour problem could be a peripheral one, such as with pitch perception and production, manifested in emotional and certain forms of linguistic prosody. Perceptual deficit is consistent with Tompkins and Flowers' finding impaired discrimination. Ryalls figured that expressive aprosodia in some cases of RHD is a phonatory disorder (Ryalls and Behrens, 1988). This argument over whether RH dysfunction includes a prosodic "language disorder" contains agreement that emotion is not the only source of prosodic problems.

Linguistic prosody may be impaired as a component of aphasia. LHDs were impaired in recognizing linguistic tones in Thai and Chinese (Gandour and Dardarananda, 1983; Hughes, Chan, and Su, 1983). Persons with Broca's aphasia had difficulty comprehending lexical stress and resolving syntactic ambiguity with stress cues (Baum, et al., 1982), and fluent and nonfluent subjects were impaired comprehending lexical contrasts, while RHDs were not (Emmorey, 1987). Yet, others recognized lexical stress successfully (Blumstein and Goodglass, 1972). LHDs had less difficulty than RHDs with Bryan's (1989) tasks, and her aphasic subjects were impaired only on lexical stress comprehension. Thai aphasic subjects produced linguistic tones normally, in contrast to their impaired comprehension (Gandour, Petty, and Dardarananda, 1988). In general, aphasic processing of linguistic prosody has been variable.

To determine an affective-linguistic double dissociation, few researchers compared linguistic and affective prosody with both RHDs and LHDs. They tended to study either type of prosody or compare them with one group. Also, there is the task-effect to consider. Deficits with RHD and LHD indicate that each hemisphere has a role in the tasks used to study linguistic prosody, not

necessarily in linguistic prosody itself. Bryan (1989), studying linguistic prosody, and Tompkins and Flowers (1985), studying emotional prosody, both found that RHD impairs discrimination, and both found that LHDs had no deficit of discrimination. Thus, perception can be a problem for RHDs.

Finally, another reason for receptive and expressive aprosodia has been relatively ignored. Pitch and rhythm are musical qualities of speech exploited by poets. When someone with RHD complains that "I talk like a robot," the problem may be associated with failed music recognition and flattened singing. Sacks' (1985) patient who heard music in her head also lost her ability to carry a tune after her stroke. Researchers tend not to examine musical functions when considering dissociations of prosody.

SUMMARY AND IMPLICATIONS

The stature of the right hemisphere has grown well beyond the idea that it is a stupid spare for the left (Galin, 1976). To those who think that their workshops and audiocassettes will expand our mental powers, the RH is the source of our imagination and creativity. Research shows that, while we may enhance our imaginations, we need not attribute our self-improvement solely to exercising the right hemisphere. Nevertheless, people with RHD have particular primary disorders, and research refines the identification of these disorders, such as discovering the perceptual basis for errors of recognition. Many of these disorders are listed in Table 7–3.

Sacks (1985) gave us another way of summarizing problems with RHD. Dr. P., "the man who mistook his wife for a hat," was a music teacher with a tumor in "visual parts of his brain." He possessed clinical signs of RHD with left neglect, abnormal reflexes on the left side, and "no trace of dementia in the ordinary sense." When asked to imagine a stroll through a familiar part of town, he mentioned buildings on his right but not on his left. Describing pictures, he "failed to see the

TABLE 7–3 A sample of disorders according to usual site of lesion.

Usual Lesion Site	*Impaired Function*	*Terms for Dysfunction*
Left Hemisphere		
Perisylvian	Language functions	Aphasia
Parietal	Calculation	Acalculia
	Construction	Constructional apraxia
	Right-left discrimination	Finger agnosia
Right Hemisphere		
Temporal	Continuous sounds; music	Amusia
Parietal	Complex perception; mental rotation (object-centered)	Apperceptive agnosia Transformation agnosia
	Unfamiliar face perception and recognition	
	Spatial orientation and construction	Topographic and geographic disorientation Constructional apraxia Dressing apraxia
Parietotemporal	Visuospatial attention	Left neglect/hemi-inattention Neglect dyslexia
Bilateral		
Temporal	Sound recognition	Auditory agnosia
Occipital	Object perception (viewer-centered)	Apperceptive agnosia
	Object recognition (good perception)	Visual object agnosia/ associative agnosia
Occipitotemporal	Color perception	Achromatopsia
	Familiar face recognition	Prosopagnosia

whole, seeing only details, which he spotted like blips on a radar screen. . . . He had no sense whatever of a landscape or scene" (p. 9). Sacks (1985) sensed that Dr. P. "faced me with his *ears*." He approached familiar faces as if they were "abstract puzzles or tests." He did not recognize himself in a mirror and knew a student only by the sound of his voice. He saw faces when there were none, as "he might pat the heads of water-hydrants and parking-meters, taking these to be the heads of children" (p. 7). When Dr. P. decided that the neurological examination was over, he looked around for his hat and tugged his wife's head.

Neurologists and neuropsychologists diagnose these disorders, and speech-language pathologists are interested in understanding how these disorders interfere with linguistic and communicative abilities. We may administer an aphasia test, and we may find a few errors here and there. Theoretical issues are addressed to what we would assume to be the underlying basis for these errors and, thus, the target of rehabilitation. In this regard, there is some difference of opinion. According to some, a goal would be to improve the lexical-semantic system. For others, goals include improving the shifting of visuospatial attention and/or enhancing imagery. Improving recognition and expression of prosody may depend on whether symptoms are caused by a problem with emotion or a problem with music. Once a disorder is diagnosed properly, a rehabilitation team may divide tasks. Speech-language pathologists may concentrate on tasks involving language and communication; others may work on activities of daily living that involve visuospatial processes. Regarding language behavior, we should not forget the domain of pragmatics and discourse (Chapter 8). Moreover, treatment has theoretical implications. Does work on musical skills lead to improved prosody? Despite all the possibilities, some patients do not see much reason for treatment because they do not believe they have a problem. Clinical psychologists think that neurologically intact people cannot be helped until they want to be helped, and the same principle may apply to RHD.

CHAPTER

8
PRAGMATICS AND DISCOURSE

Previous chapters focus on a within-sentence or microlinguistic level of language. With tests for aphasia, an examiner is oriented to look for lexical and syntactic aspects of stimuli and expression. Deficits within sentences are thought to be indicative of an impaired language system operating within the left perisylvian region of the brain. However, closed head injury and right-hemisphere dysfunction motivate us to attend to features of language that link sentences at a macrolinguistic level. This is the level at which language is used in everyday situations. This chapter surveys the study of natural language use, especially at a level most commonly known as discourse.

AN INTRODUCTION TO PRAGMATICS

Since Audrey Holland (1975) spoke at a convention about how aphasic individuals communicate better than they talk, the rehabilitation of language disorders in adults has undergone some adjustments according to two related perspectives. The **functional communication perspective** emphasizes getting the message across as the main objective of a language user. Deviant and devious language behaviors have some value for this purpose, and other modalities such as gesture also help to get the idea across. A similar **natural language perspective** was brewing in psycholinguistics as a concern for the "ecological validity" of research. What messages are really conveyed between persons? How does the language system comprehend and get a message across in natural situations? A few aphasiologists feared that the functional perspective was steering us away from treating the aphasic person's impairment, but the natural language perspective forced us to look at language in a different way.

Language and Context

Like any research, ecologically valid research involves manipulation of variables. The problem is to identify variables of natural language use that are missing from traditional laboratories. These variables are identified generally under the heading of "context," and **pragmatics** pertains to the use of language in relation to context. Pragmatics is not merely the presence of context. Language is mixed with context for conveying messages. When a functional treatment goal entails requesting items in a drug store, we should be cognizant of whether a little language and the situation together succeed in getting the message across. Context resides in two locations. **External contexts** exist in a situation and are independent of linguistic stimuli in the environment. **Internal contexts** are independent of the language system and include world knowledge, beliefs, episodic memories, and emotional states. It is in this sense that plausibility of sentences is a pragmatic variable in the assessment of comprehension. Conversation tends to be *situation-dependent,* because referents exist in surroundings. Reading is *knowledge-dependent,* because meaning depends mainly on activation of semantic memory. "Rarely can we look around the room to make sense of what we have just read in a book" (Smith, 1982, p. 82). Pragmatics considers interaction of cognitive systems dealing with representations of language and contexts, and interaction of responsible neural systems.

The Communication Contract

When we enter a conversation, we function as if we make a tacit agreement or "social contract" with conversational partners based on a **principle of cooperation.** Grice (1975) suggested that conversation follows "maxims" in which a speaker tries to be informative, truthful, relevant, and concise, and a listener assumes that this is what the speaker is trying to do. For example, the informativeness maxim states that a message-sender tries to convey *new* information in conjunction with

given information known by the receiver of the message. Comprehension can be considered to be a process of relating new information to given (or "old") information. A speaker helps a listener identify what is new and old with certain linguistic devices. A pronoun, for example, is a specific signal that says we are referring to information in previous utterance, the situation, or the listener's world knowledge. When following the cooperative contract, a message-sender assumes the point of view of the message-receiver by estimating what the message-receiver knows about the topic.

Context and Cooperation in Cognition

As listeners/readers, we are not interested in just computing the linguistic meanings of single sentences produced by speakers/writers. We are not just matching sentences to pictures. We "read between the lines" by supplementing what someone is saying from our experience and knowledge. Interpretation extends to connotative overtones that are conjured by an utterance and may also contain unstated concepts called **inferences.** Given the sentence in *1,* we might wonder if activation of semantic memory spreads to a concept node for an instrument such as [spoon]. This would be an **elaborative inference,** which adds to the information explicit in a sentence.

(1) PRIME: The woman stirred the coffee.
     TARGET: SPOON

Inferencing was assessed with priming tasks involving stimuli like *1* (Dosher and Corbett, 1982). If the sentence activated [spoon], then response to the target should have been facilitated. However, there was no priming effect for implicit instruments. Elaborative inference is not automatic and appears to be activated when task instructions or the situation calls for it.

Pragmatic psycholinguistics seeks to determine the messages computed inside the heads of participants in a real communicative exchange (Figure 1–3). Sperber and Wilson

(1986) explained that "there is a gap between the semantic representations of sentences and the thoughts actually communicated by utterances" (p. 9). In a notorious murder case, a defendant's life hinged on interpretation of a speaker's intent behind "Let him have it, Chris." A speaker may refer to referents rather than linguistic sense, such as making a plea about a gun rather than the concept [guns]. Literal or **sentence-meanings** usually differ from communicated thoughts or **speaker-meanings** (Searle, 1979). Communication occurs when a listener figures out a speaker's intent; that is, when listener-meaning corresponds with speaker-meaning. The sign "Handicapped Entrance" is interpreted in relation to the situation rather than linguistic structure. We reject sentence-meanings because we assume that message-senders want to be truthfully or appropriately informative. In real communication, we often misinterpret or fail to figure speaker-meaning.

"Is someone sitting here?" We want to be polite or gentle. We make statements that can have an interpretation differing from sentence-meaning, and context dictates this difference. An example is the polite **indirect speech act**, such as an indirect request (e.g., "Can you open the door?"). Searle (1969) contended that the basic unit of communication is the speech act beneath the surface of a sentence. Speech acts include asserting, greeting, warning, and requesting. Researchers tried to specify contextual conditions that determine the form of indirect requests (Francik and Clark, 1985; Gibbs, 1986). They concluded that we are likely to formulate the greatest obstacle to meeting a request. We would not go to McDonalds and ask, "*Do you have* Big Macs?" Utterances are formed from assumptions about situations. According to the social contract, a listener assumes that a speaker is making these assumptions. When someone expresses a literal falsehood, we look for the truth. When sentence-meaning is inconsistent with a situation, a listener is said to make an inference (Sperber and Wilson, 1986) or a conversational implicature (Grice, 1975) to derive speaker-meaning. Inference is the means for

dealing with instances in which what is said is not what is meant (see Tannen, 1986).

"He has snakes in his head." Communication is strewn with literal foolishness and falsehood. We want to be vivid and entertaining. We want to express a feeling. Metaphor or figurative language is a treasure trove of nonliteral meaning for the pragmatic researcher. Phrases like "bury the hatchet," "shoot the bull," and "pop the question" may come to mind. Despite the frequency of such language in conversation and books, Pollio, Smith, and Pollio (1990) had the impression that there is an aversion to studying this phenomenon. "There is a strong, pervasive, and continuing distrust among people of analytic temperament (e.g., linguists, cognitive psychologists, logicians) for any method of knowing other than that based on principles of, or derived from, logical analysis" (p. 162). Pollio's survey of literature indicated "that cognitive psychology has dealt with figurative language as less important than literal language largely because of an implicit bias towards rationalistic philosophy and because of an unwillingness to deal with issues of ambiguity, novelty, beauty, and context; precisely those issues made salient by current research on figurative language" (p. 141).

Nevertheless, research has been done. Metaphoric meaning might take longer to comprehend than literal interpretation because of additional time needed to relate literal meaning to context (e.g., Glucksberg, Gildea, and Bookin, 1982). Yet, with idiomatic metaphor, nonliteral interpretation is more common in everyday usage, and nonliteral meaning comes to mind regardless of context (Gibbs, Nayak, and Cutting, 1989). The interdependence between language and context may be illustrated with more creative metaphor. The following situation-dependent statement takes on a unique meaning, when a baby-sitter is trying to control unruly children: "Regardless of the danger, the troops marched on" (Ortony, Schallert, Reynolds, and Antos, 1978). Other statements may be knowledge-dependent and situation-dependent, as when a photographer requests of a subject, "Please, do a Napoleon for the camera" (Clark and Gerrig, 1983). Original or unconventional requests and metaphors require more cognitive work. In communicative exchanges, speaker-meaning and listener-meaning usually differ from sentence-meaning, and communication requires that language be related to context.

PRAGMATIC LANGUAGE IN LANGUAGE DISORDERS

Indirect requests and metaphor are two of the devices used to examine language-context interactions in cases of brain damage. Most subjects have been persons with left or right focal lesions, which presents interesting possibilities when associating the left hemisphere with the language system and the right hemisphere with important context-processing responsibilities. On this basis, we might anticipate that language use in aphasia is based on an impaired language system interacting with a spared context-processing system. Someone with RHD might be communicating with an impaired context-processing system interacting with an intact language system.

Aphasia

Let us consider whether interpreting situations remains intact with aphasia. Previous chapters told of relatively intact conceptualization of objects except for severe aphasia, especially Wernicke's aphasia. Aphasic persons recognize emotion or humor depicted in a picture (Cicone, et al., 1980; Gardner, et al., 1975). The ability to derive implicit meaning of situations was studied by asking subjects to group pictures according to a theme or "gist," such as despair or love (Myers, Linebaugh, and Mackisack-Morin, 1985). Aphasic subjects who could sort objects had a slight deficiency when sorting situations according to theme. Implicitness of themes (e.g., hugging as explicit, love as implicit) had no effect on normal or aphasic ability. Patients made errors sequencing picture sequences of rou-

tines and stories representing common knowledge in semantic memory (Cohen and Woll, 1981). Errors were frequent in patients with global and Wernicke's aphasias; this ability, however, was close to normal with Broca's and anomic aphasias (Huber and Gleber, 1982). Patients with pronounced comprehension deficit can have some difficulty in processing situations.

The role of context in linguistic performance was explored initially with respect to realism of nonverbal stimuli. For word comprehension, referents were shown in a realistic situation which was detrimental for nonfluent subjects when four or more objects were pictured (Pierce, Jarecki, and Cannito, 1990). Chapter 4 indicated that realism of objects does not have much impact on naming. The Token Test of sentence comprehension has patients follow instructions with "tokens" of various shape, color, and size (Chapter 10). Following these instructions with houses and flowers was easier than pointing to tokens (Kreindler, Gheorghita, and Voinescu, 1971). Pointing similarly to varied common objects was also easier (Martino, et al., 1976). Other researchers found that performance did not improve with common objects (Lesser, 1979; Lohman and Prescott, 1978). Use of realistic objects was thought to create a functional situation, an idea that led to the *Functional Auditory Comprehension Test* (FACT). Patients were asked to do things like "Give me the key, point to your pajamas, and pick up the paper" (LaPointe, Holtzapple, and Graham, 1985).

Pierce and Beekman (1985) presented a context to determine if it would influence literal comprehension of a sentence. Aphasic subjects were asked to identify thematic relations in reversible active and passive sentences. A target sentence was presented alone or was preceded by a related statement or related picture. Like primes, both types of context facilitated target comprehension for low-comprehending subjects but not for high-comprehending subjects. Later, Pierce (1988) wondered if following the target with a context would also facilitate thematic comprehension:

(2) TARGET: The man was kicked by the woman.
 CONTEXT: The man has a sore leg.
 TEST: Who was kicked?

Both contexts facilitated comprehension. Pierce decided that this shows an ability to integrate contextual and target information, because the context provided a clue for answering the test questions. However, looking at the target and context independently, we can see that either one could be the basis for answering the test question. Subjects could have ignored one or the other and been successful. Situation-dependence is studied best when neither context nor target by itself could lead to interpretation.

Language comprehension depends on context when dealing with indirect requests. In one study, video vignettes contained a situation followed by a request (e.g., "Can you open the door?"). Another actor made either an appropriate response to speaker-meaning or a pragmatically inappropriate literal response (i.e., "Yes"). A mixed group of aphasic subjects preferred the nonliteral response, indicative of an ability to relate the situation to the utterance (Wilcox, Davis, and Leonard, 1978). This ability to interpret intent was unrelated to literal comprehension measured by a collection of standard comprehension tests. Later, this method was focused on Broca's aphasia and conventional requests (e.g., "Can you . . . ?"). Interpretation of literal meaning, when it was appropriate, was impaired, whereas nonliteral interpretation continued to be intact (Hirst, LeDoux, and Stein, 1984). In another study, subjects were presented a pictured situation with an indirect request printed beneath. Two pictured response options depicted literal and nonliteral responses. Normal controls and aphasic LHDs preferred nonliteral choices (Foldi, 1987).

The ability to deal with appropriate nonliteral interpretation has also been demonstrated in studies of connotative and metaphoric meaning. When choosing the most similar pair of words in a triad, aphasic LHDs relied on connotation (e.g., *loving-warm*) more than denotation (e.g., *loving-hateful*).

Normal controls used both meaning components (Brownell, Potter, Michelow, and Gardner, 1984). Study of metaphor comprehension began with presentation of phrases like *heavy heart* and *colorful music* (Winner and Gardner, 1977). Aphasic subjects chose nonliteral meanings more often than literal meanings and scoffed at the absurd literal options. Aphasic LHDs had less difficulty comprehending idioms (e.g., *He turned over a new leaf*) than novel sentences (e.g., *He's sitting deep in the bubbles*) (Van Lanker and Kempler, 1987). This research at simple linguistic levels indicates that aphasic people are better equipped to understand nonliteral than literal meanings. Pragmatic capacities reflect a retained ability to process contextual information and an ability to integrate these cues with remnants of language capacity.

Right Hemisphere Dysfunction

Considering the attentional and perceptual problems caused by a stroke in the right hemisphere, we should have an inkling that interpreting situations can be disrupted. Patients have difficulty interpreting emotion in faces, scenes, and the tone of utterances. RHDs made more errors than LHDs when sorting pictured situations according to a theme (Myers, et al., 1985). Unlike the aphasic subjects, RHDs had more difficulty with implicit themes than with explicit themes. In comprehension of nonliteral meaning, RHDs often exhibited a pattern that was the reverse of the aphasic pattern. RHDs could paraphrase intent of phrases such as *heavy heart* and *colorful music*, but still chose pictured literal meanings much more often than aphasic subjects (Winner and Gardner, 1977). RHDs had a great deal of difficulty defining single-meaning idioms (e.g., *out of character*) and dual-meaning idioms (e.g., *out of the woods*) (Myers and Mackisack, 1986). In another study, idioms were harder than novel sentences, and LHDs displayed the opposite pattern (Van Lanker and Kempler, 1987). When presented indirect requests, RHDs strangely preferred literal over nonliteral response (Foldi, 1987). Whatever is responsible for literalness on these tasks may also be responsible for social behavior that is out of place for the situation.

When pairing words in a triad, RHDs relied on denotation more than connotation, in contrast to aphasic subjects (Brownell, et al., 1984). Then, Brownell wondered if deficit includes the lexical-semantic domain (Brownell, Simpson, Bihrle, Potter, and Gardner, 1990). He compared RHDs to LHDs with his connotative/metaphoric triads and a similar semantic task. Semantic noun-triads included a polysemous target noun (e.g., *suit*), a synonym related to the less frequent meaning (e.g., *trial*), and a word related to the more frequent meaning (e.g., *tailor*). Subjects were asked to choose "the two words which mean almost the same thing." The correct answer was the target and its closest synonym. Both groups were impaired on each task. RHDs were more impaired in the metaphor task, whereas LHDs were equally impaired in both tasks. Brownell and his colleagues concluded that RHD causes "a pervasive dysfunction limiting interpretation of both literal and more figurative alternative meanings" (p. 381).

Following up Brownell's 1984 study of word triads, Tompkins (1990) asked if the difference between automatic and effortful processing matters when dealing with metaphoric interpretations. She employed an auditory lexical decision task in which a target (e.g., *sharp*) was preceded by a metaphoric prime (e.g., *smart*), a literal prime (e.g., *dull*), or an unrelated prime (e.g., *warm*). Both related primes facilitated target recognition for RHDs and LHDs. Experimental groups performed equally and like normals except for overall response latency. Tompkins concluded that the divergence from Brownell's finding pertains to his use of a strategic task. Her priming task indicated that RHDs access nonliteral meaning automatically; disorder lies in controlled operations for choosing pictures or giving definitions. This is consistent with a previous indication that metaphoric intent is understood, but problems arise when decisions must be made regarding situations presented along with an utterance.

AN INTRODUCTION TO DISCOURSE

"Discourse" has been used to refer to conversation (Scherer and Olswang, 1989); language in use (Brown and Yule, 1983; Stubbs, 1983); or sentence-strings in monologue, dialogue, and text (Kintsch and van Dijk, 1978). In this book it refers to sentence-strings. "Conversation" means conversation. Discourse differs from a series or list of sentences because of interrelationships among statements known broadly as **coherence**. Even if conversational participants alternate in making one statement at a time, conversation makes sense because of a coherence among these statements. Discourse is studied at two levels. The local or microstructural level pertains to connections between sentences and can be studied with sentence pairs. Broad themes and structural schemes appear at the global or macrostructural level. First, however, we should become familiar with the basic unit of discourse, which is not a sentence.

Units of Discourse

For experimental or clinical analysis, discourse is commonly divided into units. A sentence is a grammatical unit and, in text, is specified somewhat arbitrarily according to a writer's choice of punctuation. Instead of the sentence, the basic unit of discourse is informational and corresponds to the **proposition**. In theories of semantic memory (Chapter 3), a proposition is a connection among an action concept and related objects. In discourse, it is a predicate and its arguments. Propositions express the actions and states in a discourse and are thought to be units of encoding for processing. Coherence is established across two propositions illustrated in 3.

(3) Bill saw Susan, and he crossed the road.

This sentence could be two sentences. Coherence is achieved with a pronoun in one proposition referring back to another proposition. Clinical investigators may divide discourse into sentences according to pauses and intonation (e.g., Mentis and Prutting, 1987). Others utilize syntactically specified **T-units** containing a main clause and attached subordinate clauses (e.g., Brenneise-Sarshad, et al., 1991; Liles, Coelho, Duffy, and Zalagens, 1989; Ulatowska, Freedman-Stern, Doyel, Macaluso-Haynes, and North, 1983). The difference from a proposition can be seen with the following T-unit: *The heroic policeman who apprehended the thief turned over his weapon before the investigation began.* This sentence has three propositions conveying three events in a story. A story told with one sentence or many is the same story.

Levels of Discourse

At the microstructural level of analysis, we can focus on devices that establish an overlap of meaning between sentences. We produce lexical forms that mean nothing unless we find meaning for them elsewhere. Some of these devices either contribute to coherence of a discourse or serve to reference something in the situation. A pronoun is one of these devices. *Endophora* are elements that refer to information elsewhere in a discourse and provide a connectiveness known as **cohesion.** The most common endophoric elements are **anaphora,** which refer to information presented previously. Anaphora, such as the pronoun in 3, are said to refer backward in a text. *Cataphora* refer forward (e.g., "He is a strange man. Dr. Davis irons his socks"). *Exophora*, on the other hand, refer "outward" to external context (Brown and Yule, 1983). *Deixis* also stands for pronouns and words like "here" and "now" that point to the communicative situation. Anaphora and exophora serve the pragmatic function of denoting information that a speaker assumes is known to a listener who retains previously stated referents or is aware of surroundings.

Macrostructure is the "upper limit of structural organization," where stories differ from lecture or conversation (Stubbs, 1983). The overt structure of a discourse is guided by our knowledge of the world. Semantic or declarative memory is thought to be built of propositional relations that are interwoven into knowledge of situations called **schemas** (Figure 3–3). Knowledge of making a sandwich or going to a restaurant is contained in the intricate structure of semantic memory in a form known as **scripts** (also *routines*) (Abbott, Black, and Smith, 1985). We also possess knowledge of organizational forms in which discourse is produced. For example, part of our communicative competence is knowledge of conversational conventions, such as turn-taking and topic-initiation. **Exposition** on work or a hobby has a particular form. A fairly rigid format is required of research writing, in which information is organized into background, method, results, and discussion. In the terminology of discourse studies, **narrative** is another form of discourse more commonly known as a story.

Narrative is studied often because of its apparent structure. Knowledge for story-telling is formalized in so-called **story grammars.** These grammars specify functions for telling a story, such as establishing characters and stating a conclusion. Story functions are organized roughly into a beginning, middle, and end. Thorndyke's (1977) "macro-rules" began with *story* as the top node in a hierarchical structure of functions. *Story* was rewritten into major components of *setting, theme, plot,* and *resolution.* Then, *plot* consisted of multiple *episodes,* which were rewritten into *subgoal, attempt,* and *outcome.* Stein and Glenn's (1979) grammar had a plot-starter called the *initiating event.* We may recognize a beginning such as, "Once there was a wily fox who lived in a forest." The plot is initiated when "one day the fox left the forest to explore a nearby village." We know the story is over when "the disheartened fox returned to the forest, swearing that he would never leave again." While it is apparent that narration follows a characteristic schema, story grammars have suffered criticism for modeling phrase structures of linguistics (Black and

Bower, 1980). Yet, studies of reading time and recall support the notion that story grammar has psychological reality as a knowledge structure (Mandler, 1987).

DISCOURSE COMPREHENSION

The limited capacity of working memory presents the main problem for comprehending a speech, lecture, or story. Only small chunks of information can squeeze into the cognitive work space at one time. In psycholinguistic studies, researchers often present text by showing one sentence at a time on a computer screen. When a sentence is understood, subjects press a button, which causes the sentence to disappear and the next one to appear. A text may appear one word at a time, called the "moving-window" paradigm (Haberlandt and Graesser, 1990). Processes are inferred from *subject-paced reading* time (SPR), and eye fixation time (Rayner, Carlson, and Frazier, 1983), or recognition times for particular words (Dell, McKoon, and Ratcliff, 1983).

Making Connections Between Propositions

Elements of discourse comprehension can be detected in establishing cohesion between propositional statements. Chang (1980) presented sentence primes such as 4 and asked subjects simply to recognize a subsequent target (e.g., BILL or MARY) as to whether it appeared in the sentence.

(4) Bill and Mary went to the store and he bought a quart of milk.

While both names appeared in the sentence, recognition time for the pronoun antecedent was faster than time for the other name. This result indicates that *he* enhanced activation of the antecedent (e.g., *Bill*) so that it facilitated recognition. Thus, a pronoun acts like other words in the sense that it activates meaning. However, meaning was in a previous proposition rather than semantic memory. This suggests a number of things about comprehension. Previous information has to have been retained in the short-term buffer. The backward-pointing anaphor signals the need for **backward scanning** of information in the buffer to find the antecedent (Malt, 1985). Also, 4 has two possible referents for a personal pronoun, but pronominal cues, such as gender, guide selection of the referent. Other research shows that latency of pronoun processing increases with increasing distance between a pronoun and referent, which is indicative of increasing scanning effort as the buffer becomes more crowded (e.g., Ehrlich and Rayner, 1983). This distance effect may be exacerbated by aging. The elderly have difficulty assigning referents when two sentences intervene between a pronoun and referent (Light and Capps, 1986).

How do we assign referents to a personal pronoun when the options are ambiguous with respect to pronominal cues (e.g., *5b*)?

(5a) Steven blamed Jane because she spilled the coffee.

(5b) Steven blamed Frank because he spilled the coffee.

Subjects pressed a button labeled with an antecedent to indicate the meaning of a pronoun appearing in sentences like 5 (Ehrlich, 1980). Assignment times were faster for sentences like *5a* than for *5b*, indicating that gender ambiguity can delay assignment. As when faced with semantically ambiguous nouns (Chapter 3), additional time may be taken for automatic activation of both antecedents and subsequent integration of other information leading to sensible assignment. Plausibility based on world knowledge leads to assigning a referent to an ambiguous pronoun.

(6a) Henry spoke at a meeting while John drove to the beach. He brought along a surfboard.

(6b) Henry spoke at a meeting while John drove to the beach. He lectured on the administration.

In an antecedent-choice task, subjects assigned antecedents to *6a* and *6b* based on plausibility and took longer to choose when information was neutral (Hirst and Brill, 1980).

Called a lexical anaphor, a superordinate term may be used to refer back to a referent, especially when preceded by the definite article *the*.

(7) A robin/goose would sometimes wander into the house. The bird was attracted by the larder.

For stimuli like 7, reading time for the second sentence was longer when there was greater semantic distance between anaphor and antecedent (e.g., bird-goose) (Garrod and Sanford, 1977). Thus, activation in the semantic network operates across sentences as cohesion is established in concept comparison. Lexical coreference also occurs with a **bridging inference,** when the referent is not explicitly stated in a previous statement.

(8a) The hostess seated Jack and Chris at the table. The table was near the window.

(8b) The hostess seated Jack and Chris. The table was near the window.

(8c) Jack and Chris walked into the dining room. The table was near the window.

These sentences were part of a story, and the lexical anaphor in the second sentence was considered to be a peripheral detail in the story (Walker and Yekovich, 1987). In the second sentence, *the* signaled that the lexical item refers to given information. Time to read the second sentence increased from *8a* to *8c*; that is, from an explicit referent to a "deeply implicit" referent. The longer times were considered to occur in order to establish an elaborative inference bridging the two propositions. A bridge is often needed when a distant antecedent in a discourse has vanished from the short-term buffer holding previous information.

Comprehending a Narrative

When listening to a story, or when reading this chapter, we can process only a little at a time. According to van Dijk and Kintch (1983), we encode at three levels: a *verbatim* form for the segment being confronted at the moment, a *propositional textbase* in the buffer for holding information from previous statements, and a *situation model* or schematic representation of the whole story. The situation model must be deposited gradually into long-term memory, and the final representation is reflected in what we remember a month later even when we did not plan to remember. Narrative comprehension is an ongoing process of making connections. A connection between segments can be established only when both segments are in working memory at the same time (Fletcher and Bloom, 1988). The buffer holds information so that a verbatim statement can be related to previous statements. This is called **text-level buffering** (Haberlandt and Graesser, 1990). Composing a situational model is thought to be done in a succession of **cycles** in working memory (Fletcher, 1981). A cycle contains an active verbatim statement, processes of the moment (e.g., backward scanning), and previous information in the buffer.

Text-level buffering cannot hold all that came before. Segments of a story are forgotten or put into the situation model in LTM. Therefore, the cognitive system must be selective for information maintained in the buffer. The most prominent or salient information tends to be retained (e.g., main characters, setting). Recency of appearance is another factor (e.g., Schustack, Ehrlich, and Rayner, 1987). Selecting prominent information for the buffer is called **foregrounding** (Fletcher, 1986). Devalued segments are assigned to the background (i.e., dropped from the buffer). Anaphoric bridges to implicit concepts are established as quickly as links between lexical repetitions when the lexical anaphor refers to "central concepts" (Walker and Yekovich, 1987). This indicates that we buffer concepts most likely to be antecedents for subsequent anaphora. Recalling that connections can only be made between concepts alive in working memory, we may wonder how connections are made when an anaphor refers to information that has been dropped from the buffer. One mechanism is to establish bridging inferences to concepts implied by information in the buffer. Another mechanism is a *reinstatement search*, which involves activating a portion of the expanding story representation in LTM as a referent for the anaphor being processed (Fletcher and Bloom, 1988).

DISORDERS OF DISCOURSE COMPREHENSION

Brownell (1988) compared patient groups by suggesting that "aphasic patients often appear to understand more of a conversation or story than one would expect given their impairments with words and sentences, and RHD patients appear to understand less than one would expect given their intact linguistic skills" (p. 249). This section considers how research might lead to this conclusion, beginning with right-hemisphere dysfunction.

RHD and "Missing the Point"

The study of discourse comprehension after RHD began with some general observations. After improving their previously reported methods for comparing explicit and implicit content in narratives, Nicholas and Brookshire (1986) found that RHDs remembered explicit details better than details that had to be inferred. In other studies, RHDs recalled details verbatim but were poorer than aphasic subjects in recalling the moral and reporting unstated emotions and motivations of characters (Gardner, Brownell, Wapner, and Michelow, 1983). RHDs were said to "miss the point" of proverbs and narratives.

Two investigations focused on inferring relations between propositions. McDonald and Wales (1986) presented items involving spatial (*9a*) and nonspatial (*9b*) inferences.

(9a) The bird is in the cage.
    The cage is under the table.
    TEST: The bird is under the table.

(9b) The woman held the little girl's hand.
    Her daughter was only three years old.
    TEST: The woman held her daughter's hand.

After hearing the two statements and engaging in a brief distractor task, 22 RHDs were tested as to whether they had heard a statement before. Normal controls recognized true inferences as often as true facts (e.g., *The cage is under the table*). RHDs matched normals in recognizing true facts and inferences. Another study exposed a deficit (Brownell, Potter, Bihrle, and Gardner, 1986). RHDs made true-false judgments about sentence pairs (*10*).

(10) Barbara became too bored to finish the history book.
    She had already spent five years writing it.
    TRUE-FALSE TEST: Barbara became bored writing a history book.

RHDs made more errors with inferences (31.2 percent) than with factual statements (13.1 percent), indicating a deficiency in combining information between sentences.

Jokes were among the first devices used to study detection of coherence in stories. A conclusion becomes a punch line because of surprise relative to expectations in the body of a joke and its coherence relative to a theme (Brownell, Michel, Powelson, and Gardner, 1983). After hearing the body of a joke (e.g., *11*), subjects selected a conclusion from choices containing a punch line, a surprising non sequitur, and two coherent conclusions. If RHDs do not choose punch lines, do they err in favor of surprise or coherence?

(11) BODY: The neighborhood borrower approached Mr. Smith on Sunday afternoon and asked if Mr. Smith would be using his lawn mower. "Yes, I am," Smith answered warily. The neighborhood borrower then replied:

CORRECT: "Fine, then you won't be needing your golf clubs. I'll just borrow them."

SURPRISE: "You know, the grass is greener on the other side."

NEUTRAL COHERENCE: "Do you think I could use it when you're done?"

SAD COHERENCE: "Gee, if I only had enough money I could buy my own."

Asked to pick the funny conclusion, RHDs chose the punch line 60 percent of the time. Normal controls got the joke 81 percent of the time. RHDs were deficient but not devoid of a sense of humor. In their errors, they chose surprise over coherence. This study was expanded by using cartoons and adding a humorless story condition (Bihrle, Brownell, Powelson, and Gardner, 1986). Again, RHDs preferred surprise when they made mistakes, whereas LHDs chose coherence over surprise.

Another paradigm is to present a few sentences portraying a situation, called a vignette, and then to conclude the vignette with a target statement that, to be understood, requires integration with the vignette. Targets have been indirect requests or sarcasm. In one study, short vignettes ended with a conventional indirect request (e.g., "Can you . . . ?") or a request worded to favor literal interpretation (e.g., "Are you able to . . . ?") (Weylman, Brownell, Roman, and Gardner, 1989). Both vignettes established situations in which the most appropriate response was to indirect meaning, so that the study would examine use of linguistic context. RHDs could use context to comprehend an indirect message, but they were impaired relative to normal controls. RHDs also preferred conventional wording. Later, RHDs answered questions about vignettes that ended with one person praising or deriding another about a good or poor performance (e.g., golfing) (Kaplan, Brownell, Jacobs, and Gardner, 1990). Subjects were given information about whether the characters liked or disliked each other. The closing comment could be interpreted literally or sarcastically (e.g., *You sure are a good golfer*). RHDs accurately judged conclusions when literally true. Yet, when conclusions were literally false, RHDs had difficulty detecting sarcasm based on the characters' relationship. Patients thought a sarcastic positive statement makes a person feel better.

A few studies addressed sensitivity to structure of discourse. RHDS had difficulty arranging sentences into a story (Delis, Wapner, Gardner, and Moses, 1983) and sequen-

cing frames of cartoons (Huber and Gleber, 1982). Is there a loss of schema knowledge? RHDs who had difficulty telling stories retained script knowledge accessed with a variety of tasks (Roman, Brownell, Potter, Seibold, and Gardner, 1987). Individual variability indicated that disorders of processing are varied. In another study, RHDs were compared to LHDs in recalling main ideas in narratives (Hough, 1990). In a manipulation of central theme, the crucial thematic statement was put at the beginning or end. Delayed location of a theme was presumed to model a speaker's attempt to clarify preceding discourse. For normal controls, there was no effect of delayed theme on recalling main ideas. RHDs scored 13.88 of 16.00 when the theme was early (LHDs 12.68) but scored 8.35 when the theme was delayed (LHDs 11.88). Anterior RHDs showed a more pronounced effect than posterior RHDs. If we can be confident in identifying the processes assessed with this task, then we may say that RHDs can have a problem with an exceptional demand on integration but can use early thematic information to foreground ideas.

Little attention has been given to studying whether nonverbal disorder has a role in discourse disorders. Benowitz, Moya, and Levine (1990) compared narrative comprehension and constructional skills using 41 RHDs. Significant correlations were found between recall of narrative elements and drawing skills. Some of these correlations were weak. Recalling narrative details related to drawing details ($r = 0.36$), but recalling inferences had a stronger relationship to visuospatial organization ($r = 0.64$). When the group was divided into subgroups, a younger and better-educated group had correlations between inferences and constructional skills ranging from 0.75 to 0.83. Benowitz concluded that narrative and visuospatial functions are connected by a common mental representational system that is impaired in RHD.

We can draw a few conclusions about the status of discourse processing. Better retention of salient ideas may be indicative of intact foregrounding for the buffer. Dysfunction usually occurs with integration among sentences. Brownell (1988) pointed to impaired "backwards inferences." If vignettes model communicative situations, then integrating a situation with language is suspect as well. Deficit with sarcasm was interpreted as reduced sensitivity to beliefs and desires of others (i.e., taking another person's point of view) (Kaplan, et al., 1990). The automatic-strategic distinction was considered again with the recognition of prosodic emotion in a neutral sentence after a paragraph (Tompkins and Flowers, 1987). The paragraph was congruent or incongruent with the prosodic pattern. Deficits were small but statistically significant, and RHDs were helped by context. Effects were attributed to a retained automatic integrative capacity, and previously observed impairments were attributed to the demands of strategic processing. Yet, Tomkins and Flowers utilized the slow task of choosing labels of emotions, so the factor of automaticity needs to be examined further.

Aphasia

Paragraph comprehension has been examined for decades for the purpose of diagnosing subtle aphasic deficits. Yet, many test questions in aphasia batteries can be answered without having heard or read the paragraphs, and the unique features of discourse have seldom been addressed (Nicholas, MacLennan, and Brookshire, 1986). When more care was taken to address this level of comprehension, aphasic LHDs were discovered to recall main ideas better than details, indicating that they, like RHDs, can foreground salient information for subsequent processing. LHDs recall explicit details better than implicit ones. Slowed rate of presentation improved retention in a first session but not a second session (Nicholas and Brookshire, 1986). In the study that delayed the thematic statement in a narrative, LHDs, like normals, were not seriously reduced in recalling main ideas (Hough, 1990). A study of attention allocation showed that listening

to one or two persons telling a story does not matter (Katsuki-Nakamura, Brookshire, and Nicholas, 1988). Also, script knowledge is not diminished with moderate-to-mild aphasia (Armus, Brookshire, and Nicholas, 1989).

Only a few studies so far have been focused on more specific aspects of processing discourse. A pronoun disambiguation task was applied to groups with Alzheimer's dementia or confusion following cardiac surgery (LeDoux, Blum, and Hirst, 1983). In aphasiology, limited phonological encoding in working memory was thought to make it difficult for someone with conduction aphasia to relate widely separate elements in stories (Vallar and Baddeley, 1987). Another study indicated that aphasia can disrupt the ability to find an antecedent in linguistic context. Chapman and Ulatowska (1989) presented four-sentence vignettes in which two characters were introduced in the first sentence and subsequent sentences referred backward with lexical repetition or a pronoun:

(12) The customer shouted angrily at the waitress that the meal was awful. The waitress was new at the job and did not know how to respond.

or

She was new at the job and did not know how to respond.

Subjects were given response cards showing the two characters and were asked questions such as, "Who was new at the job and did not know how to respond?" Such questions alone may bias pointing to waitress over customer, but aphasic subjects generally responded with less accuracy to pronouns than to lexical anaphora. Integration through backward scanning may be studied a little better with sentence pairs and controls over pronominal cues (see also Kahn, Joanette, Ska, and Goulet, 1990).

RHDs and LHDs were compared in some of the studies of indirect intent, and the most consistent conclusion was that aphasia allows for a sensitivity to contextual information not found with RHD. LHDs understood the intent of idioms when preceded by an appropriate story (Stachowiak, Huber, Poeck, and Kerschensteiner, 1977). Aphasic LHDs preferred coherence over surprise when erring in the selection of conclusions for jokes and stories (Bihrle, et al., 1986). For indirect requests at the end of vignettes, LHDs with a wide range of comprehension ability made more errors than RHDs but were sensitive to contextual variables (Weyland, et al., 1989). These findings supplement findings of aphasic ability to get the idea behind simple indirect requests in videoed situations (Hirst, et al., 1984; Wilcox, et al., 1978).

Caplan and Evans (1990) selected subjects diagnosed as having a syntactic parsing disorder according to scores on a sentence comprehension test. The researchers wanted to examine the influence of this presumed impairment on comprehension of long stories. Each narrative was composed in syntactically simple and complex versions, and we get a free writing lesson by comparing the beginnings of these stories sampled in *13*.

(13a) SIMPLE: The robber approached the quiet gas station. He looked in the window. Three women looked after the station . . .

(13b) COMPLEX: It was a quiet gas station that the robber approached. The station was looked after by three women . . .

In the study, comprehension was tested with subsequent statements to verify what happened. Patients were less accurate than normal controls, but story complexity made no difference for both groups. A significant but weak correlation between syntactic testing and story comprehension ($r = 0.52$) was the only indication of a relationship between the two levels of comprehension. Those with good sentence comprehension but poor story comprehension fit the usual building-block concept of severity of deficit. However, some patients did poorly on the sentence test but well with story comprehension, indicating that syntactic disorder can be circumvented with sense from linguistic context for the purpose of doing what subjects were asked to do in this study.

DISCOURSE PRODUCTION

Traditionally, clinical aphasiologists have elicited discourse for assessing word-finding and sentence formulation in a natural flow of continuous utterance. Discourse was not considered to possess unique characteristics except for its length and spontaneity. Pragmatics has opened the door to evaluating, for example, the manner in which word-finding difficulties affect the specification of given-new distinctions in language production. Moreover, persons with CHI and RHD are waiting for clinical research to identify specific objectives of rehabilitation at the discourse level.

Discourse Formulation

Building a theory of discourse formulation might start with Garrett's model of sentence formulation (Figure 3–9). His distinctly vague **message level** is the "locus of the inferential processes that determine structured discourse" (Garrett, 1984). Buckingham (1989) added that it is the basis on which "subsequent mental processes are 'executive driven.'" Thus, we may recognize familiar areas of function and dysfunction that are relevant to this pre-linguistic phase of production; namely, inferencing and executive planning. Also, cognitive processes keep track of contextual inputs to the message level. External contexts contributing to a moment in the process include the communicative situation and previous elements in a dialogue or story. Internal inputs already in the cognitive system include semantic memory, discourse schemas, and communicative conventions. A theory of discourse production is exhibited in Figure 8–1 (Levelt, 1987). It contains the basic components introduced in Figure 3–8 in the form of a conceptualizer, language formulator, and speech articulator. Additional components inform the message

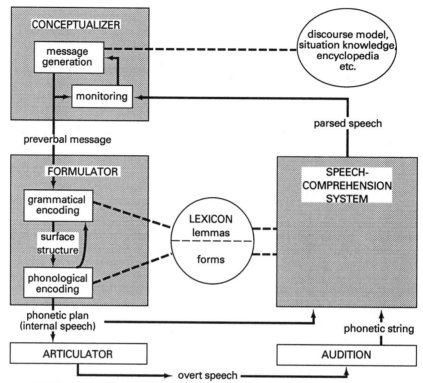

FIGURE 8–1 Another theory of systems involved in language production. The theory accounts for discourse by the inclusion of discourse schemata (e.g., "story grammar"), situation knowledge (e.g., Figure 3–3), and monitoring. (Reprinted by permission from Levelt, W.J.M., *Speaking: From intention to articulation*. Cambridge, MA: Bradford/MIT Press, 1989, p. 9.)

generator and consist of the knowledge base and an active monitoring system, based on what has been said before which is retained partly in the temporary buffer. The monitoring system should keep a speaker on the course defined by the topic of a discourse.

In a nutshell, here is how the message level drives the language formulator. We start with an intention and knowledge of pragmatic conventions and discourse forms (Clark and Clark, 1977). The intention to tell a story activates a narrative structure to guide the ordering of statements to be formed at the functional level of the language formulator. The intention to inform motivates inferences about a listener's knowledge of settings and episodes, which may determine the content to be constructed at the functional level. Inferencing continues as we monitor what has been said. Delineation of given and new information motivates the selection of linguistic devices for establishing cohesion with previously introduced settings and characters of the story. That is, saying "the dirty rat" instead of "a dirty rat" is based on an assumption that the listener knows which rat is being mentioned. Thus, given-new inferences inform lexical selection. We are considerate of the listener's status and beliefs so that content is conveyed tastefully.

Clinical Investigation

When the goal was simply to elicit a spontaneous display of grammatical capacities, clinicians paid little attention to macrostructure. Also, classifying discourse has been inconsistent. Depending on instructions, a pictured scene can elicit description or narration. Ehrlich (1988) asked subjects to tell "everything you see happening..." and called the result "narrative discourse." Others instructed patients to "tell me a story about the picture" (Liles, et al., 1989). Procedural discourse is obtained upon request to report everyday routines such as how to change a tire or bake a cake, which Mentis and Prutting (1987) called narrative. Exposition has not been studied explicitly. It may occur in an interview about family and work, with "minimal interviewer involvement" (Glosser and Deser, 1991). Tasks also vary in input to the message formulator, especially when eliciting stories. Narration can be spontaneous from episodic memory (i.e., "Tell me a favorite story"), can be retold after listening to a story, or can be elicited from the visual mode with cartoon-sequences or filmstrips. Pictures can be removed, and this puts a demand on recall. When pictures are present, pronouns can be used for pointing outward to a situation rather than backward to an antecedent in the narration. This is difficult research that takes time to mature.

Most researchers attend to cohesion, an attribute of any discourse. The first thing to look for is the presence of **cohesive elements,** such as personal or demonstrative pronouns or *the* tagging lexical coreference. Then, we look for an antecedent that forms what investigators call a **cohesive tie.** The following types of cohesive ties were presented by Halliday (1985) as part of his functional grammar:

reference, a semantic binding between anaphoric pronouns and preceding portions of a discourse (e.g., *3, 4, 5*);

lexical coreference, in which content words refer to the same referent as previous words, as in repeating a word or using superordinate terms (e.g., *7, 8*);

ellipsis, a link to previous information according to what is left out (e.g., *She did?*);

conjunction for linking sentences, such as starting a sentence with *Consequently.*

Investigators count the number of elements per cohesive category and employ a new category indicative of "error": the **incomplete cohesive tie.** In an incomplete tie, an antecedent for a cohesive element cannot be found in previous discourse. Cohesion analysis has been most explicitly reported in studies of closed head injury.

Story grammar has been mentioned as a framework for the less frequent study of global structure (e.g., Stein and Glenn, 1979). One analysis was a rating scale, including no points for "unrelated statements," 3 points for "reactive sequences," and 6 points for a "compound or complex episode" (Bottenberg, Lemme, and Hedberg, 1987). Methods have been general, such as recording the number of complete episodes defined according to three major story functions rather than specifying deviations of organization with respect to the many functions in the grammars (Liles, et al., 1989).

The most problematic clinical issue for the study of discourse pertains to the identification of deficit. This problem plagues the entire domain of pragmatics, in which investigators are deciding what is "inappropriate" with respect to a situation. Whose culture, experience, and value system are we to follow in making judgments of propriety? On what basis are we to say that a narration is too much or too little? One person's embellishment is another person's ingenuity. One person's digression is another person's interesting side trip. Discourse style varies with the condition. Mentis and Prutting (1987) found that normal controls used relatively more ellipsis and reference in conversation and more lexical and conjunctive cohesion in procedural discourse. Neurologically intact persons are highly variable story-tellers. A group of 23 college sophomores used as normal controls had a range of 1.25 to 4.20 cohesive ties per T-unit for telling a story, whereas four closed head-injured subjects ranged from 2.38 to 2.92 (Liles, et al., 1989). Finally, discourse production seems to change with aging (Ulatowska, Cannito, Hayashi, and Fleming, 1985). We should expect that researchers will be sensitive to the problems of interexaminer reliability and diagnosis of deficit.

Aphasia

Aphasic persons should tell stories with a crippled language formulator driven by a relatively intact conceptualizer (Figure 8-1). Conceptual capacity and episodic memory should facilitate analysis of situational input. At least, this should be true for moderately to mildly aphasic patients. Severely impaired aphasic persons were noted earlier to have difficulty arranging cartoon frames into a story. Ulatowska and her colleagues examined moderately aphasic subjects for story-retelling and cartoon elicitation. Subjects maintained narrative form by ordering elements of stories. Aphasic subjects did not differ from controls in the number of actions they told but were deficient in producing setting, resolution, and evaluation statements (Ulatowska, Freedman-Stern, et al., 1983). Subjects produced essential elements of everyday routines (Ulatowska, Doyel, Stern, Haynes, and North, 1983). When retelling stories, aphasic subjects foregrounded salient information like controls (Ernest-Baron, et al., 1987). One study indicated that mild aphasia can make it hard to formulate logical relations between events (Bottenberg, Lemme, and Hedberg, 1985).

In early work on cohesion, two patients with aphasia changed in their conversational use of cohesive ties during recovery (Piehler and Holland, 1984), and the condition for eliciting stories did not affect cohesion for ten mildly impaired subjects. Later, fluent subjects produced as many cohesive elements as normal controls during an interview but produced more incomplete cohesive ties with respect to personal and demonstrative pronouns and definite articles (Glosser and Deser, 1991). Because pragmatic sensitivities are coded in language, expressive language deficiencies can mask capacities at the message level. It can be difficult to find antecedents for the vague terms used by individuals with anomic aphasia. In studies of discourse parameters, aphasic subjects are often intact

with respect to "macrolinguistic" discourse-level factors in the midst of reductions in "microlinguistic" parameters, such as number of words, content efficiency, and syntactic complexity.

Closed Head Injury

People with CHI may have trouble telling a story from periods of amnesia. Executive dysfunction may disrupt the realization of goals, action-lists, and conclusions in a story. Investigators have been interested in CHI beyond the acute phase at Levels V to VIII of the scale of cognitive function (Table 6-1). These patients can put words into grammatical sentences and score at high levels on language tests. Yet, they have problems comprehending complex language and expressing complex ideas. "Conversational problems may take the form of rambling talk that moves unpredictably from topic to topic, lack of social initiation, or lack of inhibition which may result in language that is inappropriate or offensive" (Gobble, Dunson, Szekeres, and Cornwall, 1987, p. 369). Rambling verbalization is thought to be a manifestation of impairment of executive control.

Disorganization may be specified in cohesion. The first study was an unpublished doctoral dissertation by Wyckoff in 1984. She studied 11 severely injured subjects (i.e., coma of five to 90 days) from one to 20 months after injury. She elicited a routine (i.e., how to buy groceries) and two narratives (i.e., cartoon-elicited and story-retelling) and found a deficient number of cohesive ties and an additional problem with accuracy of content in narration (cited in Hartley and Levin, 1990; Mentis and Prutting, 1987). Hartley and Levin (1990) analyzed Wyckoff's data and decided that it contained three general profiles: *confused* discourse, which comes soon after injury and contains frequent repetitions, revisions, and a large amount of inaccurate content; *inefficient* but cohesive discourse, which is accurate but sometimes excessive; and *impoverished* discourse, with short utterances, little cohesion, and limited content.

Other early clues to the nature of traumatic discourse came from persons with focal pre-frontal lesions. In a study of patients with tumors, picture description and expositions were elicited about concrete and abstract topics (Kaczmarek, 1984). Subjects with left dorsolateral lesion were inhibited in initiating discourse, and those with left orbitofrontal lesion rambled with digressions and confabulations. Patients with right frontal lesions misinterpreted pictures and misplaced statements. Novoa and Ardila (1987) included cases of trauma among their subjects and portrayed discourse broadly as containing immature or concrete thoughts. As in Kaczmarek's study, lack of initiation occurred more with left lesions. A free association of ideas occurred more with right pre-frontal lesions.

Mentis and Prutting (1987) assessed cohesion for three patients at or above Level VII at least one year after injury. Subjects made high scores on a test for aphasia, and syntax was judged to be preserved. Subjects engaged in ten minutes of conversation with a familiar partner, described their work or rehabilitation program, and produced routines (e.g., how to play a sport or bake a cake). CHIs used fewer cohesive ties than three normal controls for description and routines. The two groups did not differ in number of ties for conversation. CHIs produced pronouns without clear reference, which differed from controls. Use of cohesive elements also differed. Controls used more lexical cohesion. CHIs used more ellipsis. One patient produced little reference. Pattern of use varied according to conditions, which, as indicated earlier, is a normal feature of discourse. Glosser and Deser (1991) obtained a different result. Nine CHIs were not impaired in cohesion. Glosser and Deser studied lower levels of function (V–VII), used an older control group (age 55), limited discourse to interviews, and looked for ties only within the preceding three "verbalizations." These studies are too different to find compatibilities. In general, some high-level CHIs can be deficient in cohesion, and symptoms depend somewhat on the type of discourse examined.

Liles and her colleagues (1989) were curious about the effect of the procedures used for eliciting narration. They examined four CHIs at Level V or above who recovered a high level of language use. College students provided a frame of reference. Two stories were elicited with pictured stimuli. One story was told after viewing a 19-frame filmstrip. The other story was told about a Norman Rockwell painting that remained in view during narration; this was called a "generation task." Two CHIs were deficient in cohesion, and all CHIs presented cohesive styles that differed according to condition. Relative to recalling the story in a filmstrip, the generation task decreased CHIs' use of pronoun reference and increased use of lexical cohesion, a reversal of the normal pattern. The diminished cohesion was attributed to the requirement of translating a static representation into a dynamic series of events. Liles dismissed the factor that a situation was present while telling the Rockwell story so that pronouns could reasonably refer outward instead of backward.

Macrostructure was addressed in two of these investigations. Eliciting exposition about family and work, Glosser and Deser (1991) studied thematic coherence by judging topic maintenance through the whole discourse. CHIs were distinctly impaired, contrary to their good cohesion and sentence form. Thus, deficit was described as being greater for "global" coherence than for "local" coherence. Fluent aphasia had the opposite pattern: intact coherence but deficient lexical and syntactic features of sentences. Liles and others (1989) took advantage of the narrative structure and studied completeness of episodes with respect to presence of an initiating event, actions, and a consequence marking the attainment of goal. Three of four subjects produced no complete episodes for telling a story from a Rockwell painting. The report did not say whether CHIs deviated from story structure in a particular way.

Signs of difficulty appear in samples obtained with a six-frame cartoon called the Flower Pot story. In Huber and Gleber's (1982) cartoon, a man is walking his dog when a falling flower pot hits him on the head, making him angry (i.e., theme, initiating event). The man storms into a building, and a female culprit responds to his rap on the door. She is nice to his dog, and he tips his hat without mentioning the bump on his head. A patient at Level VII gave the following version:

(14) "Looks like the guy got hit on the head with a flower pot, and he's probably swearing or something. He's gonna go up and paste the guy one. He's bangin on the door, and the woman goes up, 'Oh, nice doggie.' And he's all sucked in. And he's showin her the bump on his head. She gave the dog a bone."

We can take two perspectives in evaluating this story. One is to see how well the story stands alone, irrespective of the pictured situation. Another is to consider that the patient was looking at a sequence of pictures. The use of pronouns is fairly clear, except that when considering the story independently from the picture, *the woman* has no antecedent in previous discourse. Also, with respect to the cartoon frames, order of the last two events is reversed. Another patient at the same level told a few more details in a fairly complete and accurate version and, a few minutes later, retold the Flower Pot story with the cartoon absent from view:

(15) "The apartment of the Mrs. Jones or Mr. Jones each waving his cane up her, cause he was watering the plants and fell out the window."

RHD and "Wandering from the Point"

Misconception of a situation and conscious inferencing deficits may fill the conceptualizer (or message-level) with inadequate input to the language system. In studies, input to the formulation system is often specified in pictures from which it may be difficult for RHDs to draw implicit information (Myers, et al., 1985). Using picture descriptions, Myers (1979) examined situation-based inferencing by studying "literal" content (e.g., a woman in a scene) and "inter-

pretive" concepts (e.g., "She is the mother"). An interpretation ratio was determined from number of inferred concepts with respect to total concepts produced. Subjects had deficient interpretation ratios. In another study, subgroups of RHDs producing many or few concepts did not differ in interpretation ratios (Trupe and Hillis, 1985). When input was a cartoon sequence, RHDs omitted information that can be inferred from transitions between pictures (Joanette, et al., 1986). The following example shows how literalness and a focus on detail contributes to description of events in the Cookie Theft picture:

(16) "Well, it's on 8 1/2 × 11 inch paper overall covered by plastic. Looks like it may have been done with drawing pens and India ink on white paper. It's less than 20 pound paper. Else you wouldn't have used black to keep it from shining through. I see window and curtain somebody has pulled back and hospital-type curtains exposing a window and utensils on table, pan or a pot, curtains drawn back with strings tied. Kitchen curtains, no particular design on them. A valance at the top of the curtains with an ordinary angular design. The rest of the curtains only called curtains because of their placement and overall lack of color. There's evidence that the paper was punched for a three ring binder before it was made. The room seems to be filled with air since the curtains have a billowing effect" (Trupe and Hillis, 1985, p. 94; reprinted by permission of the publisher, BRK).

RHDs may also wander from the theme when telling stories (Gardner, 1982). Conceptualizing narrative structure may be elusive, indicated by poor cartoon sequencing relative to Broca's and anomic aphasia (Huber and Gleber, 1982). Autobiographical stories and story-retelling included event-sequence errors, confabulations, digressions, and embellishments (Gardner, et al., 1983; Myers 1979; Rivers and Love, 1980; Trupe and Hillis, 1985). RHDs varied widely in script production; some were tangential, and others terminated too soon (Roman, et al., 1987). Twenty-two RHDs were compared with 20 normal controls in telling a story from a nine-minute video (Uryase, Duffy, and Liles,

1990). RHDs were deficient in cohesion and number of episodes told to a naive listener.

Attributes of narration are revealed in telling the Flower Pot story while looking at the cartoon.

(17) "The guy got hit over the head with a flower pot, and he's mad as a hatter. And he's gone in the house mad and carryin' the dog after him. And he's knockin' at the door to complain to the lady that the pot fell off, I guess. And she's givin' the dog a bone and sends him away happy. But the guy gotta lump on his head."

Story 17 is told somewhat cohesively, with an accurate theme and an approach to the point, seeming to say that the man's or dog's happiness is incongruous with the lump on the man's head. Stories 18 and 19 have more serious problems.

(18) "It looks like the man is out walking his pet dog, and it looks kinda like he's lost, and he's looking for help. So he goes banging on one of the doors, and a lady opens her door, and out runs her pet. Looks like he's asking her for directions, and she gives 'em to him."

(19) "The first one it looks like he's returning home with a stray dog. He takes him in. The third one. Fourth one, he's banging on the door. Fifth one, he's giving the dog a bone. Sixth one, he seem to be pleased with him. And the dog is taking off with his bone."

Story 18 is a good story with a theme, characters, motivated events, and relevant resolution. Yet, it is the wrong story, divorced from the theme and point, and with an incorrect detail about the pet. Story 19 is also the wrong story and has inaccurate details and less logical coherence than 18. Story 19 begins with vague reference to the main character. Poor pronominal reference clouds and changes the story. There is no motive for banging on the door.

Dementia

Studies of comprehension indicate that individuals with Alzheimer's dementia are defi-

cient at discourse levels. There were preliminary reports of problems recognizing nonliteral intentions (Bayles and Kaszniak, 1987). There were problems in all conditions for identifying pronominal antecedents with gender ambiguity (LeDoux, et al., 1983). For assessing production, elderly persons with DAT were interviewed (Glosser and Deser, 1991; Ripich and Terrell, 1988) and were asked to describe a picture (Nicholas, et al., 1985). Listeners judged the discourse of DATs as being incoherent, while healthy elderly subjects were judged as coherent (Ripich and Terrell, 1989). All studies indicated that syntax was intact, but subjects used indefinite words excessively (also Smith, et al., 1989). Glosser and Deser found no impairment of cohesion, but the other investigators had difficulty finding referents for pronouns. Glosser and Deser's impression was that the greatest deficit is in maintaining a topic through an interview, in contrast to subjects with mildly fluent aphasia who are not impaired in global coherence. The investigators concluded that DAT affects a macrolinguistic level, whereas aphasia is damage to a microlinguistic level of language use.

SUMMARY AND IMPLICATIONS

In cognitive terms, our traditional focus on aphasia means that we have been focused on operation of the language system. Yet, in order to deal with this system as it operates for natural communication, it has to be examined in relation to external and internal contexts. External contexts include the linguistic environment of an utterance. Aphasia places constraints on the language system as it struggles to function in conjunction with more intact operations on contexts. RHD makes it difficult to connect a relatively intact language system to more impaired processing of external and internal contexts. For some individuals with CHI, disrupted attentional and executive mechanisms make it difficult to operate a slightly impaired language system. For others with CHI, a genuine aphasia impairs communicative abilities. We bring these broad expectations to the diagnosis and treatment of language deficits in these clinical populations.

In evaluation, we may test the assertion that aphasia is a within-sentence disorder. Each clinical group has displayed some crossover into the other's domain. Aphasic people have some problems with between-sentence integration or inferencing. RHDs have some problems with sensing semantic relations and thematic relations in sentences. Some capabilities may be surprising. RHDs displayed an ability to infer by drawing from context. After comparing theme locations, Hough (1990) decided that "adults with right hemisphere brain-damage appeared unable to utilize the macrostructure as an organizer in apprehending the paragraph" (p. 271), despite success when the theme appeared early. When a score is above-chance and statistically inferior to normal controls, the glass is half full and half empty. Someone with a weakened sense of humor may develop a reputation for being humorless.

The clinical study of natural language use was a relatively new endeavor through the 1980s, motivated by the immediate needs of patients. The few researchers willing to tackle the difficult problems of discourse were indeed pioneers. Investigation has been based on intuition, clinical logic, and some cognitive theory. In the study of comprehension, there has been little use of on-line paradigms, and only a few scattered studies of production have been conducted. When we compare the extent of this research to the extent of the study of within-sentence language in aphasia, we should simply have a healthy humility regarding what we do not know. Research will continue to be less elaborate for aphasic patients than for mild CHIs and RHDs who do not have aphasia holding them back in comprehension and production. Pragmatics and the discourse level appear to be particularly appropriate places to search for language problems with CHI and RHD, but they are also appropriate places for finding communicative capacities in people with aphasia.

9

COMPREHENSIVE TESTS FOR APHASIA

Head (1920) was one of the first to do something about the informal evaluation in case reports of the late nineteenth century. Certain features of aphasia made it mandatory to create special conditions for determining the extent of deficits. He wrote: "An inconsistent response is one of the most striking results produced by a lesion of the cerebral cortex" (p. 89). An aphasic person names an object one moment and fails to name it the next. We cannot determine a reliable level of ability with just one observation and could misdiagnose this ability altogether. Head decided that a type of response had to be observed at least three or four times in what he called "serial tests." He would place a set of common objects on a table (e.g., knife, key, matches) and would ask a patient to point to them after hearing a word and after reading the word. The patient would try to name the objects orally and write the names. Head noted accuracy and speed. He recorded exactly what was said. His procedure was quite similar to methods of today. This chapter surveys current strategies for comprehensive clinical assessment of the language system.

VALID ASSESSMENT

The most important attribute of any test is that it assess what it is supposed to assess. To achieve "content-oriented test construction," a test is built according to an external standard containing the best understanding of the target domain (Lieberman and Michael, 1986). Language has been tricky in this regard. If we think we are assessing someone's language abilities, current understanding would inspire a construct that helps us shed light on processes and size up knowledge. The manual would tell us how to compare scores and analyze errors in order to infer disorder(s) after stroke, closed head injury, and Alzheimer's disease. When we evaluate prevailing batteries on this basis, we should keep in mind that our models for assessment were developed only as psycholinguistics was getting started. Aphasic people could not wait for us to find a basic science. In those days, assessing language after brain damage was nearly the same as looking for aphasia. There was little recognition of closed head injury. People with right-hemisphere stroke were volunteering merely to serve in control groups in studies of aphasia.

Advocates of a cognitive neuropsychological approach to aphasiology have been critical of mainstream aphasia batteries, saying they "were not designed primarily with the aim of elucidating the underlying nature of language disorder" (Byng, Kay, Edmundson, and Scott, 1990, p. 72). Actually, some tests were designed to elucidate the *neurological* nature of disorder, just not the underlying *cognitive* nature of disorder. Authors of the tests responded. Goodglass (1990), who was sympathetic with the principles of componential analysis, noted that "a painstaking array of experimental procedures is required—one that would be quite impractical in the ordinary course of clinical testing" (p. 94). Kertesz (1990) added, "No doubt recent advances in psycholinguistics and cognitive psychology will find their way into practical aphasia tests, modifying the existing batteries" (p. 100). With an awareness of the labor that goes into developing comprehensive test batteries, we can understand why basic research races ahead of the development of such clinical tools.

The tests reviewed in this chapter were designed to diagnose aphasia, so their content is skewed toward the defining features of this disorder. Content has been selected to *minimize the influence of external and internal contexts*. Deficits should be due to language-specific disorder instead of extraneous factors, such as amount of world knowledge (i.e., education) or reasoning skill (i.e., intelligence). The test should be free of cultural bias; if it is not, we take this factor into consideration when interpreting results. To expose the centrality of aphasia, we *assess all modalities of language use independent of each other*. With this strategy, modality-specific disorders can be distinguished from aphasia. Within each modality, *severity of deficit is examined* in two ways. One approach relies on having a sufficient number of subtests graded according to linguistic level. Another orientation does not rely on as many subtests and emphasizes measuring parameters of response.

This chapter spotlights the four test batteries that have been used most widely in the United States and that have provided models for the development of some tests elsewhere. Each test also happens to be unique, as each emphasizes one of three basic objectives of assessment:

Minnesota Test for Differential Diagnosis of Aphasia (MTDDA): created to facilitate planning for treatment by assessing many abilities;

Porch Index of Communicative Ability (PICA): designed to be a sensitive measure of degree of deficit and a patient's progress;

Boston Diagnostic Aphasia Examination (BDAE): designed to diagnose clinical syndromes of aphasia and other signs of focal neuropathology;

Western Aphasia Battery (WAB): created in the image of the BDAE but for diagnosis of syndrome based on scores that also measure progress.

Each test can be employed to meet each objective; the batteries just differ in orientation. Other tests have appeared throughout the history of clinical aphasiology. Some are historically significant, such as Eisenson's (1954) *Examining for Aphasia* and Wepman and Jones' (1961) *Language Modalities Test for Aphasia*. Others are not used widely, such as Spreen and Benton's (1977) *Neurosensory Center Comprehensive Examination for Aphasia* (NCCEA). Other comprehensive batteries have been developed in other countries, such as the *Aachen Aphasia Test* (AAT) in Germany (Huber, Poeck, and Willmes, 1984).

Some legal issues call for a standardized basis for the identification of impairment (Udell, Sullivan, and Schlanger, 1980). One issue pertains to *competency*, which involves whether patients are able to function in the best interests of themselves or those for whom they have been responsible (Porch and Porec, 1977). Competency questions include capacities to stand trial, assume parental responsibilities, live independently, conduct business and personal affairs, and simply the ability to drive. Ability to understand one's will, called testamentary capacity, is indicated by assessment of receptive language. A second issue deals with *compensation*, which involves determining how much impairment has been sustained. A patient may be seeking compensation from an employer or the government or may be suing a physician or hospital because of a surgical accident.

MINNESOTA TEST FOR DIFFERENTIAL DIAGNOSIS OF APHASIA (MTDDA)

Hildred Schuell's MTDDA has been around longer than the others. It is oriented toward the determination of strengths and weaknesses in language functions within all modalities as a guide to planning treatment. While the test has no formal devices for differentiating among language disorders, it does contain devices to facilitate diagnosis of perceptual and motor disorders that might accompany aphasia. Development of the "Schuell test" is a model of the care that can be taken in inventing an assessment device. It evolved from seven revisions over 17 years, beginning with the first version in the summer of 1948 (Brown and Schuell, 1950). The sixth form was made available in 1955 on a limited basis for experimental use. At the Minneapolis Veterans Administration Hospital, this research edition was administered to 155 aphasic patients and 50 nonaphasic patients between 1955 and 1958. The marketed form in 1965 was the eighth version, consisting of only minor revisions of the research edition. After Schuell's death in 1970, the test

and manual were revised slightly by Sefer (Schuell, 1973).

Description and Administration

The MTDDA is the most comprehensive of the aphasia batteries. For example, it contains 505 items, whereas the PICA contains 180 items. Its 46 subtests are distributed among five sections: auditory, visual and reading, speech and language, visuomotor and writing, and numerical relations and arithmetic processes. The four modality sections contain from nine to 15 subtests graded from easy to difficult. Visual perception is assessed early in the reading section, and motoric abilities are examined early in the two expressive sections. A confounding reliance on spoken response occurs in the last two subtests of auditory and reading sections. The Schuell test takes two to six hours to administer, three hours on average. Schuell recommended that it be given in more than one session to minimize influence of fatigue. Clinicians are often flexible in selecting subtests to administer for maximum efficiency given limited time. Method of scoring varies among the subtests. Most involve plus-minus scoring. Schuell left plenty of room in the scoring booklet for notation that would describe a patient's behavior.

Short Versions

Because the complete MTDDA takes so long, Thompson and Enderby (1979) asked, "Is all your Schuell really necessary?" They noted that clinicians "tend to avoid any procedure which is cumbersome or seems redundant. . . . Over many test administrations they eventually learn which items seem useful to them. However, because this is done on an intuitive basis, and looks like a lazy approach . . . clinicians are often embarrassed by the fact that they do not give the full test" (p. 196). Thompson and Enderby decided to create a short form by determining the subtests and items that are too easy or too difficult. They arrived at a version with only five items per subtest. Another short form was developed by Powell, Bailey, and Clark (1980). Schuell's (1957) short version of the research edition was intended to take 30 to 35 minutes. Then she decided that any short test is inadequate. Counting on gradations of difficulty in each section, Schuell (1966) suggested a method for establishing a baseline and ceiling within each section with the complete MTDDA.

Standardization

The research edition was given to aphasic and nonbrain-injured patients described in Schuell's text (Schuell, et al., 1964). Reviews have noted that the test was standardized on 157 aphasic patients, but only a few subtests were actually given to all of them. Eighty percent of subtest means were obtained from only 75 patients. From this smaller group, mean subtest errors are reported in the manual with respect to Schuell's own diagnostic categories. The MTDDA was also administered to 50 nonaphasic hospitalized patients, who had no difficulty with most of the subtests. However, for paragraph reading, 74 percent of the nonaphasic group made an average of 1.86 of eight possible errors. Around 1.5 errors were made on written and oral spelling, although only 36 percent and 26 percent of the group, respectively, made these errors. This data is probably indicative of the dependence of reading and writing on educational and, perhaps, cultural background.

Validity was demonstrated with content and construct analyses. The test was developed from Schuell's assumptions about the unidimensional nature of aphasia (Chapter 5). She used a Guttman scaling of 18 subtests to support her view that aphasia varies in degree and not in kind (Jenkins and Schuell, 1964; Schuell and Jenkins, 1959). Construct validity was analyzed with two factor analyses, and both were supportive of her views (Powell, Clark, and Bailey, 1979; Schuell, Jenkins, and Carroll, 1962). Reliability was not investigated during test development. The "test-retest" series reported in Schuell's text involved retesting upon termination of treatment, with test intervals ranging from one to 13 months (Schuell, et al., 1964). Thus, the idea was to measure progress.

Interpretation

Diagnosis of deficit is based mainly on the presence of errors. Degree of impairment is based on a percentage of correct responses. Clinicians refer to linguistic level of impairment, such as whether problems begin with words, sentences, or paragraphs. Differential diagnosis of aphasia, confusion, or dementia depends on medical history and careful analysis of symptoms. In the manual, patterns of deficit are related to Schuell's classification, in which disorders are identified according to whether someone has aphasia plus sensory and/or motor impairments. Schuell did not recognize qualitative differences among aphasias, and the manual does not provide guidelines for diagnosing syndromes. The short version revealed differences among aphasia, apraxia of speech, confusion after head trauma, and intellectual impairment of dementia (Halpern, Darley, and Brown, 1973). Recovery has not been studied with this test on the scale achieved with the PICA and WAB. The test has been ignored for this purpose because of its length and its susceptibility to inconsistent administration and scoring. The manual has general guidelines for prognosis based on the author's influential clinical experience.

PORCH INDEX OF COMMUNICATIVE ABILITY (PICA)

When Bruce Porch's test was published in 1967, it took some time for many experienced clinicians to adjust to its demands for consistency, which were inconsistent with the MTDDA's flexibility. Porch wanted us to portray our patients' problems with numbers. It was startling that a 40-hour workshop was needed to learn the test. Yet, other speech-language pathologists, especially in Veterans Administration hospitals, were looking for a steady precision, and they welcomed the test with open arms. Angst still follows the PICA around, as when Lincoln (1988) asked, "Are we flogging a dead horse?" She felt the test is more useful for research than for clinical endeavor. Among the responses to her commentary, Crockett and Purves (1988) advised that "the fact that the PICA is not all things to all practitioners should not be used as a rationale for recommending that it be eliminated from the clinical shelves, where in fact it may sit all too often" (p. 509). This perspective applies to any test.

The PICA is oriented toward measuring severity of language disorder by conforming to psychometric axioms that maximize reliability. Use of the initial test as a basis for prognosis has also been explored quite seriously. From "what was to be a nine-month study" and a doctoral dissertation in 1959, Porch standardized the basic battery and scoring system during a six-year period. The manual was published in two volumes. Volume II, *Administration, Scoring and Interpretation*, was revised in 1971 and 1981. The current manual includes supplements for the scoring procedure and, most notably, a change in summary categories. The scoring

system has been applied widely, having been incorporated, for example, into the *Revised Token Test* (McNeil and Prescott, 1978). Porch (1986) interpreted results according to a cybernetic theory.

Description

The PICA contains 18 subtests of the four language modalities and other functions. Similar to Henry Head's serial tests, each subtest utilizes ten common objects arranged neatly on a table. The objects are a cigarette, comb, fork, key, knife, matches, pen, pencil, quarter, and toothbrush. Order of subtest administration differs from other batteries (Table 9–1). The test is not sectioned according to modalities. Auditory, reading, and speech tasks are mixed together in subtests I through XII. Graphic subtests are together at the end. Order of subtests proceeds roughly from difficult to easy, as opposed to other batteries that start with easy subtests. In the revised version, subtests are classified so that scores can be summarized according to meaningful functions. For many years, subtests were cat-

TABLE 9–1 Order of administering PICA subtests. (Adapted by permission from Porch, B. E., *Porch Index of Communicative Ability: Theory and Development, Volume 1*. Palo Alto, Calif.: Consulting Psychologists Press, 1967).

Test	Output (1967)	Function (1981)	Task
I	Verbal		Describes function of object
II	Gestural	Pantomime	Demonstrates function of object
III	Gestural	Pantomime	Demonstrates function in order
IV	Verbal		Names objects
V	Gestural	Reading	Reads function and position
VI	Gestural	Auditory	Points to object, given its function
VII	Gestural	Reading	Reads name and position
VIII	Gestural	Visual	Matches picture to object
IX	Verbal		Completes sentence with object name
X	Gestural	Auditory	Points to object, given its name
XI	Gestural	Visual	Matches object to object
XII	Verbal		Repeats name of object
A	Graphic	Writing	Writes function of object
B	Graphic	Writing	Writes name of object
C	Graphic	Writing	Writes name to dictation
D	Graphic	Writing	Writes name when spelled
E	Graphic	Copying	Copies name of object
F	Graphic	Copying	Copies geometric forms

egorized according to modality of response; namely, gestural, verbal, and graphic performances. Auditory and reading functions, because they involved "gestural" response, were collapsed into a summary score that included object manipulation. We had to qualify reports of this score so that auditory and reading abilities could be addressed distinctly. Now performance is summarized into more readily interpretable categories shown in Table 9–1: pantomime (i.e., object manipulation), auditory, reading, visual, verbal, writing, and copying.

The rationale for organization lies in Porch's psychometric goals. The ten objects are used across each subtest in order to compare functions without changes in content. Word comprehension and retrieval can be compared with respect to the same vocabulary. Because of the lexical constant, tasks are ordered to minimize a "learning effect." If word comprehension were to come before naming, as in other batteries, a patient would have heard the word before the naming test. Minimal linguistic information about the objects is given early, with maximum information deferred until later. Also, keeping the number of items per subtest constant permits comparison of scores from the same sample size. However, comparing auditory comprehension and reading is confounded with an addition of prepositions in the reading stimuli (e.g., "Put this card under the fork"). A study indicated that most of the difference in scores between these two functions is due to the complexity of reading stimuli rather than a modality difference per se (Sanders, Davis, and Wells, 1981).

Administration and Scoring

Administration is constrained by explicit guidelines to maximize the likelihood that a patient is assessed the same way each time the test is repeated. These prescriptions apply to the physical conditions of testing as well as to what a clinician is to say and do for each subtest. Completing the battery in one session is preferred. It takes an average of about one hour for a well-trained clinician to give the PICA, a range of 22 to 143 minutes. Subtests I through XII usually can be administered in 20 minutes, while the six graphic tests take much longer. Comparable scores can be obtained whether writing is done by hand or on a computer (Selinger, Prescott, and Katz, 1987).

A multidimensional scoring system of 16 scale points was conceived so that several dimensions of impaired responding could be quantified (Table 9–2). It is intended to be descriptive and yet manageable. The scale-points reflect degrees of correctness and incorrectness and, therefore, provide more sensitive scores than a plus-minus system. Each of 180 responses is assigned a score, which leads to a single *overall score*, indicative of general ability and especially useful for studies of recovery. The scale is based on five dimensions of response. The most inclusive dimension is *accuracy*; 8 to 16 represent degrees of correctness, and 7 to 1 stand for variation of error. Correctness is divided according to four other dimensions: *responsiveness* (amount of information needed by a patient to complete a task), *completeness* of response, *promptness* (time to respond), and *efficiency* (motoric facility). There are subtle variations among subtests in the definition of scale-points. Assigning these scores quickly is learned from extensive practice in the 40-hour "PICA workshops." Mean scores are used for characterizing severity and pattern of deficit. An average such as 12.25 for a subtest or category of subtests is called a *response level*. In the 1981 revision, diacritical markings provided additional notation for characterizing a response.

Short Versions

There has been an increasing demand for assessment taking less than an hour. Would an overall score from a shortened PICA be the same as an overall obtained from the complete test? A regression analysis of 222 administrations of the complete test determined that ten subtests and five objects per subtest produces the overall score that is obtained from the complete test (DiSimoni,

TABLE 9–2 Multidimensional scoring system of the PICA (Adapted by permission from Porch, B. E., *Porch Index of Communicative Ability: Theory and Development, Volume 1*, Palo Alto, Calif.: Consulting Psychologists Press, 1967).

Score	Level	Description of Response
16	Complex	Accurate, complex, and elaborate
15	Complete	Accurate and complete
14	Distorted	Accurate, complete, but with reduced facility
13	Complete-delayed	Accurate, complete, but slow or delayed
12	Incomplete	Accurate but incomplete
11	Incomplete-delayed	Accurate, incomplete, slow or delayed
10	Corrected	Accurate after self-correction of error
9	Repetition	Accurate after repetition of instruction
8	Cued	Accurate after specified cue
7	Related	Inaccurate but related to correct response
6	Error	Inaccurate
5	Intelligible	Intelligible but not related to test item
4	Unintelligible	Unintelligible, differentiated
3	Minimal	Unintelligible, not differentiated
2	Attention	Attention to item but no response
1	No response	No awareness of test item

Keith, Holt, and Darley, 1975). A similar version was used by Wallace and Canter (1985) for selecting subjects for a study. Two other short versions had similar results (DiSimoni, Keith, and Darley, 1980). One of these, called the "SPICA," has been used in one clinic for years (Holtzapple, Pohlman, LaPointe, and Graham, 1989). Only subtests I, VI, VII, and D are presented with the ten objects, but the overall score from the SPICA is significantly different from the overall obtained with the PICA. Another SPICA with five objects was reliable but had less sensitivity to recovery over four weeks than the complete test (Lincoln and Ells, 1980; Phillips and Halpin, 1978). A shortened PICA may be merely efficient for a single assessment and may not be the best means of measuring change.

Normative Information

Performance of 130 normal adults was obtained by Duffy, Keith, Shane, and Podraza (1976). It is discussed here in some detail because the report is out of print. Whereas an average of one hour is needed for most aphasic patients, the normal subjects breezed through the PICA in about 30 minutes. The normal subjects had some difficulty in areas that can be influenced by education. Ninety-five percent averaged 12.95 on the graphic subtests, with a mean of 9.63 on writing sentences. Also, in demonstrating function of objects, they averaged 11.52 (subtest II) and 12.79 (III). Most of the sample averaged 12.05 on the first verbal subtest, which requires a spoken description of object function. Therefore, a score of 15 indicates a level defined by the test and does not necessarily indicate normality (see Table 9–3).

Conversion tables were developed for right-hemisphere-damaged patients (RHD) according to the 1967 subtest categories (Deal, Deal, Wertz, Kitselman, and Dwyer, 1979a). Porch and Palmer (1986) revised the tables from another sample of RHDs so that tables would relate to revisions of the test. Porch thought the original sample might not have been representative of all RHDs. His revised response levels turned out to be considerably lower than the earlier scores. If Deal's higher scores were used, "a patient with minor deficits would be described as being at a low percentile level and more impaired than his actual symptoms suggest" (Porch and Palmer, 1986, p. 275). Table 9–4 contains a few scores compared with LHDs. As deficit increases (i.e., percentiles), the dif-

TABLE 9–3 Normal adults (Duffy, et al., 1976) and aphasic adults (Porch, 1971a, 1981) compared according to classification available when the normals were studied. Aphasia scores illustrate the impact of sample expansion between 1971 (N = 280) and (N = 357).

	Overall	*Gestural*	*Verbal*	*Graphic*
Normal Adults				
Range	13.40–14.99	13.73–15.00	13.48–15.03	11.18–15.03
Average	14.46	14.66	14.55	14.12
Left-Hemisphere Damage				
95th percentile (1981)	14.44	14.74	14.62	13.91
50th percentile (1981)	10.89	12.96	10.77	8.22
50th percentile (1971)	10.64	12.73	11.20	7.50

ference between aphasia and RHD becomes more pronounced. A difference in auditory comprehension does not appear until severe overall impairment at the 25th percentile, whereas a difference in verbal expression becomes pronounced at a higher level or around the 50th percentile. Relative deficit is reversed for copying shapes (subtest F), as RHDs have lower scores than aphasic patients. RHDs' difficulty is striking, considering that persons with RHD are not likely to have paralysis of their preferred (right) hand, while many aphasic people attempt to draw with their weakened preferred (right) hand.

Validity and Reliability

Content concentrates on language instead of a broader communicative ability. Construct validity was investigated by Clark, Crockett, and Klonoff (1979b) to determine whether the test measures the dimensions of communicative function that were intended. Several factor analytic procedures were applied to Porch's correlation matrix of subtest means. One analysis exposed three factors that did not correspond precisely to the three output categories in the original test. A general factor was revealed in another factor analysis. Results supported the notion that the PICA measures three dimensions of language and a general dimension related to the test's overall score.

Criterion-related validity has been evaluated by several investigators in cross-validation with respect to other tests. Correlations were 0.93 with the *Aphasia Language Performance Scales* (Keenan and Brassell, 1975), 0.89 with Kertesz's *Western Aphasia Battery* (Sanders and Davis, 1978), and 0.93 with *Communicative Abilities in Daily Living* (CADL) (Holland, 1980a). Correlation with Holland's CADL is interesting, because this test measures communication in a much different way (Chapter 10). Holland also used a measure of communication in natural environments as a criterion for comparison with the CADL and the PICA. The PICA correlated at 0.55 with Holland's naturalistic measure. Therefore, the PICA has been demonstrated to possess strong criterion-related validity with respect to standardized tests but may fall short of reflecting natural communicative abilities in daily life.

To determine reliability, Porch (1967) reported interexaminer and test-retest correlations. Relationships among three workshop-trained scorers of 30 patients were 0.93 or higher for subtests and 0.97 or higher for the original response categories. Upon retest two weeks or less after initial testing, stability for a group of 40 patients was 0.90 or higher for all but five subtests. Stability in response categories was 0.98 (overall), 0.96 (gestural), 0.99 (verbal), and 0.96 (graphic). All shifts between first and second subtests involved a mean improvement of 0.38 points. This indicates that a *subtest shift* of 0.40 or more is likely to represent real change. A change of 0.38 or less could simply be random variation that occurs between two test sessions. Mean *overall shift* was about the same.

TABLE 9–4 Response levels from 94 right-hemisphere-damaged patients (Porch and Palmer, 1986) compared with 357 left-hemisphere-damaged aphasic patients (Porch, 1981) at percentiles determined for each group. Copying shapes is subtest F, in which RHDs have lower scores than LHDs.

		Overall	Auditory Comprehension	Verbal	Writing	Copying Shapes
90th	RHD	13.99	15.00	14.59	13.21	13.8
	LHD	14.04	15.00	14.35	13.18	14.5
75th	RHD	13.47	15.00	14.24	11.94	12.8
	LHD	12.89	15.00	13.50	11.05	14.0
60th	RHD	12.95	14.87	13.92	10.66	12.1
	LHD	11.71	14.60	12.30	9.23	13.3
50th	RHD	12.60	14.80	13.73	9.82	11.7
	LHD	10.89	14.25	10.77	8.22	13.0
40th	RHD	12.34	14.66	13.45	8.90	11.2
	LHD	9.96	13.60	8.90	7.33	12.4
25th	RHD	11.32	14.15	12.56	7.50	9.9
	LHD	8.38	11.70	6.04	6.29	11.1
10th	RHD	9.33	11.30	10.30	5.63	7.3
	LHD	6.15	8.05	3.75	4.98	8.0

Interpretation

The mean response level scores (i.e., raw scores) for each subtest, the function categories, and overall performance are starting points in using the PICA for differential diagnosis, prognosis, and treatment planning. The formatting and analysis of scores are hastened with a program for computers developed by Porch and Katz called PICAPAD (cited in Mills, 1986).

Diagnosis. Aphasic deficit at the 95th percentile includes scores of 14.44 overall, 15.00 for auditory and reading comprehension, 14.62 for verbal subtests, and 13.46 for written language. Table 9–3 shows that these scores are similar to normal, leaving diagnosis of mild aphasia to clinical judgment. **Percentiles** depict severity of deficit with respect to a standard population of aphasic people. Different forms are used to display patterns of response levels and to facilitate interpretation. Modality-specific conditions, such as motor speech deficits or illiteracy, are revealed by depressions of the relevant modalities beyond what would be expected with respect to the typical aphasia pattern among modalities. For example, a patient with agrammatic aphasia and apraxia of speech might display verbal scores that are depressed below written language scores. Consistent with issues discussed in Chapter 5, someone with conduction aphasia might have a similar pattern, so attention to qualitative features of expression should be considered. In a report of a case of conduction aphasia, "we did not see the oral, nonverbal posturing—starts, stops, and reattempts—and inconsistent articulatory errors typical of the patient who suffers apraxia of speech" (Wertz, Bernstein-Ellis, and Roberts, 1989, p. 142).

The manual contains a conversion table and graphed profiles for persons with bilateral or diffuse brain damage (also see Porch, 1978; Watson and Records, 1978; Wertz, 1985). Porch (1981) has noted three exceptions to aphasia displayed by this group, called **three bilateral signs:** (1) a visual-auditory reversal with either auditory subtests VI or X higher than the visual matching subtests VIII or XI, (2) high verbal ability near levels of receptive modalities, and (3) unusually low copying subtests E and F. The second and third signs in particular are also seen with RHD (Table 9–4). A pattern from right-hemisphere damage includes the visual-auditory reversal and unusually low copying. Porch has investigated patterns in neurosis and psychosis and cases of malingering in which aphasia is feigned (Porch and Porec, 1977; Porec and Porch, 1977). A "nonaphasia profile" shows poor scores on easy tasks and a random up-and-down pattern of response levels.

Traumatic brain injury was studied with 15 cases, with most having been comatose from one day to four months (Bernstein-Ellis, et al., 1985). A discriminant analysis showed a different deficit pattern from that of aphasia after focal LHD. Differences were seen in visual matching (VIII, XI), object naming (IV), auditory comprehension of object function (VI), and writing sentences (A). Significant differences were observed, with visual matching being worse and written language being better after head injury. The three bilateral signs did not distinguish the two groups. Ten of the head-injured patients showed one sign, five showed two signs, and none displayed all three. Therefore, cause of bilateral damage may be an important variable with respect to the PICA's diagnostic clues.

There has been some curiosity about the PICA's capacity to identify syndromes of aphasia and, consequently, sites of lesion (Porch, 1978, 1981). Factor analyses have shown that this test is capable of differentiating aphasic persons into distinct groups (e.g., Clark, Crockett, and Klonoff, 1979a). Metter, Riege, Hanson, and others (1984) wondered if these groups are related to the syndromes as identified by the Boston Diagnostic Aphasia Examination. They discovered that five PICA-derived groups did not correspond to the syndromes, and the test was less predictive of lesion site than the BDAE. It appears that the PICA measures abilities that are irrelevant for syndrome identification and localization of lesions, which may be expected because the test does not measure sentence repetition and does not distinguish certain verbal symptoms in its scoring.

Recovery and Prognosis. The PICA has been used extensively to measure progress. Reliable *change scores* (i.e., differences between a test and retest) can be determined for general and specific abilities. A 10 percent increase in the overall score is a reasonable treatment goal, and 5 percent "has a limited effect on communicative ability" (Porch, 1981, p. 105). One patient, who improved from 55 to 80 points on another test, improved by eight percentile points on the PICA (Wertz, et al., 1989).

Mean scores, especially the overall, form the basis for predicting later levels of language function. A few studies were undertaken to determine the predictive potential of PICA scores. Porch (1974) correlated early overall scores with later overall scores using a relatively small group of aphasic subjects with mixed etiologies. Later, the predictability of summary scores and age was examined using 144 patients with occlusive CVAs (Porch, Collins, Wertz, and Friden, 1980). Porch looked for the best combination of these factors obtained at one, three, or six months post onset for predicting overall scores at three, six, and 12 months. The most consistent predictor was the now defunct gestural mean, and the least successful predictor was age. The conclusion was that statistical prediction is possible, supported also by Deal, Deal, Wertz, Kitselman, and Dwyer (1979b). Porch and his colleagues (1980) warned that clinical application of a predictive formula was premature until the original study is replicated and other factors are considered. Nevertheless, statistical prediction has been tried based on assumptions about a patient's range of performance one month after onset (see Chapter 11).

The Controversies:
Questions and Answers

1. Does the order of subtests disturb a patient in a manner that confounds assessment of language ability? Emerick and Hatten (1979) felt that starting with the most difficult verbal task often overwhelms patients and disrupts subsequent performance.

Dumond, Hardy, and Van Demark (1978) used PICA subtests to investigate a general question about the effect of order of task difficulty. There was no difference in performance between hard-to-easy and easy-to-hard ordered tasks. We should be concerned about the initial difficulty of the PICA, a concern that is lessened with the realization that early subtests II and III are quite easy for many patients. A sensitive examiner can minimize early frustration and still follow the rules of psychometrics. A patient may be advised of this structural feature prior to beginning the test. If the first three items of a subtest produce failure so striking that it is likely to be maintained for the rest of the subtest, then the three items can suffice for obtaining the mean for that subtest.

2. Does the formality of administration weaken rapport established with a client? Keenan and Brassell (1975) suggested that aphasia batteries in general are too time-consuming, too restricted as to where they can be given, and too rigid in administration. They argued that tests "have been so formal that they have served to break down the rapport which clinicians spend so much time and effort to establish" (p. 2). Emerick and Hatten (1979) thought that clinicians respond mechanically to patients when using the PICA, breaking down the clinician-client relationship. Indeed, we might be concerned about moments during the test when we have to ask an adult whether he or she has ever used a fork or a toothbrush. Naturalness is sacrificed to achieve reliability. For another perspective, we might consider that a client's reaction to any test is related to a clinician's handling of the situation as much as it is related to the test itself. The PICA does not cause a clinician to be mechanical and need not be given mechanically. A clinician can be warm and consistent, too. Also, these 60 minutes need not be harmful to a relationship that begins before testing and develops over several weeks of circumstances that differ from testing. The PICA can be presented and taken with a smile.

3. Is the scoring system valid in its ranking of responses? Clinicians wonder whether a 12 (incomplete) is really better than a 10 (self-correction), because more information may be conveyed in the latter. Duffy and Dale (1977) and McNeil, Prescott, and Chang (1978) questioned whether the scoring system represents a response hierarchy and, therefore, a truly ordinal scale. Ordinality means that a 12 is better than an 11 and a 6, but a 12 is not necessarily twice as good as a 6. The distance between 12 and 11 need not be the same as the distance between 6 and 5. In the two studies, students not familiar with the PICA were asked to develop their own rankings of the scale-point definitions based on judgments about functional communicative adequacy of the definitions. Both studies showed that repeats (9) and self-corrections (10) were considered to be better than incomplete responses (12). The multidimensional system may not entirely reflect what people consider to be more or less effective communication. McNeil and others (1978) also discovered that students' rankings varied from subtest to subtest, indicating that ordinality depends on the situation. A test with different 16-point scoring systems for different subtests would be unwieldy at best. However, these studies indicate that borrowing the PICA system for research should be done with caution and that a clinician's interpretation of subtest performances should be tempered with pragmatic considerations.

4a. Are subtest means accurate in their description of a patient's behavior? Silverman (1974) raised a couple of issues concerning mean scores. He argued that subtest means can be inaccurate because a 10.0 could be obtained from a variety of responses well above and well below a 10. The same mean may also be derived from responses that vary minimally around 10. The question of representativeness of a mean was raised by Caramazza regarding subject groups, and Zurif noted that the same problem exists for depicting an individual's performance (Chapter 5). Silverman suggested that the mode, the most frequent response, would be more descriptive in many instances. Porch (1974) replied that one mode can be difficult to obtain, while we can always compute a single mean. He added that mean scores were not intended to be descriptively precise but, instead, were intended to be a convenient quantification of performance level with certain advantages for statistical analyses. For clinical reports, Van Demark (1974) recommended including the individual cell scores, especially when they are not reflected in the mean.

4b. Are the PICA's means appropriate for statistical analysis? Silverman (1974) noted that there are technical assumptions underlying the use of a mean score statistically. A mean is most appropriate when it is derived from an interval or ratio scale, not from an ordinal scale. Porch (1974) countered with some disadvantages in using a mode statistically and some advantages to using a mean. He concluded that a mean provides a valuable compromise. Duffy and Dale (1977) decided to investigate this issue. They compared Porch's ordinal scale with an interval scale derived from the 16 levels of response in the PICA. From tests of 50 patients, correlations between the ordinal scale and the derived interval scale were above 0.99 for all 18 subtest means and all summary means. Duffy and Dale concluded that the PICA scoring system functions as if it were an interval scale.

BOSTON DIAGNOSTIC APHASIA EXAMINATION (BDAE)

The "Boston Exam" is oriented toward sampling behaviors that are crucial for identification of clinical syndromes. These behaviors include spontaneous extended verbalization and repetition. The test has been used by researchers as a basis for grouping subjects according to syndrome. It follows an orientation to clinical neuropsychological assessment called the "process approach," which shuns scores and prefers description of apparently strategic behaviors (Kaplan, 1988). This is indicated by the absence of broad summary

scores and reliance on pattern of deficit for depicting a patient's disorder. For planning treatment, it is a relatively comprehensive battery. Its 27 subtests place the BDAE between the PICA and the MTDDA in length.

Harold Goodglass and Edith Kaplan started developing the test in the early 1960s, coincident with their pioneering studies of extended utterance and previously neglected linguistic aspects of aphasia. Subjects were described in these early studies according to something called the "Boston VA Hospital Aphasia Test." Some of its components were part of this research. A rating scale profile of speech characteristics was seen in an analysis of spontaneous utterance (Goodglass, Quadfasel, and Timberlake, 1964), and other portions devoted to peculiarities of word comprehension and naming were introduced by Goodglass, Klein, Carey, and Jones (1966). The Boston Exam was published first in 1972, but a new normative sample of patients was obtained between 1976 and 1982. The test was revised in a royal blue edition (Goodglass and Kaplan, 1983).

Description of the BDAE

The first section is distinctive in its assessment of *conversational and expository speech.* Conversation is elicited with an interview and discussion of familiar topics. Then a patient is asked to describe the previously mentioned **Cookie Theft** picture: a kitchen setting in which a child, perched on a tilting stool, is reaching for a cookie jar in a cupboard while a woman, appearing unaware of the crime, is washing dishes over a sink with water running over onto the floor. This picture has commonly been used in studies of discourse production.

Formal testing begins with the *auditory comprehension* section. For understanding words, patients point to objects, actions, letters, numbers, colors, and shapes. Body parts are used to test left-right discrimination as a left parietal lobe function. The *oral expression* section includes subtests for apraxia, automatic sequences, singing, repetition, naming, and reading aloud. Subtle apraxias of speech are sought by having a patient repeatedly produce "huckleberry" and "caterpillar." A unique feature is the systematic examination of repetition with sentences of increasing length and decreasing probability (e.g., "I got home from work" and "The phantom soared across the foggy heath"). Naming is assessed with the categories and items used for word comprehension. A word fluency subtest requires production of as many animal names as possible in 90 seconds. The *understanding written language* section contains five fairly brief subtests. The *writing* section contains seven subtests for assessing mechanics, spelling, naming, and narrative production.

The manual includes suggestions for supplementary testing of verbal and nonverbal functions. The *psycholinguistic explorations* are aimed at auditory comprehension of prepositions, passive sentences, and possessives, and repetition of constructions "that may not have occurred in free conversation." One recommendation originated in Goodglass' story completion studies of grammatical elements in Broca's aphasia (Chapter 5). Three examples for eliciting verb tense markers are provided, and the examiner is free to create others. In the nonverbal realm, the *spatial-quantitative battery* shows how a clinician can search for constructional apraxia with drawing tasks, finger agnosia with finger naming, and acalculia with basic arithmetic.

Administration and Scoring

The Boston Exam can be administered in one to three hours. Initial conversational and expository speech is described with a simple *aphasia severity rating scale* and a *rating scale profile of speech characteristics*, shown later in Figure 9–2. Scoring differs among subtests, as there are plus-minus scoring, four-point scales, and frequency counts of paraphasias in most of the oral expression subtests. The possible score varies from 8 or 10 points on some subtests to 105 points on confrontation naming. Therefore, clinical reporting of scores should be in terms of ratios. For classifying symptoms, "jargon" in the 1972 edition

was replaced with *paragrammatism* (see Chapters 1, 5). A *subtest summary profile* provides a format for depicting performance (Figure 9–1). Besides cosmetic adjustments, the subtest profile differs from the 1972 version in positioning of paraphasia scores and the rating for graphic descriptions of the Cookie Theft "because of the experience that the 1972 scale ratings did not adequately reflect clinical assessment of performance" (Goodglass and Kaplan, 1983, p. 45).

Standardization

A new set of norms was developed for the second edition. Performance by 147 normal adults, determined in a study by Borod, Goodglass, and Kaplan (1980), is now shown in the test manual. This data includes means, standard deviations, and ranges for each subtest. In the Borod article, moreover, performance is differentiated as to age, with scores reported by decade. The manual also contains normal scores for the spatial-quantitative battery, distributed according to age and education. The normative sample of 242 aphasic persons replaces the sample obtained for the first edition. The second sample was loaded with patients who had focal lesions. Data from the new group was used to relate raw scores to **percentiles** across the top of the subtest summary profile (Figure 9–1). The percentiles replace the obscure z-score method of analysis in the first edition.

It has been difficult to compare the BDAE to other tests statistically because of its lack of summary scores. Criterion-related validity as a measure of communicative ability was investigated by Holland (1980a) and Ulatowska, Macaluso-Haynes, and Mendel-Richardson (1976). Holland found that the BDAE correlated at 0.84 with the CADL and at 0.49 with her measure of communication in natural circumstances. Ulatowska compared the Boston Exam to an assessment of functional communication skills at patients' homes. She did not find a significant relationship between BDAE scores and home-visit scores with 12 subjects. Again, we find a strong relationship between formal tests but

SUBTEST SUMMARY PROFILE

NAME: **J.M.**   DATE OF EXAM: **12-9-68**

Category	Subtest	0	10	20	30	40	50	60	70	80	90	100
PERCENTILES:		0	10	20	30	40	50	60	70	80	90	100
SEVERITY RATING			0	(✱)				2		3	4	5
FLUENCY	ARTICULATION RATING		1	2		5	6		7			
	PHRASE LENGTH				3	4	5	6	7			
	MELODIC LINE			2	4			6	7			
	VERBAL AGILITY		0	2	5		8	9	11	13	14	
AUDITORY COMPREHENSION	WORD DISCRIMINATION	0	15	25	37	46	53	60	64	67	70	72
	BODY-PART IDENTIFICATION	0	1	5	10	13	15	16	17	18		20
	COMMANDS	0	3	4	6	8	10	11	13	14		
	COMPLEX IDEATIONAL MATERIAL	0		2	3	4	5	6	8	9		12
NAMING	RESPONSIVE NAMING			0	1	5	10	15	20		27	30
	CONFRONTATION NAMING		0	9	28	43	60	72	84	94	105	114
	ANIMAL NAMING			0	1	2		3	4	6		23
ORAL READING	WORD READING			0	1	3	7	15	21	26	30	
	ORAL SENTENCE READING					0	1	4	7	9	10	
REPETITION	REPETITION OF WORDS			0	2	5	8		9		10	
	HIGH-PROBABILITY			0	1		4	5	7	8		
	LOW-PROBABILITY						1	2	4	6	8	
PARAPHASIA	NEOLOGISTIC	40	16	9	4	2	1					
	LITERAL	47	17	12	9	6	5	3	2	1		
	VERBAL	40	23	18	15	12	9	7	4		1	0
	EXTENDED	75	12	5	3	1						
AUTOMATIC SPEECH	AUTOMATIZED SEQUENCES			0	1	2	3	6	7	8		
	RECITING				0					2		
READING COMPREHENSION	SYMBOL DISCRIMINATION	0	2	5	7	8	9					
	WORD RECOGNITION	0	1	3	4	5	6			8		
	COMPREHENSION OF ORAL SPELLING					0	1	3	4	6	7	8
	WORD-PICTURE MATCHING		0	1	4	6	8	9				
	READING SENTENCES AND PARAGRAPHS		0	1	2	3	4	5	6	7		10
WRITING	MECHANICS	1		2				4		5		
	SERIAL WRITING		0	7	18	25	30	33	40	43	46	47
	PRIMER-LEVEL DICTATION		0	1		6	9	11	13	14	15	
	SPELLING TO DICTATION						1	2	3	5	7	10
	WRITTEN CONFRONTATION NAMING				0	1	2	6	7		9	10
	SENTENCES TO DICTATION							1	3	6	8	12
	NARRATIVE WRITING					1	2			3	4	5
MUSIC	SINGING		0			2						
	RHYTHM		0					2				
SPATIAL AND COMPUTATIONAL	DRAWING TO COMMAND	0	6	7	8	9	10	11	12			
	STICK MEMORY	0	3	4	6	7	8	9	10	11		14
	3-D BLOCKS			0	2	4	5	6	7	8	10	
	TOTAL FINGERS	0	54	70	81	93	100	108	120	130	141	
	RIGHT-LEFT	0	1	3	4	6	8	9	11		16	
	MAP ORIENTATION (OMITTED)	0		2	5	6	9	11	13	14		
	ARITHMETIC			0	2	4	8	11	14	17	21	27	32
	CLOCK SETTING	0		3	4	6		8	9	12		
		0	10	20	30	40	50	60	70	80	90	100

FIGURE 9–1 The *BDAE*'s subtest summary profile of scores in relation to percentiles for the aphasic population. This is an example of Broca's aphasia with good auditory comprehension, few paraphasias, and expressive problems mainly in repetition. (Reprinted by permission from Goodglass, H., & Kaplan, F., *The Assessment of Aphasia and Language Disorders*. Chicago: Riverside, 1983, p. 78).

not between a formal test and naturalistic observation.

Several factor analyses were carried out on the sample of 242 aphasic patients and on smaller groups. The manual presents the various results without strong conclusion. The BDAE was shown to measure several language factors with factor rankings varying subtly depending on the analysis that was done. Discriminant analysis was also conducted "to provide the user of this test with an improved basis for deriving diagnostic classifications from test score configurations" (Goodglass and Kaplan, 1983, p. 23). Formulas were proposed for computing diagnosis of Broca's, Wernicke's, conduction, and anomic aphasias. The formulas involve selected raw scores and weights. While they exhibited a 90 percent hit rate for 41 selected cases, the authors stated that further validation of the formulas is needed.

Validity of the BDAE as to its classification of aphasias was questioned by Wertz (1983). There are two distinct issues: (a) whether syndromes of aphasia are valid entities, as discussed in Chapter 5, and (b) if syndromes do exist, whether the Boston Exam is accurate in identifying them. If we assume that syndromes are valid entities, then validity of the BDAE can be determined by comparing its classification to another method for classifying patients. Wertz, Deal, and Robinson (1984) made such a comparison to the more recently developed Western Aphasia Battery (Kertesz, 1982), which was designed to identify the same clinical syndromes. Forty-five aphasic patients with single left-hemisphere occlusive lesions were given both tests. There was only 27 percent agreement as to classification of these patients into 11 categories. There has also been some study of the relationship between test patterns and site of lesion (Naeser and Hayward, 1978; Metter, Riege, Hanson, Kuhl, and Phelps, 1984). Naeser, in particular, found agreement between independent classification with the test and predicted site of damage determined with CT scans for 19 subjects.

For interexaminer reliability of the profile of speech characteristics, three judges listened to tape-recorded conversations of 99 aphasic patients. Correlations were 0.85 and above for rating melodic line, phrase length, articulatory agility, and grammatical form. Correlations of 0.79 and 0.78 were found for paraphasias and word-finding, indicative of the "subjective uncertainty" of the judges, according to the authors. Goodglass and his colleagues (1964) examined interexaminer reliability with the severity rating. There was full agreement among three examiners on 38 percent of the cases, and two judges agreed on 57 percent within one point. Ulatowska and others (1976) studied interexaminer reliability with 12 BDAE subtests and two speech rating parameters. She found complete agreement among three testers on 76 percent of the test items and a one-point discrepancy in scoring on another 22 percent of the items.

Interpretation

Cutoff scores were derived from the studies of normal adults. Lowest scores tended to be made by persons over age 60 with fewer than nine years of education. Exceptions to cutoffs for people 60 years of age and older were recommended for measures of nonverbal agility and word fluency (i.e., animal-naming). In assessing an elderly client, the cutoff score should be relaxed before it is concluded that performance is disordered.

Diagnosis of syndrome is accomplished by examining pattern of results on the rating of speech characteristics and the subtest summary profile. The manual provides examples and ranges of performance that are typically seen in cases of Broca's, Wernicke's, anomic, and conduction aphasias. Data shown with the *rating scale profile of speech characteristics* is a convenient guide for classification (Figure 9–2). The profile describes extended expression according to the telltale signs of the syndromes. Six dimensions of extended utterance are compared with auditory comprehension deficit determined during formal testing, and repetition was added in 1983. Figure 9–2 shows the range around mean

RATING SCALE PROFILE OF SPEECH CHARACTERISTICS (a)

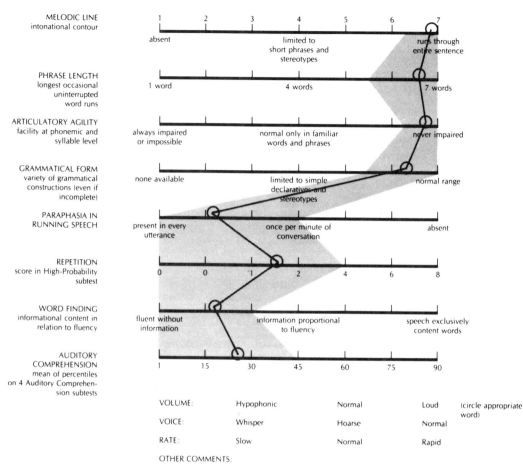

FIGURE 9–2 The Boston Exam's rating scale profiles of speech characteristics for (a) Wernicke's aphasia and (b) anomic aphasia. These syndromes are similar in melodic line, phrase length, articulatory agility, and grammatical form (i.e., fluency). Differences

performance for two fluent aphasias: Wernicke's and anomic aphasias. In Chapter 5, some concern was expressed with respect to criteria often used (or not used) in selecting representatives of these syndromes for research. The rating scale profile is seldom reported.

The BDAE does not contain a formal basis for predicting recovery. Its use for this purpose depends on identification of syndromes and application of research in which syn-

drome was a factor (Chapter 11). This test has not been used very much for documenting recovery in published studies, perhaps because of its undemonstrated reliability and lack of summary scores. A few studies of treatment involved reporting progress in portions of the Boston Exam (e.g., Helm and Barresi, 1980; Sparks, Helm, and Albert, 1974). Progress in a case study was described with the profile of speech characteristics by Helm-Estabrooks, Fitzpatrick, and Barresi

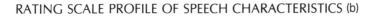

RATING SCALE PROFILE OF SPEECH CHARACTERISTICS (b)

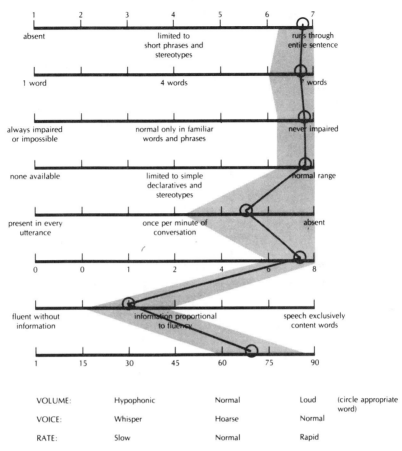

occur with paraphasias, repetition, and auditory comprehension. (Reprinted by permission from Goodglass, H., & Kaplan, F., *The Assessment of Aphasia and Language Disorders.* Chicago: Riverside, 1983, p. 81, 85).

(1981). The entire test was used for investigating recovery by left-handed aphasic patients (Borod, Carper, and Naeser, 1990).

WESTERN APHASIA BATTERY (WAB)

The WAB was developed by Andrew Kertesz at the University of Western Ontario, and it has attained wide use in studies of recovery and treatment efficacy. When it was intro-

duced, it was described as a modification of the Boston Diagnostic Aphasia Examination (Kertesz and Poole, 1974). The WAB is similar in content and purpose. However, Kertesz hoped to minimize the subjectivity of pattern recognition by identifying syndromes according to specific test scores. Also, "the Western's" summary scores made it attractive as a measure of progress. The test was known for some time from studies of aphasia taxonomy (Kertesz, 1979; Kertesz and Phipps, 1977) and recovery (e.g., Kertesz and McCabe, 1977). The complete test was published in 1982.

Description of the WAB

The basic battery examines *oral language abilities,* which include auditory comprehension and spoken expression. This part of the test is divided into four sections corresponding to the areas that have been most important in identifying aphasia syndromes: (I) spontaneous speech, elicited through interview and picture description; (II) auditory verbal comprehension, which includes tasks that are similar to the Boston Exam but with more yes/no questions and instructions to follow; (III) repetition, of single words, phrases, and sentences; and (IV) naming, in a variety of circumstances. This portion of the test can be given within an hour to most aphasic patients. *Visual language and other subtests* is an additional section consisting of (V) reading, (VI) writing, (VII) apraxia, and (VIII) constructional, visuospatial, and calculation tasks. The entire test could take as long as the MTDDA, and Kertesz (1982) recommended dividing it into segments across sessions.

WAB Scores

Calculations from test performance and summary scores set this test apart from the Boston Exam. Scores are obtained for the four sections of the oral language test. The spontaneous speech section is rated with two ten-point scales, one for *information content* and another for *fluency.* Kertesz (1979) felt that the information content rating is a good estimate of functional communication. The fluency scale is used in classification. For example, 0 to 4 represents levels of nonfluency, and 5 to 10 depicts levels of fluency. The following summary scores have been calculated:

Aphasia Quotient (AQ): Used with the test since 1974, the AQ is the summary score for the four sections of auditory-spoken language. Forty percent of the score is derived from the sponta-

neous speech rating scales. Possible score is 100 (see Shewan and Kertesz, 1980).

Language Quotient (LQ): This is the most recent score developed for this test (Shewan and Kertesz, 1984). The LQ is a composite of all language sections, including reading and writing. It is more similar to the PICA overall than the AQ.

Performance Quotient (PQ): For a while, reading, writing, apraxia, and construction tasks were combined into this score (Kertesz, 1979; Appell, et al., 1982).

Cortical Quotient (CQ): The is the only score besides the AQ that is mentioned in the test manual. The CQ represents performance on all subtests, verbal and nonverbal. The CQ and AQ are the only summary scores examined in reliability and validity studies (Shewan and Kertesz, 1980).

A regression analysis of subtests led to a suggestion for a *short version* of the WAB that would predict the AQ (Crary and Gonzalez Rothi, 1989). It would consist of sequential commands and repetition subtests and the two scales for rating spontaneous speech.

Standardization

Norms were reported initially by Kertesz and Poole (1974) from samples consisting of 150 aphasic persons, 21 nonbrain-injured subjects, and 17 people with unilateral hemisphere damage without aphasia. The aphasic sample included varied etiologies, such as CVA, tumor, head injury, and degenerative disease. Typical scores were reported again for 215 aphasic subjects, 63 normals, and 53 nonaphasic brain-damaged patients (Kertesz, 1979). Normals in the two samples had mean AQs of 98.4 and 99.6. The two samples of nondominant (mostly right) hemisphere damage differed somewhat, with an AQ of 97.1 in the first group and 92.9 in the larger group. Kertesz also reported mean AQs for the different aphasia syndromes. The tendency for anomic and conduction aphasias to be mild and moderate impairments is indicated in mean AQs of 83.3 and 60.5, respectively. Broca's and Wernicke's aphasias scored means of 31.7 and 39.0, respectively. Broca's aphasia had the widest standard deviation of all the aphasias. Persons with global aphasia had a mean AQ of 10.5.

In the manual, criterion-related validity was supported by a comparison with the *Neurosensory Center Comprehensive Examination for Aphasia*. Sanders and Davis (1978) found a 0.89 correlation between the AQ and PICA overall score. Subtests were shown to be highly correlated with each other and with the AQ (Crary and Gonzalez Rothi, 1989). Shewan and Kertesz (1980) also reported high internal consistency of test items, and they presented strong test-retest reliability for 38 chronic patients and strong interexaminer reliability for ten patients. Interexaminer consistency of the content and fluency scales was investigated by Trupe (1984), who found weak reliability even after clarification and revision of scoring criteria. She concluded that it is difficult to use one fluency scale to characterize behavior consisting of multiple dimensions and recommended that independent dimensions be rated separately, as in the speech characteristics profile of the Boston Exam.

Interpretation

Diagnosis and measurement with the WAB have depended on the AQ, with diagnosis of syndrome based primarily on pattern of performance with respect to the fluency scale and scores from auditory comprehension, repetition, and naming subtests. Presence of a language disorder, or of "aphasia" according to Kertesz, is identified with an AQ cutoff score of 93.8 (Kertesz and Poole, 1974). In a study of prognostic indicators, aphasic people who surpassed the 93.8 score were considered to be "recovered" (Holland, Greenhouse, Fromm, and Swindell, 1989).

Aphasia syndromes are identified according to patterns shown in Table 9-5. Conduction aphasia, for example, is recognized by scores that are low in repetition relative to higher scores in spontaneous speech fluency and auditory comprehension. One perspective on diagnosis according to these criteria is illustrated in Figure 9-3. The test is being used increasingly to characterize patients in cognitive neuropsychological case studies.

Construct validity for the purpose of classification, which is essential for interpretation, was examined with 144 cases of infarction (Kertesz and Phipps, 1977). A cluster analysis indicated that mathematically generated groups correspond to clinically defined syndromes. However, Wertz found 27 percent agreement between the WAB and BDAE in classification of patients (Wertz, et al., 1984). Swindell, Holland, and Fromm (1984) compared WAB classification to clinical impressions based on understanding of neoclassical syndromes. The clinical impressions were recorded by clinicians trained in giving the WAB. Swindell found that the test agreed with clinical impression in 54 percent of 69 left-hemisphere-damaged patients. Agreement was greater for nonfluent

TABLE 9–5 Criteria for classifying aphasias based on scores from the Western Aphasia Battery. (Reprinted by permission from Kertesz, A., *Aphasia and Associated Disorders: Taxonomy, Localization, and Recovery*. New York: Grune & Stratton, 1979).

	Fluency	Comprehension	Repetition	Naming
Global	0–4	0–3.9	0–4.9	0–6
Broca's	0–4	4–10	0–7.9	0–8
Isolation	0–4	0–3.9	5–10	0–6
Transcortical motor	0–4	4–10	8–10	0–8
Wernicke's	5–10	0–6.9	0–7.9	0–9
Transcortical sensory	5–10	0–6.9	8–10	0–9
Conduction	5–10	7–10	0–6.9	0–9
Anomic	5–10	7–10	7–10	0–9

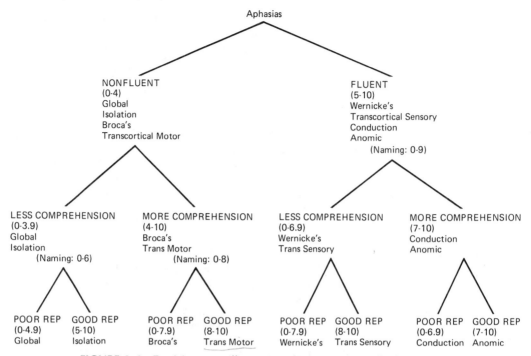

FIGURE 9–3 Decision tree illustrating the manner in which the *WAB* classifies aphasias according to scores for fluency, auditory comprehension, and repetition.

aphasias than for fluent aphasias. The studies by Wertz and Swindell may reduce our confidence in the WAB or BDAE as a basis for classifying aphasic patients. Swindell suggested that we use description to supplement scores for confirming a syndrome.

The WAB has been examined with two other patient groups. It was given to 15 bilaterally damaged head-injured patients (Bernstein-Ellis, et al., 1985). The AQ classified 14 as having a language impairment, and 12 were consistent with the profile for anomic aphasia. This score has been used to determine language impairment in persons with Alzheimer's disease (Appell, et al., 1982; Bayles, et al., 1989). When pattern of language impairment was compared with aphasias, it was shown that nonfluent aphasia patterns were absent from those studied. Appell's subjects were similar to those with Wernicke's and transcortical sensory aphasias.

ASSESSMENT OF BILINGUAL CLIENTS

People who use two or more languages in their daily lives present special problems for monolingual and bilingual clinicians. Aphasia may be manifested in each language differently. Cross-linguistic research indicates that this difference may result partly from the nature of the languages in addition to the relative use of languages. Grosjean (1989) had some suggestions for the evaluation of bilingual aphasic persons.

First, we should determine the following information about a patient's bilingualism prior to brain injury, perhaps by interviewing a family member:

Relative ability in each language (linguistic level, style, reading, writing);

Situations and purposes for which each language was used (home, work, recreation);

Persons with whom each language was used (family, friends, colleagues);

Situations and people when in a monolingual mode;

Situations and people when in a bilingual mode;

Amount and kind of mixing when in the bilingual mode (code-switching, borrowing);

Translation abilities.

This information leads us to assessment and treatment that are appropriate for a particular language used by the bilingual patient. We should not assess for aphasia in reading and writing in a language not used for these purposes. We should employ work-related content with the language used at work.

When evaluating aphasia in each language, we obtain samples of language behavior in conversation and formal tests. Each language should be examined in each interactional mode, remembering that the abilities of a bilingual person in each language are not the same as the abilities of two monolingual persons. In the **monolingual mode,** conditions should lead to a deactivation of the language not being used, which is likely to occur when the examiner does not know the other language. Pretending not to know the other language "is rarely foolproof" (Grosjean, 1989). For an English- and Spanish-speaking patient, a monolingual English-speaking person should do one evaluation and a monolingual Spanish-speaking person should do the other evaluation. A family member may be enlisted to translate and administer the aphasia test in the language not known by the clinician (e.g., Paradis and Goldblum, 1989). In a study of object-naming in English and Spanish, clinicians placed 30 minutes to two days between tests (Vogel and Costello, 1986). The clinicians claimed that 15 to 20 minutes seemed too brief to minimize interference (or maximize deactivation of one language). Thirty minutes to one hour was sufficient for most subjects.

For obtaining behavior samples in the **bilingual mode,** the patient should feel comfortable about code-switching and borrowing. Again, a bilingual family member or friend may be sought. Grosjean (1989) recommended that we learn about how aphasia has affected the special skills used in this mode,

such as whether the patient uses the "wrong" language when speaking to a bilingual family member or friend, mixes languages to the same extent as before, and mixes in the same way as before. Has ability to translate languages changed? We know relatively little about aphasia in bilinguals when evaluated this comprehensively, so clinicians have an opportunity to contribute to our knowledge in this area through clinical research.

COMPARISONS AND INTERPRETATION STRATEGIES

Different ideas about aphasia and the purpose of assessment shaped the major aphasia batteries. Schuell, who was not interested in localization, put shape copying and figure reproduction in the "visuomotor and writing" section, perhaps thinking in terms of visuomotor prerequisites for writing skills. Setting a clock and using arithmetic were placed in a separate section as somewhat different functions that had been recognized as being disturbed in some cases of aphasia. Because neurological studies showed that a site of damage pulls down apparently different functions together, Goodglass and Kaplan placed shape copying and arithmetic together in a supplemental battery that was originally intended to assess effects of parietal lobe damage. This battery includes tests for finger agnosia and right-left discrimination. Goodglass and Kaplan changed their classification of these tests from "parietal lobe battery" to "spatial-quantitative battery," indicating that lesions causing impairments in some of these areas need not be found in a particular lobe.

In clinical practice, a test is seldom used to diagnose aphasia, in the sense that a clinician has no idea as to what the disorder is until a test is analyzed. A radiologist's localization of lesion and a neurologist's cursory overall evaluation of function establish that a patient is likely to have aphasia. Having read a patient's chart, an experienced clinical aphasiologist need only talk to a patient before reaching an initial conclusion about not only the presence of aphasia but also the type of aphasia.

Nevertheless, substantiation for these conclusions, such as distance of a test score beneath a cutoff, supports a recommendation for treatment. The initial test is also a baseline for measuring progress to support a recommendation to continue treatment. Testing can resolve some genuine ambiguities of diagnosis. With closed head injury, for example, the primary basis for language behavior may be in doubt until testing exposes the contribution of perception, memory, and so on. A specific aphasic disorder can be obscured by pragmatic and systemic adaptations occurring in conversation. Auditory comprehension ability is especially difficult to discern in informal interaction. Mild aphasia may become evident only in assessment of reading and writing. The main clinical purposes for initial assessment, however, are to substantiate recommendations for treatment and to provide direction for starting treatment. Refinements of diagnosis, especially borrowed from basic research, can be a problem-solving component of the treatment process.

Beginning with definition of aphasia in Chapter 1, a clinical implication of previous lessons is that *any level of diagnosis is based on a comparison*. Deficit is indicated by a comparison with the norm, and aphasia is indicated in verbal deficiency relative to performance in nonverbal tasks. Memory for events and spatial orientation are considered in interviews and addressed in the medical chart. The MTDDA and the PICA contain a few shape-matching and copying tasks for simple perceptual and constructional skills. The BDAE and the WAB have supplemental tasks for these abilities. Also, from the start, this book set a foundation for the idea that dysfunction occurs in cognition. Diagnosis is a hypothesis about impairment underlying task performances. Research tells us which disorder(s) we should be looking for with the batteries we happen to have. Chapter 4 indicated that we may look for short-term memory impairment or a disruption of a language process to account for comprehension disorder. We want to know if perceptual or conceptual deficits underlie tasks that entail lexi-

cal retrieval. In Chapter 5, several disorders were contemplated as underlying agrammatism, jargon, and phonemic paraphasia. Where research is indecisive, we can only be indecisive, too, and must fall back upon the fickle signals of behavior to specify the aims of treatment procedure.

Disorders should not be identified with respect to one task, as Davis (1983) suggested with the notion of "pure task blindness." Especially with a focal lesion, a patient is likely to have one or two disorders underlying test scores. If we were to diagnose in terms of a task (e.g., "naming disorder," "repetition disorder"), then we would have to say that the PICA allows us to discover 18 disorders, whereas the MTDDA allows us to discover 46. We can be lured into a trap of thinking of a task as having a purpose specified by its location in a battery. Schuell focused on the stimulus by putting repetition in the auditory section and reading aloud in the reading section of the MTDDA, in spite of the fact that both have a speech component. Goodglass and Kaplan put repetition and reading aloud in the oral expression section of the BDAE. This orients the examiner to focusing on the speech component of these tasks. We avoid the trap of task blindness by remembering that we are trying to figure out the status of a few cognitive systems. We need not be paralyzed by the datedness of standardized batteries for aphasia. The strategies of task-comparison and error analysis, introduced at the end of Chapter 2, are the means by which we try our best to figure out the meaning of performances on a comprehensive aphasia battery. In fact, everything from the first page of this book has something to tell us about assessment and diagnosis.

Like drawing on command (Chapter 2) and object-naming (Chapters 4, 7), any task should be viewed as involving several processing components, beginning with processing the stimulus and concluding with generating response. **Task-comparisons** are required for examining these components, and some basic comparisons are discussed in previous chapters. We look for a "common thread" among tasks in which a patient has particular difficulty (Gardner, 1974). Deficit only on tasks with linguistic stimuli or response is suggestive of aphasia. Deficit only on tasks with a speech component is suggestive of motor speech disorder. Misnaming only to visual input is suggestive of a visual perception or recognition problem. Comprehension errors only when there are competing stimuli are suggestive of impaired attention, not impaired comprehension. We may have to deal with implications of a patient having much more difficulty with comprehension tested by following instructions than by pointing to pictures. The problem lies in a difference between the tasks. This strategy is facilitated by changing one task-related variable at a time, a rather fastidious approach achieved in a limited fashion with the PICA which controls for content across tasks.

Another strategy is **item-comparison,** which is inevitable when a clinician notices a common thread across the items missed within a task: "He has problems only with long sentences or only with words beginning with /k/." Detecting common threads among difficult items leads to more specific diagnosis and, thus, a more focused treatment. The possibility of detecting such problems depends on the items presented. Some subtests in our batteries contain a jumble of items that do not allow item-specific disorders to be revealed. One of the MTDDA's tests of sentence comprehension consists of questions ranging from *Are towns larger than cities?* to *Is it a policeman's duty to enforce the law?* These items vary not only in length but also in features of linguistic structure that may be important for some patients. In general, we use standardized tests to get us started, and further analysis may become part of the treatment process. A main objective of initial assessment is to determine if a patient has a deficit in a general area, not to diagnose a specific disorder (except for those that a test was designed to detect). A trend in the expanding market of supplemental assessment, surveyed in the following chapter, is an increased attention to item-comparison.

CHAPTER

10

SUPPLEMENTAL TESTS AND MEASURES

Other tests and analytical strategies are invented for clinical problems that the comprehensive batteries do not solve. Clinicians often do not have time to give one of these batteries, but they still want to substantiate diagnosis with a standardized evaluation. Another problem is posed by patients at each end of the severity continuum. A test may be so difficult for the most severe aphasia that it does not expose capabilities. We depend on successes for a starting point in treatment. Conversely, for a seemingly intact patient with brain injury, a test may not be difficult enough to expose deficits that would point to goals of treatment. Also, we may replicate psycholinguistic methods to see if our patients have disorders found in research. Traumatic brain injury and other etiologies present impairments that aphasia batteries were not prepared to examine. Finally, legislators and payment providers are asking for evidence of functional progress not indicated in traditional batteries.

SCREENING EXAMINATION

To minimize cost of hospitalization, a patient's stay in the acute-care setting is as brief as needed to ensure survival. This can take 30 days or usually much less for someone who has suffered a stroke. Speech-language pathologists are as busy as physicians and would like to get to treatment as soon as they can. The *Halstead-Wepman-Reitan Aphasia Screening Test*, a precursor to the *Language Modalities Test for Aphasia*, was used by physicians as a quick evaluation of patients at bedside (Halstead and Wepman, 1949). Two hundred were distributed to military neurologists and neurosurgeons during World War II. One version, Form M, could be carried in a shirt pocket, and another version was absorbed into the Halstead-Reitan neuropsychological battery (Chapter 6). Short versions of the MTDDA, PICA, and WAB were suggested (Chapter 9). The Boston Exam may be given partially to obtain the most crucial information about a language disorder. Other tests have been developed for speedy evaluation:

Sklar Aphasia Scale (SAS) (Sklar, 1973): The SAS assesses the four modalities in about an hour. It is a "test of fives," because each modality is tested with five subtests and each subtest contains five items. The 100 items in this test contrast with *The Aphasia Screening Test* (Whurr, 1974), which has 50 subtests of five items each. In the SAS, a five-point scoring system starts with zero for normal response and four points for an incorrect effort. A higher score means greater impairment.

Aphasia Language Performance Scales (ALPS) (Keenan and Brassell, 1975): The ALPS provides an informal standardized assessment in 20 to 30 minutes. The examiner can utilize objects in pockets and a patient's room for assessing comprehension and expression. Modalities are tested with four "scales," each containing a series of items increasing in difficulty.

Bedside Evaluation Screening Test (BEST) (Fitch-West and Sands, 1987): The BEST comes in a portable kit with a magnetic display board, a few objects, and forms for instant reporting once the test is completed. The test should take less than 20 minutes including the report, and it assesses auditory comprehension, reading, naming, repetition, and conversational skills.

Acute Aphasia Screening Protocol (AASP) (Crary, Haak, and Malinsky, 1989): The AASP, like the ALPS, depends on objects found consistently in a patient's room, such as a pillow, window, and TV. It should take around 10 minutes. The AASP begins with a quick check of attention and orientation, and then it assesses auditory comprehension and basic expressive abilities. It includes a score for conversational style. Validity and reliability are reported in the journal *Aphasiology*.

Brief Test of Head Injury (BTHI) (Helm-Estabrooks and Hotz, 1990): With the BTHI we are introduced to tests created for a neuropathological group rather than for a function or set of functions. The test is designed to take 20 to 30 minutes to evaluate orientation, memory, and visuospatial skills as well as a variety of language functions.

We do not need one of these tests to evaluate a patient's language abilities at bedside. All we need is a concept of what needs to be assessed, a few common objects, a pen, and some paper. We have the patient answer some yes/no questions, point to things, and name and describe some other things. If the patient cannot converse, we want to see if he or she can count or recite the days of the week. The published tests become valuable when their standardized administration maximizes consistency in diagnosis, supports a diagnosis, and facilitates convenient measurement of progress.

AUDITORY COMPREHENSION

Without complicating sensory deficits, the auditory language modality is usually the least impaired in aphasia. The auditory sections of the PICA and the BDAE were found to have low ceilings for aphasic patients, meaning that the challenging end of the tests does not leave enough room for mildly impaired patients to show deficit (Morley, Lundgren, and Haxby, 1979). More demanding supplemental tests explore deficiencies and establish baselines for mildly impaired patients. Also, new strategies are inspired by psycholinguistics and especially by the study of agrammatic aphasia.

Token Test

Mild comprehension deficits are found in anomic, conduction, and Broca's aphasias and in patients with RHD, CHI, and early dementia. Ennio DeRenzi and Luigi Vignolo at the University of Milan felt that it was difficult to identify these deficits with routine methods in the 1950s. They created the Token Test to detect subtle deficits and to measure progress when the ceiling effect of other tests prevents such measurement. The test was introduced in a journal (DeRenzi and Vignolo, 1962), where incomplete description left it open to modifications. Its deployment has expanded to studies of comprehension and assessment of any aphasia. It has been incorporated into batteries such as the *Aachen Aphasia Test* (Huber, et al., 1984).

Description. The Token Test was designed so that correct response would be based on the processing of language without clues from a situation, props, knowledge of a topic, and extraneous verbalization. With contextual factors cleared away, it provides a focus on the influence of length and complexity in the comprehension of commands. A client is instructed to manipulate tokens of different shape, color, and size. In publishing a complete list of commands, Boller and Vignolo (1966) contributed to consistency of administration.

The 1966 version became the basis for most subsequent Token Tests. The test has five parts. Parts I through IV contain ten items each, and they differ according to information given about the tokens and length of command. Part V contains 22 commands of varying syntactic construction, and items are generally more complex than the items in previous sections. The following illustrates each part of the 1966 version:

I. Touch the yellow rectangle.
II. Touch the large blue circle.
III. Touch the red circle and the yellow rectangle.
IV. Touch the small yellow circle and the large green rectangle.
V. (1) Put the red circle on the green rectangle.
  (11) Touch the white circle without using your right hand.
  (20) After picking up the green rectangle, touch the white circle.

The tokens are arranged in rows. Ten tokens are used for Parts I, III, and V, and 20 are used for Parts II and IV. The first version in 1962 had patients "pick up" the tokens in I and II and "take" the tokens in III and IV. Use of the verb "touch" in 1966 simplified re-

sponse and increased consistency across parts. Example (11) was added to Part V. Most applications of the complete test contain a total of 62 items.

Subsequent Variations. Some tinkering was done with the 1966 test. The most frequent modification was recommended first by Spreen and Benton (1977), who replaced *rectangle* with *square*, which has more common usage and is more comparable to the original *circle*. Then, *blue* was replaced with *black*. The elimination of *blue* was prompted by problems that elderly adults have in discriminating between blue and green (DeRenzi and Faglioni, 1978). When giving the test to children, Whitaker and Noll (1972) changed the words for size to *big* and *little*. This modification was not adopted as regularly as the others.

Some clinicians replaced tokens with common objects (e.g., Tompkins, Rau, Marshall, Lambrecht, Golper, and Phillips, 1980). Tokens were supposed to minimize contextual cues from the manipulative features of objects so that testing would focus on processing of linguistic input. Several researchers examined this variable and found mixed results with respect to ability to follow the commands (Chapter 8). The *Functional Auditory Comprehension Test* (FACT) is a "Token Test" with objects (LaPointe, et al., 1985). The most consistent Token Test has been the 1966 version, with squares instead of rectangles.

A "configurational" Token Test was created as a means of isolating components of test performance and distinguishing between aphasic patients and persons with RH dysfunction (Brookshire, 1978b). A patient pointed to one of four arrangements of tokens drawn on a card, thereby minimizing the motoric complexity of response. Aphasic subjects found the configurational version to be easier than the standard version, while RHD subjects experienced equal success on both versions of the Token Test. A similar strategy, called the "Three-Figures-Test," involves pointing to shapes on a card (Peuser and Schriefers, 1980).

The first **shortened Token Test** became the "Identification by Sentence" subtest of the *Neurosensory Center Comprehensive Examination of Aphasia* (Spreen and Benton, 1977). There are 39 items instead of 62. A sixth part was added at the low end to provide an easier section so that application can be broadened beyond the original goal of assessing mild deficit. It involves identification by shape or color (e.g., *Show me a square; show me a red one*). A 16-item version was equally capable of deficit identification (Spellacy and Spreen, 1969). Norms were developed for a 36-item Token Test that absorbs most of the changes to the original test (DeRenzi, 1979; DeRenzi and Faglioni, 1978). DeRenzi's short test also contains six parts.

Administration and Scoring. Tokens are arranged in two or four rows, depending on the part being given. Several arrangements have been recommended to enhance standardization. DeRenzi and Vignolo (1962) suggested a circles-first arrangement. When all 20 tokens are displayed for Parts II and IV, the top two rows should be circles, large and then small; the bottom two rows should be rectangles (or squares), large and then small. On the other hand, Spreen and Benton (1969) used a large-small arrangement: large circles and squares formed the first two rows, and small circles and squares formed the last two rows. Scoring systems have also been variable. Originally, errors were counted for each element of each command, with total possible errors being 250 (DeRenzi and Vignolo, 1962; Hartje, et al., 1973). Boller and Vignolo (1966) recommended scoring each command as correct or incorrect and then adding the total correct, with the best score being 62 (e.g., Swisher and Sarno, 1969; Gallaher, 1979).

Norms and Standardization. Normative information must be pieced together from several studies. Seventy-eight normal adults had a range of 48 to 62 of 62 possible points. In one study, the mean score was 57 (Swisher and Sarno, 1969), and another was 59.7 (Noll and Randolf, 1978). Patients with RHD were equivalent to normal subjects (Boller and Vi-

gnolo, 1966). A sample of mildly impaired aphasic subjects, the original target group of the test, ranged from 18 to 59, with an average of 43.5 in Noll's study. With mild comprehension deficit, patients did well with Parts I through III and poorly on Parts IV and V in Boller's study. An unselected sample of patients ranged from 0 to 58, with an average of 23, indicating that the Token Test is very difficult for a wider range of aphasic persons (Swisher and Sarno, 1969). DeRenzi (1979) used a cutoff score of 29 for identifying aphasic deficit with his 36-item test.

The Token Test was significantly correlated with other tests, such as the *Functional Communication Profile* (Swisher and Sarno, 1969), tests of semantic and syntactic comprehension (Parisi and Pizzamiglio, 1970; Pizzamiglio and Appicciafuoco, 1971), a clinical test of comprehension (Needham and Swisher, 1972), and comprehension subtests of the PICA and the Boston Exam (Morley, et al., 1979). The Token Test may be unrelated to functional comprehension, as it failed to correlate with Holland's test of communicative abilities described later in this chapter (LaPointe, et al., 1985). Scores were also unrelated to a measure of nonverbal cognition (Boller and Vignolo, 1966). However, the Token Test correlated with a picture-matching task, indicating that visual perception might be involved. Education was implicated as a factor (Boller and Vignolo, 1966; DeRenzi, 1979), which is often an intrusion in the assessment of language at a high level.

The original aim was to expose auditory problems in patients that seem to be in good shape with standard batteries. DeRenzi and Vignolo (1962) found that 13 "motor" aphasic patients and six recovered "sensory" patients, all with adequate comprehension in standard tests, had pronounced difficulty with Parts IV and V (also Boller and Vignolo, 1966). Noll and Randolph (1978) studied patients with mild or no impairment on the MTDDA or the PICA. These subjects scored much worse than normals, indicating that initially undetected deficit can be revealed with the Token Test. Average errors by section were as follows: (I) 1.0 of ten items, (II) 4.1, (III) 6.1, (IV)

9.8, and (V) 11.5 of 22 items. Morley and others (1979) concluded that the PICA auditory tests provide little information at high levels of comprehension ability, whereas Parts IV and V of the Token Test elicit a range of scores.

Interpretation. Although not widely used for this purpose, the Token Test may be sensitive to aphasic deficit. Aphasic groups performed much worse than RH-damaged groups (DeRenzi and Faglioni, 1978; Hartje, et al., 1973; Lesser, 1976; Martino, et al., 1976; Swisher and Sarno, 1969) and had lower scores than LH-damaged nonaphasic patients (DeRenzi and Faglioni, 1978; Hartje, et al., 1973). Problems with Part V in LHD nonaphasic subjects led to a diagnosis of "latent aphasia" (Boller and Vignolo, 1966). Nonfluent and fluent aphasias did not differ in average score (DeRenzi, 1979; Poeck, Kerschensteiner, and Hartje, 1972), which was of interest to those wishing to prove that clinical syndromes do not exist (Chapter 5). When more specific syndromes were studied, there was a difference among groups (Poeck and Hartje, 1979); and Wernicke's aphasia produced more errors than nonfluent aphasias (Mack and Boller, 1979).

The major emphasis has been the identification of peculiar disorders of processing that would not be revealed in an overall score. An analysis of **error location within commands** might expose a particular type of problem. The Token Test was used extensively by investigators wondering if disorders of auditory processing and short-term memory account for language comprehension deficit (Chapter 4). Lesser (1976, 1979) found that scores are correlated with auditory STM, visual STM, and motor sequencing. A gradual increase of errors from Parts I to V may indicate that reduced STM capacity is the primary deficit (Noll and Randolph, 1978). However, increased length is accompanied by changes in linguistic features. A large increase of errors from IV to V is suggestive of good STM capacity and problems with syntactic operations for V. Noll and Randolph

(1978) found that patients with mild comprehension deficits make many more syntactic errors (e.g., wrong relationship between tokens) than semantic errors (e.g., wrong shape or color). Finding specific syntactic problems in Part V is impeded by the variety of structures that are presented only once or twice (Poeck, Orgass, Kerschensteiner, and Hartje, 1974). Revised Token Tests have been created in which certain structures are presented repeatedly for analysis of error location (Mack and Boller, 1979; McNeil and Prescott, 1978).

Revised Token Test (RTT)

The RTT is what we get when administrative and scoring strategies of the PICA are applied to the Token Test. McNeil and Prescott (1978) wanted to replace the inconsistencies in the family of Token Tests. They also wanted to provide more information by applying multidimensional scoring to each element of each command and by reconstructing the presentation of certain syntactic structures from Part V. Two colors differ from the original version. The RTT consists of green, blue, and black, despite the suspected perceptual problems between blue and green. Yellow was eliminated. This "black-and-blue" version has been employed in the study of auditory processing in aphasia (Brookshire and Nicholas, 1984; Hageman and Lewis, 1983).

The test contains ten sections with ten commands per section. Subtests I through IV are constructed on the same basis as Parts I through IV in the original Token Test. The remaining six subtests concentrate on nine of the original Part V items and, thus, offer an expansion of the strategy of item-comparison. Subtests V and VI present several **prepositions** for placing tokens in spatial relationships to each other. Subtests VII and VIII involve placing tokens to the **left or right** of each other. Subtests IX and X contain a variety of **conditional clauses** (e.g., *Unless you have touched the white square, touch the green circle*). Like the PICA, a protocol booklet specifies each command and instructions for repeating and cueing. A 15-point scale is applied to each element of each command (McNeil, Dionigi, Langlois, and Prescott, 1989). The score for one command is derived from averaging the scores for its elements. A subtest score is the mean of all element scores, such as the 60 elements of III. After giving the test, computations include 100 item scores, ten subtest scores, and an overall score. Percentiles can be derived for patients with LHD or RHD.

The RTT takes an average of 30 minutes to administer in a range of 13 to 75 minutes. Because administration and computation take considerably longer here than in other supplemental auditory comprehension tests, a project was undertaken to determine if a **shortened RTT** yields the same information (Arvedson, McNeil, and West, 1985). With the first five items from each subtest, a "five-item" version was predictive of the overall score from the complete test. Arvedson suggested that the 50-item version is substitutable for the 100-item version in order to obtain the overall score, but she was cautious about more specific analyses with the short RTT.

More specific analyses pertain to profiling patterns of performance. McNeil and Hageman were interested in patterns of scores **across items in a subtest** (e.g., *tuning-in*, gradually improving from the first to tenth item; *intermittent*, fluctuating across items; *tuning-out*, declining across items). They also watched for patterns **across subtests** (e.g., poorer performance from I to IV, as indicative of tuning-out). At first, only one pattern was clearly evident: intermittent success across items (McNeil and Hageman, 1979). Distinctive performance was unrelated to severity of deficit, site of lesion, or other factors, so we cannot anticipate who would have a particular problem with respect to the factors chosen for study. When the RTT was given again in two days, within-subtest patterns were consistent for individuals; those who were intermittent were consistently intermittent. Between-subtest patterns were inconsistent (Hageman and Folkestad, 1986;

Hageman, McNeil, Rucci-Zimmer, and Cariski, 1982). The kinds of deficit that can be logically determined by this test have not been shown to occur consistently in aphasic patients. Moreover, findings with the RTT have not been associated with disorders implied in psycholinguistic studies of agrammatic comprehension and so on (Chapter 5).

Auditory Comprehension Test for Sentences (ACTS)

Shewan's (1979) ACTS was inspired by psycholinguistic studies of the 1960s, which examined the influence of grammatical transformations on ease of comprehension (Shewan and Canter, 1971). An error analysis was developed so that type of deficit could be revealed (Shewan, 1976). The test takes ten to 15 minutes to determine contribution of sentence length, vocabulary, and syntax on auditory comprehension. The ACTS contains 21 test sentences that are read to a patient who responds by pointing to one of four pictures. The three foils are based on changes of semantic elements in the test sentence. The score is number of correct sentences, and error type is defined relative to position of semantic change in the sentence (i.e., first or second half) and grammatical category (i.e., primarily nouns or verbs).

Norms were obtained from 150 aphasic patients and 30 normal controls. A cutoff score of 18 became the basis for diagnosing disorder. A score of 17 was used for those with under eight years of education. Aphasic syndromes were ranked in severity (Chapter 5). Shewan's (1976) research showed that position of error did not distinguish syndromes. However, grammatical class of error appears to differentiate syndromes (Klor and Mlcoch, 1984). More errors on nouns than verbs and prepositions were found with anomic aphasia, whereas patients with Wernicke's aphasia made more errors with pictures that contain a different verb or preposition. The ACTS was used in studies of aphasia treatment effects (Shewan and Kertesz, 1984) and comprehension with Alzheimer's dementia (Bayles and Kaszniak, 1987).

Caplan's Batteries

Considering psycholinguistic issues raised in ongoing research, Goodglass and Kaplan (1983) attached supplementary language tests to their Boston Exam. One task is for assessing comprehension of passives, and one example is the following: "If I tell you, 'The lion was killed by the tiger,' which animal is dead?" (p. 52). Other items consisted of a boy slapped by a girl and a car damaged by a motorcycle. Violence seems unavoidable. Chapter 4 introduced Caplan's application of linguistics for constructing sentence stimuli and his use of toy animal manipulation for

testing comprehension of sentences such as, "It was the monkey that the elephant kicked" (Caplan, et al., 1985; Caplan and Hildebrandt, 1988). He has wanted to identify specific types of comprehension disorder with two general batteries (Table 10–1). The idea is to get away from general evaluation with a list of varied structures and expand on item-comparison by defining a subtest according to syntactic structure rather than according to type of task.

The **Thematic Role Battery** assesses ability to assign thematic roles to NPs in reversible sentences. A core set of structures is invariably employed, and batteries are some-

TABLE 10–1   Selected types of sentences in Caplan's Thematic Role and Coreference Batteries (Butler-Hinz, Caplan, and Waters, 1990; Caplan, Baker, and Dehaut, 1985; Caplan and Hildebrandt, 1988).

Thematic Role Battery

Active (A)
  The frog hit the monkey.
Passive (P)
  The monkey was hit by the frog.
Cleft-subject (CS)
  It was the frog that hit the monkey.
Cleft-object (CO)
  It was the monkey that the frog hit.
Dative (D)
  The frog gave the monkey to the goat.
Dative passive (DP)
  The monkey was given to the elephant by the frog.
Dative cleft-object (DCO)
  It was the monkey that the frog gave to the elephant.
Conjoined (C)
  The frog hit the monkey and patted the elephant.
Subject-object relative (SO)
  The monkey that the frog hit patted the elephant.
Object-subject relative (OS)
  The frog hit the monkey that patted the elephant.
Subject-subject relative (SS)
  The frog that hit the monkey patted the elephant.

Coreference Battery

Simple active pronoun (AP)
  The old man tickled him.
Simple active reflexive (AR)
  The old man tickled himself.
Empty NP, object control (OC)
  The boy convinced the old man to wash.
Empty NP, subject control (SC)
  The boy promised the old man to wash.

---

times added to explore function even more thoroughly (e.g., Hildebrandt, Caplan, and Evans, 1987). Toy animals include a monkey, frog, elephant, goat, cow, rabbit, and sometimes a bear and donkey. A pre-test verifies ability to identify the animals. Twelve sentences are used for each structure. In one study, 14 structures generated a battery of 168 items (Waters, et al., 1991). Items are presented in a pseudo-random order so that no more than two examples of each type are consecutive. A sentence is read once. With numbers designating NPs, an examiner records enactment of agent, theme, and goal. For the simple active sentence in Table 10–1, frog is 1 and monkey is 2; the correct answer is 1–2, and an error is 2–1. Comparison is made according to number correct per sentence type.

What clues to deficit might be uncovered with this assessment? As stated in Chapter 4, sentences that preserve canonical order are easier than those that do not (Caplan, et al., 1985). Thus, a patient may perform at a high level for types conforming to English canonical order, such as the ones coded as (A), (CS), and (D); but the patient may perform at a low level for structures not conforming to canonical order, such as (P), (CO), and (DP). Canonical and noncanonical sentences vary in surface complexity, so this hypothetical patient can be said to be able to process a variety of syntactic complexity. The problem lies in difficult mapping of thematic roles onto computed phrase structure.

Only a few structures used in the **Coreference Battery** are illustrated in Table 10–1. In Chapter 4, some of these sentences are shown in example 9. This test examines the ability to assign antecedents to pronouns, reflexives, and empty NPs. Empty NPs are the so-called gaps where an NP is implied, as in comprehending who is washing; a pronoun is a kind of gap that must be "filled" in comprehension by locating an antecedent. Materials consist of four male dolls, labeled as boy, father, grandfather, and friend, and four female dolls, labeled as girl, mother, grandmother, and friend. Some assessments label the dolls with proper names (Hildebrandt, et

al., 1987; Waters, et al., 1991). A pre-test verifies ability to identify the dolls according to these labels. In the battery, half the items involve the male dolls and the other half involve the female dolls. Eleven types of sentences have been used (Waters, et al., 1991). With 12 items per structure, a battery contains 132 sentences. The interpretation of performance on both batteries becomes quite sophisticated linguistically, and one should study Caplan's articles carefully for further information about these tests.

READING COMPREHENSION

For more thorough examination of a patient's reading capacities, clinical aphasiologists have created printed versions of auditory comprehension tests (e.g., Waters, et al., 1991), borrowed reading batteries from the field of education (see Brookshire, 1986), or created their own batteries of silent and oral reading tasks (e.g., Webb and Love, 1983). The **Reading Comprehension Battery for Aphasia** identifies silent reading abilities (LaPointe and Horner, 1979). The test contains ten subtests that progress from word to paragraph levels of difficulty. Unique sections include subtest IV for functional tasks such as reading common signs, a checkbook, and a phone directory. A patient must read a sentence-length instruction in order to carry out each item. Subtest IV was found to be among the most difficult subtests for aphasic subjects (Van Demark, Lemmer, and Drake, 1982). Subtests VIII and IX involve questions about explicit and implicit information in paragraphs. They also contain some humor, and the examiner is instructed to note the patient's reaction.

Aphasic patients are often meticulous readers, making administration of the RCBA take over an hour in some cases. Van Demark and others (1982) measured an average time of about 45 minutes for the first administration. They also determined that the test has strong reliability and correlates at 0.80 with a test of silent reading and 0.87 with reading subtests of the PICA. In gathering data on 26 aphasic subjects, Van Demark compared 19 nonfluent and seven fluent patients. Both groups had PICA scores indicative of moderate impairment, probably with few global aphasias in the nonfluent group and few Wernicke's aphasias in the fluent group. With a maximum score of 100, the nonfluent group averaged 70.73, and the fluent group averaged 77.85. The mean and range for all subjects were 71.34 and 31 to 97.

LANGUAGE PRODUCTION

Several methods for eliciting and analyzing language are presented in previous chapters as research on aphasic language production. Convergent and divergent tasks are described for the study of word-finding (Chapters 4, 6). There are measures of speaking rate and information efficiency and strategies for describing features of discourse (Chapter 8). This section is a reminder of some of these methods and adds to our selection of possibilities.

Boston Naming Test (BNT)

Naming is a convergent task that isolates lexical retrieval from other components of sentence production. Equipped to detect mild naming deficit, the BNT contains 60 line drawings representing words of varied familiarity (Kaplan, Goodglass, and Weintraub, 1983). It can be obtained along with the BDAE. An earlier 85-item version, available in 1976, was used in research (Kohn and Goodglass, 1985; Table 5–1). The BNT begins with *bed* and *tree* and presents *trellis, palette, protractor,* and *abacus* at the end. The score is derived from total correct, and the maximum is 60. A patient who appears not to recognize an object gets another chance when a function cue is presented. If a response does not occur in 20 seconds, a phonemic cue is presented. It is recommended that a clinician begin with item 30 (i.e., *harmonica*) for adults but work backwards if middle items turn out to be too difficult. Testing stops after six consecutive failures.

"Provisional norms" from 84 normal and 82 aphasic adults are included in the scoring booklet. Normals in their 50s averaged 55.82 in a range of 49 to 59, and a range of 42 to 60 was found across all adult age groups. Scores for aphasia were separated according to severity level. For mildest levels, scores were derived from small groups of less than ten, leading to some unusual ranges. The range for the mildest aphasia was 2 to 58; but the range for somewhat more impairment was 33 to 58, perhaps leading to the warning that the norms are provisional. Thirty-five severely impaired subjects averaged 1.4 with a range of 0 to 30. Many researchers have used the original BNT to correlate whatever they are investigating with naming ability. In addition, some researchers have begun to use a 63-item **Action Naming Test** by Obler and Albert (e.g., Nicholas, et al., 1985).

Nicholas and Brookshire were concerned about some of the features of the BNT and administered the test to 60 neurologically intact persons (Nicholas, Brookshire, MacLennan, Schumacher, and Porrazzo, 1989). Some of the pictures seemed ambiguous, capable of eliciting names other than the one considered to be correct. Administration and scoring procedures seemed vague. Reliability was not reported by the test designers. Nicholas and Brookshire decided to make some changes. They wrote more explicit instructions for administration, developed a more elaborate response coding and scoring procedure, and established a cueing procedure following certain types of incorrect response. The subjects, with a mean age of 56, averaged 54.5, which is close to the mean reported by Kaplan. Some of the items starting with number 50 elicited more than 25 errors from this group of 60. The new procedures produced strong reliability, except for coding relatedness of errors and distinguishing "don't know" from "off-task" categories. Some items elicited a name consistently that was not specified as correct in the test. The investigators recommended caution in interpretation of performance on this test, especially with respect to attributing errors to brain damage.

Eliciting Sentences and Discourse

Sentences are often elicited by asking a patient to describe an object's function or a simple pictured event. Specific syntactic forms can be targeted in **short story completion** (Gleason, et al., 1975) and with **elicited imitation**, is in the *Northwestern Syntax Screening Test* (Lee, 1971), which has been used with agrammatic patients. The Token Test was turned around to create the **Reporter's Test** for measuring mild and moderate disorders of verbal expression (DeRenzi and Ferrari, 1978). The patient reports an action that a clinician performs with tokens. In a procedural twist, the clinician shields the tokens from an imaginary listener. The patient is instructed as follows: "Imagine that a person is sitting beside you, but is prevented from seeing what I am doing by a curtain. . . . Your task is to describe what I am doing as carefully as possible, so that this person would be able to repeat exactly my performance on another set of tokens. . . ." (p. 281).

Procedures for eliciting discourse were presented in Chapter 8. Let us review the main procedures, because the literature contains some inconsistency in reporting the type of discourse elicited by particular types of stimuli.

Descriptive discourse is often obtained by presenting a picture of an elaborate set of events, and a patient is asked to state everything that is going on in the picture. Such pictures are favored because they standardize input for comparison of patients. Researchers make frequent use of the Cookie Theft picture from the Boston Exam, mentioned often in previous chapters. The MTDDA and the WAB provide different versions of a "kite-flying" scene. A gender bias was detected in a comparison of these pictures. The Cookie Theft was strongly "female," and the MTDDA picture was slightly "male"-oriented (Correia, Brookshire, and Nicholas, 1989). Also, the Cookie Theft elicited more action than the others; the WAB and MTDDA pictures elicited more names and less action. Many researchers claim that these pictures elicit *narrative*. This demonstrates a possible confusion of terminology: not realizing that "narrative" refers to a particular discourse structure. A patient may be instructed explicitly to tell a story from one of these pictures.

Narrative discourse is elicited by asking a patient to tell a story spontaneously. To standardize input, a patient may retell a story or relate a story in cartoon-style picture sequences or filmstrips.

Procedural discourse involves telling how to do common tasks, as in, "Tell me how you make a sandwich." The task taps into knowledge of routines or schemas. It does not assess procedural knowledge, which is realized only when someone is actually doing these things.

Conversational discourse occurs when a clinician and patient take turns exchanging information. Free-wheeling exchanges are avoided in research, because of the likelihood of inconsistency between repeated conditions. A study reported in Chapter 4 indicated that spontaneous conversation and elicited descriptions of object functions differ in the characteristics of language produced (Roberts and Wertz, 1989). Therefore, it is valuable to examine discourse under different conditions. An *interview* is sometimes said to elicit conversation, but this depends on the extent of a clinician's passivity or control, which may minimize turn-taking. Complaints about ambiguity of reports of such procedures should heighten awareness of the variables in such interactions. The manner in which a conversation or interview is conducted is not self-evident.

Linguistic Analysis

Linguistic description of aphasic language began with identification of form class or grammatical class of words (Jones and Wepman, 1967; Spreen and Wachal, 1973). Transformational grammar was then applied to the structural relationships among words (Myerson and Goodglass, 1972). Since then, various approaches to analysis of grammar in agrammatism have been employed in research (Chapter 5). Crystal, Fletcher, and Garman (1976) developed "a procedure for analyzing the syntactic character of language disorders, capable of being used routinely by anyone involved with the diagnosis, assessment, and remediation of language disability" (p. 20). They called it LARSP, for *Language Assessment, Remediation, and Screening Procedure*. This procedure leads to a profile of word classes and syntactic structures appearing in spontaneous verbal expression. Also, constituents are classified according to stage of language development, which was compared to examining aphasia at different severity levels. Case studies were presented by Crystal and by Kearns and Simmons (1983). LARSP was also used to assess closed head injury, confirming preservation of syntax (Mentis and Prutting, 1987). Kearns and Simmons worried about the procedure's taking "several hours" and its limited usefulness for severe aphasia. However, it helped them specify treatment goals and identify linguistic compensatory strategies.

Measurement of Linguistic Features

Quantification of sentential elements is useful for measuring subtle progress in natural discourse production. Because counting number of units is biased by size variations among speech samples, most researchers utilize **ratios.** A traditional device for measuring diversity of vocabulary is the *type-token ratio* (TTR). The TTR is the number of different categories of items (i.e., types) relative to the total number of items produced (i.e., tokens). For lexical diversity, it is the number of different words relative to the total number of words. As variety of vocabulary increases, this TTR increases; we want to see this increase in someone with anomic aphasia. The TTR can be applied flexibly, such as number of different content words relative to total content words or number of different function words relative to total function words. However, the ratio is sensitive to sample size; "generally speaking, the smaller the number of words spoken the larger the type-token ratio" (Fillenbaum, Jones, and Wepman, 1961). A noun-pronoun ratio might be much lower in anomic discourse than agrammatic discourse (Wepman and Jones, 1966). An "anomia index," a slightly different type of noun-pronoun ratio, was used in a study of Alzheimer's dementia (Chapter 6).

Prins, Snow, and Wagenaar (1978) measured progress in 28 variables of spontaneous speech, with a substantial exploitation of ratios (Table 10-2). A computer program initially developed by Miller and Chapman for children was adapted for analysis of adult-adult interactions (Holland, Miller, Reinmuth, Bartlett, Fromm, Pashek, Stein, and Swindell, 1985). Called *Systematic Analysis of Language Transcripts,* or SALT, this system combines linguistic description and measurement. It computes a type-token ratio and mean length of utterance as well as use of auxiliaries, inflections, negatives, indefinite words, conjunctions, and more. SALT also contains a measure of the length of speaking turns in conversation.

Profiles of General Parameters

Another approach to description is to profile parameters of aphasic language expression, as is done with the BDAE (Figure 9-2). Shewan (1988b) drew from Prins' measures, Yorkston and Beukelman's communicative efficiency measures (Chapter 4), and some other precedents, and she combined them into a more elaborate profile called *Shewan Spontaneous Language Analysis* (SSLA). In her data collection, the analysis was conducted for descriptive discourse elicited by the kite-flying picture from the WAB. The SSLA profile is derived from measures of the following 12 parameters: (1) number of utterances, (2) total speaking time, (3) rate, defined as number of syllables per minute, (4) length as a percentage of utterances containing five or fewer words with respect to total number of utterances, (5) melody rating, (6) articulation rating, (7) percentage of complex sentences, (8) syntactic and morphological errors, (9) number of content units, (10) percentage of paraphasias, (11) percentage of repetitions, and (12) communication efficiency computed as number of content units divided by total speaking time. Shewan's (1988b) article presents the complete method in an appendix. The profile looks much like the rating scale profile for the Boston Exam, except that the SSLA refers scores to z-scores for interpretation with respect to a normative sample. The profile appears to be used mainly for planning treatment and depicting a pattern of progress.

TABLE 10–2 Twenty-eight variables used in the spontaneous speech analysis

Variable	Method of Calculation
Speech tempo	Number of words produced in 6 minutes
Communicative capacity	Average of the evaluations of each 2-minute sample
Melody	Average of the evaluations of each 2-minute sample
Articulation	Average of the evaluations of each 2-minute sample
Utterance production	Number of utterances produced in 6 minutes
Utterances shorter than six words	Number of utterances shorter than six words expressed as percentage of total number of utterances
Mean length of utterance (MLU)	Number of words divided by number of utterances
Complex utterances	Number of complex utterances expressed as percentage of total number of utterances
Seconds incomprehensible	Number of seconds of speech which were incomprehensible in 6 minutes
Self-corrections	Number of self-corrections expressed as percentage of total number of utterances
Automatisms	Number of automatisms expressed as percentage of total number of utterances
Imitations	Number of imitations of the test assistant expressed as percentage of total number of utterances
Literal paraphasias	Number of literal paraphasias expressed as percentage of number of content words
Verbal paraphasias	Number of verbal paraphasias expressed as percentage of number of content words
Neologisms	Number of neologisms expressed as percentage of number of content words
Literal perseverations	Number of literal perseverations expressed as percentage of number of utterances
Verbal perseverations	Number of verbal perseverations expressed as percentage of number of utterances
Function-word substitutions	Number of substitutions of function words expressed as percentage of number of function words
Function-word deletions	Number of deletions of function words expressed as percentage of number of utterances
Content-word deletions	Number of deletions of content words expressed as percentage of number of utterances
Syntactic mixtures	Number of syntactically confused structures expressed as percentage of number of utterances
Content-word/function-word ratio	Ratio of number of content words to number of function words
Nouns	Number of nouns expressed as percentage of total number of words
Personal pronouns	Ratio of personal pronouns to number of nouns
Pronouns	Ratio of all pronouns to number of content words
Word-order mistakes	Number of word-order mistakes expressed as percentage of number of utterances
Tense mistakes	Number of tense mistakes expressed as percentage of number of utterances
Unclassified mistakes	Number of all other kinds of grammatical mistakes expressed as percentage of number of utterances

(Reprinted by permission from Prins, Snow, and Wagenaar (1978). Academic Press, publisher.)

GESTURAL BEHAVIOR

Communicative needs of our clients have heightened awareness of nonverbal behavior as a means of compensating for language difficulties. Communication entails the use of several types of symbols and signals (Chapter 4). Research demonstrated that some aphasic patients have difficulty with recognition and production of pantomimic gestures, whereas signals, such as conversational regulators and affective displays, tend to be intact in nearly all cases. One constraint on nonverbal expression, in addition to the symbolic problem that may be part of aphasia, is the motor impairments that can accompany aphasia.

Limb Apraxia

Limb apraxia, like apraxia of speech, is a general term for disorders of motor function that cannot be explained by paralysis or other impairments in the execution of movement. As in apraxia of speech, there are conditions in which a limb movement is carried out normally, indicative of normal capacity for execution. Traditionally, a distinction has been made between ideational and ideomotor apraxia. While we like to subclassify disorders, this is one distinction that has been inconsistently defined and is just plain confusing. It may be best for now to be aware of factors that contribute to individual variation of impairment. There are three conditions in which limb movement is observed: (1) natural or spontaneous movement in the home environment or when the movement would normally occur, (2) requests to imitate a movement, and (3) requests to perform a movement from procedural knowledge (i.e., "from memory"). Another factor is whether the movement is performed with or without an object or objects. Another factor is complexity: whether a single movement (e.g., drinking) or a sequence of movements (e.g., making coffee) is involved. Early subtests of the PICA involve demonstrating the function of an object in hand (Table 9–1). Disorder tends to be observed in the clinic when a person is instructed to perform an action (DeRenzi, et al., 1980). However, disruption of various kinds can occur in movements performed when called for naturally or "spontaneously."

Duffy and Duffy (1989) worked on developing the *Limb Apraxia Test* (LAT), which was used in earlier research (e.g., Duffy and Duffy, 1981) and was described more recently at the annual Clinical Aphasiology Conference. Imitation is employed in order to spec-

ify response parameters precisely, minimize reliance on verbal instruction, and minimize the influence of the so-called symbolic deficit that may be the basis for difficulty making movements on command. The LAT consists of eight subtests with ten items each. Subtests are constructed according to some of the factors mentioned previously: object and no-object subtests, simple (i.e., one to three components) and complex movements (i.e., four to six components), and sequenced (i.e., imitation after examiner completes the movement) and segmented (i.e., imitation of one component at a time) movements. The PICA scoring idea is applied again with a 21-point scoring scale. Data is presented for normal controls and for left- and right-hemisphere damaged persons. The control group showed that there is no difference between left- and right-hand performance of the tasks. Sixty-eight percent of LHDs performed below the range for normal controls, and 27 percent of RHDs were below the normal range. A shortened version with a simplified scoring system was consistent with findings with the long version (Duffy, Duffy, and Uryase, 1989).

Another assessment device is the **Test of Oral and Limb Apraxia** (TOLA) (Helm-Estabrooks, 1991). Administering the TOLA should take ten to 15 minutes. The section on oral apraxia instructs a patient to perform nonrespiratory actions with the mouth, such as "Lick a lollipop," and respiratory actions, such as "Cough" and "Blow out a candle." The patient performs the movement on command and then by imitation. The limb apraxia subtests, compared to the LAT, show how differently the notion of limb apraxia is conceptualized in the clinical community. For example, in the TOLA, movements are observed upon command and with imitation. Transitive gestures (i.e., pretended actions on objects) are compared to intransitive gestures (i.e., actions not involving objects) that are proximal or distal with respect to the trunk of the body. The transitive category includes "Dial the phone," and intransitive movements include "Make an 'Okay' sign." The latter includes conventional symbols, an area that Duffy and Duffy (1989) wanted to avoid, especially with gesture on command. Thus, two tests of limb apraxia assess different things. An early version of the TOLA's limb apraxia test was compared to a rating of gesturing in natural circumstances to determine if a test is functionally valid. Correlation was higher for an aphasic group without global aphasias (0.80) than for a group that included global aphasias (0.66). While strength of these relationships is open to varied interpretation, both correlations were statistically significant (Borod, Fitzpatrick, Helm-Estabrooks, and Goodglass, 1989).

Pantomime

The **Pantomime Recognition Test** (Varney and Benton, 1978) was available from the Laboratory of Neuropsychology at the University of Iowa. It was part of the *Multilingual Aphasia Examination* (Benton and Hamsher, 1978). Thirty pantomimes of a simple movement without an object are presented via videotape to ensure consistency. A patient points to one of four pictured objects to identify each pantomime. Three foils are controlled so that type of problem might be revealed in error analysis. One foil is a semantically related object, another is an object that is pantomimed elsewhere in the test, and the third is an "odd" foil of an object unsuitable for pantomime (e.g., a tree). The test was used in a few studies of pantomime recognition in aphasia (e.g., Varney and Benton, 1982).

A more ambitious measure was first called the *New England Pantomime Tests*, which the publisher renamed the **Assessment of Nonverbal Communication** (Duffy and Duffy, 1984). It contains two tests of pantomime recognition and two tests of pantomime production. For recognition, the clinician demonstrates each gesture according to descriptions in the manual. A videotaped demonstration can be obtained for maximizing consistency. Response is made with a choice of four pictured objects. One test, Form A, contains three foils unrelated to the correct object, and Form B consists of foils

semantically related to the correct object. One expression test models the naming task. The examiner shows a picture of an object, and the patient demonstrates its use. A modified PICA scoring system is recommended. Finally, in a "referential abilities" test, the patient's gesture is evaluated by a third person, who must decide what was conveyed by choosing one of four pictures. One foil is an object that would be used in the same location in space as the correct object, thus requiring a precise gesture. Norms are provided for aphasic patients and persons with RHD for the first three tests.

If a pantomime is to replace speech as a communicative mode, it should be intelligible, although clues come from the situation and common knowledge. Flowers and Wyse (1985) examined intelligibility of pantomimes produced by normal adults who used only their nonpreferred hand. A receiver, familiar to the sender, wrote the name of an object that was demonstrated. This open-ended response contrasts with the forced-choice method in Duffy and Duffy's referential abilities subtest. Subjects' gesturing was highly variable, with a 46 to 91 percent level of transparency to receivers outside a natural situation. Like playing charades, clear pantomiming does not come naturally, but the forced-choice method probably functions like a natural situation that narrows the possible meanings. In data available for the Duffys' referential abilities test, four normal subjects were 97 percent accurate (R.J. Duffy, et al., 1984).

FUNCTIONAL ASSESSMENT

Application of pragmatics to assessment made sense if we are to have a valid examination of natural language abilities and if we are to help a patient to communicate by any means. Now, functional assessment is being mandated by legislation and payment providers (Frattali, 1992). The main idea is to ensure that services are helping a patient progress in activities that are essential for daily living and, therefore, that maximize independence from the health care system. For clinical aphasiology, functional assessment is a special notion that pertains to how well a patient can perform everyday tasks that depend on language skills. Payment for services is more likely to hinge on whether a patient is progressing in self-care tasks such as shopping than on whether the patient can repeat words or name things.

Functional Independence Measure (FIM)

Rehabilitation programs are experimenting with various quick methods for keeping track of a patient's progress in a wide range of domains. Areas of a FIM evaluation include self-care, sphincter control, mobility, locomotion, communication, cognition, and social skills (State University of New York at Buffalo, 1990). Communication includes comprehension and expression. Each domain is rated on a seven-point scale, recorded by a professional for his or her area of responsibility. The FIM becomes a vehicle for reviewing a patient in regular meetings of a nurse, physical therapist, occupational therapist, social worker, neuropsychologist, speech-language pathologist, and other members of a rehabilitation team. Specialists share information about a patient's progress in a domain. Six to ten patients may be reviewed in an hour. This general monitoring does not replace and may actually be based on the speech-language pathologist's independent measures of functional progress.

Functional Communication Profile (FCP)

The FCP is a rating scale for language functions of "everyday urban life" (Sarno, 1969). It was designed in 1956 by Martha Taylor Sarno to be part of a battery of tests to be used at the Institute of Rehabilitation Medicine, New York University Medical Center. Functional performance is defined for this measure as the ability to use language "without assistance, cues, or artificial conditions" (Sarno, 1969, p. 15). The FCP was employed extensively in Sarno's investigations of recovery from stroke and head injury. In comparisons with a traditional aphasia test, it

was found that the aphasia test detected language recovery during the first six months post onset that was not detected by the FCP; but the FCP detected improvement not measured by the aphasia test for the six- to twelve-month period (Sarno, et al., 1971; Sarno and Levita, 1979).

The examiner estimates level of ability in 45 communicative behaviors in five categories: movement (e.g., gestures), speaking (e.g., saying nouns, verbs, noun-verb combinations, and sentences), understanding (e.g., of object names and action verbs, in conversation and for television and movies), reading, and other (e.g., writing and calculation). Estimates are obtained from an informal interview prior to formal testing, and test performance is used for some writing functions. While the interview is fresh in the rater's mind, each item is rated on a nine-point scale, with major categories of normal, good, fair, and poor. Goodness is judged with respect to knowledge of the patient's premorbid abilities. The score for each section is converted into a weighted score in order to arrive at an overall percentage of retained natural language ability. Interexaminer reliability was 0.95 for the overall score and 0.87 to 0.95 for the section scores. Test-retest reliability was described in the manual as significant, but correlations were not reported.

Communicative Abilities in Daily Living (CADL)

With the CADL, we assess aphasia with an ear and eye toward whether an intended message was conveyed. An innovative feature is that behavior is evaluated according to its communicative adequacy. The test is also unique in presenting familiar situations for eliciting behavior, such as making an appointment with a doctor and shopping at a store. In addition to examining interpersonal interaction, many items pertain to the numerous visual symbols and signs that we rely on in everyday life. Holland (1980a) wanted "to incorporate both more natural language activities and a more natural style in an effort to more closely approximate normal communication" (p. 47). The test takes a perspective on an aphasic person's communicative skills that differs from the linguistic adequacy demanded in traditional aphasia tests.

The CADL contains a series of 68 items that are not sectioned according to modalities. Instead, items are organized within a series of situations; and, within each situation, items are arranged according to the natural sequence in which behaviors would occur normally. The test begins with two items for social greetings between a patient and clinician occurring away from the test site. It proceeds to a brief interview; then, in the only truly simulated situation, a trip to the doctor's office is role-played. Twenty-one items follow from arrival at the office to being interviewed by a "doctor." Subsequent situations are presented with drawings, photographs, and props. Functional problems include driving, shopping, and using a telephone.

The test takes 35 to 40 minutes. Other than the pictures and a scoring booklet that come with the test, props must be obtained by the examiner. These include a white lab coat and stethoscope, a shoelace, soup packages, and so on. The clinician is reminded to be relaxed and friendly; but, in role-playing and using props, Holland (1980a) advised, "If you are able to do this with a flourish, or with humor, we believe this is both relaxing and helpful in terms of the informal mood we are trying to create, and we urge you to do so" (p. 49). The examiner should act the role of doctor. Scoring is done with a three-point scale applied to each item. A score of 2 is given when the patient conveys a message in any manner. A clearly inadequate communication is scored 0. A 1 is a broad category between correctness and incorrectness, an "in the ballpark" response. The maximum score is 136 points.

Two studies were conducted for standardization. In study I, validity and reliability were examined for an early version of the test that contained 73 items. For study II, Holland removed five items and obtained norms on 130 normal adults and 130 aphasic persons with the current version. Twelve cutoff scores, used to identify aphasic deficit, were developed for groups defined according to sex, age, and living environment. For example, the cutoff is 128 for noninstitutionalized males under age 46. It is 111, however, for institutionalized females over age 65 and below 80. Patterns of performance are provided for five syndromes of aphasia. For criterion-related validity, correlations with three measures of natural behavior were 0.60 to 0.62. The CADL correlated at 0.93 with the PICA, 0.84 with the BDAE, and 0.87 with the FCP. Interexaminer reliability with 20 subjects was 0.99. This reliability is achieved with a training procedure that comes with the test.

Item scores are distributed among ten categories of communicative behavior to facilitate interpretation of performance. More than one category may be addressed by an item; 22 of the 68 items sample a single category. A patient's profile is based on the following communicative areas:

Reading, writing, using numbers, and judging time (e.g., What can you buy for 85 cents?)
Speech acts (i.e., items that call for informing, explaining, negotiating, requesting, and warning)
Utilizing verbal and nonverbal context (e.g., What do you do when the gas gauge reads empty?)
Role-playing (i.e., the visit to the doctor's office)
Sequenced and relationship-dependent behavior (e.g., dialing a phone number; cause-effect problems, such as relating a speed limit sign to a speedometer)
Social conventions (e.g., near end of test, reaction to clinician's saying, "I'm sorry this all took so long")
Divergences (i.e., creative elements in response, including humor and metaphor items)
Nonverbal symbolic communication (e.g., recognition of facial expression)
Deixis (i.e., movement-related or movement-dependent behavior)
Humor, absurdity, metaphor (e.g., Look at these cartoons. Which one is funny?)

As with any test that samples different types of behavior in a rather large domain, we may want to supplement areas covered in the CADL with further testing. Some specific areas that have become increasingly important for pragmatic assessment are sampled with only two or three items. One of these areas is metaphor, which is useful for assessing persons with RHD, a group for which the CADL was not originally intended.

Across most of the ten categories, aphasic groups could be ranked as to level of ability from most ability to least: anomic, Broca's, Wernicke's, mixed, and global aphasias. This ranking corresponds with findings from most language measures. With respect to within-syndrome patterns, only two groups had clearly differential capacities among the ten categories. In global aphasia, social conventions and utilization of context were stronger than many of the other categories. Reading and writing, speech acts, and relationship-dependent behavior were especially weak. These patients had pronounced difficulty with role-playing. Persons with mixed aphasia were also strong in social conventions and were particularly weak in reading and writing, speech acts, sequenced behavior, and nonverbal symbolic behavior. Later, persons with mild and moderate levels of Alzheimer's dementia were shown to have deficits with the CADL (Fromm and Holland, 1989).

Profiling Natural Behavior

The CADL's stronger correlation with the PICA than with naturalistic observation may reflect the fact that the CADL is still a test. No matter how jovial the examiner might be, it may produce test-anxiety; and, except for the role-playing items, it does not provide for observing natural interactions. In order to determine how well clients are really doing outside the clinic, we should be able to arrange and analyze naturalistic observation. Holland (1982a) reported a system for recording behavior in a patient's natural environment. Unfortunately, natural situations, besides their logistic challenges, suffer from inconsistency of stimulus conditions. There is a trade-off between tests and naturalistic observation. The CADL may be better for measuring progress in general communicative adequacy, while naturalistic observation provides im-

portant judgments about progress as well as identification of communicative strengths and weaknesses.

Profiles became popular guides to observation of pragmatic behavior. Gurland, Chwat, and Wollner (1982) created one for conversation. They looked for communicative acts and conversational acts. Conversational acts included topic initiation, maintenance, and termination. Communicative acts centered around intentions or speech acts. Similar categories went into a checklist developed for children and later applied to adults with CHI by Mentis and Prutting (1987), who noted that the protocol was being revised. The revised pragmatic protocol addresses 30 features of conversation in sections for *verbal aspects* (e.g., topic selection and initiation, a variety of turn-taking behaviors), *paralinguistic aspects* (e.g., intelligibility, prosody), and *nonverbal aspects* (e.g., proximity, posture, gesture) (Prutting and Kirchner, 1987). These behaviors are evaluated as being appropriate, inappropriate, or not observed. Results are reported for 11 LHDs and ten RHDs in 15 minutes of conversation with a familiar partner. In general, we should be reminded of the dilemma for assessment presented by cultural variation in what is considered to be "appropriate" communicative behavior.

Communicative Effectiveness Index (CETI)

The CETI is a questionnaire intended to extend evaluation into daily life (Lomas, Pickard, Bester, Elbard, Finlayson, and Zoghaib, 1989). A spouse, other family member, or friend is asked to rate communicative ability for 16 situations that were determined in development of the questionnaire to be most important to family members. Situations include getting someone's attention, giving yes/no answers, having coffee-time visits and conversations, conveying physical problems such as aches and pains, starting a conversation with people not close to the family, and conversing with strangers. It is a list of real-life situations to be aware of for any evaluation and for orienting treatment to functional activities. Ratings are based on a scale that states "not at all able" at one end and "as able as before stroke" at the other end. Test-retest results revealed a stable mean score for a group, but some individuals displayed considerable variation. Developers of the test have used it for measuring progress.

Everyday Language Test (ELT)

The ELT was suggested in a journal article (Blomert, Koster, Van Mier, and Kean, 1987). The device is now called the *Amsterdam-Nijmegen Everyday Language Test* (ANELT), and versions in other languages are being developed (Blomert, 1990). As reported in 1987, the idea is to identify pragmatic verbal sensibilities for 15 scenarios of everyday life. The scenarios are presented verbally, and response is evaluated with respect to communicatively necessary elements (N-scale) and socially conventional elements (C-scale). The examiner says, "You have an appointment with the doctor. Something else has come up. You must change the appointment. What do you say to him?" (Blomert, et al., 1987, p. 466). An N-scale reply is to say something about not being able to come to the appointment. Social adornment includes "hello" and the implied request to make a new appointment. Another scenario is to say, "You see your neighbor walking by. You want to ask him/her to come visit sometime. What do you say?" (p. 466). The necessary response is to ask the neighbor to come by. Adornment may include a reason or time for the visit. Maximum performance is to communicate 19 N-scale elements and 28 C-scale elements. Scores include number of elements produced in each category and the total number of elements produced. Among 17 subjects with Broca's aphasia, none was severely impaired on an independent auditory comprehension test (Blomert, et al., 1987). Among 12 so-called Wernicke's aphasic subjects, most had moderate comprehension deficit and two had mild deficit. With respect to the N-scale, both groups were only slightly below normal controls and did not differ from each other; they had higher scores with the N-scale than the C-scale. Modifications in scoring were mentioned later by Blomert (1990).

Referential Communication

Another approach to pragmatic assessment is to adjust traditional tasks so that they incorporate a previously ignored dimension of natural language use. The dimension comes from assumptions in the cooperative principle as it applies to conversation (Chapter 8). The specific assumption is that speakers convey a mix of given and new information. Traditional naming tasks, for example, expose the meaning to be verbalized to the listener as well as the speaker so that producing the name conveys given information. However, if the listener is not privy to the meaning, then the name can be thought of as new information. The condition in which the speaker's meaning is hidden from the listener creates a situation for the speaker called referential communication. This notion is broadened to considering the role of the listener's knowledge of a topic. The new information condition is a feature of the *Reporter's Test* (DeRenzi and Ferrari, 1978) and the *Assessment of Nonverbal Communication* (Duffy and Duffy, 1984). A basic procedure is to provide the patient and a listener with their own set of four pictures of slightly differing simple events. A barrier of some kind is usually placed between the patient and listener. The patient conveys enough information about one picture so that the listener selects the same picture. The patient's communicative effectiveness is determined by the listener's accuracy. Aphasic subjects were very good at verbalizing information distinctive enough for listeners to choose the picture (Busch, Brookshire, and Nicholas, 1988). Those with mixed and anomic aphasias were less efficient than nonfluent aphasic subjects.

A few investigations were undertaken to determine whether referential communication matters with respect to what an aphasic person says. If it does matter, then it should be considered for inclusion in a battery of functional assessment. Brenneise-Sarshad,

Nicholas, and Brookshire (1991) addressed this question, not with the simple events of Busch's study but with 13-frame picture sequences that elicit a story. This time, the investigators created two listener conditions and evaluated various parameters of discourse production. Aphasic subjects told stories to a familiar person assumed to be familiar with the stories and to a stranger believed to be naive about the stories. The two listener conditions made no difference with respect to content efficiency, T-unit length, and percent of successful cohesive ties, which is the parameter most related to the linguistic devices that are used to distinguish given and new information. Bottenberg and Lemme (1990) also found no effect of shared knowledge on cohesion and structure of narratives told from six-frame picture sequences. Both studies indicate that referential communication has little effect on telling stories with respect to the parameters studied. However, we should recall the model of narrative comprehension in Chapter 8; that is, a listener is building given information while listening to a story. Listener knowledge of story themes evolves, and a pragmatically sensitive speaker should be aware of this while telling a story. Referential communication made a difference in assessing gestural ability in severe aphasia, because patients did much better than they did with a formal test of limb apraxia (Feyereisen, Barter, Goossens, and Clarebaut, 1988).

SPECIAL POPULATIONS

The beginning of this chapter noted the need for assessment at the ends of the aphasia severity continuum. However, most of the tests and measures are more appropriate for the mildest aphasias than the most severe aphasias. The problem with severe or global aphasia is to discover areas of ability upon which a rehabilitation program might build. These areas might be found in the evaluation of gesture and other functional communicative behaviors. A test targeted for this group is the **Boston Assessment of Severe Aphasia** (Helm-Estabrooks, Ramsberger, Morgan, and Nicholas, 1989). The BASA is designed to take 20 to 30 minutes at bedside for patients in the early acute phase. It contains a series of 61 items, beginning with "Good morning/afternoon" and ending with "Good-bye." The clinician records gestural and verbal responses to these and other items between. Performance can be summarized in categories of auditory comprehension (e.g., "Take the penny"), praxis (movement), oral and gestural expression (e.g., identifying a picture of Hitler or Marilyn Monroe), reading comprehension (e.g., matching a word to a coin), gesture recognition, and writing, which is tested only by requesting a signature on a form. A few items assess visuospatial abilities such as drawing.

Within-sentence comprehension and expression, the domain of aphasia, has been the traditional domain of clinical aphasiologists. It made sense that our evaluation of people with closed head injury and right-hemisphere dysfunction should be aimed at determining their abilities in this domain. We give these patients aphasia tests and deal with their results. With a screening test, we substantiate diagnosis of the absence of aphasia, and with a comprehensive battery, we illuminate aphasia occurring with traumatic brain damage. The discovery of other communicative problems with CHI and RHD expands the domain of assessment for clinical aphasiologists. Diagnosis of primary disorders is accomplished with clinical neuropsychological evaluation, but the clinical aphasiologist may supplement this evaluation with tests of pragmatic language and related communicative abilities.

Many aspects of verbal behavior, not addressed in aphasia batteries, can be impaired in persons with RHD (Chapters 7, 8). A few tests are available as initial attempts to fill this void. Perhaps the first is the **Rehabilitation Institute of Chicago Evaluation of Communication Problems in Right Hemisphere Dysfunction,** or RICE (Burns, Halper, and Mogil, 1985). This evaluation covers the following areas: general behavior patterns, visual scanning and tracking, writing, pragmatic communication, and metaphorical language. General behavior includes orientation examined in an interview. Writing is an opportunity to look for neglect dyslexia and linguistic problems with sentences. Pragmatic communication is profiled with very general rating scales for intonation, gesture, a few conversational skills, and narrative abilities. Metaphoric language is examined by asking a patient to explain proverbs and idioms (e.g., "Look before you leap," "Beat around the bush"). Areas not covered include the comprehension of prosody as well as comprehension and production of discourse with respect to the features surveyed in Chapter 8. Another offering is **The Right Hemisphere Language Battery,** first reported in an article by Bryan (1988). The test controls for visual perceptual deficits in assessing the following areas: lexical-semantic comprehension, metaphor appreciation in listening and reading, verbal humor appreciation, comprehension of inferred meaning, production of emphatic stress, and conversational discourse.

Other strategies of evaluation can be modeled after research, which has provided many ideas for the formal assessment of comprehension and production of prosody (e.g., Cancelliere and Kertesz, 1990; Schlanger, et al., 1976; Ross, 1981). Questions to be answered are discussed in Chapter 7. We can ask whether someone with RHD has a deficit in comprehension and/or production, whether the problem includes linguistic prosody, and whether the problem is related to muted emotion or damage to the music processor. Comprehension is tested by presenting neutral sentences in varied emotional tones and having a patient point to a face expressing the emotion. Besides noting intonation in conversation, we can have someone with RHD repeat neutral sentences in the emotion presented and produce a sentence in a requested emotional tone (also, as a statement and question). We should ask the patient to sing a familiar song. These tests are supplemented with nonverbal tests, such as

recognition and expression of facial gestures and recognition and reproduction of music, especially music that cannot be put into words. To diagnose the disorder in emotion or music, we look for common threads among the deficient performances.

CLOSING COMMENTARY

The clinical crucible will continue to create tests and measures. New methods will serve traditional objectives with more efficiency and will follow the latest research with, perhaps, less efficiency. Clinicians will ask to be convinced of the need to spend an hour to determine a detail and the need to labor into the evening over impressive analytical systems. However, we should support research that starts with a thorough and valid procedure and takes the time to whittle the method down to something workable in the contemporary clinic. Supplemental tests will respect the widening functional communication perspective and will assess natural language so that we can identify the communicative disorders of closed head injury and right-hemisphere dysfunction with the validity and reliability that has characterized tests for aphasia. For aphasic patients, clinicians will demand measures of functional progress that can be validated by family and friends. For studying the effects of treatment, clinical researchers will invent measures of progress in conditions not necessarily presented in the treatment.

Publication of clinical tests has become a big business. Clinicians can purchase a test at considerable expense before standardization is completed. There are products for problems for which research has only begun to provide some understanding. Speech-language pathologists are inventing tests for areas of cognition that are not required topics of study for professional training (e.g., visual perception, attention, orientation). A catalog hails a new test for head-injured persons: "At last, here is a battery of subtests to assess cognitive abilities of head-injured patients..." Yet, the battery evaluates functions that have been examined for decades by neuropsychologists (e.g., Lezak, 1983). Advertising does not say who should be giving some of these tests. Understanding that language comprehension is a cognitive function is not an intrusion into the domain of clinical neuropsychology, but assessing attention and orientation may be such an intrusion. Moreover, we should contemplate the justification for tests aimed at a clinical population as substitutes for tests of functions appropriate for many populations. Clinical aphasiologists should understand the impact of primary deficits on language and communication, and we should be evaluating this impact.

11
RECOVERY, PROGNOSIS, AND EFFICACY OF TREATMENT

Families ask questions: *Will my wife get better? How much better? Will my husband be like before?* Payment providers ask similar questions. Medicare pays for services based on expectations for diagnostic categories called **DRGs,** or diagnostic-related groups. Expectations should be based on research, but the study of recovery is an arduous job. Researchers are challenged by the many factors that influence progress and by many functional domains that could be measured. Payment providers are interested in whether treatment influences recovery, and expectations of treatment are still made of a curious brew of belief and fact. Beyond prognosis, our minimal task is to determine if a patient is progressing. Because impressions of improvement must be substantiated, assessment does not stop with the initial treatment plan. We want to know whether a patient is meeting our treatment objectives.

Let us think for a moment about some basic notions and terminology. The difficult reality is that the permanence of brain damage limits the amount of improvement that can occur. To the extent that "recovery" implies a cure, there is an uneasiness in use of the term. Some clinicians prefer "progress" or "improvement." In this chapter, all three terms are used interchangeably because "recovery" is still used often, hopefully, with a mutual understanding of the constraints imposed upon it. Also, we may be confronted with the notion of "significant progress"; sometimes we use the term ourselves. Some clinical researchers distinguish between *statistical significance* of differences between mean scores and *clinical significance* of these differences. A quantified change may or may not be a valued change. This concern relates to a distinction between *clinical improvement* (i.e., progress in many tasks used in treatment) and *functional improvement* (i.e., progress in the activities of daily living). Sarno, Sarno, and Levita (1971) contended that "improvement which is not reflected in the patient's daily life is not improvement in fact" (p. 74).

RECOVERY OF LANGUAGE WITH STROKE

One distinctive aspect of recovery with stroke is that patients improve regardless of whether they receive treatment. This is called **spontaneous recovery**. When this chapter gets to discussion of treatment efficacy, the key issue will be whether treatment causes more improvement than the progress that occurs spontaneously. For a while, however, this chapter focuses on recovery per se as a basis for prognosis, and we should distinguish studies of treated subjects from studies of untreated subjects.

The Influence of Stroke

After a stroke, an acute phase is followed by a chronic phase. At onset, a patient often has serious reduction of a broad range of functions. It is as if the entire brain has been impaired. A patient is likely to be paralyzed, confused, disoriented, and unable to talk. Some of these functions improve rapidly during the acute phase, and many of the deficits nearly disappear within two or three weeks. A person with LHD becomes oriented to surroundings but still is unable to talk. The rapid improvements may continue into the chronic phase and can be attributed to immediate consequences of focal brain damage. Diaschisis acts as a cloud that hangs temporarily over regions beyond the site of infarction (Chapter 2). It is caused by edema, swelling, and a generalized hypoperfusion that continues to some degree through chronicity. Thus, much of the progress observed in the acute phase is due to a diminishing diaschisis and not to response of the brain to the specific infarction (Laurence and Stein, 1978). This early rapid progress is related partly

to the *sparing* of regions of the brain from infarction rather than recovery from the infarction.

A general impression of recovery was obtained from 92 patients with ischemic CVA. They were followed for two to three years post onset (Skilbeck, Wade, Hewer, and Wood, 1983). Averaging about 68 years of age, this group consisted of survivors from an initial group of 162, balanced for gender and hemisphere that was damaged. Everyday function was measured with the Barthel scale for *Activities of Daily Living*, which rates ten functions including feeding, bathing, dressing, and ambulation. The scale produces a single overall score. Statistically significant progress occurred during the first three months post onset. Progress was not significant when measured between three and six months, and no change was measured after six months. The FCP measured language ability mainly for subjects with left-hemisphere damage, and again, significant progress occurred across the first three months, with gradual but nonsignificant improvement thereafter. The researchers had the impression that no improvement occurred after one year. One of the expectations affecting payment for services is that "significant progress" is unlikely after the first year post onset. Also, some of our substantiation of recovery refers to generalized scores, irrespective of whether they are representative of each function tested. Do ambulation and feeding have the same recovery curve?

Proportion of Patients That Improve

What is the likelihood that language abilities improve at all? In the days before standardized measurement of deficit, the main dependent variable in research was the proportion of subjects making some estimate of progress. Improvement had to be reasonably obvious, and rating scales or test scores contributed to these judgments. Subjects were categorized as much improved, moderately improved, or unchanged (Butfield and Zangwill, 1946; Wepman, 1951), or excellent, good, fair, or poor (Marks, Taylor, and Rusk, 1957).

Marks and others (1957) studied 205 cases of CVA and concluded that 50 percent made some improvement. In another study, 37 percent were rated as improved (Godfrey and Douglass, 1959). Estimates vary with respect to specific language functions. In a study of the effectiveness of treatment, 59 percent of all subjects made "clinically relevant" or "remarkable" progress in auditory comprehension, but only 36 percent made this progress in oral expression (Basso, Capitani, and Vignolo, 1979). Without addressing the effect of treatment, these figures indicate that only half of patients with a CVA get demonstrably better. Yet, according to PICA measurement, 90 percent of untreated patients were found to improve over the first ten weeks post onset (Lendrem and Lincoln, 1985). This percentage dropped to 79 between ten and 22 weeks. Unfortunately, this research did not specify what constituted improvement, because a small amount of change can be random variability. Still, reliable measurement paints a more hopeful picture than cautious judgment.

Measures of Communicative Behavior

Utilizing a scientific basis for prognosis entails coming to grips with the variations in the manner in which research can be done. Studies differ in subject attributes, dependent variables, and tests used to measure a dependent variable. Subjects vary in etiology, age, and gender. Progress of untreated subjects has been followed frequently with the WAB. Treated subjects have been measured often with the PICA and increasingly with the WAB. Other batteries were employed in Europe. A few investigators followed functional progress with Sarno's FCP and Holland's CADL. However, the database is more likely to address clinical progress than functional progress.

Some data is from untreated subjects, but most of it is from treated subjects. Conditions for examining spontaneous recovery have been variable. In one study, "patients were prevented from attending therapy by extraneous factors, such as family or transporta-

tion problems, but were willing to come back once again to the unit after six months or more in order to take the second examination" (Basso, et al., 1979, p. 191). In another study, "all subjects were seen daily (6 days/week) for 15 minutes. . . . The daily visits consisted of semistructured conversational interactions and systemic scoring of the patient's communicative behaviors" (Holland, Greenhouse, Fromm, and Swindell, 1989, pp. 233–34). Some explanations of untreated groups are mysterious; "inclusion of a no speech therapy group was considered ethically acceptable because there was considered to be reasonable doubt whether the speech therapy service available to these patients was effective" (Lendrem and Lincoln, 1985, p. 744).

Amount. Amount of improvement is determined by subtracting an earlier test score (i.e., pre-test) from a later score (i.e., post-test). The result is a "difference-score" or "change-score." In research, an **initial score** may be obtained at different times post onset. Sarno and Levita (1971) gave FCPs to 28 patients at bedside within two days post onset, when some had "a total lack of responsiveness and, quite probably, total absence of consciousness" (p. 177). Some investigators obtained a few initial scores between four and 19 days post onset (Bamber, 1980; Hanson and Cicciarelli, 1978). Aphasic people often make substantial linguistic progress in the first 14 days (Hartman, 1981). In other studies, the first test was conducted an average of 16 days post onset (Demeurisse, Demol, Derouck, Beuckelaer, Coekaerts, and Capon, 1980) or at discharge from acute care with a median stay of 20 days (Holland, et al., 1989). Researchers and many clinicians often prefer to wait until medical condition stabilizes and pattern of language deficit is apparent before giving the first comprehensive test. Therefore, the first score may be obtained around one month after onset (e.g., Lendrem and Lincoln, 1985; Wertz, Collins, Weiss, et al., 1981), sometimes depending on the time of admission to a rehabilitation center (Pickersgill and Lincoln, 1983).

The **post-test** may not always be taken at the point of maximum recovery. In studies of spontaneous recovery, investigators tend to give this test at three or four months post onset. In one study, the WAB's Aphasia Quotient (AQ) progressed 16.64 percentage points in 36 mostly untreated subjects (Kertesz and McCabe, 1977). One subgroup improved 5.16 points; another, 36.80 points. Ten subjects, measured initially with the PICA within one month post onset, improved an average of 1.30 overall response level points until the final test at 12 months post onset. The variability of improvement ranged from 0.34 to 2.72 (Deal and Deal, 1978). In another study, improvement between one month and over five months was significant for 52 untreated aphasic patients, and, when testing was extended to over eight months post onset, average overall change with the PICA was 1.98 with a range of –0.49 to 5.18 (Lendrem and Lincoln, 1985). Research on spontaneous recovery introduces us to the wide variability in recovery among aphasic persons.

In studies of patients in rehabilitation, the final test may be given around one year post onset. Three small-sample studies show some agreement in amount of change measured with the PICA (Table 11–1). Hanson and Cicciarelli (1978) and Bamber (1980) each studied 13 cases resulting from infarction. Initial tests were given at an average of one month post onset. Change-scores were based on *peak scores* achieved during treatment, at nine or 13 months post onset, respectively. Improvement averaged 3.24 and 3.25 in overall mean response level, representing a change of 35

percentile points. In a study of 17 cases, Deal and Deal (1978) obtained *final scores* at termination of treatment around one year post onset and found a similar average improvement of 3.38 overall points. Wertz and others (1981) found smaller progress of 29 percentile points for 18 subjects after a year. These studies tantalizingly indicate that treated aphasic persons improve around 3.30 points in a year. Unfortunately, we cannot promise this improvement for everyone. A treated aphasic client may improve between 0.10 to 7.16 response level points.

A change-score is problematic in studies in which aphasic groups are compared. Although groups may differ in initial severity of aphasia, we may think that we can still compare amounts of progress. Yet, because severity of deficit may be a determining factor in recovery, an equal amount of progress between groups may be misleading. A group with the smaller initial score may be restrained in its progress by its severity of deficit. If this group were to start on an equal level, it might make more progress within the experimental conditions. Statistical analyses of covariance have been used to compensate for initial differences among groups. In a comparison of spontaneous recovery among four groups, Lomas and Kertesz (1978) reported modified change-scores and "thereby had any artifacts due to initial severity reduced" (p. 393). In a study of treatment efficacy, Shewan and Kertesz (1984) analyzed outcome-scores instead of change-scores.

Outcome. What will an aphasic person be like at the end of recovery? In terms of a test

TABLE 11–1 Amount of change in PICA overall scores from three studies of mixed aphasic groups. Ranges show that amount of change is quite variable. Initial scores are compared to Porch's initial scores at one month post onset.

	N	*Initial*	*Final*	*Change*	*Range of Change*
Porch, et al. (1980)	103	9.23			
Hanson and Cicciarelli (1978)	13	9.48	12.72	3.24	0.98–4.29
Deal and Deal (1978)	17	9.14	12.52	3.38	0.51–7.16
Bamber (1980)	13	8.40	11.65	3.25	0.10–6.18

score, the endpoint has been identified with the final score at termination of treatment (Deal and Deal, 1978; Keenan and Brassell, 1974) and the peak score late in a rehabilitation program (Hanson and Cicciarelli, 1978). Final and peak scores may not represent the same assessment. The end of recovery is usually demonstrated with a series of measures showing a plateau of slightly variable scores. The length of plateau may be related to clinical decisions independent of the recovery process per se. Treatment may be continued in order to maintain a stable level of function or enhance pragmatic skills. The scores themselves may not differ much if at all. The distinction is worth considering with respect to studies involving the time to reach outcome. A peak may be reached any time along the plateau, often prior to the final score upon termination of treatment for whatever reason.

In their study of spontaneous recovery within four months post onset, Kertesz and McCabe (1977) reported that 21 percent of 93 subjects attained levels above the WAB's cutoff AQ of 93.8. That is, one-fifth of the group attained a normal level of function. Yet, this group had mixed etiologies, as 20 percent also had subarachnoid hemorrhages and traumatic injuries. The investigators categorized outcomes of 47 mostly untreated patients with AQs taken at an average of two years post onset. Then Kertesz (1985) tabled outcomes with 20 more subjects. He placed 27 percent in the excellent category (75–100 AQ); 24 percent attained good (50–75); 24 percent were fair (25–50); and 25 percent ended up in the poor category (0–25).

The PICA has represented outcomes for thromboembolic patients treated until a year post onset. The final scores in Table 11–1 are indicative of the average. Again, variability is more pertinent clinically, and outcomes ranged from 8.69 to 14.88 across the three studies. A reference for normal is drawn from a large neurologically intact group that scored between 13.40 and 14.99 overall (Duffy, et al., 1976). About one-third of the aphasic subjects represented in the table reached into this range. The brain does not return to nor-

mal, but it is tempting to believe that cognitive function does in a few cases. The latter is unlikely, too, not only because of the permanence of cortical lesion but also because of continued deficiency in difficult verbal and writing functions hidden by an overall score. In the research, highest levels after a year were auditory comprehension and word repetition, around or above 14.50. Verbal subtests averaged 12.52, with describing the function of objects at 10.87 (Hanson and Cicciarelli, 1978).

Outcome may be considered with respect to the number of patients that eventually return to school, enter vocational training, or obtain employment (Schuell, et al., 1964). In Schuell's youngest and least impaired group with "simple aphasia," 14 percent entered school or vocational training, while 19 percent resumed employment. Success was greater in a group with a diagnosis similar to Broca's aphasia: 33 percent entered vocational training and 27 percent found employment. Schuell explained that the less impaired aphasic clients had more difficulty accepting employment that was less demanding than their previous jobs. The more successful group seemed more determined to improve and to adjust realistically to deficit. Among the most impaired groups, no one entered vocational training or employment. Many were persons who had retired before suffering a stroke. These goals are more common in rehabilitation of traumatic brain injury.

Rate. Rate refers broadly to the time it takes a patient to reach different levels of progress. Reports of amount of progress usually include the time intervals from which change-scores were obtained, so some information about rate is available. Certain time frames are frequently employed in the study of recovery rate: onset to three months, three to six months, six to 12 months, and beyond 12 months (e.g., Kertesz and McCabe, 1977; Sarno and Levita, 1971). Time to outcome may be based on different endpoints, depending on whether peak or final scores are used.

One of the most consistent findings is that progress is more rapid in the first two or three months post onset than in any period thereafter. This recovery curve is illustrated in Figure 11-1, obtained from Lendrem and Lincoln's (1985) study of spontaneous recovery in 41 PICA overall scores until eight to nine months post onset. When comparing intervals within the first year, the most change occurs within the first three months. Lendrem and Lincoln found statistically significant progress between four and 22 weeks. Changes after ten weeks were not significant. This curve applies to spontaneous recovery (Kertesz and McCabe, 1977; Sarno and Levita, 1971) and progress during rehabilitation (Demeurisse, et al., 1980). For patients receiving language treatment until 11 months post onset, 65 percent of their progress occurred within the first four months (Wertz, et al., 1981).

Duration of spontaneous recovery has been an important question with respect to the efficacy of treatment. For patients receiving treatment of language function, researchers and clinicians sometimes conclude that progress can be attributed to the treatment when the improvement is observed after spontaneous recovery is assumed to have run its course. A longstanding belief is that spontaneous recovery lasts around six months (Butfield and Zangwill, 1946), but the belief is difficult to substantiate because of the reluctance to withhold treatment after three or four months. The belief is supported by Lendrem and Lincoln's (1985) study that stretched to over eight months. Yet, Kertesz and McCabe (1977) discovered progress after six months. Wernicke's aphasia showed substantial gains between six and 12 months. Recovery in terms of overall function may mask progress that continues for specific functions (e.g., Hagen, 1973). With statistical analysis of change-scores, the magnitude of difference is a function of the interval between measures. An amount of progress achieved in three months may be achieved again over the next 18 months. Very little is really known about spontaneous recovery.

The shape of the recovery curve in Figure 11-1 is the most consistent feature of recovery rate. In studies of peak outcome for treated patients, one patient took over seven months to improve 4.01 overall on the PICA, whereas another took about eight months to improve only 0.98 points (Bamber, 1980;

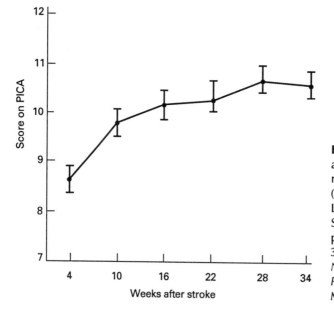

FIGURE 11-1 Progression of means and standard errors for overall PICA response levels by 41 patients. (Reprinted by permission from Lendrem, W. & Lincoln, N.B., Spontaneous recovery of language in patients with aphasia between 4 and 34 weeks after stroke. *Journal of Neurology, Neurosurgery, and Psychiatry*, 48, 1985, p. 747. British Medical Association, publisher.)

Hanson and Cicciarelli, 1978). The duration of progress may be quite different between patients improving the same amount. Two patients improved almost 3.00 points, but took about four and 19 months, respectively, to do so. Two who improved 4.84 and 5.22 points took 7.7 and 30.4 months, respectively. The data indicates that recovery rate is quite variable, which is shown later with respect to syndromes of aphasia. Such data also hides the shape of recovery and is a function of when peak scores happen to have been obtained.

The recovery curve of Figure 11–1 underlies a relationship between *time post onset of initial test* and *amount of recovery*. That is, the later the first test is given, the smaller the amount of improvement that is measured. Pickersgill and Lincoln (1983) examined patients initially from one to 36 months post onset, an average of about five months post onset at the time of admission to a rehabilitation program. The post-test was administered to 24 moderately impaired aphasic subjects after eight weeks. Average overall progress measured with the PICA was 1.01 points, much less than the change-scores in Table 11–1, representing initial tests around one month post onset. Pickersgill and Lincoln found a relationship between time of initial test and overall change. When the first test is given between one and six months, time post onset is also related to verbal outcome (Marshall and Phillips, 1983). Yet, when given within the first two months, time of first test is unrelated to change measured over a year, as indicated in Bamber's (1980) study and an analysis of data reported by Hanson and Cicciarelli (1978). Thus, the relationship between time of initial test and progress is evident across a broad expanse of time over which an initial test might be given.

Based on little data, the belief is that an aphasic patient's progress reaches a chronic plateau by one year after onset. Few studies have extended measurement well beyond the first year, but substantial progress has been found in some cases receiving treatment (e.g., Broida, 1977; Sands, Sarno, and Shankweiler, 1969). A group of 35 patients with infarcts, hemorrhages, and one trauma was given the PICA at three, six, 12, 24, 35, and 55 months post onset (Hanson, Metter, and Riege, 1989). These patients were receiving varied amounts of individual treatment until 24 months and mostly group treatment after 24 months. Many patients showed steady and substantial improvement in the overall score until 24 months. After this point, patients either held steady or declined. Those that declined tended to have the mildest aphasias, and contributing factors included declining health and depression.

Pattern. Relying on an overall measure of language for substantiation of recovery may be misleading and is certainly less informative than attending to specific functions. A patient may progress substantially in one function while regressing in another, but this result would balance out in a score for the test as a whole. Caramazza's concern about the representativeness of subject-group means applies to the representativeness of function-group means, as suggested earlier for a measure of activities of daily living. A clinician probably attends to such distinctions when following a client. In research, most comparisons have been between auditory comprehension and oral expression. In anticipating findings, it is helpful to recall that auditory comprehension is usually less impaired than oral expression soon after onset.

Spontaneous recovery for the four months post onset was differentiated according to eight subtests of the WAB (Lomas and Kertesz, 1978). The observations included two auditory comprehension tasks, one repetition test, and five expressive tasks, mainly requiring word retrieval. Yes/no questions improved significantly more than the other functions. Categorical word fluency (i.e., animals) was the only expressive task that did not show early progress. The investigators concluded that comprehension fares better than verbal expression in early spontaneous recovery. Auditory comprehension has had a better outlook for treated patients, also (e.g., Basso, et al., 1979; Prins, et al., 1978). One exception was Ludlow's (1977) ten subjects who improved more on sentence production within three months post onset.

The PICA is supposed to have one advantage over other tests, in that functions can be compared because of the similar content and scoring across subtests. Following recovery to its peak, Hanson and Cicciarelli (1978) found that verbal functions improved more than auditory functions. Object-naming (IV) and description of object function (I) improved 5.29 and 6.36, respectively, whereas pointing to objects by name (X) and by function (VI) improved 2.56 and 3.30. These auditory functions reached their peaks sooner, at 5.7 and 5.4 months post onset, than the expressive functions, at 7.8 and 8.6 months. This data is compatible with a comparison by Demeurisse and others (1980), indicating that comprehension and expression start at different levels and then improve at similar rates for six months, which could be called a "differential synergistic" pattern (e.g., Paradis, 1977). Amount of progress in auditory functions is smaller, because the less impaired auditory function reaches the ceiling of testing, indicated in the discussion of outcome of PICA scores. In effect, standard tests keep us from observing further progress, and verbal expression eventually overtakes auditory functions in measured amount of improvement over a long period of time.

Progress in features of spoken expression (Table 10–2) was detected by Prins, Snow, and Wagenaar (1978). Shewan (1988a) used her SSLA profile to summarize a picture description obtained twice from 47 subjects. The first sample was obtained within the first month, and the second sample was obtained at an average of 9.6 months after the first one. Of the 12 parameters in this profile, significant recovery was measured for number of utterances, speaking time, syllable rate, number of content units, content efficiency, melody, and articulation. Length of utterance did not change for the whole group, but severely impaired subjects had a significant increase. Complexity did not have a significant change. Deterioration was not observed for any variables.

Recovery was examined in a patient with an LH seizure disorder, who was admitted to a hospital severely aphasic and was near normal on the WAB 15 days later (Holland, et al., 1985). This was an opportunity to examine recovery in "fast forward." Fifteen-minute daily conversations were analyzed with SALT (Chapter 10) and the researchers' own coding of conversation. Elements of conversation were classified as "facilitators," such as queries, repairs, and social remarks, and "tanglers," which were likely aphasic difficulties in conversation. Usage was compared with the conversational partner. Rapid improvement was measured for mean length of utterance, bound morphemes, and conjunctions. These parameters overlapped with the patient's partner in the ninth day. Conversational facilitators increased while tanglers decreased steadily across the 13 days of observation. Holland emphasized the value of measuring both increases in normal usage and decreases in aphasic features of verbal expression. Crary and Kertesz (1988) monitored errors in repetition and naming at regular intervals over the first year post onset. Early types of error decreased, but during recovery, when patients were verbalizing more, new errors would mix with the declining old errors. The basic idea with these studies is that there is more to learn about recovery with respect to specific aspects of linguistic and pragmatic behavior.

Bilingual Speakers

What is the pattern of recovery of the languages known and/or used by multilingual aphasic persons? Paradis (1977) reviewed 138 cases of bilingual aphasia reported in the literature and found many possibilities. Nearly half the cases (i.e., 67 out of 138) improved in a **synergistic** pattern, in which progress in one language is accompanied by comparable progress in the other language. Most of these, or 41 percent overall, were *parallel*, in that two languages were similarly impaired at the beginning and recovered at the same rate; recovery curves overlapped or were nearly identical. Another synergistic pattern is *dif-*

ferential; that is, two languages are impaired to different degrees at the start but improve at the same rate. Recovery curves are separate but parallel. Paradis discerned this pattern in 8 percent of the cases. We should most often expect parallel synergistic recovery in the languages used by bilinguals.

Other patterns are compatible with equal initial severity of deficit. **Selective** recovery occurs when one language improves but the other does not improve, a pattern detected in 27 percent of Paradis' (1977) 138 cases. In **successive** recovery (6 percent), one language recovers after another; one language seems dormant while another is progressing, and the dormant language starts improving weeks or months later. Selective and successive recovery may occur in multilingual persons when one language does not improve and two languages progress in succession. In **antagonistic** recovery (4 percent), one language progresses but the other regresses. The sixth category is **mixed** in two systematically intermingled languages. Subsequently, Paradis and others (1982) described a new category in one case caused by head injury and another caused by surgery. In **alternate antagonism,** or "seesaw recovery," "for given periods of time, the patients could speak only one language, and the available language would alternate for consecutive periods" (p. 56) (see also Nilipour and Ashayeri, 1989).

Exceptions to equivalent recovery of two languages have been associated with the "rules" of Pitres and Ribot (Chapter 4). The rules had explanatory overtones and indicated that a difference has something to do with which language is the native tongue and/or which is the most familiar language. The *rule of Ribot* ("primacy rule") states that the first learned or native language should recover first. The *rule of Pitres* states that the most frequently used language recovers first. Obler and Albert (1977) observed that the rule of Pitres describes recovery more often than the rule of Ribot. That is, the most recently used language more often recovers faster than other languages, including the native language if it is different. The degree to which this pattern occurs depends on age.

Patients over 60 were less likely to recover the most recent language than younger patients. This pattern is also more likely to be followed in multilingual than bilingual persons. We should note that both rules appear to apply to a relatively small proportion of bilingual aphasias. Moreover, these ideas are confounded by definition of "most frequent/familiar language," partly because functional bilinguals use two languages depending on the situation.

PROGNOSTIC VARIABLES

Three strategies of prognosis were discussed by Porch, Collins, Wertz, and Friden (1980). Given that brain-damaged persons are highly variable in amount and rate of recovery, we may still be able to make predictions based on factors contributing to this variability. The **prognostic variable approach** is the most common strategy. We compare "a patient's biographical, medical, and behavioral characteristics against how these variables are believed to influence change in aphasia" (p. 312). The **behavioral profile approach** entails "evaluating the aphasic patient with a variety of listening, reading, speaking, and writing tasks; constructing a profile of his performance; and comparing this profile with the change made by previous patients with a similar profile" (p. 313). This approach is not used often except for the extent to which syndrome of aphasia, as a prognostic variable, is known to imply a pattern of recovery. Finally, **statistical prediction** is the use of test scores to predict subsequent test scores, perhaps with a mathematical formula. While there is considerable overlap in these approaches, the third one is identified with the PICA and is presented later.

The prognostic variable approach is carried out by making a judgment for each patient about the collective impact of several factors. *Endogenous factors* are attributes of patients, many of which are present at the time of evaluation soon after onset (e.g., severity of deficit, age). Some of these factors are two sides of the same coin, depending on whether the neurological side or the functional side is addressed (e.g., site of lesion and type of aphasia). *Exogenous factors* are external to patients and are a function of clinical decisions or circumstances. The main exogenous factor is treatment for language impairments, which is considered later in the chapter. What follows is the knowledge base from which we utilize endogenous factors.

Etiology: Type of Stroke

There is some indication that recovery differs depending on whether a stroke is ischemic or hemorrhagic. The features of gradual recovery described so far are derived mainly from thromboembolic infarction. Clinical experience with hemorrhage indicates that a patient has alternating periods of progress and plateau (Rubens, 1977a). In Kertesz and McCabe's (1977) study, the few subjects with hemorrhage were quite variable with respect to the observations considered. Some patients had large and rapid recovery, somewhat like people with traumatic brain injury. Other patients had little or no recovery. Holland and others (1989) conducted a multivariate analysis of recovery for 50 LHDs and RHDs who engaged in "semistructured" conversation at the hospital for three months after onset. Patients were given the WAB at hospital discharge and at one and two months after discharge. The median length of hospital stay was 20 days, with a range of nine to 58 days. Type of stroke had a moderate influence, with hemorrhage being more favorable than ischemia.

Size of Lesion/Severity of Aphasia

When lesion size was studied, it had a nonsignificant correlation to amount of recovery based on WAB-AQ difference scores, hinting that larger lesions are related to less recovery (Kertesz, 1979). It is easier to determine initial severity of dysfunction than size of cerebral lesion. When patients were tested two to seven days after onset, there was no relationship between an early measure of severity and recovery (Gloning, Trappl, Heiss, and

Quatember, 1976; Sarno and Levita, 1971). Severity measured this soon may not be a factor because of the unstable medical condition and generalized acute effects of CVA. The early severity of dysfunction from an infarction itself may not be revealed until three or four weeks after onset.

Initial severity around one month after onset, measured with the PICA, was unexpectedly correlated in a positive direction with amount of recovery by patients with thromboembolic CVA (Bamber, 1980; Hanson and Cicciarelli, 1978). Patients with the most severe disorders tended to change the most. This finding contradicts the conclusion "that there is a negative correlation between severity of aphasia in the early recovery period and the amount of improvement which occurs during the recovery process whether or not speech therapy is given" (Sands, et al., 1969, p. 204). The research may not damage Sands' conclusion if we consider that the lowest initial overall scores in both studies were 5.85 and 6.63. Inclusion of more severely impaired patients may leave a different impression. Also, aphasic subjects with initially mild impairment will have small amounts of recovery against the ceiling effect.

Considering more specific functions, Lomas and Kertesz (1978) studied spontaneous recovery with 31 aphasic subjects divided into four groups based on initial levels of comprehension and verbal fluency. These subjects were tested initially with the WAB within one month post onset and were retested two-and-a-half to four months later. The relative amounts of progress, weighted for a statistical analysis of covariance, are shown in Figure 11–2. The low-fluency/high-comprehending group made the most progress. The low-fluency/low-comprehending group (i.e., "global aphasia") made the least amount of progress. The two high-fluency groups (i.e., "posterior aphasias") made moderate amounts of progress. This study also indicated that pattern of improvement among language functions varies among these groups (Figure 11–3). In general, subjects with low comprehension improved mainly in receptive functions, whereas subjects with

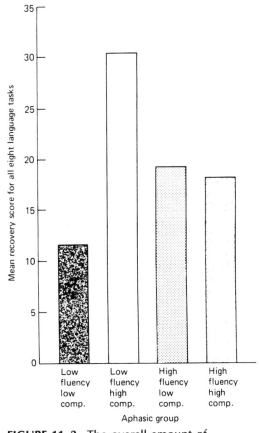

much more recovery of *expressive language* than low-comprehending subjects. However, for severe aphasia, initial severity of comprehension deficit may not be predictive of recovery in *comprehension* (Gaddie, Naeser, Palumbo, and Stiassny-Eder, 1989).

Severity of aphasia has often been identified with respect to *initial test,* which is not necessarily soon after onset. The "intake score" was used in one study in which over half of the 30 subjects started treatment after three months post onset (Sands, et al., 1969). The five patients making the greatest improvement had an average intake FCP score that was over twice the intake score of the five with the least improvement. This finding supports the impression of the negative relationship between severity of deficit and amount of recovery. This relationship was also supported with respect to incidence of progress in an aphasic sample, when initial test was obtained at unspecified times within six months post onset and sometimes after six months post onset (Basso, et al., 1979; Butfield and Zangwill, 1946). Initial test may be a more realistic predictor for speech-language pathologists, because an intake score can usually be obtained, whereas severity of aphasia within one month after onset is determined less often.

With respect to measurement of overall language ability beginning at one month post onset, Porch (1981) predicted that small amounts of progress would be measured for the mildest aphasias because of the ceiling effect, and very small amounts of progress would also be measured for the most severely impaired patients, especially starting with an overall score less than 5.00. Studies of the most severely impaired aphasias tend to support this generalization. However, pockets of improvement in specific functions have been reported for patients receiving treatment. Within one year post onset, seven severely impaired patients made significant gains in auditory language comprehension and gesturing, and most of this progress occurred between six and 12 months post onset (Sarno and Levita, 1981). During early spontaneous recovery, low-comprehending patients im-

FIGURE 11–2 The overall amount of spontaneous language recovery differs among groups defined according to level of comprehension and fluency. These amounts are from the first four months after onset. (Adapted by permission from Lomas, J., and Kertesz, A., Patterns of spontaneous recovery in aphasic groups: A study of adult stroke patients. *Brain and Language,* 5, 388–401, 1978)

high comprehension improved receptively and expressively. One exception for low-comprehending subjects was that those with high fluency made significant progress in answering questions with nouns. Reflecting the unique nature of word fluency, no group improved in this skill in the early months post onset. Initial **severity of auditory comprehension deficit,** in particular, has been of interest. High-comprehending subjects made

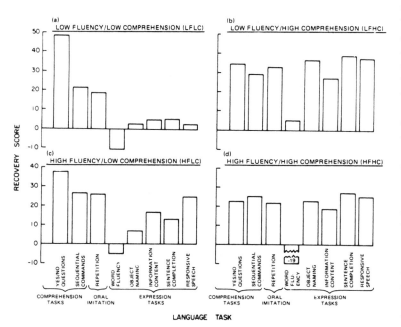

FIGURE 11-3 Pattern of spontaneous recovery among eight language tasks differs somewhat among groups defined according to level of comprehension and fluency. This pattern is from the first four months after onset. Other research suggests that amount of recovery in verbal expression would be relatively higher when measured six months or later. (Reprinted by permission from Lomas, J., and Kertesz, A., Patterns of spontaneous recovery in aphasic groups: A study of adult stroke patients. *Brain and Language*, 5, 388–401, 1978)

proved in comprehension but not expression (Lomas and Kertesz, 1978).

Site of Lesion/Syndrome of Aphasia

In Holland's multivariate analysis, RHDs had a moderately favorable advantage over LHDs for spontaneous improvement of language ability (Holland, et al., 1989). Within the left hemisphere, site of lesion has a pronounced effect, depending on whether it is in the primary language zone around the Sylvian fissure or in the borderline or marginal areas encircling the primary language zone. The latter tends to cause the transcortical aphasias. Several patients with penetrating traumatic damage to marginal zones made rapid and complete recovery, and recovery occurred more often in these patients than in those with perisylvian damage (Luria, 1970b). The rapid and total or near total recovery of a few transcortical aphasias has been observed by Rubens (1977b) and Kertesz and McCabe (1977).

Site of lesion is a factor if we consider deficits caused by subcortical lesion (Chapter 2). Hemorrhages in the thalamus were followed by complete disappearance of aphasic symptoms by the end of the second month (Rubens, 1977b). Later, four cases with capsulostriatal hemorrhage were assessed with the WAB, the BNT, and other measures at three, six, and 12 months post onset (Kennedy and Murdoch, 1991). Contrary to Rubens' thalamic hemorrhages, each case had some aphasic symptoms at three months, but two of these cases had AQs above the 93.8 cutoff for aphasia in five of their six assessments. Another case had global impairment that changed little. The fourth case had AQs of 47.6, 73.2, and 78.6 for the three tests. A single characterization of recovery could not be rendered for these cases.

Diagnosis of major clinical syndromes is said to imply different sites of lesion in the perisylvian region. We may be tempted to associate Lomas and Kertesz's (1978) groups with syndromes (e.g., Davis, 1983). That is, a low-fluency/high-comprehending group is consistent with Broca's aphasia. The high-fluency/high-comprehending group could contain conduction and anomic aphasias. Several studies relied on broad classification. The earliest research examined "receptive" and "expressive" categories. A consistent conclusion was that those with expressive aphasia make the most progress (Butfield and Zangwill, 1946; Godfrey and Douglass, 1959; Marks, et al., 1979). With respect to NCCEA subtests, Broca's and fluent aphasias differed in pattern of improvement during the first three months post onset (Ludlow, 1977). However, nonfluent and fluent aphasias have been shown not to differ (Prins, et al., 1978; Sarno and Levita, 1979).

Kertesz and McCabe (1977) compared spontaneous recovery among syndromes. Data on subjects within each group represented varying time intervals after onset, and some subjects were followed much longer than others. Amounts of recovery were reported for 36 of 93 subjects. Lendrem and

Lincoln (1985) also compared four major syndromes with the PICA overall score, and Shewan (1988a) compared syndromes with respect to her SSLA profile of descriptive discourse. In general, Shewan found nonfluent groups improving mainly in verbal output and articulatory-prosodic parameters and fluent groups improving in content-related variables. Results of these studies are summarized as follows:

Broca's aphasia: Four subjects improved an average of 36.8 AQ points. This syndrome had the greatest amount of recovery and varied outcomes of fair, good, and excellent. Figure 11–4 shows the variability of PICA overall scores over eight months post onset.

Global aphasia: In contrast to Broca's aphasia, these patients changed by an AQ of 5.16. Shewan found that those with global aphasia improved significantly on several parameters. However, a significant impairment of communicative efficiency several months after onset

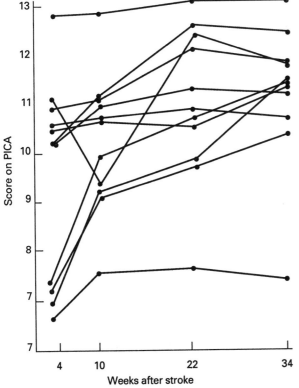

FIGURE 11–4 Spontaneous recovery of persons with Broca's aphasia. (Reprinted by permission from Lendrem, W. & Lincoln, N.B., Spontaneous recovery of language in patients with aphasia between 4 and 34 weeks after stroke. *Journal of neurology, Neurosurgery, and Psychiatry,* 48, 1985, p. 745. British Medical Association, publisher.)

indicated that abilities had not progressed satisfactorily for functional purposes.

Anomic aphasia: Starting at a mean AQ of 85.5, this group was similar to global aphasia in having the smallest amounts and slowest rates of progress, which is consistent with portrayal of the mildest and most severe aphasias.

Conduction aphasia: These patients had an amount of recovery comparable to Broca's aphasia and reached nearly maximum AQs in some cases. Most anomic, conduction, and transcortical aphasias had excellent outcomes, and many rose above 93.8 for the AQ. In Shewan's study, patients with conduction aphasia distinguished themselves by decreasing in number of utterances and speaking time.

Wernicke's aphasia: These patients displayed a bimodal distribution of recovery in Kertesz's study. Some improved little. Others improved by at least 20 AQ points. Some untreated Wernicke subjects made substantial gains between six and 12 months post onset. Some of those

making the greatest progress, however, took six months to do it. Patients with higher initial test scores and less jargon did better than others. Outcomes were as varied as Broca's aphasia but with none in the excellent category and a few in the poor category. Lendrem and Lincoln also found that Wernicke subjects had poorer outcomes at eight months than Broca's, conduction, and anomic aphasias. With PICA overall scores, a varied picture is also evident for Wernicke's aphasia (Figure 11–5).

With the WAB, Kertesz and McCabe (1977) tabulated "evolution of aphasic syndromes and the patterns of transformation from one clinically distinct group to another as defined by the subscores on subsequent examinations" (p. 15). Thirty-three percent of their subjects were noted to have ended up with a syndrome that differed from the initial diagnosis. Fifteen of 68 initially nonanomic subjects had anomic aphasia at final testing,

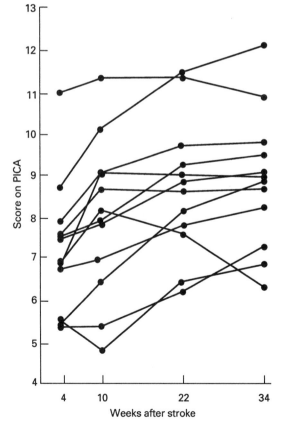

FIGURE 11–5 Spontaneous recovery of persons with Wernicke's aphasia. (Reprinted by permission from Lendrem, W. & Lincoln, N.B., Spontaneous recovery of language in patients with aphasia between 4 and 34 weeks after stroke. *Journal of Neurology, Neurosurgery, and Psychiatry,* 48, 1985, p. 746. British Medical Association, publisher.)

prompting a conclusion that anomic aphasia is a common end-stage of recovery. Kertesz (1979) wrote that "often global aphasia evolves to Broca's aphasia; Broca's, conduction, and Wernicke's aphasics usually become anomic aphasics when recovery reaches a plateau" (p. 99). Yet, "often" and "usually" should be interpreted with respect to the proportions just cited; four of 13 Wernicke subjects ended up in an anomic category. Kohlmeyer (1976) found that type of aphasia changed in 13 percent of 303 cases during the first four weeks post onset, indicating that symptom patterns are stable early and may change over a few months.

Age at Onset

Because of aging, age may be a predictor of progress. Chronological age by itself may not explain much (Tompkins, Jackson, and Schulz, 1990). Growing older is accompanied by changes in biological function, susceptibility to disease, and cognitive and social changes. There has been a mixed experimental substantiation of age as a factor in recovery of language. Correlations between age and amount of spontaneous recovery were not significant in two studies (Kertesz and McCabe, 1977; Sarno and Levita, 1971). It was also not a factor in studies of treated patients (Basso, et al., 1979; Keenan and Brassell, 1974; Sarno, et al., 1971; Sarno, 1981). Younger adults made more spontaneous recovery than older adults in Culton's (1969) study of 11 subjects. Sands and others (1969) called age "the most potent variable influencing recovery" (p. 205), because the five subjects making the most change averaged 47 years of age and the five making the least change averaged 61 years of age. Holland and others (1989) found age to be a strong predictor in their study of 50 LHDs and RHDs over two or three months post onset.

Gender

Gender would be suspected to be a factor if males and females differ in the distribution of functions between the cerebral hemispheres (Chapter 2). Based on theory of functional asymmetry, women might progress more because of some language ability spread to the undamaged right brain. This issue has been difficult to address because of the amount of research done in male-dominated veterans' hospitals. Gender was found not to be a factor in several studies (Gloning, et al., 1976; Kertesz and McCabe, 1977; Lendrem and Lincoln, 1985; Sarno and Levita, 1971). In a study of nearly 400 patients, females did improve more than males in spoken language but not auditory comprehension (Basso, Capitani, and Moraschini, 1982). In cases of severe aphasia, women had more improvement than men (Pizzamiglio, Mammucari, and Razzano, 1985). Holland found that gender was a moderate predictor, but it favored males; however, the prediction about gender does not clearly apply to this study because of its mix of LHDs and RHDs in an examination of language behavior (Holland, et al., 1989). More research needs to be done before a clinician can rely on this factor with confidence.

Handedness

For similar reasons, handedness could be a clue because of differences in cerebral organization between right-handed and left-handed people. However, as noted in Chapter 2, these differences apply to half of left-handers at the most. The factor is of particular interest with respect to right- and left-handed people getting aphasia after damage to the left hemisphere. The influence on recovery would be related to the tendency for left-handers, like females perhaps, to have more bilateral representation of language functions than right-handers. The scarcity of data on this question results partly from the scarcity of left-handers and also from the tendency of investigators to control for the potential of this factor by studying only right-handers. In a study of young adults with traumatic injuries, Luria (1970b) found an effect of familial left-handedness in right-handers; that is, pure right-handers did not recover as quickly. Borod, Carper, and Naeser (1990) simply followed the progress of 19 left-handed aphasic subjects, most of whom had lesions in the left hemisphere. In this retrospective study, most subjects had been tested twice and at various times post onset, so there were few controls. BDAEs indicated patterns of change that were similar to right-handers.

Using Prognostic Variables

Before considering what we do with the variables just discussed, there are other patient variables that have not been studied much. There may even be a reason to think that some of these variables influence recovery or are readily observable signs of other factors. In Holland's multivariate study, she found that **race** and **history of previous stroke** did not matter in the early progress made by her subjects (Holland, et al., 1989). **Length of hospital stay** was a moderate predictor, as 20 days or less was more favorable than 21 days or more. This is one of those indicators of more direct influences, such as the reasons for the short stay (e.g., less severe deficit, good medical condition). Some probable factors have been tough to measure. Few clinicians would argue with the notion that **motivation** to improve has something to do with improvement. Other possible factors include **education,** which has been seldom studied. Tompkins and others (1990) complained that investigators continue to examine the same old variables with the same old measures. They recommended that researchers consider the influence of auditory processing, personality and attitude, and social support system. Holland (1980a) found that institutionalized people with aphasia performed less well on the CADL than did aphasic people living at home.

A "real factor," which should lead to a theory that explains recovery, is not necessarily the same as a predictive variable. A real factor is the pathophysiology of etiology. A predictive variable could be a clue such as chronological age and length of hospital stay; it is related to progress with respect to statistical probability and, therefore, has utility for making a prediction. In considering the clues presented so far, we can say that not much is known about age, gender, and handedness. Age is a clue to the extent that it corresponds with a patient's health and sense of well-being. The most solid clues are the ones that are most likely to be directly influential, and include etiology, size of lesion/severity of aphasia, and site of lesion/type of aphasia. Other factors, such as motivation and social support, are compelling with respect to common sense and clinical experience. We simply weigh the strength of each factor in an individual patient and present the possibilities in terms of whether large or small amounts of improvement are possible and the rate at which this progress should occur.

STATISTICAL PREDICTION

With the Porch Index of Communicative Ability, one aim has been to make a fairly precise prediction of progress, especially for six months post onset. Several analytical devices were created for establishing a patient's recovery potential. One device, called the *high-low gap,* is derived by determining the difference between averages of the nine high subtest scores and the nine low scores. This gap is considered to represent a *dynamic range* between the most serious impairments and current maximum processing capacities. Methods of prediction were largely based on the concept that maximum capacities exhibited soon after onset represent a patient's potential for overall recovery. That is, the nine high scores one month after onset represent a look into a patient's future five or six months later. Therefore, narrowing the high-low gap over the next few months would be indicative of whether a patient is reaching his or her potential.

Porch recommended three approaches to prediction based on assumptions surrounding dynamic range. The *high-overall prediction* (HOAP) relies on a table of high- and low-score percentiles (Porch, 1981). The overall score at one month post onset is converted into the high score that is usually obtained with this overall. This high score establishes the overall outcome at six months (see also Wertz, Deal, and Deal, 1980; Darley, 1982). Porch (1986) referred to this method as an "interim approach" that is "reasonably accurate and simple to use" (p. 297). It is simpler to use a derivative method with *HOAP slopes*, which are graphic representations of the HOAP method. Six-month outcomes are found directly on a graph. The third suggestion is based on intrasubtest variability, another version of dynamic range called the *peak-mean difference* (PMD). The PMD is determined with a formula utilizing differences between the highest score and mean score of each subtest. These three predictive devices provide such specific information that they have been enticing as an apparently empirical basis for prognosis, perhaps because the predictions are made up of numbers. Families were advised that the PICA is capable of early predictions for six months post onset (Broida, 1979).

Clinicians wondered if the six-month predictions are accurate, especially because of the apparent lack of empirical foundation for the three methods. These devices are based on the logic of dynamic range, and the HOAP method is figured from a table derived from the standardization sample rather than from actual measures of progress for six months. As noted previously, Porch has found that early scores correlate with later scores; but other investigators set out to evaluate the HOAP and PMD methods. In a study of 85 patients, Wertz, Deal, and Deal (1980) concluded that the HOAP methods are inadequate as predictors. Actual progress was off the predicted target at enough distance and with enough frequency to trouble these clinicians regarding how much we should trust the HOAP approach. Aten and Lyon (1978) studied the PMD with 24 aphasic subjects and concluded that this method is also unreliable. Porch and Callaghan (1981) advised that variation in recovery around a prediction should be expected. Actual outcome at six months should vary like a normal curve around the prediction. Also, anterior

and posterior patients differ as to PMD changes over time; thus, pooled data would show disappointing results. More research is needed if such predictive devices are to be used with confidence.

EFFICACY OF TREATMENT

Clinical aphasiologists often work in an atmosphere in which others do not believe that treatment for aphasia makes any difference in a patient's recovery. That is, "most neurologists are skeptical of applying these methods to patients and, in general, believe the extent of long term recovery from a lesion is a function of the individual's capacity to realize repair and has little to do with external therapy" (Gazzaniga, 1974, p. 204). This is a dated quote, but it is a belief that clings. There is a "deeply entrenched and widely taught adage ... that the improvements gained through formal therapy merely represent the anticipated spontaneous recovery" (Benson, 1979b, p. 187). One neurologist looked at the evidence at the time and changed his mind, saying that "language therapy has a demonstrated effectiveness in the treatment of aphasia and, as such, occupies a place in the therapeutic armamentarium of the neurologist" (Benson, 1979b, p. 189). This section presents major group studies of the effectiveness of treatment for aphasia, which has been truly an international effort. Along the way, the difficulties in doing this research and its limitations should become evident.

The Meaning of Efficacy

Bloom and Fischer (1982) wrote of the "three eff's" of **accountability** in clinical practice. Administrators maintain measures of *effort*, such as the number of patient visits and length of visit. Clinicians know how hard they work on planning and reporting. Another "eff" is *efficiency*, which, in part, is a measure of effort with respect to time (e.g., visits per day). Finally, of most importance to the client and payment providers is *efficacy*, or the difference that the efficient effort makes in a patient's life. This term can be tossed around rather loosely, as if effort is confused with efficacy. Also, many procedures are commercial products, and publishers market these products with claims such as, "Finally! A method that works!" Data may even be provided to show that patients made progress while being treated with the method. Two somewhat different points are being introduced here. One is that effort needs to be backed up with independent evidence that basic method in the treatment of aphasia is generally effective. Thus, we would not be spinning our wheels if we give it a try. The second point is that there are times when we consider the purchase of methods or materials for which claims of efficacy are made and there are times when we want to make such claims ourselves. We should know what it takes and what it has taken to demonstrate efficacy so that our claims are draped in a recognition of their limitations.

If we want to be scientifically correct about claims of efficacy, then we should begin with the realization that measuring progress does not by itself demonstrate efficacy of a treatment. The notion of efficacy should be viewed with the same respect that nags answers to any question of cause and effect: What is the effect of deodorant spray on the atmosphere? What is the effect of cueing on naming? Determining efficacy conforms to rules of investigation applicable to any question of *What is the effect of X on Y?* (Davis, 1986). In designing a study to answer such questions, X is an independent variable, and Y is a dependent variable. Treatment is an independent variable, and progress is a dependent variable. The reason for challenging measurement of progress during treatment as evidence for efficacy is that other factors could account for progress at any time post onset (e.g., neurological adjustments to damage, adjustments in medications or motivation). Effects of some of these factors are known as spontaneous recovery. We cannot know that language treatment is "efficacious" unless we control for the possible effects of other factors in some way. Thus, to demonstrate efficacy, measurement of Y must be accompanied by a manipulation of X to separate treatment from other factors. Researchers have shown through monumental efforts that this is easier said than done.

Evidence That Language Treatment Works

The aim of group studies is to determine the effects of a broad treatment methodology on parameters of recovery. The principal control for intrusion of other factors is to compare a treated group with a *comparable group* that is *not treated*. Ideally, the only difference between the groups is that one is receiving a treatment for aphasia and the other is not. Unfortunately, one of the first comparisons fed traditional beliefs of neurologists by showing that treated subjects did not progress differently from untreated subjects (Sarno, Silverman, and Sands, 1970). Before waving this publication in our faces, physicians should have considered characteristics of the study. All subjects were severely impaired, so conclusions could be generalized only to that subset of the aphasic population. Also, treatment was administered at 27 to 41 months post onset for these patients, a time when progress for any reason is tough to come by.

The study that moved Benson to change his mind was conducted in Italy. It was published fully by Basso, Capitani, and Vignolo (1979; Basso, et al., 1982). Most of their subjects had aphasia caused by CVA; a few had traumatic injury. The researchers minimized obstacles to group comparison by accumulating groups large enough to be comparable. Ethical concerns were minimized by selecting subjects for the no-treatment group who "were prevented from attending therapy for extraneous factors, such as family or transportation problems" (Basso, et al., 1979, p. 191). It took 30 years to complete the study by these rules; but, in spite of this effort, the comparability of groups was weakened by the nonrandom selection. The reasons for selecting untreated subjects made them differ from treated subjects in other respects. Nevertheless, Benson (1979b) was impressed with similarities in educational and socioeconomic levels, and distribution of types of aphasia, etiology, and gender. Other variables were studied, such as the time of initial test after onset, corresponding to the variation of periods in which treatment occurred relative to onset.

The dependent variable was the percentage of subjects making at least a two-point improvement relative to a five-point scale. During the first two months, when most spontaneous recovery occurs, more of the 162 treated subjects (59 percent) than the 119 untreated subjects (33 percent) improved in oral expression. For those assessed for auditory comprehension, more of the 107 treated subjects (88 percent) than the 86 untreated subjects (50 percent) progressed the required amount. For the two- to six-month period post onset, 39 percent of the treated subjects and 9 percent of the untreated subjects improved in expression; 65 percent of the treated subjects and 48 percent of the untreated subjects progressed in comprehension. Percentages were lower, but the differences between groups were still pronounced, after six months. The study showed that treated subjects are more likely to make substantial improvement than untreated subjects, but the study did not indicate relative amounts of progress with respect to measures that were developed long after this major undertaking had begun.

In Canada, Shewan and Kertesz (1984) compared three treatment groups to an untreated group of subjects "who did not wish or who were unable to receive treatment" (p. 277). The groups ranged from 28 to 23 subjects with ischemic or hemorrhagic CVAs. The treatment approaches consisted of language-oriented treatment (LOT), stimulation-facilitation therapy (ST), and an unstructured support therapy provided mainly by nurses (UNST). LOT was a decision-making process for treatment developed by Shewan (Shewan and Bandur, 1986), and ST was associated with Schuell's methods (Duffy, 1986). Differ-

ences between these two procedures were not reported in detail. Treated subjects received three hours of treatment per week for a year. Progress was measured with the WAB's LQ and CQ and with the ACTS at regular intervals beginning within the first month and then at three, six, and 12 months post onset. With an analysis of covariance for the "last LQ," treatments together produced a better outcome than choosing not to have treatment. Both treatments by speech-language pathologists had a better outcome than no treatment, whereas the unstructured group did not differ significantly from no treatment. There was no difference between LOT and ST. The treatment effect occurred mainly in the six- to 12-month period post onset.

Poeck, Huber, and Willmes (1989) followed the progress of 68 treated German aphasic patients with the *Aachen Aphasia Test*. The treated subjects were compared with the spontaneous recovery of 92 subjects in 17 departments of neurology where aphasia treatment was not available at the time. Treatment was said to be similar to Shewan's LOT, but it was three times the amount. It was given in five 60-minute individual sessions and four 60-minute group sessions per week. Treatment periods lasted only six to eight weeks. The treated group was divided into an early group (N = 23), receiving treatment between one and four months post onset, and a late group (N = 26), treated between four and 12 months post onset. For some in the late group, treatment occurred beyond the final measurement of spontaneous recovery. A "chronic" group started after 12 months (N = 19). The progress of each treated subject was computed by correcting for spontaneous recovery. That is, treatment effects were determined by "subtracting" the control group's spontaneous recovery from the progress that occurred. With these corrections, significant treatment effects occurred for 78 percent of the early group and 46 percent of the late group. Poeck and his colleagues thought that these estimates were low because of the strictness of the correction. No correction was made for the chronic group; however, 68 percent showed significant improvement, which should be of interest to those who believe that progress cannot occur after the first year.

Veterans Administration Cooperative Studies

In the United States, a massive project was undertaken to explore several variables of treatment without an untreated group. First, a group receiving individual treatment was compared to a group receiving group treatment, and in these circumstances subjects were randomly assigned to groups (Wertz, Collins, Weiss, et al., 1981). Several VA Medical Centers participated in a fastidious effort to match groups according to several criteria. For over three years, over 1,000 patients were screened, and 67 met the criteria. Eight hours of treatment per week was started at one month post onset. Twenty-nine patients per group received treatment for 11 weeks, or until about four months post onset. Because of attrition, a total of 34 subjects were followed for 44 weeks, or until about a year post onset. The PICA was one of many measures of progress. The only difference between methods was that individual treatment had greater progress in the PICA overall score. Otherwise, both methods were similar in being accompanied by significant progress. The only suggestion of treatment efficacy per se was a common one. That is, significant improvement occurred after six months, the point at which spontaneous recovery is believed to have ceased.

The next report from the VA project addressed a comparison between two other categories of treatment (Wertz, Weiss, Aten, et al., 1986). One type was treatment in the clinic by a speech-language pathologist ($N = 38$). The other was a home-based treatment by a volunteer who had received six to ten hours of training ($N = 43$). The treatments began about seven weeks after onset. Eight to ten hours per week were devoted to the treatments for 12 weeks, a longer period than was studied in Germany. Comparisons to periods

of no treatment were introduced partly by using these groups as their own controls. That is, treatment was followed by 12 weeks without treatment. Yet, because the spontaneous recovery curve biases this design to favor the period of treatment, a deferred-treatment group was added ($N = 40$). This group, beginning about eight weeks post onset, had 12 weeks without treatment followed by 12 weeks of clinic treatment. The progress made by the clinic-treatment group was significantly greater than that made by the deferred-treatment group over the first 12-week period. The home-treatment group was between these groups, not differing significantly from either one. The three groups did not differ from each other at the end of the 24-week study period, or about eight months post onset, indicating that delaying treatment for a while does not matter ultimately.

Evidence That Treatment Does Not Work

The first study to try random assignment of patients to treated and untreated groups stirred the world of clinical aphasiology (Lincoln, McGuirk, Mulley, Lendrem, Jones, and Mitchell, 1984). A large pool of 327 patients was chosen six weeks post onset when group membership was assigned, but 134 dropped out before the study began at ten weeks. The no-treatment group was compared to a group that was to receive two hours of treatment per week for 24 weeks for a total of 48 hours of treatment. There was no difference between groups at the end of the study period, over eight months after onset. This result was inconsistent with other studies and naturally motivated a close inspection of Lincoln's report. For one thing, it seems that only 26 percent of the treated subjects received the intended 37 to 48 hours of treatment, and 37 percent received zero to 12 hours of treatment.

One response to Lincoln's study was a letter printed in *Asha* magazine (Wertz, Deal, Holland, Kurtzke, and Weiss, 1986). Wertz and others noted that there were no selection criteria to ensure that subjects had aphasia and that there was no evidence that random assignment resulted in a match between groups according to prognostic factors. Moreover, it appeared that around 74 percent of the treated subjects were dropouts at some point in the study. Also, the amount of treatment scheduled was "considered minimal" for most clinics. The letter concluded that "the results indicate that when one does not treat patients who may or may not be aphasic, those patients do not improve" (p. 31). Parsons (1987b) recommended ignoring Lincoln's study: "If clinicians are ignoring poorly conducted research then they are doing what they have been trained to do as consumers of research" (p. 83). Lincoln and McGuirk (1987) responded by saying that "No-one has yet done the perfect study" (p. 442), and that their finding should generalize only to two hours per week of treatment. They even redid the statistics and had the same result. Parsons (1987a) replied, "don't try to mislead me," showing that original wording claimed broader implication; "there are so many violations of basic research methods (threats to validity) in the *Lancet* study that the use of statistics would yield meaningless information" (p. 444). Perhaps our lesson from this is that some studies are more imperfect than others.

Studies on a Smaller Scale

Several studies with smaller groups and/or less experimental control have been reported. Control for spontaneous recovery or other factors was achieved either with untreated subjects or with a *post-spontaneous recovery comparison*, in which progress after six or 12 months is compared to an assumption that progress would not have occurred without treatment. Wepman (1951) found that 68 aphasic patients, whose treatment had begun at least six months post onset, improved in grade level from 3.8 to 9.1. Fourteen cases reported by Broida (1977), where treatment was started at least 12 months post onset, improved an average of ten overall percentile points on the PICA. Three patients improved as much as 19 and 22 points. Hagen (1973)

compared treated and untreated groups in a study that "commenced when all subjects were discharged from the physical rehabilitation program six months post-onset" (p. 456). The treated group had substantial progress in language functions, for which the untreated group had no improvement. Other investigators have found impressive progress in patients whose treatment was not started until four to seven months after onset (Butfield and Zangwill, 1946; Deal and Deal, 1978).

Holland (1980b) bumped into some data pertaining to treatment efficacy during standardization of the CADL. Twenty-eight subjects were retested at intervals varying from eight to 15 months, and the first test was given no sooner than four months post onset. Many patients improved in their test scores. Thirteen who received treatment had significantly more improvement than the 15 who did not receive treatment. Holland discovered that the groups were comparable in several prognostic factors. This "post hoc" study had its weaknesses; but if Holland had not known the basic principles of designing efficacy research, then she would not have recognized her accidental study.

Principles of Single-Patient Experimental Evidence

Some remarkable investigations have shown that treatment influences an aphasic patient's recovery of language abilities. Some of the limitations of group studies, however, should be evident by now. The main problem lies in achieving the no-treatment control with a group comparable to a treated group. This problem constrains the number of studies that can be done. These studies substantiate the value of treatment in a general sense for aphasic people in general. For more specific information, the research has shown mainly that intensive individual treatment does not differ greatly from intensive group treatment (Wertz, et al., 1981) and that two similar language treatments administered by a speech-language pathologist are equally effective with respect to tests of language ability (Shewan and Kertesz, 1984). Yet, few of the programs studied may be typical or applicable to a particular clinical setting. Intensity (hours per week) and duration (number of weeks) varied widely in the studies. A comparison of schedules or methods still requires that a no-treatment condition of some kind be instituted if an investigator wants to make a conclusion about efficacy of the schedules or treatments. Considering the monumental demands of group research, clinicians have turned to single-case experimental designs as a means of accumulating data on some fairly specific features of treatment.

Introduction to Designs. Single-subject designs can be carried out by any clinician with any patient. So far, there is no requirement that speech-language pathologists do this. The minimal obligation is to provide evidence that a patient is progressing; any doubt about whether treatment is the cause of this progress is minimized with knowledge of the major group studies. A clinician may also interpret progress occurring after six months as resulting from something other than spontaneous recovery. The scientifically correct view, however, is that until independent variables are controlled, there could be factors besides treatment that are responsible for someone's progress. Thus, an even stronger argument for substantiating an effect of treatment is to address whether other events occurred in the treatment period that could account for improvements. Treatment may be the only known factor. Claims of efficacy can be supported with serendipitous design conditions or clinical plans that are also design conditions for suggesting cause and effect. Knowledge of designs also helps a speech-language pathologist to be a better consumer for treatment products that are purported to be substantiated with single-subject experimentation.

All single-subject experiments are designed so that a manipulation is performed on X (i.e., treatment) and a suspected dependent variable Y is measured (i.e., progress). The question that can be answered is restricted to the domains of X and Y. That is, one could not claim for certain that an effect

of treatment on PICA performance is also an effect on conversational ability at home. There are two basic strategies of investigation, and more elaborate strategies are detailed in several books (e.g., Barlow and Hersen, 1984; Kazdin, 1982; McReynolds and Kearns, 1983) and in a tutorial for the *Journal of Speech and Hearing Disorders* (e.g., Kearns, 1986a).

One basic design was indicated in the comparison of clinic treatment and deferred treatment (Wertz, et al., 1986). The **ABAB design** entails alternating periods of baseline/no treatment (A) with periods of treatment (B). It is common clinical practice or accident to use a "baseline" prior to instituting treatment, and sometimes a patient wants to stop treatment for a while. An AB or ABA design is not enough to nail down treatment as the cause of behavior unique to the treatment period. A key feature of single-case research, which is often ignored, is that several data points should be collected for the one subject. Measures should be obtained regularly during a phase to determine the trend during that phase. The practice of "bordering" phases with pre- and post-tests does not establish the nature of change during a phase. Such occasional measures may simply be showing random variation. Because aphasic people often progress in both phases and because it is difficult to withhold treatment, ABAB designs are seldom used intentionally in clinical aphasiology.

The more frequent strategy is **multiple baseline design.** The idea is to compare effects of a treatment on different behaviors or on a behavior in different settings. A treatment is administered to each behavior, one at a time or in sequence. This happens in the normal course of treatment. We stimulate spoken language for a while and later start with writing using the same approach. The main difference between this and an experiment is that, when following multiple baseline design, measurement of writing is obtained while spoken language is being treated. One complication with this design is that different dependent variables should be functionally independent, and the functional independence of aphasic behaviors is a theoretical uncertainty. Functional connections among behaviors have been defined in basic research according to assumptions about underlying cognitive mechanisms.

A straightforward example of multiple baseline design is Thompson and Kearns' (1981) study of a treatment for naming deficit with a patient who had anomic aphasia. Figure 11–6 shows that the design was actually a series of ABA designs applied sequentially to four dependent variables. These Ys were four different lists of words elicited in naming tasks which, behaviorally speaking, are "independent" behaviors. Two lists were from one semantic category and thus were semantically related (i.e., A1 and B1). The other two lists were from another semantic category and were semantically related (i.e., A2 and B2). The difference between the A phase and B phase was that treatment added a cueing procedure to the naming task. Treatment was applied to one list and then another. Data shows that trend changes for each behavior occurred only when treatment occurred. What are the odds that these shifts result from something else happening at these times?

Measuring Dependent Variables. If we are to follow these designs in a scientifically correct manner, then we are faced with the prospect of losing valuable treatment time for measurement time. Needs for clinical measurement have been discussed with respect to substantiation of progress. Many single-subject experiments in clinical aphasiology are filled with ideas regarding the investigators' administration of continuous **probes** (i.e., brief recording of observations) during treatment sessions. This is a strategy for determining trends with respect to specific objectives of treatment. One solution to the time problem is to measure behavior during a treatment task and to chart progress over time. The data in Figure 11–6 was obtained during treatment by recording responses before feedback was provided. Such data can easily be inserted into monthly reports of progress. One question that we should ask ourselves, however, is whether this convenience tells us much about functional progress.

One of the important issues surrounding treatment is addressed mainly in single-subject research. The issue pertains to **generalization,** and the question is whether progress recorded in the clinic generalizes or transfers to conditions and behaviors beyond the treatment or the clinic (Thompson, 1989). In most of the group studies, efficacy was demonstrated with respect to standard test batteries administered in a clinic. Thus, we may question generalization of treatments to other treatments, and we may question the generalization of effects to other conditions or dependent variables. The study by Thompson and Kearns (1981) produced good news and bad news. The good news was that treatment had an effect on behavior. The bad news was that the demonstration of this effect also showed that progress with one list of words was not transferring to other lists of words, not even to words in the same semantic category (Figure 11–6). It seemed the treatment in the study would have to be applied to every word the patient would use in his daily life.

There are two interrelated features of the dependent variable at work here. One is the functional validity of the dependent measure, and the other is the difference between the treatment and the condition of measuring the dependent variable. Let us focus on this difference. To show that a patient is improving in a functional sense, we assess behavior in conditions outside the clinic. Minimally, functional progress should occur in a situation that differs from the treatment. The notion of difference may be thought of as the **distance** between clinical behavior and functional behavior (Davis, 1986). Sometimes a treatment (e.g., naming objects) is a considerable distance from the activity in which we want to observe progress. Measuring behavior of the treatment, in effect, is not measuring the behaviors that are consistent with our functional objectives. We may address the likelihood of functional progress if we can show simply that a patient is progressing in "something else"; namely, something with

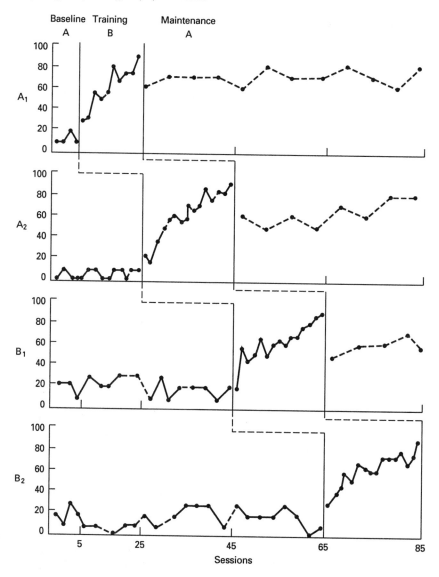

FIGURE 11–6 Probing an anomic patient's progress according to a multiple baseline design. Clinicians obtained percent of naming across four sets of words during periods of baseline and treatment. (Reprinted by permission from Thompson, C.K. & Kearns, K.P., an experimental analysis of acquisition, generalization, and maintenance of naming behavior in a patient with anomia. In R.H. Brookshire (Ed.), *Clinical aphasiology conference proceedings.* Minneapolis: BRK, 1981, p. 39.)

some distance from the treatment. A battery like the PICA or the WAB is a little distant from a treatment; functional assessments in Chapter 10 may be considerably distant from the treatment. As discussed in the chapters on treatment, there are times when we narrow the distance between clinical and functional activity by making the treatment more functional, which may shorten the distance that transfer has to travel.

TRAUMATIC BRAIN INJURY

"The major problem in studying recovery phenomena after traumatic brain injury is that there is *great variability* in the type and severity of actual brain pathology associated with these injuries" (Prigatano, 1987, p. 604). In following aphasia resulting from stroke, assessment has targeted an especially measurable function. Aphasia, however, is not often transparent with head injury, and other cognitive disorders may be a primary concern. In studies of TBI, parameters of recovery are frequently related to psychosocial status and vocational adjustment and are recorded with broad rating scales. Some of the research has been like early studies of aphasia, a morass of obfuscation that is disorienting to someone used to diagnosing a syndrome and specifying an 11.43 level of ability. There is a reliance on descriptors such as "mild," "moderate," and "severe" to characterize a patient's or group's neuropathology or dysfunction. These descriptors are often presented as if we should know what they mean. We can find mild, moderate, and severe subcategories of severe head injuries; there are also mild and moderate subcategories of mild head injuries.

Luria (1970b) found differences in progress made with penetrating/open head wounds and nonpenetrating wounds from World War II. Most of the 73 cases (93 percent) of penetrating injury to language areas continued to be clinically aphasic after two months post onset. However, 63 percent of 16 cases of nonpenetrating injuries to language areas remained aphasic after two months. The extreme difference of sample size weakened the impact of this comparison, but data on damage to marginal language areas also showed that nonpenetrating injury had a higher frequency of "total recovery." This study also does not strictly apply to the spectrum of blunt or closed head injury caused by falls and vehicular accidents. It is suggestive of the rapid and large recovery that sets closed head injury (CHI) apart from CVA.

Cripe (1987) described four general phases in recovery from CHI: (1) the **coma phase,** or a loss of consciousness lasting hours to weeks, (2) the **post-traumatic amnesic phase** (PTA), beginning when consciousness is regained and ending when the patient can remember day-to-day events on a continuous basis, (3) the **rapid recovery phase,** during which patients make significant progress over a few months, lasting three to six months depending on severity, and (4) the **long-term plateau phase,** in which residual deficits persist and progress is painstakingly slow. Outcome, especially regarding success of rehabilitation, is often represented in terms of whether a patient has returned to independent functioning or to previous employment. Cripe (1987) associated treatment strategies with each phase. During PTA, assistance with attention and orientation is provided, but complicated cognition is avoided. During rapid recovery, treatment is focused on basic skills, and patients are helped to minimize unrealistic expectations of returning to school or work. The long-term phase emphasizes compensatory adjustments to disabilities.

All severe injuries, with coma of at least 24 hours, have a PTA exceeding one day. A family member may identify the conclusion of this phase when the patient begins to remember previous conversations. In more than 90 percent of cases, it lasts more than a week; it lasts more than four weeks in 60 percent (Jennett and Teasdale, 1981). The longer PTA lasts, the more difficult it is to recognize exactly when it ends, and identification can be one or two weeks off. The length of this period is sometimes used as an indication of severity of injury. PTA less than ten minutes is a very mild injury; ten to 60 minutes is a mild injury; and one to 24 hours is moderate injury. Duration of PTA is also related to severity of dysfunction. A strong relationship was found between increasing PTA and decreasing scores on the *Wechsler Memory Scale* (Brooks, 1976).

A sense for recovery rate in cognitive functioning was obtained in a cross-sectional design in which different groups were evaluated at different periods post onset (Bond, 1975; cited in Prigatano, 1987). An overall IQ score from the WAIS was followed. Most improvement occurred in the first six months after injury. Progress was slower thereafter until two years post onset. With measures of memory in a longitudinal study, Lezak (1979) found significant improvement extending to six to 12 months post onset but no significant change thereafter. In another study, relatives rated changes in personality ten to 15 years post onset (Thomsen, 1984). Childishness had declined but sensitivity to stress and loss of interest in surroundings increased in some patients.

Patients with CHI have been observed to recover language to a functional level by four months post onset (Groher, 1977) and to normal levels on an aphasia battery by six months (Levin, Grossman, Sarwar, and Meyers, 1981). Persistent deficit was associated with persistent hematomas in the left hemisphere. After reviewing studies, Levin (1981) found "an overall trend of improvement that may eventuate in restoration of language or specific defects ('subclinical' language disorder) in naming or word finding in about two-thirds of the patients who are acutely aphasic" (p. 441). Adolescents with CHI still had deficits of verbal expression one year after onset (Campbell and Dollaghan, 1990). Luzzatti and his colleagues (1989) followed 18 patients with an Italian version of the Aachen Aphasia Test and some other language and neuropsychological tests. The time periods were highly variable. The first test was given at a median of five months post onset and the second at a median inter-

val of 17 months, ranging from four to 36 months. Progress was more evident in most of the aphasia battery subtests and in a categorical word-fluency task than in supplemental naming and neuropsychological measures. Findings were probably influenced by the early recovery that was not observed and ceiling effects with certain tests.

In developing a foundation for prognosis, Luria's (1970b) findings with penetrating and nonpenetrating injuries indicated that type or severity of head injury is probably a factor. Patients with only diffuse swelling have a better level of neuropsychological recovery than those who evidence diffuse axonal injury (Uzell, Dolinskas, Wiser, and Langfitt, 1987). Severity of injury estimated by duration of coma and/or PTA has been considered. "Most mild injuries . . . show substantial recovery and are often back to work within 3 to 6 months postinjury," noted Prigatano (1987, p. 603). "Patients with moderate injuries . . . and severe injuries . . . are quite *variable* in their recovery course." Bond (1983; cited in Prigatano, 1987) focused on duration of PTA. When PTA was under three weeks, overall IQ improved from 94 to 100 in six months. When PTA was four to six weeks, IQ improved from around 80 to 92 in six months and reached 100 after 12 months post onset. When PTA was eight to 11 weeks, a pattern of recovery was evident. The verbal scale improved faster than the performance scale over the first six months (Table 4–1). Afterward, the performance scale progressed slowly to two years post onset. In general, PTA less than seven weeks is accompanied by the early, rapid recovery associated with CHI. If PTA is longer than 12 weeks, progress is not so promising.

A study of 84 children and adolescents with CHI was conducted with a variety of tests (Tompkins, Holland, Ratcliff, Costello, Leahy, and Cowell, 1990). Patients were followed for a year post onset. The first test was one month after hospital discharge, and the second and third tests were at six and 12 months post onset for all subjects. Multiple regression analysis showed that for adolescents, severity of injury and existence of premorbid disorders were predictive of performance one month after discharge. Also for the older subjects, poor performance at one month after discharge was associated with poor performance one year post onset. Severity of injury or dysfunction has been the most consistent prognostic sign.

One team of clinicians ventured into the world of statistical prediction based on PICA-theory with 13 subjects, mostly with CHIs (Fleming, Hubbard, Schinsky, and Datta, 1982). The subjects were said to have aphasia. Fleming focused on the peak-mean difference (PMD), a computation of intrasubtest variability. A large PMD was thought to be predictive of good progress for persons with aphasia. Seven of the patients exhibited a "C-pattern," in which PMD declined over several months post onset, while the test's overall score increased. A declining PMD should happen with recovery, as subtest variability should decrease. The other patients showed no coherent relationship between PMD and the overall test score. The authors concluded that the PMD has little value for prognosis with CHI. They recommended a direct comparison of the peak score and mean score for each subtest, supposing that the peak score is a clue to potential for improvement.

SUMMARY AND CONCLUSIONS

Important decisions about supporting services for people with aphasia are based on notions of recovery from stroke and efficacy of treatment. These notions have stuck from the early period of research and are quite general. It is thought that recovery is greatest and swiftest during the first two or three months post onset and slows down until about six months after onset. At this point, treatment has its clearest effect until around 12 months post onset for most patients. The generalization ignores the considerable variation that seems to occur as a function of severity and type of aphasia and some other factors that are not understood very well. This variability may result in more variable support for service if we could predict the variation to the satisfaction of health system managers. We know that patients in the middle range of severity one month post onset improve the most, but the capabilities of mildly impaired patients have been hidden by ceiling effects. Mildly impaired patients have the best outcomes. However, most of this information is based on measurements within the first year after onset. The same amount of data is not available for the period after 12 months. No one can say much for sure about this period. There is evidence to show that aphasic patients in treatment improve well beyond the first year, but there is little research that tells us the type of patients and conditions that produce this change.

The scientific foundation for clinical decisions is also based on standard tests of clinical language ability. This data is represented mainly as overall scores or scores for comprehension and verbal expression. Further differentiation of skills that may be important to an individual's quality of life has not been brought to the forefront of decision making based on prognosis. Continuing in this direction, we should realize that the foundation for prognosis says little about the recovery rate for functional abilities. This is a curious situation, considering that payment providers want progress to be measured with functional assessments. We have an idea that eight to ten hours of treatment per week is more effective than two hours per week. Yet, we know little about effects of new treatments or treatments specialized for particular disorders. We do not know if general knowledge of treatment efficacy applies to pragmatic treatments, especially when the distance between treatment and functional assessment is minimal. Our actuarial tables are not very complete. As Wertz (1987) concluded after his review of what is really known, there is work to be done.

CHAPTER

12

PRINCIPLES OF LANGUAGE TREATMENT

Treatment of aphasia has matured into a multidimensional enterprise. It has multiple objectives and approaches. An aphasic patient may benefit from different approaches at different phases of recovery. The domain of language impairment has expanded beyond the sentence, and speech-language pathologists have become integral members of rehabilitation teams. So-called **cognitive rehabilitation** addresses disorders of attention, perception, memory, and reasoning. This term is associated with head injury; but when "cognition" is aligned with cognitive neuropsychology, aphasia treatment is technically an example of cognitive rehabilitation. Principles of research and treatment are similar across these patients. We may aim treatment at impaired processes when someone has a stroke or trauma. Principles of goal-setting, behavioral modification, and functional generalization are applicable across disorders.

This chapter maintains this level of general applicability while considering mostly the language problems of aphasia. Implementation for specific deficits is the theme of Chapter 13.

THE HELPFUL CLINICIAN

Rehabilitation is supported by the relationship between a clinician and a client, which may have to be sustained for several months. Rapport, trust, and motivation are factors that contribute to the therapeutic process. A comprehensive approach to rehabilitation involves intruding on a person's thoughts, feelings, and home life to some degree. We establish an atmosphere in which our clients can comfortably tell us of extraneous events that may be interfering with the treatment process or the likelihood of generalization. This information may help us make an appropriate referral to a professional who can help with the problem (see Kennedy and Charles, 1990). Our technical skills are not enough for a constructive therapeutic relationship to flourish for a long time. If a patient is uncomfortable with a clinician, the patient quits. Our "people skills" are an integral part of language rehabilitation.

Unconditional Positive Regard. A stroke does not discriminate according to beliefs, values, and attitudes. Some patients have not heard of feminism. Head injury may have ended a drunken spree in a stolen Camaro. Some patients keep smoking while trembling with a violent cough. Emotions may be hard to control, and profanity is unwittingly produced. We wait for responses while the next patient is waiting at the door. We think we understood something and then find out later we were wrong. An aphasic adult detects body language and prosody conveying attitudes about all of this. Sacks (1985) stated that "one cannot lie to an aphasic person." In a survey by Skelly (1975), patients "cited numerous subtle signs of impatience from those around them which were deeply discouraging—audible sighs, tightening of the mouth muscles, shoulder and eye movements, and drumming fingers" (p. 1141).

In creating a positive climate for therapeutic change, a clinician must have unconditional positive regard for a patient. The influential clinical psychologist Carl Rogers (1961) defined it as "an outgoing positive feeling without reservations, without evaluations" (p. 62). The impact of positive regard was expressed by Wulf (1979) when she commented on her first contact with her therapist, who wore a "radiant smile": "And this was the first miracle speech therapy wrought for me. No word was needed—it was the magic of a look—an instantaneous rapport partly because my innermost messenger had told me that it would be that way" (p. 50). "The notion of an accepting atmosphere in the clinic should not be misconstrued to mean that 'anything goes,' that there are no boundaries within which the patient must

function to achieve the goals of language treatment. It does mean, however, that the patient's depression, frustration, or anger is allowed in the clinical setting without reservation or evaluation by the clinician" (Davis and Holland, 1981, p. 218). The magical smile means that a patient in a hospital is never an intrusion and is always welcome in the clinician's office.

Empathic Understanding. Wulf (1979) also wrote that "speech therapy's rare talent is this: being able to hop on anybody's wave length and stay there until the aphasic has learned how to climb the unending tortuous crag facing him" (p. 50). In a survey of clients who evaluated attributes of a good clinician, "empathetic-genuineness" ranked second to technical skill (Haynes and Oratio, 1978). Empathy is a capacity to sense the feelings and personal meanings that another person is experiencing at each moment (Rogers, 1961). We cannot walk in an aphasic person's shoes, but we can convey that we understand the problems created by brain damage. Rapport is enhanced when expertise and sensitivity are established at the first meeting. Experienced clinicians are familiar with the soothing of frustration that comes with statements such as, "I know, you know what you want to say but just can't think of the words to say it." Sometimes a speech-language pathologist is the first person to convey this understanding. A client discovers someone who knows that he or she is not stupid and suddenly believes there is someone in the hospital who can help with the exasperation of trying to talk. Empathetic genuineness breeds hope and motivation. A client is inclined to accept the rigors of clinical advice when he or she knows that the helper understands the problem.

Rogers (1951) also advised that "it is the counselor's function to assume, insofar as he is able, the internal frame of reference of the client . . . to lay aside all perceptions from the external frame of reference while doing so, and to communicate something of this empathic understanding to the client" (p. 29). An external frame of reference includes stereotypic conceptions according to gender, age, race, or religion. Ageism, for example, may entail a fear of the elderly that interferes with addressing a client as an individual (Davis and Holland, 1981). Prospective clinical aphasiologists should evaluate their attitudes regarding these attributes so that they can keep them out of clinical interactions and can attain unconditional positive regard and empathy for their patients.

BASIC OBJECTIVES OF TREATMENT

The objectives of treatment are dictated by the nature of impairments and their impact on a patient's daily life. For anyone with a cerebral injury, the main goal is **to repair or restore cognitive processes.** For someone with aphasia, the main goal is **to repair or restore language processes.** This class of objectives follows the spirit of repairing what is broken or reviving what seems to be lost. For someone with closed head injury, the goal may be to repair systems of attention or memory. A speech-language clinician tries to repair language systems battered either directly or indirectly. Goals can be stated with respect to different domains of the problem:

Neurological: to restore operation of inefficient parts of the brain.
Cognitive-general: to repair sentence comprehension.
Cognitive-specific: to repair the syntactic parser.
Behavioral: to achieve 95 percent accuracy of pointing to pictures in response to spoken sentences with reduced relative clauses.

Speech-language pathologists concern themselves with each domain except for the neurological goal, which might be achieved with medication.

By thinking of aphasia as a communication disorder, we acknowledge its impact on everyday life. We want to reduce the frustration in exchanging messages, and so we want **to improve a patient's adaptive capacities.** Our repairs of a language system should contribute to this end, but the idea of adaptation expands our goals into areas involving a client's spared skills and environmental influences on interpersonal interaction. Communicative goals are compatible with being realistic about the constraints on restoration or repair because of a permanently damaged brain. With mild head injury, capacities are tantalizingly close to pretraumatic levels, and the patient is anxious to return to school or work. A realistic approach to language disorder is driven by the following objectives:

to improve the efficiency of residual capacities, which include the working parts of an impaired language system;
to develop augmentative or alternative modes of communication, which include residual capacities outside the language system.

Identification of retained capacities depends on how we identify impaired capacities. When function is divided according to cognitive processes, we may identify retained and impaired processes within a modality (e.g., word retrieval, syntactic formulation). For Broca's aphasia, a goal may be to improve the efficiency of a residual word-finding process. When treatment is directed to other cognitive functions, such as memory, we remember that these functions are multidimensional as well. Objectives include improving the efficiency of retained memory capacities and developing alternative means of remembering.

Linguistic and communicative skills can be improved within a clinical task but may not extend to life outside the clinic. We stretch our primary goals **to transfer repaired processing and improved residual capacities to a client's daily life.** Some speech-language pathologists distinguish between acquisition and generalization. *Acquisition* refers to reestablishing a behavior/function in the clinic. That is, a client can name things that could not be named before. *Generalization* is the transfer of a new behavior or repaired process to conditions beyond the treatment. If word-finding is improved for naming, then it should also be improved when conversing at the dinner table. When remembering names of foods is improved in a list-recall task, it should also be improved when shopping at a grocery. When pointing to items on a menu is practiced in a hospital, it should also be used when ordering in a restaurant. In rehabilitation from head trauma, generalization is a component of goals for **community reintegration.** Until improvement is shown in natural communicative situations, the job is not done.

Other considerations pertain to the contexts in which the language system functions. The helpful clinician cannot ignore the struggle to adjust to a new life with stroke or traumatic brain injury. A patient's psychological state and support system may provide either a constructive or a destructive atmosphere for improving the language system. A speech-language pathologist assists a rehabilitation team **to maximize psychological adjustment to the realities of disorder.** Moreover, goals so far are aimed at changing the patient. A patient's crisis becomes a crisis for the family, too. A speech-language pathologist is often involved in trying **to facilitate adjustment by significant others to changes in their lives attributable to someone with aphasia.** Pursuit of this objective can be viewed as a means of helping the patient by improving the contexts in which the language system is used.

AN APPROACH TO APPROACHES

An approach to treatment begins with an objective, such as the desire to repair a language subsystem or enhance a residual capacity. Then it articulates principles for administering procedures that meet the objective. It may add a method of measurement to determine whether the goal is met. An approach may be shown to stand on theoretical assumptions about function, dysfunction, and/or recovery. Because rehabilitation has multiple complementary goals, it has multiple approaches.

Basic Repair of Language Functions

Reviews of aphasia treatment have presented us with imposing lists of "approaches."

Some approaches address aphasia generally, and others dictate procedures for specific impairments such as agrammatism. A specific approach may be one version of a general approach. Lists refer to linguistic, cybernetic, psycholinguistic, cognitive neuropsychological, behavioral, functional, and pragmatic approaches. Also, approaches are identified with individuals, such as "Schuellian treatment" (Rosenbek, et al., 1989), or they have officious names, such as Language-Oriented Treatment (Shewan and Bandur, 1986) or Promoting Aphasics' Communicative Effectiveness (Davis and Wilcox, 1985). Clinicians seem to have nine or ten options when sitting down to help an aphasic client. Some terms merely represent variants of the same thing (e.g., functional and pragmatic). Classifications may emphasize a discipline that shaped a clinician's thinking, although procedures turn out to be similar to other approaches. Some of the labels point to parts of a large therapeutic elephant. A linguistic approach may emphasize structural features of content found in another approach that prescribes the same tasks. A basic approach may draw upon many sources, each being a valuable tributary to a main stream of methodology.

One of the broadest classifications of approach was Wepman's (1972) distinction between direct and indirect treatment. **Direct approaches** focus the aphasic patient on specific language skills and behaviors. The skills, such as naming things, are practiced with a highly structured task. **Indirect approaches** may be aimed at language but do not restrict a patient to a specific skill or behavior. They are portrayed as being "unstructured" and include conversation or social activities. Direct approaches have been explicitly designed to repair an impaired function. Indirect approaches have been justified variably as improving a function, expanding its use to natural situations, and facilitating psychosocial adjustment. Currently, the direct-indirect distinction is too vague to characterize the many dimensions of rehabilitation. Improving a language skill can be achieved indirectly, and generalization can be addressed directly.

The main orientation of clinical aphasiology has been to try to repair the damaged language mechanism with direct methods. Generally, a clinician finds a functioning level of language behavior during initial assessment and then creates tasks or drills that allow a patient to practice using language at the functioning level. The tasks are similar to those employed in basic research and assessment. Brookshire, Nicholas, and others (1978) studied 40 videotaped treatment sessions conducted in various regions of the United States. The clinicians may have considered themselves to vary in approach, but they did basically the same thing when administering treatment. In any task, a clinician presented a **stimulus;** a patient made a **response;** and the clinician provided **feedback** to the patient's response. Tasks are structured according to this standard framework in order to allow a patient to practice verbal expression or language comprehension.

The functional components of a treatment task include a **target-stimulus** and a **target-response.** In a comprehension task, the target-stimulus is a word or sentence. The response may be pointing to one of a set of pictures. A target-stimulus such as an object or object description may be supplemented with cues to elicit naming as the target-response. A task contains several stimulus **items** such as words or objects; and, using the terminology of experiments, presenting each item is called a **trial.** A task consists of multiple trials, as few as ten or as many as 30. An item may be presented once or repeatedly as in blocks of ten items three times to create 30 trials. Fastidious attention to these components guides clinical investigators in considering the variables of a treatment and in explicitly describing the treatment being studied.

Reviewers have settled on two variants of direct treatment that make a difference in conducting stimulus-response-feedback interaction (LaPointe, 1985; Sullivan and Brookshire, 1989). The **cognitive stimulation** approach is traced to Hildred Schuell's techniques developed in the 1950s and emphasizes presentation of the stimulus (or antecedent event) as the mechanism for improving an aphasic language system. **Operant conditioning** is traced to principles practiced broadly in speech-language pathology beginning in the 1960s, and it relies on feedback (or the consequent event) as the primary mechanism for changing language behavior. Table 12-1 summarizes the contrasts between these approaches, and the following sections provide brief explanations of the main features of each orientation.

Cognitive Stimulation

Cognitive approaches originated in what has been called a **stimulation-facilitation** methodology. Stimulation is what a clinician does, and facilitation is the presumed effect of stimulation on central processes. A clinician stimulates a patient in order to facilitate comprehension and formulation. Schuell's

TABLE 12–1 Comparison of cognitive and behavioral approaches to treatment of aphasia.

	Cognitive Stimulation	Operant Conditioning
1.	Beliefs that aphasia involves impaired mental processes	No theoretical assumptions about the nature of aphasia
2.	Goals expressed in terms of mental processes	Goals expressed solely in terms of observable events (i.e., response to stimuli)
3.	New behavior established using *antecedent event* as facilitator	New behavior established by using *consequent event* as reinforcer
4.	Large amount of content (e.g., lexicon) varying from session to session	Items often restricted and constant from session to session
5.	*Restimulation* as feedback upon error	Punishment in response to error

therapeutic insights have been associated with other clinicians of her time such as Wepman (1953) and Eisenson (1984). These clinicians influenced Darley (1982), Brookshire (1978a, 1986), Duffy (1986), Shewan and Bandur (1986), and Rosenbek and others (1989). They extended Schuell's principles based on studies that systematically explored effects of antecedent events on aphasic behavior (Chapter 4).

Theoretical Assumptions. In a posthumous publication of her lectures, Schuell stated that "what you do about aphasia depends on what you think aphasia is" (Sies, 1974, p. 138). By remembering that aphasia is a language disorder, we establish goals that differ from those in the treatment of speech disorders. The acquired nature of the disorder has implications that differ from developmental language disorders, especially with respect to the extent that learning language is required. Theories of the brain's recovery from injury also motivate our approach in that we may emphasize training residual capacities. Finally, we base our treatment on assumptions about how cognitive functions are supposed to operate normally. Assuming that we still have much to learn about the nature of aphasia and natural language processing, we should assume that our approaches to treatment will develop as theories of language capacity and aphasia develop.

The primary assumption underlying Schuellian treatment is that "aphasia is not a loss of language, but is the result of impairments in processes which underly speaking, listening, writing, and reading" (Brookshire, 1986, p. 127). Schuell had said that "I do not teach aphasic patients words. I stimulate language processes and they begin to function. Words come out that I never used" (Sies, 1974, p. 138). We help someone "retrieve what he knows more readily than if he were left to his own devices" (Eisenson, 1972, p. 134). Brookshire (1978a) subscribed to this theme for syntax: "We do not advocate teaching the patient certain grammatical constructions. Instead, we feel that treatment should

be directed toward those basic language processes which are necessary to understand and use those grammatical constructions" (p. 147). With the cognitive stimulation approach, we speak of *retraining* a mental process rather than *teaching* linguistic forms. In Europe, clinicians speak of "reeducation." Goals are expressed in terms of cognitive processes, such as improving sentence comprehension or word retrieval.

Schuell believed in bombarding a patient with stimulation and requiring many responses in a session. Treatment was aimed at language production in a general sense, and she used all modalities to this end by having patients identify spoken and written words and repeat, copy, and read words aloud as a multifaceted activity (Schuell, et al., 1964). This was called a **multimodal approach**, mainly oriented toward improving word-finding ability in naming tasks (e.g., Howard, Patterson, Franklin, Orchard-Lisle, and Morton, 1985b). Now, researchers tend to avoid this approach when they wish to identify effects of specific stimuli on recovery of specific abilities. We also rely on the idea that aphasia is a central disorder. Work on one language modality should affect other modalities. Treatment may consist of auditory comprehension tasks, but the goal is to improve naming (Howard, et al., 1985b). In this way, stimulating comprehension is expected to infiltrate mechanisms of production in an indirect attack on impaired word finding. Following this logic, facilitation of speaking should show up in writing if the impairment underlying both modalities is the same. A clinician may devote a great deal of time to auditory-spoken language with the promise of some generalization to reading and writing.

There is another procedural implication of the rejection of teaching. The stimulation approach "is likely to lead the practitioner away from concern with specific stimuli and responses and toward concern with general processes or abilities that may underlie a given patient's tendency to respond to certain stimuli with certain responses" (Brookshire, 1986, p. 128). A task such as sentence completion may be designed to elicit 30 or 40 different words, and more than one response may be acceptable for one stimulus (e.g., "You drive a *car*," *Ford, bus,* and so on). With respect to their Language-Oriented Treatment (LOT), Shewan and Bandur (1986) suggested that the "learning of specific stimulus-response bonds is not the goal. In LOT the same stimuli are not used over and over again. . . . Different stimuli at a comparable level of difficulty are presented to elicit responses" (p. 13). A patient could say "car" in response to "You buy a ____," "You wreck a ____," and "You fix a ____." Because learning specific language forms is considered to be inconsistent with the nature of aphasia, the words or sentences to be comprehended, repeated, or elicited may vary from session to session.

Emphasis on the Stimulus or Antecedent Event.

Eisenson (1984) wrote that a clinical aphasiologist is "a stimulator or an *agent provocateur*." Schuell is known for emphasizing auditory stimulation. She said that "I am going to depend largely on auditory stimulation, because I think language is most dependent on this perceptual system" (Sies, 1974, p. 139). Darley's (1982) treatise on aphasia, dedicated to Schuell, argued for maximizing the "arousal power" of a stimulus. In reviewing Schuell's contributions, Duffy (1986) suggested that stimulation should be given with a strength sufficient to elicit a response without forcing the response (also, Wiegel-Crump and Koenigsknecht, 1973). **Unforced elicitation** depends on retention of pockets of automatic language processes such as lexical access for word recognition. Minimal stimuli, such as the first sound of a word, may arouse a dormant process. The idea is that exercising seemingly trivial processes should lubricate them and pry more complex processes loose from the restraints of injury. As Schuell discovered, "words come out that I never used."

Retained capacities become the starting points for enhancing language abilities. One basis for choosing auditory stimulation is that the auditory modality is the least impaired of the language modalities. The **success princi-**ple states that treatment "should be constructed so that the patient's performance is slightly deficient, but not mostly or completely erroneous. . . . In most cases, no more than 20% of an aphasic patient's responses in treatment activities should be errors" (Brookshire, 1986, pp. 141, 142). Brookshire (1972) discovered that erroneous naming on one trial increased the likelihood of error on the next trial. Brookshire and Nicholas (1978) found that three or four consecutive errors reduced the chance of subsequent correct response to almost nil. Success ensures that a functioning process is being practiced or that a patient is not practicing aberrant processing. Yet, the task should present a challenge. Accurate responses can be slow or incomplete. Rosenbek and others (1989) wrote that adults with aphasia sense their successes and that "this observation, combined with our feeling that good clinicians can—by their stimulus selection, ordering, and presentation—elicit responses from all but the most severe or sullen patients, causes us to emphasize antecedent over consequent events" (p. 137).

Feedback and Restimulation upon Error.

We should be responsive to a patient's efforts. Brookshire (1986) wrote about two types of feedback. **Incentive feedback** is a reward for desired responses (e.g., "good") and punishment for undesired responses (e.g., "No, that's wrong"). **Information feedback** tells the degree to which a response approximated a criterion (e.g., "It's not a complete sentence" or "Close, but you should have put 'was' in front of the verb"). This feedback may transform a stimulation task into a confusing analytical exercise. Brookshire recommended it for self-motivated clients who may be unaware of the target or the relationship between the target and an inadequate response. Discriminative feedback, such as turning on a red light after correct responses (Mills, 1977), may be considered to be informative. In general, however, "if the client (1) is motivated to respond, (2) knows the target response, and (3) knows how closely his or her attempts approximate the target, then *any* feedback may be trivial" (Brookshire, 1986, p. 147). Generally, Brookshire preferred to use encouragement that is not necessarily contingent on adequacy of response (e.g., "You're doing fine" or "You're doing much better today").

A crucial feature of cognitive stimulation is feedback provided when a response is not forthcoming or is erroneous. "The objective is to get the language processes working, not to teach the patient that whatever he says is wrong" (Schuell, et al., 1964, p. 342). Schuell suggested that, instead of correcting errors, we should stimulate the patient again. Let us call it **restimulation.** "If a response is not elicited, the stimulus was not adequate. What the patient needs in such cases is more stimulation, not correction or information about why a response was inadequate" (Duffy, 1986, p. 191). We can repeat the initial stimulus in the spirit of saying "let's try again" or may supplement the stimulus with cues such as the first sound of a word. In a study by LaPointe, Rothi, and Campanella (1978), repeating a command before a response did not facilitate comprehension, but following commands improved when the stimulus was repeated after failure on the first attempt. When planned stimulation is powerful enough to elicit a good response most of the time, there is little need for restimulation. However, when a patient starts making errors at a frequency of more than 20 percent, "the activity should be changed so that the frequency of errors decreases" (Brookshire, 1986, p. 141). This change may take the form of utilizing the restimulation as the antecedent event for the new task.

During their study of treatment samples, Brookshire and Nicholas (1978) found a strong tendency not to provide feedback subsequent to unacceptable responses. There was some negative feedback and correction. Errors tended to cluster, as if "failure begets failure." Nicholas and Brookshire (1979) studied efforts to break up these clusters occurring in tasks designed to elicit verbal responses. They found that evaluative feedback on one trial did not result in improved performance on the next trial. This

feedback included incentive feedback, informative correction, and repetition of an error. Nicholas and Brookshire then examined occurrences of stimulation with the target-stimulus of a preceding trial. Restimulation consisted of repeating, rewording, or changing the stimulus that had elicited an error. None of these strategies improved verbal response. In sum, Brookshire and Nicholas' research indicated that clinicians did not often follow Schuell's advice; however, when they did, the restimulation was ineffective. Later, the use of cues as restimulation of naming will be examined in more detail.

Instrumental/Operant Conditioning

Behavior modification has been taught as a basic methodology for varied communicative disorders, implying that underlying causes are irrelevant to methods for changing behavior (Chapter 1). "Speech modification therefore proceeds by a functional analysis of the behavior-environment interactions and the development of a program to modify the environment and thus change the behavior" (Sloane and MacAulay, 1968, p. 4). This approach was said to be chosen because aphasia was assumed to be a loss of linguistic knowledge. This misunderstanding made behavior modification appear to be inappropriate for disorders of processing (Sullivan and Brookshire, 1989). Yet, a strict behaviorist would deny any interest in the nature of aphasia and would say that, no matter what causes aphasia, the goal is to change behavior. Still, perhaps inadvertently, a clinician may speak of "teaching" language to aphasic patients.

In choosing between classical and instrumental/operant conditioning, speech and language behavior are assumed to be volitional, instead of "automatic," such as the reflexive salivation of Pavlov's dog in classical conditioning. Operant conditioning has been preferred for modifying volitional behavior. It is "a situation in which the subject responds to a stimulus and is rewarded following the response" (Mowrer, 1982, p. 204). Some of the earliest operant treatment for aphasia was provided by Brookshire (1967) and Holland and Harris (1968). Behavior modification faded from clinical aphasiology for a while and then reappeared in the early 1980s in conjunction with the introduction of single-subject experimental designs in efficacy research (e.g., Kearns and Salmon, 1984; Thompson and Kearns, 1981; Thompson, McReynolds, and Vance, 1982; Tonkovich and Loverso, 1982). Behavioral methods have also been used in cognitive rehabilitation for head injury (e.g., Edelstein and Couture, 1984).

Behavioral Objectives and Specific Content. Objectives are stated in terms of observable behaviors that can be measured. The wording of these goals identifies a stimulus and response, and the objective is a criterion of performance that may include a time period in which the criterion should be reached. One goal may be *to name eight of ten objects correctly by September 20.* Another goal may be *to point to pictures in response to sentences with 100 percent accuracy in two days.* A behavioral goal can be so specific that it describes the treatment task used to meet the goal. This type of goal takes the mystery out of vague goals (e.g., to improve language ability) or mentalistic goals (e.g., to improve language comprehension). With respect to comprehension, the planning of treatment and measurement is facilitated by our ability to translate cognitive notions into observable events that can be manipulated and counted. Clinicians are usually not afraid to speak of pointing to pictures as a behavior that is indicative of comprehension.

As indicated in the previous section, advocates of stimulation wanted us to know that this method does not focus on "teaching the patient certain grammatical constructions" (Brookshire, 1978a) or "specific stimulus-response bonds" (Shewan and Bandur, 1986). Behavioral methods have entailed the training of specific sets of responses to specific stimuli, and these sets have tended to be quite small. Thompson and Kearns (1981) trained the production of ten names to ten pictures until a patient reached a criterion.

Kearns and Salmon (1984) trained ten sentences with the auxiliary *is.* The frequently used *Base 10 Response Form* (LaPointe, 1985) is compatible with restricting a task to ten items. It contains an area for graphing scores on a task for which target-stimuli are listed below. It has been easy to chart progress with a task containing the ten stimuli that can be listed.

Emphasis on Feedback or Consequent Event. Whereas stimulation methods rely on a patient's retained capacities to respond to an adequate stimulus, behavioral methods do not necessarily rely on such capacities to help the patient produce the desired response. Operant methods rely on reinforcement as the primary mechanism of behavioral change. Without elicitation, we may wonder how a correct response is achieved initially. A laboratory rat accidentally presses a lever and then receives food, and subsequent lever pressing is thought to be an effect of the reinforcement. A brain-injured patient's first response does not occur accidentally but may be imitated through a clinician's **modeling** the correct response. "The response is emitted rather than elicited" (Leith, 1984, p. 19). It is as if a patient must learn that a response, such as a word, goes with a stimulus, such as an object. Thompson and McReynolds (1986) described an operant procedure for training question production such as "What is he drinking?" The clinician "sequentially modeled the first two words of the target response, then the remaining words of the target response, instructing the subject to repeat each portion as it was modeled" (p. 198). Unlike unforced elicitation, responses may be considered to be forced (Sullivan and Brookshire, 1989).

The previous paragraph indicated that "one of the chief features of instrumental conditioning is that the consequences of the behavior serve to control the frequency of its occurrence" (Mowrer, 1982, p. 204). Clinical aphasiologists usually use a form of verbal praise, such as *good* or *nice job.* In training production of an auxiliary verb form, Kearns and Salmon (1984) presented redeemable coupons and tokens after correct responses. For retraining attention after head injury, tokens were contingent on attending to a task for two minutes (Wood, 1986). **Reinforcement schedules** specify a rate for presenting a reward. Each correct response may be rewarded (i.e., continuous reinforcement), or some correct responses may be rewarded (i.e., intermittent reinforcement) (e.g., Thompson and Byrne, 1984). Intermittent reinforcement may be supplied according to a fixed-ratio schedule, such as every second or fourth correct response (FR-2, FR-4). With a variable-ratio schedule, reward follows correct responses at a varied rate that may average every second or fourth response (VR-2, VR-4). Contrary to the Schuellian tradition, errors may be "consequated" by **verbal punishment.** Tonkovich and Loverso (1982) administered a "verbal reproof," such as *No, that wasn't right.* Thompson and Byrne (1984) simply said *No, not quite.* Scott and Byng's (1989) computer emitted a "cheerful sound" after a correct response and a "negative tune" after an error.

CUES: MAXIMIZING COGNITIVE STIMULATION

In cognitive terms, we want to improve a client's access to information stored in long-term memory. Stimulation activates access processes and is said to facilitate a weakened or damaged process. The hub of treatment for aphasia has been the desire to improve access to lexical memory, exhibited most succinctly in the naming task. The target-stimulus may be description of an object or the object itself, although description is usually a more difficult target to name. When a patient has difficulty naming, we try to facilitate the process by adding a cue to the target-stimulus. In contrast to modeling the word, we would like the cue to be a "hint" or information that does not contain the entire phonemic form of the word, so that genuine word-retrieval is practiced. Cues are used to meet the following goals:

Cognitive: To improve retrieval of words from the mental lexicon.

Behavioral: To increase accuracy of naming objects presented by the clinician.

Cues and Cueing Strategies

Two types of cues address two points in the naming process (Figure 4–1). **Semantic cues** activate an area in the field of information about the object in semantic memory (e.g., "It's a sport"). **Lexical cues** point to the word itself in the mental lexicon (e.g., "It starts with /b/"). Stimley and Noll (1991) figured they had supported this assumption when they found that lexical (i.e., phonemic) cues tended to elicit phonemic paraphasias when there were errors, whereas semantic cues elicited semantic paraphasias as errors. Some semantic stimuli may function as either a target-stimulus or a cue. For example, a definition or carrier phrase may be presented as a primary task for eliciting words or along with an object to facilitate word finding. In a completion task, a carrier phrase may be enhanced with a phonemic cue. Other semantic cues include the sound of an object, but Mills (1977) found that it took more than four sessions for a sound to facilitate naming more than presenting the object by itself. Cues are used because they do not require training.

We may use **single-cue** presentations or **combined-cue** presentations employing multiple cues. Some combined cues can be presented simultaneously (e.g., printed word/first sound). Combined cues may also be presented sequentially (e.g., carrier phrase + printed word). A single cue may be presented in various temporal relationships with the target-stimulus (Table 12–2). In **pre-target cueing,** a cue is presented before the target-stimulus. In Mills' study, the sound was presented before the object. In **post-target cueing,** a cue is presented after the target-stimulus, differing slightly from restimulation, in which the cue is presented upon failure to name an object. The position of a cue, a factor largely ignored in research, may be important because of the sequence of access to semantic

TABLE 12–2 Interactions showing temporal arrangement of a target stimulus and cue in naming tasks mostly prescribing an object and cue in the planned antecedent event (i.e., clinician's stimulus).

	Clinician Stimulus	Patient Response	Clinician Feedback
Simultaneous	Object/cue	Name	"Good"
Pre-target cue	Cue + object	Name	"Good"
Post-target cue	Object + cue	Name	"Good"
Restimulation	Object	No response	Cue
	Object + cue	No response	Repeat/change the cue

and lexical systems in naming. In a study in cognitive psychology, neurologically intact adults retrieved words more slowly to letter + category stimuli (e.g., A + *fruit*) than to category + letter stimuli (e.g., *fruit* + A), because we must end up in the lexical system anyway for word retrieval (Collins and Loftus, 1975). Presenting an object before a lexical cue, such as the first sound of the word, may be more natural than presenting a lexical cue before the object.

Restimulation with cues has also been conceived as lowering the level of response from an initially intentional or volitional level to a more automatic level. Basso (1978) provided carrier phrases and phonemic cues upon failure to name an object. Then, a patient may be asked to try naming again without the cues. Cues are presented and then removed for each item in a task. The approach was portrayed as follows:

If an aphasic cannot bring forth an intended response by himself, it is sometimes possible to lead him to do so by eliciting a response first in a more automatic way and then in more and more voluntary ways by gradually withdrawing the facilitations incorporated in the stimuli. This passage from more automatic to more voluntary constitutes the core of rehabilitation (Basso, et al., 1979, p. 192).

Later, this principle of movement along a dimension of volitionality will be presented as a basis for planning a progression of treatment activities.

Investigation of Cueing

Supplementing an object with a cue is usually compared to a control condition in which the object is presented by itself. In some studies, a pictured object was shown before the cue was administered as restimulation; that is, a cue would be provided after a subject failed to name the object (e.g., Li and Williams, 1990; Kohn and Goodglass, 1985; Love and Webb, 1977). Other researchers examined pre-target cueing (Pease and Goodglass, 1978; Podraza and Darley, 1977; Stimley and Noll, 1991). In other studies, the cue's position was not reported in description of procedures. For example, Bruce and Howard (1988) stated that "the patients were provided once with the appropriate cue and given a further 5 seconds to retrieve the picture's name" (p. 258). Also, research has focused on cueing with objects determined to have been difficult to name. However, following the success principle, stimulation treatment tends to consist of objects that are easy for the patient to name, and restimulation should be infrequent. Despite procedural variation in the research, some fairly consistent findings have emerged.

Most studies focus on immediate effects or arousal power of cues. The most frequently studied lexical cue has been the first sound or syllable, and the most frequently studied semantic cue has been a carrier phrase conveying superordinate, functional, or locational information (Table 12–3). Either

TABLE 12–3 Common cues used to facilitate spoken object-naming. Carrier phrases create syntactic probabilities that may be helpful.

Semantic Cues	Example	Lexical Cues	Example
Definition	"It uses ink and you write with it."	Phoneme (first sound/syllable)	"puh"
Function	"You use it for writing."	Rhyming word	"It's not ten; it's a _____."
Semantic associates	"Pencil," "ink" "It's like a pencil."	Spelling	"p-e-n"
		Printed word	PEN
Carrier phrase	"A ball-point _____." "You write with it. It's a _____."	Modeling	"pen"
Location	"You find it on a desk."		

type is more effective than no cue (Stimley and Noll, 1991). In comparison of the types, the most common finding was that a phonemic lexical cue was more effective at eliciting names than semantic cues and other lexical cues, such as a printed or rhyming word. Across a spectrum of aphasias, phonemic cues elicited names about 50 percent of the time following failure to name an object, and semantic cues were effective around 30 percent of the time (Li and Williams, 1989). The arousal power of phonemic cues is evidence that impairment lies in retrieval instead of the stored knowledge of word forms (Howard, Patterson, Franklin, Orchard-Lisle, and Morton, 1985a). Semantic cues may be redundant, because the target-stimulus activates semantic memory through the object-recognition capacity of most aphasic persons. The patient, who knows what he or she wants to say, still needs help finding the lexical form. Moreover, while some cues were more stimulable than others, not even the best cues guarantee word retrieval. Cues were more effective as severity of naming deficit decreased. Some exceptions were also exposed:

(a) **Syndromes differed in level of cueing effectiveness.** Phonemic cueing was superior to seman-tic cueing in the following proportions: conduction aphasia, 62 to 41 percent; Broca's aphasia, 55 to 28 percent; and Wernicke's aphasia, 41 to 22 percent (Li and Williams, 1989). Among different studies, the highest level (e.g., conduction aphasia) was statistically superior to the lowest level (i.e., Wernicke's aphasia). Other studies left the impression that phonemic cueing is especially useful for Broca's aphasia (Goodglass and Stuss, 1979), especially for those with the most difficulty in naming (Bruce and Howard, 1988; Love and Webb, 1977).

(b) **Greater stimulability of phonemic cues did not occur for anomic aphasia,** when analysis of covariance balanced groups for severity of naming deficit. In an earlier study of pre-target cueing, phonemic cues were more powerful than semantic cues for this syndrome (around 70 percent versus 40 percent) (Pease and Goodglass, 1978). This group was the least impaired syndrome in the study. When severity was balanced for studying restimulation, phonemic and semantic cues were equally effective at a 35 percent level for anomic aphasia (Li and Williams, 1989). Even without covariance, the types of cues were comparable at 43 and 47 percent effectiveness (Li and Williams, 1990). Theorists guess that lexical memory ought to be well-connected to semantic memory so that minimal phonemic information can elicit the word that goes with an object (Bruce and Howard, 1988). This connection may be weakened in anomic aphasia.

(c) **The greater power of phonemic cues applied to nouns but not verbs.** For an action-naming task, phonemic and semantic cues were equally effective around 40 percent of the time after failure to name across all aphasic subjects (Li and Williams, 1990). Semantic cues were more effective for verbs than for nouns. For those with anomic aphasia, semantic cues were twice as effective as phonemic cues in eliciting verbs. The difference from nouns is reminiscent of the unique representation of verbs and the difficulty aphasic patients have with action-naming (Shapiro and Levine, 1990; Williams and Canter, 1987).

The arousal power of phonemic cues is quite seductive. In England, a series of studies was started for examining the duration of cueing effects (Patterson, Purell, and Morton, 1983). Eleven clients were stimulated with phonemic cues and objects that had been difficult to name. Later, eight patients were given a treatment package of word repetition, rhyme judgment, and rhyming cues (Howard, et al., 1985a). In both studies, phonemic cueing was superior to no cueing for one session; but, after a 30-minute interval "filled with general chat and a cup of coffee," trained names were retrieved no better than before treatment and no better than names that were not cued. Then, a "phonological treatment" was given to 12 patients for four days across one week or eight days across two weeks (Howard, et al., 1985b). The package was similar to the previous one but did not include rhyming cues. Cued objects were easier to name than uncued objects during the training period. A week later, the superiority of treated items remained; but after six weeks the superiority faded. This research indicates that one session of phonemic or other lexical cues is a "quick fix" that can impress through the one-way mirror. Howard's studies raise a question as to whether a few sessions of lexical cueing are enough to repair the retrieval process for more lasting use.

Self-Cueing

If an aphasic person can identify the first letter of a word in a tip-of-the-tongue (TOT) state and can retrieve words when a clinician provides the first sound, then maybe the patient can generate his or her own cues to facilitate retrieval. This would make the patient more independent of the clinician; it sounds like a good idea. It was reported first by Berman and Peelle (1967). They described training a patient to write the first letter, sound it out, and generate his own carrier phrase; but they did not submit the program to experimental scrutiny. Later, a seemingly aphasic patient with a thalamic lesion was trained to use his TOT skills to give a portable computer partial information about a desired word, and the computer would retrieve it from a lexical-semantic database (Colby, Christinaz, Parkison, Graham, and Karpf, 1981). A patient should have some reading and spelling skills to do this. Bruce and Howard (1988) studied possibilities with 20 persons who had Broca's aphasia, only half having been helped by clinician-generated phonemic cues. These researchers figured that the patients should be able to point to the first letter of a word that cannot be retrieved, sound out (or recode) the letter, and use the sound as a cue. Six patients could identify first letters upon failing to name objects. None was cued to find words when identifying the first letter. Only two could sound out letters, and none displayed all three abilities. Bruce and Howard reported that attempts to train the recoding skill have been laborious, and so the reports of compensatory self-cueing have been discouraging so far.

THE NOTION OF PROGRAMMED STIMULATION

Methodologies merge. The most prevalent merger is the use of principles of programmed learning to plan ahead for stimulation-facilitation. Compatible elements of cognitive stimulation and behavior modification combine to form what is called **programmed stimulation** (LaPointe, 1985). Thompson and Kearns (1981) elicited ten object names with carrier phrases and phonemes, as well as with modeling, and relied on reinforcing correct responses. The main idea, however, is to fas-ten stimulation tasks into a harness of stages through which treatment might proceed for the long term. We have borrowed from **programmed instruction,** consisting of principles for creating "a series of instructional items called *frames* which build cumulatively in small steps designed to help the student to reach some predetermined objective" (Mowrer, 1982, p. 286).

Initial and Terminal Behaviors

Besides identifying the start of treatment in capacities to respond, we look ahead to a conclusion identified in a goal. Treatment is a progression from "point A" (initial response) to "point B" (terminal response). The plan for this progression is called a **program,** and a patient's rehabilitation may consist of several programs and, thus, several initial and terminal behaviors. Programs may be designed for different functional systems, such as one for comprehension and another for formulation. Programs may also overlap, such as one for auditory comprehension and one for reading. Programs are tied to **short-term goals,** coinciding with steps in a program; **intermediate goals,** sighting the conclusion of a program; and **long-term goals,** identifying an endpoint of rehabilitation. For improving comprehension, an initial stimulus is likely to be single words for severe impairment, and the terminal stimulus is sentences of everyday complexity. For agrammatism, the initial response may be two-word phrases, and the terminal response is complete sentences of flexible complexity. Programming is compatible with pragmatic goals in which a terminal point is defined further as natural responses in conversation. The last step of Taylor and Marks' (1959) naming program was the use of their core vocabulary in "everyday life without the help of a picture, a word card, or a therapist" (p. 16).

One line of progression is specified on a **continuum of volitionality or automaticity.** Luria's (1970b) notion of *intrasystemic reorganization* transfers an impaired function through levels within a system such as language formulation. This is done by shifting a disturbed function to a lower level than the level at which a patient is struggling to perform. Word retrieval may be shifted to saying "seven" when counting to ten instead of answering a question with "seven." Shifting within a functional system can be done in the other direction. A "downward" shift may raise a normally automatic process to conscious awareness. That is, a patient may be struggling to verbalize with natural automaticity, and we may help the patient use conscious strategies such as self-cueing. Then, treatment becomes a gradual return to automatic use while conscious strategy atrophies. This progression is followed in learning complex motor skills. That is, a dance is divided into a sequence of steps and movements that are given names like "glissades" and "arabesques." The dancer thinks about performing and ordering steps one at a time and then drills the steps until the dance is performed without thinking and with the artist's grace and feeling. In general, starting with nonvolitional utterance is attempted with global aphasia, whereas starting with conscious strategy is attempted for agrammatism (Chapter 13).

Small-Step Progression

Treatment for aphasia is a series of little victories. The key to moving from an initial behavior to a terminal behavior is to progress gradually in small steps. The success principle of cognitive stimulation is operative, because a step is being performed at a high level of accuracy. Moreover, if the next step is similar to the current step, the capacities facilitated in the current step should transfer readily to the next step. A small step is determined by *changing only one variable between tasks,* a change that should increase the challenge in the same function. These variables exist in the clinician's stimulus, the client's response, and the clinician's feedback. Variation of programs among patients is forged by differences in initial behavior and in distances between steps. Some patients can move faster than others through an anticipated program. Slower patients may need to be moved by changing one variable at a time, but others may tolerate changes in more than one variable, thereby skipping some steps.

Steps are sequenced according to a **hierarchy of difficulty**, established with respect to certain criteria. *Logical criteria* include common sense (e.g., long sentences ought to be more difficult than short ones) or an understanding of linguistic structure (e.g., passive sentences ought to be more difficult than declaratives because of transformational complexity). *Empirical criteria* consist of data demonstrating an order of difficulty, especially for aphasic persons. Some of the research surveyed in Chapters 4 and 5 is used for recommending hierarchies of difficulty and constitutes much of the database for Shewan and Bandur's (1986) LOT. For instance, Barton and others (1969) studied tasks of sentence completion, object-naming, and naming to description and found that these tasks ranked in this order from easiest to most difficult. Yet, before we use this finding to etch this hierarchy in stone, we should know that about half the subjects did not follow the group pattern. Sometimes empirical criteria fail to confirm logical criteria. Long sentences are not more difficult to comprehend than short ones when long sentences contain informational redundancy (Chapter 4). An individualized program may be planned by discovering relative difficulty for the client.

Cueing may be sequenced according to a hierarchy of difficulty. The empirical basis for cueing hierarchies is indicated in the research presented previously. That is, phonemic cues should be easier than semantic cues for everyone except those with anomic aphasia. Combined cues are more powerful than single cues (Weidner and Jinks, 1983). Principles of programmed instruction state that progression from easy to difficult may be accomplished by **fading** stimulus cues. The easiest task would be to provide a target-stimulus along with a combination of cues, and the next task is specified by the removal of one of the cues. In an object-naming task, the faded cue may be the strongest one, such as the first sound, to determine if words can be retrieved under more challenging circumstances. Reinforcement may be thought of as

part of the environment and may be faded gradually according to a sequence of fixed-ratio intermittent schedules.

Another concept of stepwise progression focuses on the target-response. The notion of **shaping** (or successive approximation) capitalizes on starting with what a client is capable of producing. The strategy is discussed as reinforcing behaviors "already in the repertoire" of the client (Mowrer, 1982). Besides involuntary utterance, the initial behavior may be a version of the target-response that is slightly inadequate or incomplete but certainly close to the target. We selectively reinforce the approximations as versions even closer to the target are produced. In this manner, the target-response is gradually shaped.

Response Criterion

Small step progression is utilized so that mastery of one step can be easily applied to the next step. Clinicians frequently specify a criterion for mastery of a step, which serves as a criterion for increasing difficulty or moving to the next step. In Shewan and Bandur's (1986) LOT, a 70 percent criterion was recommended. A patient had to achieve this level of accuracy on consecutive blocks of ten task trials before advancing to the next level of difficulty. Others have recommended 80 to 95 percent criteria, indicating that a criterion varies depending on a clinician's judgment of a client's capacity to move on. In their multiple baseline design, Thompson and Kearns (1981) shifted to the next list of words when performance reached around 80 percent with the previous list (Figure 11–6).

The upward trends and response criterion of 80 percent in the treatment phases of Figure 11–6 appear to be inconsistent with the success principle of beginning a task at 80 percent. There is a slight difference between the cognitive-stimulation and behavioral approaches, because an operant procedure is more likely to begin at a lower level. Yet, the difference may be more apparent than real. The success principle and response criterion could be addressing different aspects of a treatment. For example, let us suppose that we use a naming task, and a patient is currently performing at around 20 percent accuracy. We want to see the patient at 80 percent before introducing a new set of words, like Thompson and Kearns' study. However, treatment may entail more, and a patient could be at 80 percent when cues and reinforcement are added to the task. The response criterion, on the other hand, is based on performance without cues and reinforcement. This is one possibility. Another way of looking at it is to select a task based on 80 percent *accuracy* but to measure dimensions of accuracy (i.e., completeness, speed) for the response criterion. A third option is that a clinician utilizes either the success principle or response criteria in taking a particular approach to treatment. There may be no measurement during a treatment activity, while progress is monitored with independent probes measuring "something else."

Computer-Assisted Treatment

We use computers for record keeping, report writing, and analyzing test results. For treatment, they have taken programmed instruction to greater heights than the "teaching machines" in the 1960s. Automated presentation of stimulus "frames" and feedback was tried by several clinicians (e.g., Brookshire, 1969; Holland, 1970; Sarno, et al., 1970). The devices were quickly reviled by Wepman (1968) as being "a devil's box which . . . comes between the therapist and the patient" (p. 103). Teaching machines provided immediate reinforcement by presenting the next item. An incorrect response was followed by repeating the same item. Now, microcomputers expand exercises beyond time spent with the clinician and analyze performance in a treatment task (Katz, 1986; Mills, 1986). Computers are used extensively in cognitive rehabilitation for disorders of attention, perception, memory, and problem solving (Fisher, 1989; Skilbeck, 1984). A patient can work autonomously, decreasing dependence on a clinician. Seron (1987) argued that "we should first develop programs that are beyond the capabilities of the clinician

and thus not comparable to current clinical practice" (p. 162).

One feared limitation was flexibility. Teaching machines could not shift content and timing of restimulation the way a clinician could. Like linguistics for some clinicians, programming is an area of special expertise for other clinicians. We tell sophisticated programmers that something cannot be done with a computer, and then they prove us wrong. Katz and Nagy created a word recognition program in which stimulus duration is increased in response to errors (see Katz, 1986). A subsequent word comprehension program varied the number and type of picture foils in response to a patient's accuracy. This program also generated a print-out at the end of a session for homework based on performance in the session. A clinician may be involved by operating a computer work station where stimuli can be controlled and type of response for a naming task can be recorded (Bruckert, Henaff-Ganon, Michel, and Bez, 1989). We may activate a "cue" function when a client fails to respond, thereby providing restimulative feedback that is not programmed.

For treatment of language disorders, computers seemed to be restricted to the graphemic code in reading and typing. This is not necessarily a weakness, because it can be a valuable supplement to interaction with a clinician that can be focused on auditory-oral abilities. Katz (1986) started with a reading assessment and treatment program called the *Computerized Aphasia Treatment System* (CATS). Other reading programs have been evaluated (Burton, Burton, and Lucas, 1988; Kinsey, 1990). Spelling and writing programs were developed (Katz, 1986; Seron, Deloche, Moulard, and Rouselle, 1980). However, three types of speech can be linked to or incorporated into a computer for comprehension tasks. *Analog speech* is tape-recorded natural speech. *Synthesized speech* is computer-generated and has a robot quality. *Digitized speech* is computer-generated with a more natural quality. Mills (1982) described comprehension training for an aphasic patient with digitized speech. Also, aphasic patients' ability to comprehend synthesized speech was studied. Comprehension was poorer than for natural or live speech, but practice with synthesized speech improved response (e.g., Huntress, Lee, Creaghead, Wheeler, and Braverman, 1990). Beginning with work by Vaughn, auditory comprehension practice has been conducted over the telephone for patients unable to get to a clinic (Fitch and Cross, 1983; Katz, 1986).

One issue accompanying the enthusiastic deployment of this captivating technology is associated with the application of educational and recreational software to cognitive problems for patients with stroke and traumatic brain injury. Educational software can be used in training reading and reasoning, and recreational software (i.e., video games) requires attention, visuospatial skills, memory, problem solving, and executive control. These packages are not developed with aphasia or other dysfunctions in mind, which leaves room to question whether considering the nature of cognitive dysfunctions would make a difference in the nature of such software (Wolfe, 1987). A program designed to "teach" vocabulary may differ from one designed to stimulate access. The computer could be a primary means of infusing experimental psychology into rehabilitation, especially with respect to automatic, obligatory processes obscured in traditional off-line tasks. Relevance is also questioned because some software designed for children may be advertised as being applicable for adults, perhaps to maximize sales. Many clinicians are bothered that a great deal of software is too childish for older adults.

Katz (1986, 1987) has suggested that the data collecting capacity of microcomputers enables a clinician to determine the "efficacy" of treatment. Computers compile an ongoing record of progress with the treatment task. If we recall the explanation of efficacy in Chapter 11, then we should look for how computer programming provides the manipulation of independent variables that determines cause-effect relationships. We need to have an indication that this treatment is improving the targeted cognitive skill beyond what can be attributed to practice with the particular task on the computer. Reviewers have been highly critical of the evidence put forth for the efficacy of computer treatment, especially with respect to the tendency to make assertions that cannot be supported by the experimental design (Loverso, 1987; Loverso, Prescott, and Selinger, 1992; Robertson, 1990). One assertion is that treatment made a difference in a patient's daily life. This assertion may be based on an anecdote rather than on measuring change in daily life and relating this change to a manipulation of independent variables. Robertson (1990) could not find evidence that perceptual and memory training had real-life effects for people with closed head injury and right-hemisphere dysfunction. More investigation, guided by experimental design, is needed from clinicians who are not involved in marketing the software being studied.

EXPANDING THEORETICAL FOUNDATIONS

Rationales for approaches to treatment come from theories of dysfunction and recovery. Theories multiply according to whether they address functional or neurological changes. People wonder if nerve cells grow back. There may be an expectation that treatment will teach language to the right hemisphere in the same way we train the left hand to write after the right side is paralyzed.

Theories of Dysfunction

A statement from Schuell is worth repeating. In founding the cognitive-stimulation approach to treatment, she said that "what you do about aphasia depends on what you think aphasia is" (Sies, 1974, p. 138). If we think of aphasia as an erasure of linguistic competence, then treatment may be a form of teaching. If we think of aphasia as impairment of linguistic performance with competence intact, then treatment is a form of stimulation or retraining. We are learning that these assumptions pertain to the status of cognition, and we may be reminded of the awkward distinction between language and cognition as we think about the domains of rehabilitation. For a long time, speech-language pathologists did not acknowledge that assumptions about the nature of aphasia were assumptions about the status of cognition. Rosenbek and others (1989) worried that such suggestions are "especially felicitous for those who would legitimize the speech-language pathologist's role in cognitive rehabilitation" (p. 10). This is mainly a terminology problem. Rosenbek's main concern was that some speech-language pathologists are getting into domains of cognition that have been beyond the domains of their training. However, the traditional domain of clinical aphasiology is maintained in terms of the knowledge and processes involved in language comprehension and formulation.

One theoretical basis for a treatment is the notion of **deblocking,** which is similar to priming (Chapter 3). Facilitative priming relies on automatic spreading activation in a region of LTM. Weigl and Bierwisch's (1970) idea was to sidestep barriers to accessing intact linguistic knowledge. Deblocking was achieved by preceding an item involving an impaired function with an item involving a relatively intact function. Tasks were associated by containing the same content. For example, with the same sentence, sentence copying was used to deblock impaired writing to dictation. This idea was extended to a strategy in which a target-stimulus such as an object is preceded by a prime, called **prestimulation** in clinical circles (Weigl, 1970). The difference from cueing is that response to a prestimulus is not expected. A patient listens or watches and then responds to the next stimulus. For an object-naming task, Podraza and Darley (1977) prestimulated with a series of words. Direct priming (e.g., *line, bee, goat*) was compared to indirect or semantic priming (e.g., *sting, honey, hive*). Direct priming was facilitative, but indirect priming was not, indicating that what the patients needed was facilitation for lexical access, not semantic access.

The most unabashed linkage of treatment to theory of dysfunction is now associated with cognitive neuropsychology (Lesser, 1987; Seron and Deloche, 1989). Howard and Patterson (1989) argued that treatment for aphasia must be aimed at components of the language system rather than behavioral symptoms (i.e., cognitive goals), because one symptom can arise for different reasons. If the reasons are not considered, treatment may be misdirected or aimed a little more haphazardly than necessary. Given diagnosis of a functional lesion, a procedure may mimic the mechanism assumed to be impaired. The logic of this approach is expressed as follows. Caplan and Futter (1986) figured that one subject's comprehension disorder was to employ an abnormal operation on sentences like *The frog was given to the elephant by the monkey.* This is the abnormal mechanism: "Assign the thematic roles of agent, theme and goal to N1, N2 and N3 in structures of the form N1-V-N2-N3, where N1 does not already bear a thematic role" (p. 128). This linear operation assigns the role of agent to *frog.* Could treatment start here and then direct another way of assigning thematic roles?

The basic idea is not entirely new. Clinicians have generally recognized that word-finding practice is not likely to be helpful for a naming problem caused by visual object agnosia. Brookshire's process-orientation, presented earlier, is consistent with the so-called cognitive neuropsychology movement. What is new is the extent to which task-related cognitive models are a frame of reference for identifying a targeted process. Treatment may be designed to fix or bypass an impaired component. If a patient is deficient in an object-classification task, "such a task would provide useful information about the presumed etiology of word retrieval difficulties that could be tied to treatment planning" (Jackson and Tompkins, 1989, p. 371). The communicative goal is to improve word retrieval, but the procedure is aimed at the cause of deficit and would entail work on semantic categorization. An assumption about the nature of word retrieval draws categorization and naming together in this way.

With task-blindness, we do not see the relationship; object-sorting would be object-sorting and naming would be naming. Behavioral goals become important for specifying the measurable manifestations of a cognitive process.

Assumptions about relationships between behaviors have been difficult to avoid in behaviorally oriented treatment. McReynolds and Kearns (1983) noted that "language responses are, it seems, organized into a variety of functional classes" (p. 217). Evidence for *functional response classes* may be obtained from a study of treatment with respect to multiple baselines. Examples of response classes are nouns and verbs. A real functional distinction between these classes is indicated in the greater impairment in verb-finding in agrammatic aphasia. McReynolds and Kearns suggested that "training a subset of responses within a class will result in generalized responding to other members of that class of behaviors" (p. 217). Generalization should not occur when treatment is applied serially to response classes that are functionally independent. "The two behaviors . . . need to be different enough from one another that treatment of one does not influence the other until it receives treatment"; however, behavior classes "cannot be so different that a single treatment is inapplicable to both" (McReynolds and Kearns, 1983, p. 52). The classification of functional response classes according to an underlying process may be one contribution of cognitive theory to treatment studies.

Modeling a cognitive process as treatment is a fine idea, but we may not know enough about complex cognitive mechanisms. Basso (1989) expressed her concern by saying that "it is not clear how a better understanding of the deficit can help in deciding what has to be done next" (Basso, 1989, p. 28). Byng (1988) figured that a patient had a thematic mapping problem underlying comprehension deficit. She imagined the mental procedure of mapping, because she was not satisfied with previous descriptions of the process: "Models for sentence processing have not

been developed as explicitly as models for processing single words" (p. 631). As indicated in Chapter 5, it should be unclear as to whether Caplan's linear assignment theory or Grodzinsky's trace-deletion models should form a basis for treatment.

Caramazza (1989), an enthusiastic contributor to cognitive theory, had misgivings over the "unfulfilled promise" of cognitively motivated treatments reported so far: "Although I would like to believe that the analysis of a patient's performance informed by cognitive theory provides a *more* useful basis for guiding therapeutic intervention than one not so informed, this belief remains empirically unsupported (p. 394). . . . We need to ask ourselves whether we would have used a different therapeutic strategy had we had a different hypothesis about the functional lesion in the patient (p. 395). . . . No convincing evidence has been presented in support of the view that it is the specifically cognitive character of the analyses of patients' performance that is to be credited for the putative successes in remediation" (p. 396). With respect to developing a "theory of therapeutic intervention," Caramazza (1989) argued that any hypothesis about the nature of deficit "is of limited use in specifying an informed therapeutic strategy because the content of our cognitive theories does not specify the modifications that a damaged system undergoes as a function of the different types of experiences with which a patient may be presented" (p. 393). These modifications may be suggested in theories of recovery.

Theories of Recovery

The words we use to characterize recovery and general goals of treatment are metaphoric at best, because we do not really know what happens inside a patient's head. We think of **restoration** as what is done with a deteriorated historic site. The structure is made to be as similar as possible to its original state, but it is not a resurrection. The notion of **repair** is similar. Like patching up a car to get it running again, repairing a function means that it is only "like new." Basically, these terms address a modification of the damaged module of a system, as opposed to enhancing an intact module.

Regarding restoration of the brain, we wonder if neurons can grow back in the crater created by an ischemic stroke, just as bruised skin repairs itself. *Spontaneous regeneration* of damaged nerves was demonstrated in animals in the 1930s and 1940s by Weiss and Sperry (cited in Rose, 1989). Sperry cut the optic nerve of salamanders. The nerve regenerated, and sight was restored. The optic nerve in mammals, however, does not regenerate, and they remain blind. So far, there is no evidence that cortical cells regenerate. Some spontaneous physiological adjustments occur in the acute phase with resolving diaschisis. Kohlmeyer (1976) found that 33 percent of patients with an occlusion in the internal carotid artery recovered completely in one month, and he attributed this to *collateral circulation* in the Circle of Willis (Chapter 2). In cases of ischemic CVA, we can assume for now that the infarct is permanent.

In addition to neurosurgery, a direct manipulation of the brain is known as **pharmacotherapy.** Speculation about the therapeutic effects of medication on cognition is most publicized for Alzheimer's dementia (Thal, 1988). Such therapy has been reported for patients with traumatic head injury (Weinberg, Auerbach, and Moore, 1987). Medication is known to assist patients with Parkinson's disease. However, there has been negligible investigation of pharmacotherapy for patients with aphasia caused by stroke, and Bachman and Albert (1990) have been exploring the possibilities. They reviewed previous attempts around the world that have had mixed and fragmentary results. At the Boston VA Medical Center, Bachman and Albert studied various agents that manipulate the dopamine system, which consists of areas in the brain in which this neurotransmitter is dispersed across synapses. This is the manipulation tried with Parkinson's disease and is known to include the basal ganglia near the thalamus. Only a "handful" of patients were examined in the late 1980s, and the only demonstrable effect on language behavior was shown by a patient with a transcortical aphasia over three years post onset.

Other ideas about recovery pertain to adaptations by intact parts of the brain. One idea is **substitution,** in which an intact area of the brain, not normally involved in the function, takes over the function. Substitution may entail accomplishing the same goal, such as sentence comprehension, the same way as before; or the substituting region may perform the function a little differently (Gazzaniga, 1974; Laurence and Stein, 1978). In aphasic persons, the right hemisphere (RH), like a "spare tire," might take over a function of the left hemisphere (LH). Replacement could occur in a number of ways, depending on the pre-onset capacities of the substituting region. In *spontaneous substitution,* an aphasic person's brain may turn to language capacities already existing in the RH. Yet, these capacities appear to be restricted to word comprehension (Springer and Deutsch, 1989). Another possibility is that the RH learns new skills either spontaneously or as a result of treatment.

A factor pertinent to substitution is the notion of *plasticity,* which was introduced with respect to the relationship between functional asymmetry and age. The substituting region should have a capacity to change, and evidence indicates that the brain is much more plastic in childhood than in adulthood. However, biologists believe that the capacity for memory is a special case of neuronal plasticity in adults (Squire, 1987). Neuroscientists have explored the capacity of the nervous system to change in response to environmental stimulation or deprivation. One type of environmental stimulation is language treatment. An influence of environment has been demonstrated in the visual cortex of animals (Rose, 1989). Rearing animals in the dark reduced protein synthesis, and exposing these deprived animals to the light resulted in increased protein synthesis in geniculate bodies and cortex. Detector cells in the visual cortices of adult cats varied as a function of the type of visual environment in which the cats were reared.

Moore (1989) reviewed evidence for shifting of language function to the RH in studies employing common techniques for assessing asymmetry of function. Dichotic listening was used in a few studies. We should expect the intact brain to be reflected in a right-ear advantage (REA) for verbal stimuli. A left-ear advantage (LEA) for verbal stimuli indicates that the RH prefers to process this material, and an LEA was found with 20 posterior-fluent aphasic subjects (Johnson, Sommers, and Wiedner, 1977). Simple verbal recognition might have shifted to the RH, if these patients were typical prior to onset of aphasia, although the RH has been shown to already possess simple recognition capacity. Pettit and Noll (1979) found increasing LEAs along with progress in language performance. In Moore's studies, aphasic patients had left-field effects for verbal material and substantial RH alpha-suppression, indicative of activation, for language at sentence and discourse levels. This evidence of RH substitution with aphasia could have other explanations, so the theory needs better substantiation.

The notion of **reorganization** states that an aphasic person accomplishes a functional goal in a new way. Neurologically speaking, an area of the brain does not change; instead, spared areas, not normally involved in a function, are recruited for the performance of a task. Also, we may speak of formation of new "pathways." This is not as if new association tracts are sprouted; it is more like taking a new route to work because a bridge has collapsed on the favorite route. The new route may just take a little longer. Luria's (1970b) theory was called **intersystemic reorganization.** Thinking about intrasystemic reorganization as well, he wrote that "we can summarize both types by the general statement that recovery is brought about by the incorporation of some new type of *afferation* into the disturbed functional system" (p. 386). For intersystemic reorganization, an intact system or process, which is not normally involved in the impaired function, is introduced into ac-

complishing the impaired function. In functional terms, reorganization may be specified with respect to intact components of a processing theory or model. The RH may contribute its own special propensities.

Several procedures for treating aphasia are thought to promote this type of reorganization and are presented in the next chapter. These procedures introduce music, gesture, or visual cues into the act of speaking. Procedures sometimes transform clinician-client interaction from a simple elicitation of response to a more complex routine of instruction in the use of cues that encourage the patient to be analytical in comprehending or formulating an utterance. Carlomagno and Parlato (1989) described treatment of the writing system that supposedly detours a hampered graphemic route to production, possibly by way of a semantically or phonologically based "lexical relay." As a client improves, reorganization may look like restoration or repair.

PRAGMATICS AND GENERALIZATION

Pragmatic treatment can be approached from a number of perspectives that address all of the objectives of treatment. We want to improve communication by any means and for real-life tasks. The problem of generalization is another way of talking about the desire to see that improvements in the clinic are also improvements in the home. When thinking about natural language, we want an aphasic person to recognize the amount of communication that can occur with a little language and a lot of context. We contemplate what we might do to modify contexts to facilitate communication for an aphasic person. The common thread underlying the various aspects of pragmatics is that they have something to do with the interaction between language and context.

Adaptive Language

Spared components of the language system provide adaptive mechanisms for conveying a message, observed in the positive symptoms of aphasia. Positive symptoms show that there is more than one linguistic approach to conveying a message. The objective of improving communication ability is addressed in terms of a more specific goal, which is to improve residual capacities within the language system. Residual language capacities are most evident in anomic and Broca's aphasias, and patients with either type of aphasia tend to make adjustments automatically without intervention from a clinician. Someone with anomic aphasia uses an ability to access semantic and lexical stores and an ability to produce sentences. Both capacities generate circumlocutions that convey the precise meaning, despite failure to access the exact word for it. A patient with thalamic anomia used a portable computer programmed to access words based on partial information provided by the patient (Colby, et al., 1981). People with agrammatic aphasia can access semantic and lexical memories to produce structurally simplified versions of an idea (Chapter 5). Thus, saying "girl tall and boy short" is pretty close to saying *the girl is taller than the boy.*

Holland (1978) argued that it is acceptable for a patient to be "in the ball park, rather than pitching a verbal no-hitter." The clinician's job is not to discourage positive behaviors. Instead, we encourage them. This strategy is not the reinforcement of an impaired act. It reinforces an adaptive act of intact mechanisms. Because patients want to come up with the right word and produce more sophisticated linguistic structure, direct treatment activities can be focused on this end. The clinician keeps track of the effects of this effort in natural situations but does not try to inhibit communication by forcing a patient to shut down crucial subsystems of language production.

Augmentative and Alternative Communication

Nonverbal modalities can be supplements to fragmentary or vague speaking or alternatives for patients with intractable expressive impairment. Facial gesture and intonation convey feeling and thought, which can be a problem for people with RHD. Many aphasic patients adapt on their own with natural signals and mime. A heightened awareness of and comfort with nonverbal modes may increase their use for other patients. Aphasic people are quite variable in receptive and expressive communicative capacities, and we should have few specific expectations of a client prior to evaluation (Feyereisen, 1991).

For patients who use augmentative modes forthrightly, we do not discourage adaptation; our job is to respond to conveyed messages as a way of reinforcing this behavior. Gestural capacity has been demonstrated in a referential communicative situation (Feyereisen, et al., 1988). Abilities that we should encourage have also been studied in conversational interactions. Adaptation was indicated, especially with Broca's aphasia, in the use of more gesture than neurologically intact persons (Le May, David, and Thomas, 1988; Smith, 1987). Communicative use of gesture was demonstrated when it decreased with a screen placed between patients and partners. Clarity and complexity of gestures was greater for mild than for moderate impairment (Glosser, Wiener, and Kaplan, 1986). Communicative abilities were not clearly related to level of language abilities in severely nonfluent patients that differed in level of comprehension. These patients indicated when they were not comprehending, and they asked for support from a clinician (Herrmann, Koch, Johannsen-Horbach, and Wallesch, 1989). Gesturing in Broca's and Wernicke's aphasias corresponds to the nature of their verbal expression. In general, patients with Broca's aphasia produce varied spontaneous gestures, and those with Wernicke's aphasia may require more training if they are to clarify some of their spontaneous gestures (Le May, et al., 1988).

Severity of aphasia motivates us to attempt training alternative modes directly following principles of elicitation and programming applied to verbal behavior. Many modes and systems have been tried (Silverman, 1989), sometimes with patients whose aphasia was questionable but who still needed a mode of communication. Training has been designed for pantomimic gesture (Coelho and Duffy, 1990; Helm-Estabrooks, Fitzpatrick, and Barresi, 1982), American Indian Gestural Code or Amer-Ind (Skelly, 1979), a manual alphabet (Chen, 1971), American Sign Language for the deaf, or ASL (Kirshner and Webb, 1981), drawing (Lyon and Sims, 1989), Blissymbols (Funnell and Allport, 1989; Johannsen-Hornback, Cegla, Mager, Schempp, and Wallesch, 1985), other gestural-assisted symbol systems (Gardner, Zurif, Berry, and Baker, 1976; Glass, Gazzaniga, and Premack, 1973), and a computer-assisted symbol system (Weinrich, Steele, Carlson, Kleczewska, Wertz, and Baker, 1989). Patients with traumatic brain injury have been trained in pantomimic gesture and Blissymbols (Coelho, 1987; Ross, 1979). Clinicians have reported acquisition of abilities in clinical tasks but have not reported convincing transfer to real-life communication (Kraat, 1990).

Programming for Generalization

Metter (1985), a neurologist, wrote a letter to *Asha* magazine in which he referred to a paradox between documentation of a patient's improvement in clinical tasks and his observation of no progress when conversing with the patient. This distinction between clinical progress and functional progress frustrates many clinicians. We want to transfer progress in clinical tasks to a patient's daily life. At the very least, we want to see generalization to "something else"; namely, to stimuli and responses that have not been part of treatment.

One explanation for Metter's observation is that treatment for aphasia, no matter what we do, does not work. Another reason may be that traditional treatment has not been sufficient to achieve transfer. Traditional treatment interaction often simply differs from situations confronted in daily life. We may call this the **clinical-functional gap.** The approaches discussed so far involve drills for specific language functions. Vocabulary is homogenized across patients when a published kit of drawings or photos is employed for naming things. Clinical settings are usually without distraction. Clinical professionals are supportive and understand the nature of aphasia. Referring to treatment for children, Stokes and Baer (1977) thought that clinicians have used a strategy of "train and hope." Aphasia treatment might be like giving a prospective airline pilot practice in pressing a few buttons and pulling a few switches and then sending him or her out to fly a few hundred people from New York to Chicago.

In treatment of aphasia, hope has been replaced by the use of indirect or group methods as a "bridge" across the clinical-functional gap (Aten, 1986). A systematic approach, however, modifies treatment so that it gradually evolves into mimicking real life. Crossing the gap in small steps can be programmed so that previous successes are applied to new stimuli and responses (e.g., Hughes, 1985). One goal is to achieve **stimulus generalization,** which is a behavior performed in the presence of stimuli that differ from stimuli in a treatment condition. Let us suppose that a patient has acquired the ability to say her husband's name with minimal cues from a clinician, but we want her to say it when she wants to in the presence of her husband. Another goal is to achieve **response generalization,** in which a response not elicited in treatment is produced in the same stimulus condition. Cues may be designed to elicit "car" to a picture of a car, but it still would be good if the patient says "Ford" or "driving" when presented with the same picture. **Maintenance** is generalization across time, such as maintaining levels after a session or beyond discharge from the clinic (Kazdin, 1982). We may think that generalization is facilitated by presenting varied stimuli and by accepting varied responses. Among those practicing the behavioral approach, this has been called *loose training* (e.g., Kearns, 1986c; Thompson and Byrne, 1984). To some degree, loose training has always been a feature of cognitive stimulation.

One assumption behind programming for generalization is that it is valuable to begin with traditional direct procedures, especially for severely impaired patients or for training nuances of linguistic skill. Initially, we may focus on a specific process in situations free of anxiety and distraction. A patient may need to become comfortable using a compensatory or alternative strategy before trying it outside the clinic. There are a couple of general directions in which initial treatment moves toward naturalness. Some settings and people outside the clinic induce anxiety or fear. These "stimuli" may not be reinforcing because of the nature of relationships before onset or because people do not know much about aphasia. The clinic becomes more natural when the patient must deal with misunderstandings and communicative failures. Another dimension leads to a positive feature of real life. Conversational participants who know each other well share knowledge that allows messages to be conveyed with the most fragmentary verbalization and gesture. A patient realizes that he or she does not have the sole responsibility for the success of communication (Feyereisen, 1991). Conversation is a collaboration between partners, not a confrontation of contrivances to force linguistic virtuosity.

Modification of Contexts

Programming for generalization enforces an explicit consideration of contextual variables of natural language use (Chapter 8). These variables are added to language-specific variables such as length, complexity, and rate. By planning steps of treatment according to linguistic variables, we focus our treatment on the language system. By planning steps according to contextual variables, we are considering the relationship between the language system and cognitive capacities for processing nonverbal parts of the world. Another perspective on contexts is that they can be modified so that a disabled language system may function in a better environment. This brings us to the last two goals stated early in this chapter.

Internal Contexts. A dispassionate perspective is that psychological state is an internal context for the language system. A patient's perspective begins with the fear and anxiety that stems from a handshake with death. For the first couple of days in the hospital, the patient can be disoriented and may experience hallucinations. He or she is not sure of what all the fuss is about. Once survival is assured, a patient discovers how a malfunction of linguistic capacity leads to frustration and inhibits social interaction.

Eisenson (1984) was one of the first aphasiologists to write extensively about the psychological characteristics of someone with aphasia. *Egocentrism* is reflected in a concern for self which reduces pre-onset considerations of the feelings and needs of others. *Concretism* accompanies ego involvement as a heightened attention to the here and now and an intense desire for routine. A patient may quickly exhibit *unproductive coping and defense mechanisms* as a shield from recognizing impairment. Withdrawal from family and friends may be one mechanism, as the patient begins to be embarrassed about what seems to be infantile abilities. Euphoria and denial are characteristic of persons with right-hemisphere lesions and seem to occur with Wernicke's aphasia. *Emotional lability* is seen in unusually frequent crying or laughing for no apparent reason. *Catastrophic reaction* occurs sometimes with an appropriate emotion.

As a patient enters the chronic phase, other emotions or moods prevail. These states may occur in a somewhat sequential fashion over a period of weeks or months. Tanner and Gerstenberger (1988) noted a typical reaction to loss known as the **grief response** and recognized four stages: (1) *denial* has been mentioned as an initial defense mechanism; (2) *frustration* comes from the continual experience of failure in meeting everyday goals, with anger as the most common reaction; (3) *depression* occurs with awareness of deficits, especially with non-fluent aphasia (Starkstein and Robinson, 1988) and is actually a positive sign of progress for the euphoric patient with Wernicke's aphasia; (4) *acceptance* is the goal of the adjustment process. Some aphasic persons have shared their experiences with these stages (e.g., Buck, 1968; Dahlberg and Jaffe, 1977; Moss, 1972; Wulf, 1979).

Clinicians have detected the strain caused by the crisis of stroke (e.g., Kinsella and Duffy, 1978), and it was disconcerting to find that patients and their families express more optimism than speech-language pathologists (Herrmann and Wallesch, 1989). The main roles of the clinician (and family) in dealing with grief responses are to recognize that they are normal and allow a patient to work through them. These are times for unconditional positive regard and empathic understanding. We may predict how well someone will deal with this crisis when we learn how the patient has dealt with other crises. Code and Muller have been working on development of a *Scale of Psychosocial Adjustment* for aphasic patients (Herrmann and Wallesch, 1990). Part of a speech-language pathologist's job is to help a patient find counseling when the patient seems to be stuck in a phase such that it interferes with recovery of functions (Kennedy and Charles, 1990).

External Contexts. External contexts include settings and people in a patient's life. Encouragement from the environment is likely to enhance transfer of what we are accomplishing in the clinic. Lubinski (1981) was concerned about settings and advocated **environmental language intervention.** The home and hospital are often supportive. However, a group residence, such as a nursing home, may depress motivation and discourage communication. Lubinski described the *communicatively impaired environment* as having the following characteristics: (1) strict rules governing communication; (2) few places for a private conversation; (3) a staff that devalues communication between residents and between residents and staff; (4) many residents with multiple problems, including dementias; and (5) physical conditions that reduce communicative efficiency, such as linear or distant seating and poor lighting and acoustics. Clinicians should employ their diplomatic and persuasive skills to effect modifications of these conditions (Lubinski, 1988). New and remodeled nursing

homes include spaces for private meetings with family and friends, attractive areas for social gatherings, and seating in the dining room that facilitates face-to-face interaction. The staff is informed by in-service education from speech-language pathologists and has unconditional positive regard for the residents.

Aphasia is a family problem. Family members can assist the patient with language recovery and adjustment to deficits. Although the family is often in a state of shock during the acute phase, physicians often do not provide the information they want and need to be helpful. The speech-language pathologist may be the first person to explain stroke. A spouse may develop unrealistic expectations for recovery. Furthermore, family members may participate in clinical activities in the transitional programming of generalization. Another orientation is to assist family members in their own adjustments to the sudden and drastic change in their lives. These purposes are mutually supportive and are not pursued by independent activities. Information about helping someone with aphasia is likely to facilitate a spouse's or child's adjustment, and an adjusting spouse or child is likely to reinforce clinical objectives.

A family member's aphasia turns family dynamics upside down (Rollin, 1987). A patient's inability to carry out customary roles causes family members to assume new roles. Regarding traditional roles of marriage partners, a male patient may no longer be able to provide income, sign the checks, and park the car; a female patient may not be able to shop for groceries, prepare meals, and sign the checks. Dalhberg noted the following: "Since I'd grown up in middle-class America, I was used to taking care of 'masculine' details. I signed into hotels, picked up the bags, gave taxi directions, and ordered in restaurants." His wife added: "I looked forward to the time Clay would be able to do the managing again. It wasn't the physical exertion I minded as much as the loss of my female enjoyment of being 'taken care of' " (Dahlberg and Jaffe, 1977, p. 52). Given revolutionary changes in these matters, a clinician should be aware of the individual's role changes and role desires, partly as a source of content for meaningful treatment activities.

Role changes are also understood with respect to shifts in the balance of ego states defined according to transactional analysis (TA). Porter and Dabul (1977) applied TA to helping spouses understand the situation and return to a balance achieved pre-onset. A spouse seems to have to respond to shifts in Adult, Parent, and Child ego states by the patient; "he acts like a child." In the aphasic person, the Adult state is often weakened and turned into the dependent state of the Child; "he just sits around all day and watches TV." Childlike ego involvement dominates as impulsivity and a continual attention to "me, me, me." The Parent state diminishes with an inability to conform to social acceptability. Other patients may exaggerate the Parent by becoming overly protective of the spouse, constantly monitoring his or her activities. We may begin to imagine the toll this takes on a spouse and children living at home. A spouse can become overly protective of a patient. Leisure and social activities are reduced, and family members become guilty about feelings that they perceive as selfishness (Kinsella and Duffy, 1978).

The wife or husband of an aphasic patient may say, "I want someone to help *me*." There are many resources for patients and family members through which to learn about disorders and share experiences with others in the same boat (Shadden, 1988). *Stroke Clubs* are often sponsored by the American Heart Association, and they include persons with varied problems (Sanders, Hamby, and Nelson, 1984). The *National Head Injury Foundation* (in Framingham, Massachusetts) and its state organizations have provided legislative advocacy and have sponsored local survivor groups. The *National Aphasia Association,* led by Martha Taylor Sarno at Rusk Institute of Rehabilitation Medicine in New York City, is promoting community awareness and encouraging the creation of similar support groups specifically for aphasic persons and their families. We find a patient with Broca's aphasia telling an audience about a cross-country trip, one word at a time, accompanied by photos. European countries have formed Aphasia Associations for families (e.g., Wahrborg, 1991). Also, rehabilitation centers have provided a place for family support groups and counseling (Rice, Paull, and Muller, 1987; Webster and Newhoff, 1981). A husband told Newhoff and Davis (1978), "It's nice to find out you're not alone. You get ideas here of ways to cope. I've learned to enjoy my wife in spite of her stroke. I feel closer to her now" (p. 324).

GROUP TREATMENT

A great deal of treatment during and after World War II was conducted with patients in groups (Huber, 1946; Sheehan, 1946; Wepman, 1951). The large number of patients in military hospitals made groups necessary, but it also came to be viewed as a valuable supplement with its own dynamics that do not occur in individual treatment. The VA cooperative study showed that eight hours per week of group work is effective past six months post onset (Wertz, et al., 1981), although few rehabilitation programs provide group treatment of this intensity. A problem with pitting group treatment against individual treatment is that most clinicians do not use groups as a substitute for individual treatment. Many form groups to supplement individual treatment; thus, an efficacy study should compare individual treatment with and without group treatment. Group treatment has had a reputation of being an unstructured social hour for sipping tea, munching crumpets, and hoping for talk. If not devalued, it has been thought by payment providers to be obscure for computing its cost per patient. An appreciation for group treatment has suffered from ambiguity of definition and ambivalence of support.

There is no single entity for which the label "group treatment" suffices. The label says that it involves two or more clients. Otherwise, it is done for varied purposes and with equally varied methods, surveyed thoroughly by Kearns (1986b). Brookshire (1986) stated that goals of groups pertain to treatment, maintenance, transition, and support. Three of these areas overlap with the individual goals of repairing skills and maximizing generalization. Memory and orientation activities can be conducted for patients with head injuries and right-hemisphere dysfunctions (Wilson and Moffat, 1984). Elderly persons may participate in reminiscence groups (Barr, 1988). Maintenance refers to holding onto skills after discharge from regular treatment. Psychological support can be an element of these groups, but other groups are designed for the purpose of counseling. Let us think of group work with respect to what it can contribute to the basic goals of treatment listed early in this chapter. The importance of this connection is that group treatment need not be seen as extraneous to communicative rehabilitation. Groups can be designed mainly for generalization of acquired skills, and they provide a uniquely empathic environment for patients to practice without a clinician's intrusion into the interaction (Davis and Wilcox, 1985).

CAN ANYONE (OR ANYTHING) CARRY OUT APHASIA TREATMENT?

Despite the knowledge, sensitivities, and skills that go into a clinical aphasiologist's work at a rehabilitation center, several investigations have been devoted to comparing speech-language pathologists and volunteers in the administration of aphasia treatment. These studies have been focused on the part of a clinician's job description that involves providing direct treatment of language deficits, and they have had the apparent objective of contributing converging evidence to answer the question of whether traditional treatment of language is efficacious. As noted previously, the second VA cooperative study found that home-based treatment by volunteers produced nonsignificant results between professional treatment and no treatment (Wertz, et al., 1986). An additional

report showed that a spouse or friend trained by a speech-language pathologist can conduct effective treatment at home (Marshall, Wertz, Weiss, et al., 1989). Three other studies found no difference in progress when treatment was provided by professionals and volunteers (David, Enderby, and Bainton, 1982; Meikle, Wechsler, Tupper, Benenson, Butler, Mulhall, and Stern, 1979; Quinteros, Williams, White, and Pickering, 1984). In these studies, a no-treatment control group was not considered to determine whether progress in either condition resulted from the treatment. Also, professionals performed all evaluations and trained the volunteers, indicating that volunteers may be helpful under the direction of a speech-language pathologist.

As if there are forces determined to see if speech-language pathologists can be replaced, we have been pitted against computers also. One study simply showed that aphasic patients made fewer errors when reinforced by a computer than when reinforced by a clinician alone or a computer and a clinician (Kinsey, 1990). In another study, an alternating-treatments/multiple baseline design showed that a clinician required fewer sessions than computer-assisted treatment for an aphasic patient to reach some of the levels in a treatment program (Loverso, Prescott, Selinger, Wheeler, and Smith, 1985). Then, with a similar design and ten subjects, this finding was repeated in a comparison between a clinician alone and computer-clinician-assisted treatment (Loverso, Prescott, Selinger, and Riley, 1989). In providing one of the "effs," the computer was effective but less efficient than clinicians. Relative efficiency of treatments has become a crucial concern in the modern rehabilitation hospital. Seron (1987) suggested that equating the tasks administered by a clinician and a computer is less interesting than using a computer for things that a clinician cannot do. Moreover, computers have not yet been shown to be responsive to a patient's emotional lability.

SUMMARY AND CONCLUSIONS

The multiple objectives of treatment point to a number of approaches, such as repetitive drills, group activities, front-line counseling, and referral. This chapter proceeded from direct treatment intended to repair the language system to pragmatic approaches for promoting generalization and expanding communication. This may be the sequence of treatment for some patients. For others, drills and pragmatics may operate in tandem, with one making immediate contributions to the other. Targets of aphasia rehabilitation correspond to a framework used in Yorkston, Beukelman, and Bell's (1988) text on dysarthrias: *impairment*, which, for aphasia, is the impaired cognitive process and its direct manifestations; *disability*, which is the effects of language impairment on communication; and *handicap*, which is the effects of the communicative disability on activities of daily living, work, play, and personal relationships. Comprehensive rehabilitation addresses each level. An integrated comprehensive approach recognizes that addressing the handicaps can provide therapeutic mechanisms for the impairment. Transfer should not be something we hope happens; transfer is something a clinician does.

CHAPTER

13

IMPLEMENTATION OF TREATMENT FOR LANGUAGE DYSFUNCTIONS

Principles of treatment for language-specific disorders are implemented for patients with stroke or closed head injuries, for the aphasia syndromes, and for different levels of severity. The principles are implemented in the contexts of different settings and different needs of individual patients. This is not to say that procedures are the same for everyone under all circumstances. The principles are general enough to be flexible, so that the next consideration for treatment may be the ingenuity of clinicians. The procedures presented are examples of what has been done and what can be done, but they should not be taken as examples of what *must* be done.

THE BUSY CLINICIAN

Basic treatment approaches in the United States were developed in the wide-open

spaces of Veterans Administration Medical Centers in the 1950s and 1960s. (They were called VA hospitals then.) Schuell was at the Minneapolis VA Hospital, and Brookshire replaced her in the 1970s. Porch was in Albuquerque, and Goodglass and Kaplan were at the renowned Boston VA Hospital. Many speech-language pathologists work in different circumstances in the 1990s. Acute care does not necessarily lead imperceptibly to chronic care in the same facility. Hospitals and rehabilitation centers rely on Medicare or Medicaid and private insurance programs for payment of services. Speech-language pathologists are accountable for appropriateness and efficiency of service by certifying need and justifying continuation. Many clinicians have had until one year post onset to accomplish communicative goals.

Treatment goals and substantiation of progress are reported according to management systems created by payment providers. Let us consider some basic procedures required by Medicare, which is an insurance program provided by the United States federal government generally for persons over age 65. Part A of Medicare provides for necessary inpatient medical services within the first 90 days. This covers the acute phase for someone with a stroke, and DRG guidelines motivate hospitals to minimize duration of stay. Thereafter, Part B pays for physician-prescribed services in a hospital or clinic or at home. A clinician submits a short *certification* form to the physician for services under Part B. The clinician notes frequency of individual treatment according to visits per week and an anticipated maximum duration of treatment. Clinicians usually propose the fullest duration needed based on the limited knowledge base for prognosis. Certification also requires a brief statement of short-term goals that are within a patient's immediate grasp and long-term goals for the duration requested. These should be stated as measurable functional goals, and we can keep the more debatable cognitive underbelly of these goals to ourselves. After certification, a notice signifying the beginning of treatment is filed with the physician. From the date of this notice, *recertification* is required every 30 days. Progress must be documented if recertification is to be approved.

As discussed before, what we measure is a professional issue with respect to differences between clinical and functional progress. Also, there has been little enthusiasm for supporting "maintenance therapy." Functional goals are being legislated through the insistence on functional assessment (Frattali, 1992). The length of time represented by short- and long-term goals varies according to whether a clinician is reporting to the hospital or directly to an insurance company or a government agency. Often short-term goals are written according to what should be accomplished in two weeks rather than 30 days. Long-term goals may be "intermediate" to cover a three-month reporting period required in a hospital. This chapter provides some examples of behavioral goals with the assumption that they will vary depending on reporting requirements as well as a patient's disorder.

WHEN TO BEGIN

Reflecting on a patient's early confusion and diaschisis in the acute period, we may wonder about the best time to begin treatment. We consider this period when treating patients in an acute care hospital and do not have to consider it when in a strictly chronic care rehabilitation facility. Eisenson (1984) insisted that treatment begin "as soon as the patient is able to take notice of what is going on and is able to cooperate in the effort" (p. 180). Rubens (1977b), a neurologist, wrote, "I like to see aphasic patients enter therapy as early as possible, and I believe that the therapy should be as intensive as the general medical situation will allow" (p. 1). The existence of bedside examinations (Chapter 10) indicates that many clinicians begin cursory evaluation soon after onset. Physicians like to see physical therapy begin as soon as possible. The intensity of treatment is generally dictated by the medical condition of the patient.

Wepman (1972) expressed another view that differentiated between types of intervention. In the acute phase, a clinician should provide "a supportive psychological role." Because the early phase presents an evolving picture of deficit and is an emotionally delicate time, Wepman recommended delaying direct treatment of language functions beyond the acute phase. He associated early instability with spontaneous recovery and worried about adverse psychological reaction to intensive language treatment. "To be ultimately successful, it is argued, aphasia therapy should begin with the residual, permanent problem and not with the temporary one" (p. 206). Direct treatment would not begin until the patient enters a rehabilitation facility. Although it appears that he suggested delaying language drills for three months, Wepman did not dwell on a time period.

Many patients look forward to getting started with serious work on their problems as soon as possible. A speech-language pathologist's experience leads to a sensitivity to the type of activity that a patient can tolerate. Eisenson (1984) suggested that early language treatment discourages development of counterproductive communicative strategies, such as a dependence on alternative modes before it is warranted. Early treatment also should discourage development of unproductive coping mechanisms, such as withdrawal. Speech-language pathologists in an acute care facility do not have much time for a treatment program, but they provide psychological support and some language treatment, particularly when a patient is able to sit up for a while or move about the hospital. They provide valuable information for the next clinician at a rehabilitation facility.

Some research on recovery addresses the question of whether starting time makes a difference in the efficacy of treatment (Chapter 11). We know that a patient often makes much greater progress during the first two or three months than the next three months, except for those with global aphasia, who seem to make much of their progress from six to 12 months post onset (Sarno and Levita, 1981). An argument can be made that treatment is most effective while the brain is adjusting during the period of spontaneous recovery, although there is little evidence for this assertion. Two studies showed that more patients had substantial improvement with earlier than later treatment. In one study, treatment starting before and after six months was compared (Butfield and Zangwill, 1946); in another study, treatment starting before two months was compared to treatment starting between two and six months (Basso, et al., 1979). Yet, these studies did not provide comparisons of amount of progress or outcome, and the early progress of those with later treatment was not observed. Analysis of Hanson and Cicciarelli's (1978) and Bamber's (1980) data indicates that starting time did not correlate with amount or outcome of recovery. Most clinicians tend to subscribe to Eisenson's assertions and introduce treatment as soon as possible in doses adjusted according to a patient's stamina and receptivity.

GLOBAL/SEVERE APHASIA

Let us begin with patients who have deep impairment of comprehension and little verbal expression (Collins, 1986; Salvatore and Thompson, 1986). We may assume that direct repair of the language system begins with simple language and simple tasks. However, we may move quickly to augmentative or alternative modes, especially if controlled stimulation fails to elicit lasting useful verbalization.

Word Comprehension

Speech-language pathologists follow a general rule: "comprehension precedes expression." Nonverbal behavior, such as nodding "yes" or "no," is improved with progress in comprehension. Thus, short-term and intermediate or long-term goals should reflect the idea that treatment of comprehension can have far-reaching communicative consequences. With stimulation beginning at the simplest of levels, we try to raise the level of comprehension as far as we can. The following goals illustrate general points about goal-setting:

Short-term: Increase accuracy from 60 percent to 100 percent for selecting an object from four choices when given words for shopping and cooking.

Intermediate: Purchase ten items in a store with 100 percent accuracy.

Both goals are constructed with functionality in mind. Treatment should be at a level of 80 percent accuracy with a task that might be easier than the floor of initial assessment (e.g., two choices). The pointing response may have to be modeled; or, backing up further, we may need to get the patient to imitate any movement first. The intermediate goal represents what we "hope" is a consequence of meeting short-term goals. An initial baseline may be obtained in facilities in a hospital, and at least half the items should be items not trained in the clinic. Repeated probes in a real setting are taken at reasonable intervals to determine if hoped-for generalization is occurring or if the programming of more steps is needed to close the gap between a clinical task and a functional activity.

For our drills, we should have a patient's attention first. Hospitalized people working at simple levels may arrive at the clinic tired from physical therapy or in a state of depressed vigilance due to trauma. A wheelchair-bound patient may be drowsy from waiting in the hallway after being brought to the clinic too early. Collins (1986) made treatment a little more interesting by programming steps with playing cards, starting with matching and sequencing. Awareness may be heightened when the task is individualized, as in pointing to family faces when presented with family names. Especially for distractibility with CHI, **alerting signals,** such as the patient's name or "Ready?", may be presented before each stimulus item.

For word comprehension, several variables can be manipulated to decrease difficulty to a level of success or to increase difficulty toward short-term goals. The lexical stimulus may be repeated or supplemented with a printed word. We can vary familiarity or word class (e.g., noun, verb). Redundant verbal context might help in identifying an object. In addition to number of response options, pictures can be varied in semantic relatedness and can be supplemented with printed words. If a patient's brain is adjusting, no matter what the reason might be, then the patient should be moving along with almost daily shifts upward in task level. We should be on the alert for reinforcing sudden verbal response during the task. If a patient is not reaching the short-term goal, then it is not likely that much repair of the language system is possible.

Verbal Expression

One of the main principles in Schuell's method was that a patient should always respond to a stimulus. For global aphasia, it is vital that a response indicating comprehension be within a patient's expressive repertoire. When we have the urge to change tasks by asking questions, the type of response should be as simple as possible. Yet, many aphasic persons, not only the most severely impaired, are inconsistent with "yes" and "no," even to the point of nodding "yes" while saying "no." Treatment should achieve consistency of "yes" and "no" involving the simplest stimulus for the patient (e.g., "Is this four?", "red?") before this becomes a response mode for pushing the comprehension mechanism. Treatment includes response to a clinician's verbal and nonverbal affirmatives and negatives as well as practice with the various modalities in which "yes" and "no" can be expressed (e.g., speech, nodding, pointing to words).

In principle, treatment begins with what a patient can do verbally, and people with global aphasia easily produce verbal stereotypes with no relation to a situation. They can be prodded into counting to ten or singing a song. One patient, who was unresponsive to the simplest verbal input, could recite the Twenty-Third Psalm. Perhaps getting voluntary control over this speech is a start. Let us consider the following goals:

Short-term: Increase volitional word production from 0 percent to 50 percent when presented with a printed version.

Intermediate: Establish word-finding ability for conversation.

Helm and Barresi (1980) programmed what clinicians try; namely, harnessing whatever utterances are produced so that we can elicit them. The program was called *Voluntary Control of Involuntary Utterances* (Helm-Estabrooks and Albert, 1991). It began with presenting the printed form of utterances just heard. If the utterance was repeated with this stimulation, it was more volitional and potentially more under the clinician's control for subsequent practice. If a different word was produced, a stimulus card was written for that word. No treatment was pursued for any utterance that was difficult to elicit a second time. When reading aloud and repetition elicited responses, an object-picture was presented in a transition to naming tasks. Patients improved in independent testing and were reported to use some of the words appropriately in conversational interaction.

Schonle (1988) described a treatment called *compound noun stimulation* for chronic global aphasia more than three years post onset. Object-drawings labeled by compound words were presented (e.g., wheelchair, football), and the first part of the word was used to cue the second part. The goal was to elicit words. This procedure was compared with a standard naming activity in which simple words were elicited by repetition. Compound naming improved from 0 to 94 percent over four weeks, whereas standard naming improved from 0 to 12 percent. A second treatment phase advanced performance further, and only a slight drop occurred five weeks after the end of treatment. Transfer to untrained rhyming words occurred only for the compound naming method. Thus, a short distance of generalization was studied, and Schonle did not address whether word retrieval in conversation was improved. Such methods are worth a try, but we are most interested in functional improvement.

Alternative Modes

A rule of thumb for people with dysarthria (and no aphasia) is to provide them with a means of communication as soon as possible. For people without speech and severe aphasia, however, we need to refrain for a moment as we consider the influence of language disorder on the use of another mode that involves the same language or another symbol system (Chapter 4). Someone with severe verbal apraxia and mild aphasia may readily take to a small alphabetic "calculator" like the Canon Communicator (Silverman,

1989). For more severe impairment, the device simply provides another window to the depression of language skills. Collins (1986) discussed communication boards, which a hospital staff might want to provide to anyone who cannot talk. Yet, word and phrase boards can only be used by someone who understands what the words mean, and alphabet boards are very difficult with global impairment. A board or notebook with pictures and words may be within a patient's ability, but a further consideration is that some training is often required before a person will use it for functional communicative purposes. A patient is most likely to reach for a board that conveys important messages that cannot be conveyed by gesturing.

There have been a few reports on gestural skills. *Visual Action Therapy* (VAT) takes a patient through several steps involving object manipulation in order to train the use of pantomimic gestures (Helm-Estabrooks, et al., 1982). The program begins with matching tasks for perception and recognition of objects and proceeds to gesturing of function with the object in hand and then without the object. Coelho and Duffy (1987) studied acquisition of 23 Amer-Ind signs and 14 fabricated signs. The Amer-Ind Code has been enticing because it is descriptive of referents and can be used with one hand (Skelly, 1979). Coelho's training method had steps for imitation, recognition, and "naming" with each gesture. The goal for the study was to develop an ability to name referents, and stimulus generalization was measured with respect to naming untrained pictures with trained gestures. The ability to acquire these signs was negligible for patients below the 35th percentile for the PICA overall, indicating that a patient's own pantomimes may be more profitable for severe aphasia. Those above this level increased their ability to acquire and generalize signs as a linear function of severity of aphasia. In early field reports on training Amer-Ind to aphasic patients, Skelly (1979) noted that "there was almost universal dissatisfaction expressed concerning transfer from the cued retrieval/replicative stage to self-initiated use" (p. 40).

Later, Coelho (1990) reported on training selected Amer-Ind and ASL signs for four patients, and two were below the 35th percentile. The strategy for the program was based on the notion of **matrix-training,** which had been applied to training gestures to patients with Broca's aphasia by Tonkovich and Loverso (1982). Their idea was to train pairs of Amer-Ind and ASL signs for actions and objects with usual imitation-recognition-production procedures (Figure 13–1). Some items in the matrix were for training (T), and others were for assessing generalization a short distance from training (i.e., untrained combinations of trained verbs and nouns) or a longer distance (i.e., combinations with an untrained object). Coelho's stages of treatment led to varying the agent (i.e., man, woman) with two verbs (i.e., cook, eat) and eight objects (e.g., tomato, fish, egg). Conclusions from the study were that severely impaired aphasic persons do not acquire an Amer-Ind/ASL system and, for less severely impaired patients, special training is

needed to facilitate generalization. Coelho (1990) noted that "the production of sign combinations from previously acquired single signs does not occur spontaneously — that is, without training — and that even with training, at least within the context of the present experiment, the maintenance effect is weak" (p. 399).

Another mode draws from a patient's retained capacities, perhaps in the right hemisphere. Lyon and Sims (1989) tried "training expressively restricted aphasic patients to draw communicatively" (also, Lyon and Helm-Estabrooks, 1987). They encouraged the use of simple drawings such as stick figures for representing a "single event." Eight patients from the 15th to the 45th overall percentile on the PICA were trained with their method. Like any training, it started simple and gradually became more complex. It involved imitation, instruction, cueing, and encouragement. Lyon and Sims promoted transfer by having patients use drawing to convey messages in a conversational interac-

FIGURE 13–1 A matrix of verb + object pairs for training gesture and sign combinations. (T) = items trained, (I) = generalization items within the training matrix, and (E) = generalization items outside the training matrix. (Reprinted by permission from Tonkovich, J. & Loverso, F., A training matrix approach for gestural acquisition by the agrammatic patient. In R.H. Brookshire (Ed.), *Clinical aphasiology conference proceedings.* Minneapolis: BRK, 1982, p. 284.)

	MILK	COKE	TEA	COFFEE	JUICE	WATER	BEER	WINE
SPILL	SPILL MILK	SPILL COKE	SPILL TEA	SPILL COFFEE	SPILL JUICE	SPILL WATER	SPILL BEER	SPILL WINE
	T	T	T	T	E	E	E	E
DRINK	DRINK MILK	DRINK COKE	DRINK TEA	DRINK COFFEE	DRINK JUICE	DRINK WATER	DRINK BEER	DRINK WINE
	T	I	I	I	E	E	E	E
BUY	BUY MILK	BUY COKE	BUY TEA	BUY COFFEE	BUY JUICE	BUY WATER	BUY BEER	BUY WINE
	T	I	I	I	E	E	E	E
POUR	POUR MILK	POUR COKE	POUR TEA	POUR COFFEE	POUR JUICE	POUR WATER	POUR BEER	POUR WINE
	T	I	I	I	E	E	E	E

T = Training Items (7)
I = Intramatrix Generalization Items (9)
E = Extramatrix Generalization (16)

tion called PACE, presented later in this chapter. Measures showed that patients improved as a group, but the most severely impaired patients were not addressed specifically. Because interactive communication is a collaborative effort, drawings do not have to be perfect. With a vocational background in drawing and 28th percentile PICA overall at four months post onset, a patient developed some communicative use of his drawing ability (Collins, 1986). Morgan and Helm-Estabrooks (1987) presented "Back to the Drawing Board," based on copying cartoons of increasing complexity.

Speech-language pathologists have been relentless, if not heroic, in the pursuit of establishing a mode of communication for globally impaired aphasic people. This effort includes training special symbols that can be manipulated in some way. A few patients were trained to comprehend statements, questions, and commands constructed out of symbols arranged in syntactic order. Symbols in one study were cut-out paper shapes used to give chimpanzees a means of communicating with humans (Glass, et al., 1973). Another study employed a system called *Visual Communication,* or VIC (Gardner, et al., 1976). Although subjects displayed a knowledge of basic syntactic relations with an ability to respond to questions and commands, there was no sign of transfer to functional use. Blissymbols, a system of pictograms, was presented to four patients with global aphasia (Johannsen-Horbach, et al., 1985). Two patients interacted with the clinician using these symbols, and one of these used it on a limited basis while living with his mother. Another patient progressed enough in speaking that Blissymbols became unnecessary (also, Funnell and Allport, 1989). A computer-assisted nonverbal symbol system puts syntactically arranged pictures and symbols on the screen (Steele, Weinrich, Wertz, Kleczewska, and Carlson, 1989; Weinrich, et al., 1989).

A Cost-Benefit Quandary?

Marshall (1987) raised eyebrows with this assertion: "Aphasiologists spend excessive time in the treatment of globally aphasic clients but tend to dismiss the needs of the mildly aphasic person because they are less obvious" (p. 60). We should be concerned about the mildly aphasic person. For now, the issue is the benefit in relation to cost for the globally aphasic person, especially when considering prognosis for improvement in language ability and the lack of evidence for functional use of alternative modes that have been tried. Marshall "advocated that aphasiologists reapportion treatment time so as to spend more hours with mildly impaired clients, and less time with severe or globally involved clients" (p. 70).

Marshall's opinion elicited sharp responses in the "Clinical Forum" of the journal *Aphasiology.* Parsons (1987b) doubted Marshall's assumptions about the relative amount of time being spent with global and mild aphasias. Marshall's claim that clinicians are "ignoring" data on lack of recovery by treating globals assumes that clinicians are still doing the treatments that were not showing results. Edelman (1987) suggested that progress in overall scores does not tell us about progress in comprehension and gesturing seen in the last half of the first year post onset. We do not have data on spread of comprehension to other communicative functions as a function of treatment. Thus, Marshall ignored ignorance in the evidence. Edelman and Parsons also had a sensitivity for the value that a patient and family may place on any progress as opposed to the value that some clinicians evidently place on it. Sarno and Levita (1979) noted that a few words could make a remarkable difference in someone's life over an inability to produce words. Moreover, maximum effort may not have been made in programming generalization. Extending treatment beyond acquisition of skills in clinical tasks is discussed later as pragmatic programming.

BROCA'S APHASIA

Because their comprehension is usually superior to their production and patients can recognize syntactic errors, agrammatic patients appear to be most impaired in language formulation with competence preserved. Patients have been considered to have a deficit in "syntax," but treatments have varied in the extent to which syntax is the focus. Thompson, Hall, and Sison (1985) studied effects of hypnosis and imagery on naming ability for three patients with Broca's aphasia. The patients practiced imaging a set of pictured objects without naming these objects. Strong progress with trained and untrained objects was seen in one subject. There is nothing peculiar to Broca's aphasia that would suggest hypnosis and imagery training, except for the notion that imagery and hypnosis rely on the intact right hemisphere. Syntactic training of some sort is at least a logical choice.

Sentence Comprehension

Historically, treatment reflected the understanding of deficit as being a unidimensional disorder with severity graded according to the length and complexity of sentences that can be comprehended consistently. The starting point—where a patient begins to have a little difficulty—would depend on the sentences presented in initial assessment. This approach includes a few basic tasks. **Pointing to pictures** varies difficulty according to number of choices and relatedness of choices. Research gives us some ideas in this regard (Chapter 5). For example, pictures focus decisions on certain features of a sentence such as lexical items or order of agent and object, which is more problematic in Broca's aphasia. **Following instructions** has been popular, especially for addressing language forms conveying spatial relationships, and the Token Test has been a model for treatments (Flowers and Danforth, 1979; Holland and Sonderman, 1974). A similar task is Caplan's toy manipulations for assessing comprehension of thematic roles and coreference (Chapter 10). Another task is **sentence verification,** in which only one picture is needed per sentence and false decisions can be directed to a variety of differences

between a sentence and a picture. **Answering questions** has the advantage of infinite possibilities for content, and it is not much of a switch to turn questions into sentence verification and vice versa.

Luria (1970b) developed an idea that seemed to be intuitively proper for what we now call Broca's aphasia. It was called **externalization of schemas** as an example of intersystemic reorganization in the sense of employing visual images in the analysis of sentences. Diagrams that "differ little from those used in common grammar texts" (p. 441) were shown in association with a spoken or printed sentence to make relationships between words explicit, facilitating a conscious effort to integrate words into a complex concept. For example, diagrams illustrated basic spatial relations such as *above, below, on,* and *under;* they were very much like ideograms used in nonverbal symbol systems. The purpose was "to externalize the meaningful relationships implied by the constructions and compensate for the inner schemata which the patient lacks" (p. 443). Phrases like "mother's daughter" were split into parts so that a patient could analyze structure. Two pictures represented the meaning of each word. A demonstrative was added for cueing the word serving as modifier (e.g., "*this* mother's daughter"). Awareness of structure can also be raised with **metalinguistic tasks,** such as making judgments about errors in sentences.

Patients have problems making agent-object order decisions for reversible passives and other structures for which it may be difficult to assign thematic roles without semantic cues. Opinions differ as to whether disorder should be located in the syntactic parser or in mapping for semantic interpretation. Byng (1988) found two patients who erred with reversible declarative (e.g., *The man kisses the woman*) and locative sentences (e.g., *The man is beside the woman*). Byng agreed with Schwartz, believing that the impaired process was the mapping of thematic roles onto SVO structures computed by the parser. Only locatives were treated, and comprehension was measured for other types of sentences not treated. Comprehension was cued with a "meaning card" showing relations between noun phrases, which was similar to Luria's externalization of schemas and a strategy thought to facilitate mapping. One subject's progress for locatives spread to untreated active and passive declaratives, which Byng interpreted as improvement of a mapping mechanism. She concluded that locatives and declaratives are understood by the same mechanism, but as indicated in the previous chapter, Byng also had some questions about whether her procedure necessarily follows from a mapping hypothesis. After all, Luria thought of it, too, without modern psycholinguistics.

Psycholinguistic studies of neurologically intact and aphasic adults are suggestive of the facilitation of comprehension of complex structures with the presence of certain lexical and prosodic cues. For example, expanded relative clauses are easier than reduced relative clauses (Chapter 4). People with Broca's aphasia have a problem interpreting linguistic stress and juncture that may need to be addressed in treatment (Baum, et al., 1982). Aphasic patients, not necessarily with Broca's aphasia, comprehend sentences better when surface markers are added (Pierce, 1982):

1. The man has *already* caught the ball.
2. The boy is *being* hit by the girl.
3. The man takes the boy *over* to the girl.
4. The man sees the woman *who is* sitting down.

The discovery that cue redundancy improves sentence comprehension should also be of interest to clinicians (Bates, et al., 1991). Inflections, intonation, demonstratives, semantic information, and anything else we can think of should be loaded into sentences to make them easy to understand; these features can be removed to increase the challenge.

Agrammatism

Treatment of verbal expression in Broca's aphasia is viewed generally as a matter of increasing the length of utterances. It is viewed specifically as a matter of facilitating production of grammatical morphemes as a skeleton amidst the content words that can be produced. People with agrammatism still retrieve words with much effort, as if there is an upper limit on the number of content words that a person can produce in one utterance. Thus, treatment is indeed a matter of expanding facility in producing words in general, along with focusing on the peculiar grammatical difficulties so thoroughly studied in this group.

The Changing Criteria Program. A general stimulation program for Broca's aphasia was presented by Rosenbek and his colleagues (1989). "The heart of the program is a series of questions and answers using pictures as stimuli. . . . If the patient fails to answer a question about any given picture, a series of increasingly more powerful cues is provided" (p. 224). Questions address attributes of people, places, and things in pictures of simple events (e.g., "What are the persons wearing?" "What color are the clothes or objects?" "Where are they?"). Questions are not aimed at specific syntactic structures. At the first level, a carrier phrase is used as the cue. Upon success at this level, the patient is instructed to produce longer utterances for the remaining levels. Cues consist of carrier phrases or a choice of sentences to repeat. The idea is to move in steps according to the length-criterion for production, and the procedure is designed to end up with spontaneous productions.

Behavioral Methods. As indicated in the previous chapter, behavioral methods tend to train production of specific syntactic features of sentences. Multiple baseline designs have been used to evaluate training of locative phrases (Thompson, et al., 1982), the auxiliary *is* (Kearns and Salmon, 1984), and *Wh*-interrogatives (Thompson and McReynolds, 1986; Wambaugh and Thompson, 1989). Sentences are often elicited through **modeling.** One technique for lengthening utterances is **forward chaining,** in which a clinician "sequentially modeled the first two words of the target response, then the remaining words of the target response, instructing the subject to repeat each portion as it was modeled" (Thompson and McReynolds, 1986, p. 198). Another technique, **reverse chaining,** involves presenting all but the last word of a sentence as a "completion task," and then eliciting an increasingly longer version of the sentence by subtracting words from the carrier phrase toward the first word.

A rather complex ABAB experimental design was employed in a study of two cases with Broca's aphasia (Kearns and Salmon, 1984). Results for one subject are seen in Figure 13–2. The objective was to increase production of complete sentences with the auxiliary *is* (e.g., "The boy is drinking"). Treatment consisted of imitative and spontaneous production tasks designed to elicit this auxiliary in sentences; reinforcement was contingent upon complete sentence productions. Beginning with the baseline phase, probes were administered regularly to assess progress with trained and untrained auxiliary productions (upper graph). Generalization of auxiliary training to production of a different type of sentence (lower graph) was measured with a probe of untrained copula production (e.g., "The man is a cowboy"). The probes were given six times in three sessions prior to the introduction of treatment.

Efficacy of treatment was studied with reversal of training as the second baseline phase (i.e., no training) followed by reinstatement of auxiliary-is training. Reversal consisted of two parts. First, it was carried out during a period of reinforcing agrammatic productions of previously untrained copula forms, while the clinician ignored complete productions. Then, it was applied to auxiliary forms that had been trained. Performance improved with trained and untrained forms during training, deteriorated during reversal training, and improved again when auxiliary-is training was reinstated. Maintenance of progress was seen two and six weeks after termination of treatment in the retraining phase. Treatment emerged as the prominent factor because of a reversal and restoration of performance. Kearns and Salmon reported that generalization to spontaneous produc-

tion was not achieved. While they noted that such generalization is not automatic and should be programmed, it is also possible that several sessions of reversal reduced the likelihood of a wider range of generalization. ABAB-reversal may not be in the best interest of the client. "Careful consideration must be given to the consequences of reverting to baseline for the client and those who are responsible for his or her care" (Kazdin, 1982, p. 124).

With four agrammatic subjects, Thompson and McReynolds (1986) compared a "direct-production" approach and an "auditory-visual" approach to training *Wh-* question production (e.g., "What is he drinking?"). The former method was presumed to be derived from behavioral treatment, and the latter was thought to be characteristic of stimulation methods. Number of items trained and reinforcement were the same for both procedures. A session consisted of six trials for each of five items. The comparison hinged on single stimulus presentation in direct-production/behavioral treatment and multimodal presentation in auditory-visual/stimulation. However, stimulation should also be distinctive in the use of a large number of different items (Table 12–1).

An *alternating-treatments design* (ATD) was used to compare procedures. This design is also known as simultaneous-treatment or concurrent schedule design (Kazdin, 1982). As in other designs, an ATD begins with a baseline of the behavior to be treated. Then, two treatments are given in an alternating fashion. The main problem to be controlled involves sequence effects of one treatment upon a subsequent treatment. So-called "cross-over designs" simply alternate treatment periods lasting a few days (e.g., Springer, Glindemann, Huber, and Willmes, 1991). The sequence effect is minimized by providing both treatments on the same day (i.e., "simultaneous" treatments), and then, across several days, randomly alternating the order of treatments each day. Probes of the target behavior are obtained for each treatment so that a graph of the treatment phase shows two sets of data, one for each treat-

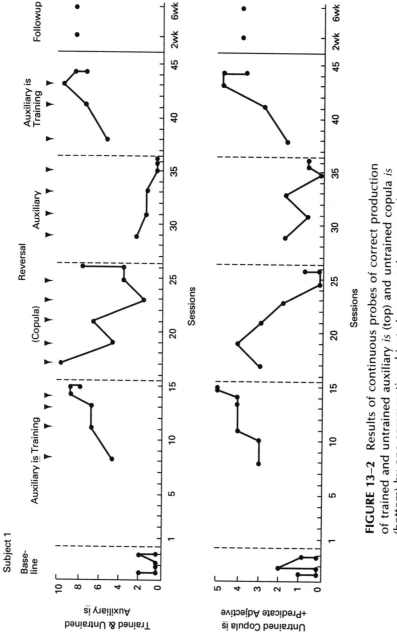

FIGURE 13–2 Results of continuous probes of correct production of trained and untrained auxiliary *is* (top) and untrained copula *is* (bottom) by one agrammatic subject. Arrows at the top mark sessions in which criterion was met for trained items. Improvement occurred for trained and untrained forms during the treatment phases. (Reprinted by permission from Kearns, K.P. & Salmon, S.J., An experimental analysis of auxiliary and copula verb generalization in aphasia. *Journal of Speech and Hearing Disorders*, 49, 1984, p. 158. American Speech-Language-Hearing Association, publisher.)

ment. In Thompson and McReynolds' (1986) study, procedures were alternated each day between morning and afternoon sessions. "To control for possible interaction effects of the two treatments, each treatment was applied to different interrogative constructions" (p. 197). The researchers found that direct-production was more effective for acquisition of trained *Wh*-question types, but the treatment did not generalize to progress with untrained interrogative types.

Response Elaboration Training. When operant training of a few specific items was not resulting in generalization, clinicians decided to modify the treatment, as opposed to declaring that aphasia treatment does not work. One change was called "loose training," which basically involves flexibility in stimuli used to elicit a particular response, flexibility in the response that is reinforced, and variability of reinforcement schedule (e.g., Thompson and Byrne, 1984). One version of loose training is Response Elaboration Training, or RET, developed by Kearns (1986c); "the clinician shapes and elaborates spontaneously produced client utterances rather than targeting preselected response" (Kearns, 1985, p. 196). RET was introduced with a patient who would refrain from initiating utterance, reducing participation in communicative interactions. The following goals are indicative of the goals for Kearns' subject:

Short-term: Increase number of utterances with at least five content words in response to pictures of actions in activities of daily living, from 10 percent to 60 percent.

Intermediate: Increase number of speaking turns initiated and mean length of utterance in conversation.

Kearns used modeling and forward chaining to elicit descriptions of pictures of simple actions. Modeling would take the form of expanding the patient's first attempt from one word to a short sentence, which the patient would repeat. *Wh*-questions would cue additions to an utterance. The patient practiced elaborated imitations. The key was to

avoid training a specific target response as in previous behavioral paradigms.

A simple multiple baseline design was used to evaluate this treatment. Treatment was initiated for one set of ten pictures and was delayed for another set of ten pictures. Probes for these sets without treatment were taken on alternate days when treatment was not scheduled (Figure 13–3). Treatment of the first set was discontinued so that it would not confound treatment of the second set. A treatment effect is observed in the upward trends of performance that begin with each treatment. The short-term goal was met between the fourth and twelfth session for the first set. The flat baselines indicate that repeated testing by itself had little effect, and it is not very likely that maturational or external events coincided with the two treatment periods. Some generalization occurred for a third set of pictures but did not occur for the second set before treatment was instituted. Whereas the patient had decreased in his verbal score on the PICA over the six months prior to this treatment (–0.35), his score improved across this period of treatment (+1.25).

HELPSS. The *Helm Elicited Language Program for Syntax Stimulation* is a program for enhancing the syntactic complexity of utterances (Helm-Estabrooks, 1981; Helm-Estabrooks, Fitzpatrick, and Barresi, 1981; Helm-Estabrooks and Ramsberger, 1986). A sequence for training syntactic forms is based on the story-completion research by Gleason and Goodglass (Chapter 5). In Level A, the target phrase is in the story so that a patient can repeat. In Level B, the patient is to complete the story with the target phrase. HELPSS has undergone some scrutiny, perhaps because it is a specific procedure that can be studied with multiple baseline experimental designs. The sequence of difficulty was not appropriate for all patients, indicating that levels should be arranged on an individual basis (Salvatore, Trunzo, Holtzapple, and Graham, 1983). In single-subject experiments, HELPSS caused little stimulus gener-

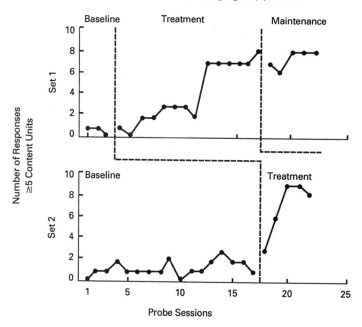

FIGURE 13–3 Continuous probes of responses containing at least five content units for the initially treated set of pictures and the second set for which treatment was delayed. Improvement with a set of pictures was contingent on treatment of that set. (Reprinted by permission from Kearns, K.P., Response elaboration training for patient initiated utterances. In R.H. Brookshire (Ed.), *Clinical aphasiology* (Vol. 15). Minneapolis: BRK, 1985, p. 199.)

alization (Doyle and Goldstein, 1985) and little response generalization (Salvatore, 1985). Doyle, Goldstein, and Bourgeois (1987) introduced a procedure modeled after HELPSS successively to baselines defined as imperative intransitives (e.g., *Stand up*), imperative transitives (e.g., *Read a book*), Wh-interrogatives (e.g., *What is your name?*), declarative transitives (e.g., *He fixes cars*), and declarative intransitives (e.g., *She dances*). As with the naming results in Figure 11–6, subjects did not progress with each baseline until treatment was applied.

Filling the SVO Frame. The verb is central to propositional structure (Chapter 3) but is more difficult to retrieve than nouns for many agrammatic patients (Chapter 5). One objective of treatment is to improve the production of verbs, which, theoretically, may pull arguments along with them. Loverso has used a "verbing strategy," or what later became known as the **cueing-verb-treatment,** as a means of improving sentence production (Loverso, Prescott, and Selinger, 1988; Loverso, Selinger, and Prescott, 1979). The procedure is used with nonfluent and fluent aphasias and is aimed at the feature of sen-

tence formulation that fills thematic slots in a complete subject-verb-object frame.

Short-term: Increase production of two-element utterances from 0 percent to 50 percent for describing pictured actions in activities of daily living.

Intermediate: Increase mean length of utterance from one thematic element to three thematic elements during conversation.

With the cueing-verb approach, we present a verb as a pivot-stimulus and then ask *who* and *what* questions to elicit agents and themes around the verb. The program has two levels. Level I is designed to elicit agent-action sentences. If a patient cannot produce SV sentences 60 percent of the time, then backup procedures include copying and repeating the sentence or choosing an agent from some choices. Level II is similar except that questions are asked to elicit an SVO sentence. A detailed example of the program was provided by Sanders (1986). The treatment can be presented with a computer, which established maintenance of levels without cues that had been achieved during treatment; generalization to other behavior was indicated in improvement on the PICA overall for eight of ten patients (Loverso, et al., 1989).

Externalization of Schemas. Luria's (1970b) intersystemic reorganization was applied to facilitate filling thematic and grammatical slots in sentences (also, Luria and Tsvetkova, 1968). The procedure was a more subtle approach to stimulation. To elicit a sentence for a simple action, sometimes all that was needed as a cue was three buttons or pieces of paper which seemed to represent a subject, verb, and object as a patient pointed to each cue. A sentence would be produced one element at a time while pointing to each cue. This was the basis for a more elaborate system of cueing tried briefly by Davis (1973). Once a sentence was elicited, the cues were faded gradually.

MIT. Melodic Intonation Therapy is a carefully crafted program developed by Sparks and Helm-Estabrooks, who had patients invoke a system not normally involved in speaking to facilitate speaking in severely nonfluent patients who were not improving by any other means (Helm-Estabrooks, Nicholas, and Morgan, 1989). The program has been described generously in books and journals (Sparks and Deck, 1986) and has been around for some time (Sparks, Helm, and Albert, 1974; Sparks and Holland, 1976). Patients should have good auditory comprehension before starting the program. We could say that MIT is an excellent example of intersystemic reorganization, and the suspicion is that the intact right hemisphere provides a kick for the speech center of the left hemisphere (Berlin, 1976). The essence of MIT is to have a patient "sing" an utterance being trained, especially because singing an utterance facilitates production for agrammatic patients with an element of verbal apraxia. Several steps lead a patient into singing language and then fade singing from the production. Patients have been reported to proceed through the program successfully (Albert, Sparks, and Helm, 1973). Performance by severely nonfluent patients can be spectacular. However, reports have been elusive for substantiating generalization beyond the last step of the program, which is to answer questions about content of the utterance being trained.

Gesturing for Reorganization

Treatment of apraxia of speech along with agrammatism is explained elsewhere (Tonkovich and Peach, 1989; Wertz, LaPointe, and Rosenbek, 1984). Apraxia may inhibit the mere initiation of utterance. When speech cannot be elicited in patients with good functional comprehension, alternative modes are considered. However, there may be one more thing we can try to elicit speech. Besides training gesture to augment verbalization (Tonkovich and Loverso, 1982), gesturing is introduced into speaking as a form of intersystemic reorganization or deblocking (Rosenbek, et al., 1989). Like MIT, gesturing may draw verbalization out of someone when other methods fail. In one study, a gesture was paired with naming in a comparison of Broca's, Wernicke's, and other types of aphasia (Hanlon, Brown, and Gerstman, 1990). Naming was better with gesture only for nonfluent subjects. Rosenbek and his colleagues (1989) stated that "our assumption is that verbal expression can be improved by the appropriate pairing of performances or with the systematic use of unique sensory inputs" (p. 218). Gestural reorganization involves pairing speaking and gesture, and Rosenbek uses Amer-Ind gestures and emblems that are readily transparent, such as cupping our hand behind our ear. The first step of training is for recognition of the gestures. The next step involves modeling a gesture and word for imitation. If a patient should spontaneously start talking while gesturing, it is likely that the patient can benefit from other treatments for language production. The goal is to maintain the verbal response after the gesture has faded.

WERNICKE'S APHASIA

Wernicke's aphasia presents some unique problems for the speech-language pathologist. Reduced awareness of deficit contributes to what Sparks (1978) called a poor therapeutic set in which a euphoric attitude creates "a rather flamboyant personality." The patient initially does not appear to comprehend the reason for being in the clinic. Studies of recovery indicate that our expectations for progress should be uncertain soon after onset, because some patients recover a great deal of language ability whereas others do not progress very much. We may have to gauge progress in early treatment as an indication of likely overall progress for an individual. Severity of auditory comprehension deficit is the main problem to be dealt with in the beginning.

Auditory Comprehension

Simple tasks are a vehicle for establishing a therapeutic set, the first goal of treatment. Patients do not understand simple task instructions. Severely impaired patients should be almost forced into a mode of cooperating with the clinician and responding to specific stimuli. The patient may be trained to point to a picture of an object in response to an environmental sound. The clinician may model the task and then indicate to the patient that it is his or her turn. When the patient gets the idea of listening and pointing, we begin to use words as stimuli with appropriate referents for response. Family names and photos may be used. Numbers may be readily recognized with response cards showing simple quantities. Response cards in numerical sequence is a cue, and the task entails responding to numbers spoken in sequence. Sequence is faded to increase difficulty. In general, we want to establish reliable responding to a verbal stimulus. Once reliable responding is established, we can work simple levels of word comprehension into the treatment.

Treatment becomes drill of auditory comprehension as we increase difficulty to push the system as far as it can go. However, the next problem, if not confronted already, is the patient's press for speech. Patients seem to prefer talking over listening, and we should

direct attention to listening. Whitney (cited in Holland, 1977) suggested a "stop strategy" for Wernicke's aphasia in contrast to a "go strategy" for Broca's aphasia. The idea was to keep the person with Wernicke's aphasia from talking during the comprehension training. A raised hand or alerting signal is often all that is needed to remind the patient to stop talking while listening to a stimulus. Improved comprehension leads to awareness of jargon, which leads to inhibition of speaking.

Meanwhile, we enhance contextual cues to compensate for limited language processing so that a patient can navigate in his or her environment as well as possible until language comprehension progresses sufficiently. Marshall (1986) recommended being sure that we have patients' attention when we talk to them, reduce our rate of speech, maximize redundancy of content in utterances, emphasize intonation, and exaggerate facial expression and gesture. This is good advice to significant others. Also, printed words are worth a try, because some patients may have a degree of modality-specific deficit in the auditory system. Reading is sometimes easier.

Jargon

Improving comprehension is the first step in dealing with the excesses of fluent jargon. When we think of the basic speech-language pathology guide of "imitation, then comprehension, then production," we are reminded that verbal expression can be modified when a patient can recognize difficulties. The improvement of self-monitoring has to be a goal when thinking about verbal expression, because people with frank Wernicke's aphasia are terrible repeaters. In a sense, we cannot enter treatment of language formulation through the front door. Comprehension training doubles as a means of setting up skills that can be used to gain control over expression. That is, a consistent yes-no response to questions and statements represents a functional responsiveness that has no chance to work in a flood of jargon. Also, we may have to wait until repetition begins to appear during the comprehension drill and then try to effect a transition to intentional repetition. Exactly how this happens and how often it happens does not appear to have been studied or, at least, reported in a systematic fashion. Whereas a great deal of research has been published for treating agrammatic verbal expression, most writing on Wernicke's aphasia is anecdotal and brief. Patients may eventually get to the point where we can use standard methods of modeling, chaining, and so on, but the crucial issue is the transition from uncontrolled jargon to volitional repetition of real words. When volitional repetition begins, we can build a program for eliciting language.

This orientation is similar to an approach Martin (1981) rejected and quite different from the approach he recommended. He wrote that "there are two ways to deal with jargon: first, to correct faulty speech itself—the thrust of most speech therapy; and second, to improve the clinician as a listener" (1981, p. 317). Martin recommended the second option, which, as a general rule, sounds like a good idea. He gave a few examples of how words and phrases in fluent aphasia can be communicative and recommended that we learn to interpret this language. Communication is disrupted by fruitless attempts to correct word-finding errors when context is sufficient to convey a message. However, the thrust of his argument was that people with Wernicke's aphasia speak their own exotic language, and we should put forth an effort to figure it out. The linguistic contexts for his examples were not provided, leaving it unclear as to whether neologistic or semantic jargon was being analyzed. Martin's recommendation still awaits evidence for the communicative value of fluent jargon. To most clinical investigators, jargon still makes little sense.

Davis (1983) suggested that research indicating that these patients have a primary deficit of semantic organization also indicates that we should be directing treatment to this diagnosis. Tasks would involve matching objects according to attributes and sorting them into categories. So far, there does not appear to have been an investigation of an effect of semantic treatment on progress in language comprehension and/or formulation in Wernicke's aphasia.

CONDUCTION APHASIA

One new development in the 1980s was the appearance of a few articles addressed to the treatment of conduction aphasia. The discovery that these patients may have sentence comprehension problems similar to those in Broca's aphasia indicates that comprehension training may be similar. In fact, embedded in a program to treat phonemic paraphasias, there were tasks for making syntactic judgments and arranging words into sentences (Cubelli, Foresti, and Consolini, 1988). The notion that conduction aphasia is a "two-headed disorder" was reflected in treatments with different orientations.

One pair of studies was devoted to treating repetition deficit (Sullivan, Fisher, and Marshall, 1986) with a consideration of the possibility of short-term memory deficit as the primary disorder (Peach, 1987). Thus, the main goal was to improve repetition. Reading aloud was the main activity used by Sullivan. Upon successful reading, the visual stimulus was removed so that the utterance could be repeated without this cue. Although basic research has led to reduced confidence in impaired "short-term memory" as the basis for repetition deficit (Chapter 5), Peach wanted to improve sentence repetition by treating memory span. The patient started with a task of pointing to pictures in a sequence spoken by the clinician. Then, the patient was asked to repeat words in the order spoken. Sentence repetition improved during the period of treatment. These researchers did not address relationships between improved repeating and functional communicative skills of any kind. Moreover, an element of repetition difficulty may be related to phonological impairment. The importance of empirically supported theory is that it points the clinician to a cognitive process as a goal (e.g., phonological encoding) rather than a task as a goal (e.g., memory span).

Another pair of studies was oriented to reducing phonemic paraphasias in verbal expression. Boyle (1989) employed a reading aloud procedure in which the patient was instructed to look at a word and think about how it sounds and then read the word again. Reading material increased in length. Cubelli and others (1988) reported a program for reducing phonemic paraphasias in three Italian patients. These clinicians made an explicit attempt to have clients confront phonemic-graphemic structure with a few metalinguistic tasks. The clients' decisions were based on this component of language rather than on other components. The first task was to choose a word to go with an object from three graphemically similar choices. This was assumed to focus attention on the sound system, as opposed to asking a patient to think about how a word sounds. A subsequent task was to give the patient a picture (e.g., table, or *tavolo*) and three cards showing each syllable of the word (e.g., TA, VO, LO), and the patient was asked to arrange the syllables in correct order. Then the patient read the word aloud. Another task was to show a picture (e.g., table) and show a letter (e.g., E). The patient had to decide if the letter belongs to the word for the picture, which requires generating a mental image of the lexical item. Although reduction in phonemic paraphasia would decrease the distraction of these errors in conversation, this study also did not address the communicative value of this treatment for the patients. Nevertheless, the study of treatment for conduction aphasia had to begin somewhere.

PRAGMATIC PROCEDURES

Perhaps the greatest challenge confronting aphasic people is the transfer of clinical gains to their daily life. A challenge for a clinician is the documentation of generalization in clinical practice and in research designed to determine if a treatment works. Thompson's (1989) review of reports of generalization indicates that we have tended to "train and hope," and this is also a concern regarding cognitive training for traumatically brain-injured patients (Webb, 1991).

Measuring Progress and Social Validation

Clinicians document a patient's progress toward short-term and long-term goals. As indicated in the previous two chapters, goals and measures usually pertain to behaviors that differ from the treatment itself. Treatment is a means to an end. A treatment may consist of imitation tasks, but the goal is to improve spontaneous verbalization. Documentation of progress toward the goal is a measure of spontaneous verbalization, not imitation. When progress occurs in a treatment but does not occur in other conditions, the difference between these conditions defines a portion of the clinical-functional gap.

Clinical aphasiologists employ three basic strategies for measurement: periodic standardized testing, frequent probing with brief tasks that are independent of treatment, and charting performance during treatment tasks. A **probe** is a measure of any behavior that is not exposed to the devices of treatment. As an independent task, a probe takes a few minutes to complete and is usually given at the end of a session, sometimes called a *post-session probe*. Post-session probes are given daily, on alternate days, or once per week. Reliability is maximized by using at least ten items. *Interspersed probes* are mingled within a treatment activity. Items without training devices are inserted among items with training devices (e.g., Kearns and Salmon, 1984). This is a common strategy that may not be recognized for its value as a probe; we wonder how a patient will do with a different or more complex stimulus or simply wonder how the client will do with an item when consistently applied cues are occasionally not presented. Another strategy is to assign a score to the first verbal response within a specified number of seconds prior to giving feedback or restimulation (e.g., Thompson and Kearns, 1981). The main limitation of an interspersed probe is that it usually is a measure of the treatment behavior and may not address a goal reported for recertification of treatment.

We want to document changes outside the climate of treatment activity. For the inpatient, the range for stimulus generalization is restricted to the boundaries of the hospital. For the outpatient, this range is much broader. Evidence of progress in real life is often anecdotal. Clinicians ask family members to report whether a behavior is occurring that had not been occurring for a long time. Holland (1982a) described a system for gathering data on patients in their natural environments, which is a logistic problem for the busy clinician. Thompson and Byrne (1984) used a probe called a *novel social dyad* to observe production of trained social conventions. The dyad was a five-minute conversation in a "comfortable, nontreatment room" with an unfamiliar person (e.g., an undergraduate student). The clinicians also administered the probe with two normal adults. These scores were a standard for interpreting peak levels of progress reached by aphasic patients. *Social validation* pertains to whether progress reaches "the demands of the social community of which the client is a part" (Kazdin, 1982, pp. 19–20). The wide range of scores exhibited by the normal controls in the study exposed a problem with interpretation of natural progress: "we really don't know what patients are supposed to do when they go out into the real world because we don't always know what non-brain-damaged people do" (Thompson and Byrne, 1984, p. 142).

Planning for Generalization

When a language process is working efficiently in a controlled drill, it still may not activate in a functional situation. Many patients may have to travel the distance between these conditions in small steps. These steps are created by making small adjustments in the contexts of treatment, leading to natural circumstances. Closing the clinical-functional gap is accomplished by bringing attributes of natural situations into the clinic and by moving the patient somewhat gradually into situations outside the clinic. This view is applied to rehabilitation for head injury as well: "For those who are making the transition to a home setting, guidelines establishing routines for spontaneous real-life situations should be developed and implemented prior to returning to independent living" (Starch and Falltrick, 1990, p. 28).

A **context analysis** is a part of evaluation. We obtain information about family, occupation, and hobbies. Contexts may be identified with respect to people and settings. In addition to home, settings include church, stores, theaters, and so on. People in these settings include a minister, clerks, and movie stars. Much of this background is *horizontal context*, which pertains to a patient's current experience. As we spend more time with a patient, we may learn more about his or her *vertical context*, which consists of past experience stored in long-term memory (i.e., an internal context). A head-injured patient may have gaps in these memories, and a severely aphasic patient cannot tell us much. Family members are a good source of information. We may guess some knowledge when we juxtapose stages of a patient's life with a timeline of events that occurred at these stages (Davis and Holland, 1981). An almanac may help us determine headline events occurring when the patient was in school, starting a family, and so on.

Because of a limited amount of time for treatment, some context targets have higher priority than others. One way of thinking about such priorities is to do a **needs-wants analysis**. *Needs* are life-sustaining, are related to functional independence, and tend to be universal among patients. For example, can the patient manage in a medical emergency? We try to direct treatment toward needs, regardless of severity of impairment. *Wants* tend to be unrelated to survival and can be quite individualized. A patient may want to be able to order in a restaurant again. Patients in the Child mode are more motivated in this direction than in meeting needs, causing the spouse to take on a Parenting role to make sure needs are taken care of. To make sure we consider the possibilities, Table 13–1 provides a list of contexts.

TABLE 13-1 Some examples of contextual components that contribute to the development of functional goals and activities. These examples are arguably arranged from *needs* on top to *wants* on the bottom.

Purpose	Setting	People
Survival	Hospital	Doctor, nurse
Shelter Central relationships	Home	Spouse, children, other residents
Essential transportation	Car, cab	Cab driver, traffic police
Spiritual nourishment	Church	Minister, friends
Essential shopping	Grocery Pharmacy	Clerks Pharmacist
Income Self-esteem	Plant, farm, office	Colleagues, boss, employees
Friendship	Another home, tavern	Bridge club, buddies
Exercise	Park, gym	Instructor, friends
Education	Television Newspapers School	Newscasters Columnists Teachers
Entertainment	Restaurants Stores Theaters Stadiums	Waitpeople Salespeople Movie stars Athletes
Travel	Airplane, airports, hotels	Attendants, strangers

For particular targets, we may want to do a **functional task analysis** of the language processes used in these targets. This is like the analysis of processes for a naming task, but now we are interested in processes needed for using the telephone or ordering from a menu. Basic language processes may be involved in most situations; but for special situations, we want to match requirements of the situation with a patient's capacities. A functional task analysis led to the *Cognitive Behavioral Driver's Inventory* for assessing cognitive skills that are essential to driving safely (Engum, Pendergrass, Cron, Lambert, and Hulse, 1988). Using a telephone requires number reading, name reading from a directory, auditory comprehension, and spoken formulation. What level of ability is required to call the fire department? The purpose for using the phone may be constrained by the level of ability in these areas. How much long-term memory is needed for particular purposes? How much concentration is needed? For ordering independently in a restaurant, one need only read and point to an item on the menu. Perhaps a patient should frequent restaurants that have menus with a lot of pictures of the food.

Programming for Generalization

After analyzing the evidence for generalization, Thompson (1989) decided that four features of treatment lead to transfer: (a) "a sufficient number of training responses," (b) responses trained in "a sufficient number of conditions," (c) activities that "incorporated aspects of the generalization environment," and (d) providing "strategies for mediating generalization" (p. 217). Presenting a sufficient number of different items in a task has been thought to be a basic determinant of generalization (Stokes and Baer, 1977). For now, we can only guess as to what is sufficient. In many of the single-subject experiments that did not show much generalization, the treatment had the behavioral orientation of drilling a small sample of the language with one task. Features (a) and (b) are attributes of cognitive-stimulation in which clinicians train a large number of different items and exercise a process with many different tasks. Cognitive-stimulation was studied mainly in the large group investigations. Yet, a repaired process (or acquired behavior) still may not transfer automatically.

Thompson's (c) and (d) are suggestive of programming that pushes transfer along. The following methods for closing the clinical-functional gap are organized according to manipulable contextual variables (Table 13–2). The order of presentation is suggestive of broad leaps in a gradual transition from traditional language exercises to real-life activities.

Some patients want to move slowly. Others are ready to dive into varied settings with different people. Reasons for being skittish about introducing some variables is that they may have always provoked anxiety for a patient and the patient is not yet prepared to deal with likely communicative failures. A mid-stage of treatment for people with CHI involves increasing "frustration tolerance" (Ylvisaker and Szekeres, 1986). Activities lead up to situations designed to include the possibility of failure.

Topic. We select words and pictures for drilling comprehension, naming, imitation, and description. Selecting content from a patient's daily life is inevitable, because published materials address objects and events in activities of daily living. We may question the adequacy of these materials merely on the grounds that many of the words we use in conversation are not picturable (Goodglass, et al., 1969). We use common words like *love, life, truth,* and *justice.* Do naming drills include these words? Topics, along with people, relate to **shared knowledge** between participants in an interaction. Some topics are well-known by most people. Other topics are well-known by a few people. Published clinical materials are designed to be well-known

TABLE 13–2 Variables for closing the clinical-functional gap, arranged in a hypothetical sequence beginning with traditional direct treatment and concluding with communication in natural situations. The example pertains to ordering at a restaurant.

Variable	Definition	Example
Topic	Content from the patient's real-life activities and interests	Pictures of things found in a restaurant for standard drill
Materials	Real-life objects or props	Menus for pointing or naming drill
Interaction	Turn-taking and other features of interaction	Conversational interaction about a restaurant (e.g., PACE)
Purpose	Real-life task or objective	Ordering in a restaurant
People	Other people	Role-playing other people; bringing other persons to clinic
Setting	Physical characteristics of a communicative situation	Model restaurant in clinic (e.g., Easy Street); Go to a restaurant

by most people, so a clinician is not usually in the awkward position of having little knowledge of what a patient is talking about. A clinician is in the position of imbalance in shared knowledge when having a conversation with a patient about some personal topics. One aphasic patient with severe apraxia of speech could write letters in the air. When his wife knew the topic was a planned vacation, he scribbled a few letters of a word and his wife recognized messages that the clinician could not fathom. Communicatively, his wife would have scored him 80 percent correct, and the clinician would have scored him 10 percent correct.

For many clinicians, selecting **personally relevant content** makes so much sense that it is naturally chosen for the first day of treatment. However, content chosen on the basis of personal relevance can conflict with content selected on the basis of psycholinguistic goals. There may be good reason to concentrate on printed words selected according to visual or sound similarity. Personally relevant content may stimulate language functions. Wallace and Canter (1985) compared personally relevant and nonpersonal content with 24 severely aphasic persons with varying syndromes. Personally relevant content was defined according to whether items pertained to self and the immediate environment. Content was compared for auditory comprehension for yes-no questions (e.g., "Is your birthday in December?" vs. "Is Christmas in December?"), reading comprehension for yes-no questions, repetition of nouns, and naming object-drawings (e.g., television vs. chicken). Performance was significantly better for personally relevant items in each task. Some personally relevant material is more "everyday" for some people than cooking utensils or plants. An artist may spend most of her time in the studio. What are the things in an artist's studio? What are they called? This patient would practice naming photographs of objects from her studio.

Materials. There is not much to say about materials beyond mentioning the practice of using real objects instead of pictures in the tasks of direct treatment. We know that aphasic patients are usually as successful with pictures as they are with real objects. Individualization of content may lead naturally to the use of photographs or props. Yet, it may be worthwhile to mention the use of certain props for certain situations. We may present a list of 15 names, three trials each, for a patient to look up in a phone book. With respect to the restaurant example, different menus can be used for the purpose of basic drill for auditory comprehension, reading aloud, and naming. We state an item, and the patient points to it on the menu. Menus are interesting, because they vary in difficulty and, thus, according to the abilities of a patient. Some menus have lots of pictures. Some menus are in another language. This is an opportunity to determine how well a patient's cognitive abilities interface with different menus. A patient may be inclined to go to only those restaurants with easy menus, or different strategies for ordering may be developed for different restaurants.

Interaction. Another step toward natural communicative conditions is to modify clinical interaction to conform to the structure of conversation with the topic areas mentioned previously. This involves some well-developed strategies known as conversational coaching (Holland, 1991) and PACE therapy (Davis and Wilcox, 1985), and these methods are explained later.

Purpose. This component pertains to interaction for a purpose, bringing **role-playing** into the treatment program. A patient is still interacting with the friendly clinician in the clinical setting. The themes employed in previous activities are retained. Transfer from the interaction phase should include the use of any available modality to get messages across. Role-playing provides an opportunity to induce the use of varied speech acts such as advising, warning, and arguing. A situation is created in which conflict is likely. The clinician and patient proceed to disagree over what to have for dinner or over how much to spend for a vacation. Schlanger and Schlanger (1970) divided "simulated life situations" into nonstress situations, such as planning a picnic, and stressful situations, such as going out to dinner. The stress situations could be pleasant (e.g., going out to dinner) or unpleasant (e.g., dealing with an emergency). In these activities, the client played a role that would normally be assumed in these circumstances. For various situations, the clinician and patient begin to anticipate communicative problems and work together to figure out how a functional goal can be achieved with the patient's communicative resources.

People. Communicative partners induce variation in the extent of shared knowledge about a topic and variation of stress in a communicative situation. A relatively minor shift from simple role-playing occurs when the clinician assumes the role of other persons in a communicative situation (e.g., a cab driver, a telephone operator, the minister, a waitperson in a restaurant). One characteristic of people in the community is their lack of knowledge of aphasia, which can be a dramatic and frustrating contrast to interacting with a clinician, even when role-playing such people. Again, the clinician can learn about the kinds of communicative failures that the patient is likely to have in such situations. Then, strategies for dealing with these failures can be developed.

Some of these strategies may be thought of as **context management.** People with very mild aphasia have difficulties dealing with natural communicative situations. A patient may have a little difficulty processing conversation at its normal rate, especially when discussing politics with friends as he or she used to do. The aphasic person starts to get lost and is too embarrassed to say so. However, instead of allowing others to restrict the aphasic person's ability to comprehend and respond, the patient can simply explain the problem and ask people to reduce their rate of speech or repeat every now and then. This mildly impaired patient may be going through a divorce and must deal with a future ex-spouse and a lawyer over the phone. In the clinic, we can play the roles of these persons so that the patient can practice asking the spouse or the lawyer to explain slowly, to repeat, or to be available if a question should come up after hanging up the phone. If the spouse and lawyer cannot agree to these conditions, then perhaps the conversation should be at another time. An opportunity to work on these strategies in the clinic with the clinician is a dress rehearsal that strengthens confidence and the likelihood that the patient will use these strategies outside the clinic.

Lyon (1989) spoke of the value of bringing other persons into the clinic so that the client can practice communicative interactions with someone else while still in the somewhat safe setting of the clinic. Our first thought would be to encourage the spouse or other family members to participate. On the one hand, the patient has practiced some situations with the clinician. On the other hand, the family member brings a genuine shared knowledge of certain topics. Although an outpatient spends most of his or her time with family members, the patient may not have produced a practiced phrase or activated a practiced process in the presence of the family member. Trying these acquired behaviors with the clinician present is a transitional opportunity in which the clinician can help out with some cues if needed. Lyon's approach was to have adult volunteers from the community spend some time with his aphasic clients as a "bridge" to facilitate generalization. His patients learned to deal with strangers. Moreover, a small segment of the community was educated about aphasia.

Settings. The setting of a treatment exercise is another component of the stimulus environment. Like people, settings influence language behavior in the extent to which they are familiar, comfortable, and demanding of the language processor. For example, driving a car involves reading simple signs quickly. After standing in line at the bank, we are expected to take care of business quickly. One step before entering these settings is to create the setting in the clinic. Hospitals have cafeterias and shops. The occupational therapy department is likely to have a model living environment. There is likely to be a driving simulator in the hospital. A few hospitals have a fairly expensive simulated little world called "Easy Street Environments" (Simmons, 1989). They are replicas of common settings in a community such as a bank, grocery, restaurant, store, and a city street with a bus and a car.

From role-playing in simulated settings, it is a relatively small step to enter the real situation. The previous steps may prove to have been vital in a number of unexpected ways, especially when we have not anticipated all of the contingencies. One example is a woman with severe Broca's aphasia who practiced pointing to items on a menu as a means of ordering for herself in a restaurant. In the clinic, she practiced with the menu for the restaurant she would be going to. However, she practiced mainly at the level of simple role-playing, in which she pretended to order while the clinician gave her feedback. When the patient got to the restaurant with a group of other patients and some clinicians and it was time to order, she was stymied by the realization that she could not use her strategy while the waitress was at the other end of the table. Before going to the restaurant, she could have worked on an additional gesture for motioning to the waitress to come to where she could see.

Conversation

Some clinicians have thought of conversation as an "unstructured" situation. The only unstructured situations, however, are those in which events occur at random. Conversation has a structure that differs from didactic treatment interactions. Recognizing this structure is a basis for managing natural interactions.

The Structure of Conversation. Most of us realize that conversation consists of two or more people alternating in producing a coherent series of utterances. Investigation of conversation tends to be an empirical endeavor in which natural interactions are recorded and patterns are uncovered (e.g.,

Stubbs, 1983). The basic unit for analysis is a **speaker-turn** in a "task" made up of alternating turns. In a transcription, two speakers may be labeled as *A* and *B* in a series of turns labeled as T-1, T-2, T-3, and so on (e.g., Levinson, 1983). Scientists are especially interested in the *local management system* for taking turns and the *overall organization* of any conversation, whether it be face-to-face or over the telephone. Speaker-turns rarely overlap (i.e., simultaneous talking), and gaps between speakers usually span less than a second. This precision stems from an inherent predictability of a speaker-turn, enabling a partner to anticipate when a switch will occur. Each turn provides a valuable "proof procedure" for the effectiveness of the previous turn. People with Wernicke's aphasia appear to be sensitive to turn-taking conventions, indicated by minimal overlap of turns and use of signs to indicate the partner's turn (Schienberg and Holland, 1980). Overall organization has been segmented into an opening section, topic slots, and a closing section.

Beyond the single turn, a larger unit for organizing conversation is the **adjacency pair,** which involves a speaker-turn (first part) followed by a predictable type of response from the other speaker (second part). A greeting is followed by a greeting; a question, by an answer. There is a rule for using adjacency pairs: "Having produced a first part of some pair, current speaker must stop speaking, and next speaker must produce at that point a second part to the same pair" (Levinson, 1983, p. 304). Usually there is a range of possible second parts, as a request may be followed by acceptance or refusal. Researchers have found a "preference organization" for second parts; that is, granting a request is preferred over rejection.

Other types of turn sequences may encompass three or four turns. One of these includes the **repair,** in which an utterance is modified because it was inadequate for conveying a message. Repair analysis is valuable for aphasiology, as repairs are frequent in conversation with an aphasic person. Lubinski, Duchan, and Weitzner-Lin (1980) referred to interaction with aphasic persons as hint-and-guess sequences, in which a patient's speaking turn is often a hint and the communicative partner makes a guess. As a typology for this behavior, a repair may be *self-initiated* (without prompting) or *other-initiated* (with prompting). It may be a *self-repair* by the speaker of the repairable utterance, or an *other-repair* by another participant. Normal adults prefer self-initiation and self-repairs. Other-repairs are rare; when they occur, they are usually modulated with prefaces such as "You mean . . . ?" or addendums such as ". . . , I think."

PACE. With adjustments to the object-naming task, interaction with a client can be modified to incorporate the structural and processing features of face-to-face conversation. One strategy for doing this is called **Promoting Aphasics' Communicative Effectiveness** (Davis and Wilcox, 1985). Procedures follow four principles representing special features of conversation (Table 13–3). Any one principle may be applied in adjusting traditional tasks, but the four principles together make the interaction like conversation. PACE still is an artificial interaction that falls short of real conversation in a progression from clinical to functional activities.

A few characteristics of PACE should be elaborated. The new information condition establishes referential communication so that a message sender need only convey what is necessary to get the idea across. PACE can be varied with respect to message-stimuli, which can be objects or simple events. Turn-taking should take us out of a directive role and place us on equal footing with the client. Our turns as sender are opportunities for **modeling** communicative behaviors that a patient is capable of using but may not be choosing. Initial tasks may train a communicative modality such as gesture or drawing, but in PACE we do not tell a client to perform in a particular way. Modeling should be an influence by showing that gesture is a reasonable "prosthetic" that gets the idea across. An adult's choices may be more likely to be maintained than a clinician's directive. Also, we should no longer be able to provide

TABLE 13–3 The four principles and essential procedures of Promoting Aphasics' Communicative Effectiveness (Davis and Wilcox, 1985).

PACE
1. **The clinician and patient exchange new information.** Instead of having a picture of an object or event (called the message) in simultaneous view of the clinician and patient, a stack of message-stimuli is placed face down to keep messages from the view of a message receiver. A client selects a card and attempts to convey the message on the card. The *Brussels modification* is to place a screen about eight inches or 20 centimeters high between the patient and clinician, and the message receiver chooses the message from options (Clerebaut, Coyette, Feyereisen, and Seron, 1984).
2. **The clinician and patient participate equally as senders and receivers of messages.** This principle puts the turn-taking feature of conversation into the interaction. The clinician and client simply alternate in drawing a card and sending messages.
3. **The patient has a free choice as to the communicative modes used to convey a message.** Contrary to training one modality such as gesture or drawing, the patient is left to choose the mode that is used for any message. We do not tell a client to perform in a particular way.
4. **The clinician's feedback as a receiver is based on the patient's success in conveying the message.** The new information condition should make this inevitable for both participants. Our feedback should let the client know if he or she got the idea across. If we already know the message, we should respond as if we did not know.

cues to a linguistic formulation as feedback, because we should not already know what the patient is trying to say. We are concerned about the message rather than linguistic virtuosity. This procedure permits the patient to practice a few skills that are unique to conversation. One is responsiveness to a receiver's attempts to interpret what the patient is trying to convey. We ask questions that a patient should comprehend. Another skill, as sender, is responsiveness to communicative failure and the use of repair or revision in trying to get the message across.

Studies indicate that there is a great deal of curiosity about this procedure in Europe. In one study, a "traditional PACE" was compared to a modified version. The two procedures were alternated for periods of five days for four aphasic subjects (Springer, et al., 1991). Three subjects were diagnosed as having "lexical-semantic" deficits. The description of PACE was incomplete, but the unstated features were reported for the other method, which included the Brussels modification (Table 13–3). Objects were used as messages in traditional PACE; the other method had the patient sort objects into semantic categories and give information about classes to the clinician. The clinician gave "corrective feedback." Measures of communicative and lexical adequacy in PACE bordered each treatment period. Results showed more progress with modified PACE by the three patients with semantic deficits on both measures and no lexical progress for the other patient. The researchers concluded that traditional PACE is not helpful for patients with certain specific linguistic impairments. Despite the lack of control for sequence effects across treatment phases, the study can be considered to be encouraging for PACE because messages had been intended to be flexible with respect to a patient's level of language ability. This research provides an ingenious suggestion for further modification.

Other investigations dealt with the responsiveness of patients to the clinician's modeling when taking a turn as message sender. Whereas modeling was mainly intended to help a patient feel comfortable about choosing modes like gesture and drawing, Glindemann and others (1991) examined the influence of modeling with respect to producing names or descriptions with objects as message-stimuli. Would the patients adapt to a clinician's modeling of these forms of verbalization? Glindemann found that the patients with mild aphasia were more likely than others to switch between names and descriptions as a function of what the clinician does as sender. Greitemann and Wolf (1991) studied this issue with respect to the use of verbal and gestural modalities. We might have a short-term goal of shifting mo-

dality use from 100 percent speech per turn to 50 percent combined use of speech and gesture. The investigators were concerned that severely aphasic patients tend to choose their most impaired modality when sending messages in PACE. The modeling function is supposed to steer a patient toward more intact modalities. Data indicated that modeling has an influence across modalities and that the use of speech does not necessarily disappear as use of gesture increases. The main goal is to maximize combined or alternating use of all available modalities by providing an accepting atmosphere in which others are doing the same thing.

PACE, as well as other pragmatic procedures, can be considered to have multiple objectives and should be evaluated accordingly. For some patients, removing pressure to perform linguistically may enhance verbal behavior, and the use of other modes may act as intersystemic reorganizers of verbalization in the manner examined by Rosenbek and his colleagues (1989). For others, the procedure's main contribution may be to facilitate transfer of trained skills to a different and more natural communicative condition. Practice in unique conversational skills may improve these skills for natural conversation. In another study, eight patients were given PACE with the Brussels modification. Referential communicative abilities improved but not language skills measured by standard language tests (Carlomagno, Losanno, Emanuelli, and Casadio, 1991). While it is not clear that we can attribute these changes to PACE per se, the investigators' conclusions point to a particular objective of the procedure. Like all of our methods, this one should receive further scrutiny.

Conversational Coaching. Holland (1991) has another approach to the training of conversational skills. Conversational coaching is relatively direct by providing a script for the clinician and patient to follow. The patient should be able to read aloud simple sentences, but a script may also be created with a few words and pictures. A script is a short list of short sentences about a topic that may be known to a listener/clinician or not known to a listener/clinician. The patient reads the script one sentence at a time, and the clinician's job is to evaluate communicative effectiveness and suggest ways of conveying the information differently. The patient then may practice with another listener, and the clinician's job is to coach the listener (e.g., "If you don't understand, it's probably better to ask him to say it another way").

Pragmatic Groups

Group treatment was introduced in the previous chapter as having several purposes that lead to different formats (Kearns, 1986b). As a mechanism for restoring linguistic and other cognitive functions, activities are similar to those employed in individual treatment. In a group, patients take turns responding to common stimuli or problems presented by a clinician. Speech-language pathologists and other specialists may conduct a **memory group** for patients with varied etiologies (Wilson and Moffat, 1984). Activities are created around themes that are functional and interesting. Patients take turns making lists of what they did earlier in the day (i.e., recent episodic memory) or what they did years before (i.e., remote episodic memory). They cooperate in making shopping lists or lists of things to do for various common routines such as doing the laundry or getting ready for bed (i.e., semantic memory). Visuospatial activities include hiding a belonging in the room and recalling its location later, or copying a movement by a patient or clinician. Patients enjoy helping each other, but they are also motivated by competition. A group is divided into teams. Team members cooperate in competing against the other teams. The whole group can develop a list of holidays, foods, cities, presidents, or movie stars. A team earns points by recalling items from the list generated earlier rather than from world knowledge. There is an electric empathic mutual support that cannot be drawn from a clinician.

Davis and Wilcox (1985) applied PACE to managing groups for the purpose of generalizing skills repaired or acquired in individual treatment. Tasks incorporate turn-taking and referential communication. We may expect that a clinician's controlling role is minimized. There are six guidelines:

1. Patients should interact with each other. To reinforce independent communicating by each patient, the clinician is not an essential participant. The clinician can be useful by helping a patient when necessary or recording generalization data.
2. The activity is designed so that communication is necessary, as opposed to having the patients do something and talk about it.
3. Materials are arranged so that patients are conveying new information to each other.
4. To avoid one patient dominating in an open-ended situation, patients take turns sending messages so that opportunities are distributed equally.
5. The activity is designed so that any communicative mode can be used for exchanging messages.
6. The activity is simple and often familiar, so that the session is not delayed by giving instructions or dominated by the nature of the task.

Card games are ideal because communication is part of the game, patients take turns, a patient's hand is held from the view of the others, nonverbal modes can easily supplement verbalization, and many games are familiar or easy to teach. For players with hemiplegia, cards are placed on a rack. One game is "two-of-a-kind" ("go fish," for kids). For functional content, the cards consist of pairs of objects or actions. Each player is dealt a hand of five cards, and the remaining cards are placed face down in the middle of the table. Patients take turns attempting to obtain matches for cards in their hands. On a turn, a player requests a card from another player. If the other player does not have the card, the initiator must draw a card from the stack. Each time a pair is obtained, the pair is removed from the hand. The goal is to obtain enough matches to be the first player without cards left in the hand.

DISCOURSE/TEXT

Discourse is a high level of language behavior in which within-sentence aphasic difficulties can be observed. Treatment may be done at this level for anomic and/or mild aphasias. Also, some cognitive impairments are observed only at this level. Problems with discourse are considered to be secondary to disorders of attention, perception, and organizational abilities. Coordinated treatments are directed mainly to restoring these cognitive functions, and the speech-language pathologist may concentrate on the manifestation of these functions and their component processes in discourse.

Anomic/Mild Aphasia

Anomic aphasia is a primary impairment of lexical access. It is often the most salient disorder when aphasia can be diagnosed in patients with head injury. Linebaugh (1983) called his strategy **Lexical Focus,** in which he used hierarchies of cueing for a convergent object-naming task (Chapter 12) and the divergent categorical word-fluency task for the mildest anomic aphasias. A hierarchy of difficulty for categories was based on "width" of exemplars in a category, from a wide *sports* to a narrow *water sports.* Head-injured patients practice organized searches through lexical memory (Ylvisaker and Holland, 1985). A client engages in controlled retrieval of subcategories of words in a personally relevant category such as *people* (e.g., family, friends, and co-workers). Encouraging adaptation with intact language systems is realized by reinforcing circumlocution. Occasionally this leads to finding the desired word. In discourse, lexical processes are stimulated in an environment of retained linguistic and other cognitive processes. As a functional level of language use, discourse provides an opportunity to determine if improvements in naming and word-fluency drills has generalized.

One challenge for people with anomic aphasia is **referential communication tasks,** in which a patient's messages are kept from view of the clinician as listener (Chapter 10).

In PACE, message-stimuli may be objects, abstract words, or proper names, and the task is to convey enough information that a listener can guess a stimulus. Guessing the stimulus precisely is a little more demanding than expectations for more impaired patients. Turn-taking and modeling may not be necessary, and precision in conveying information can be practiced with a barrier between patient and clinician. Messages can be simple events or spatial relations, and language must be accurate enough that the clinician can make an accurate choice from among similar pictures (Busch, et al., 1988). Following the pragmatic principle of varying participants in a communicative exchange, narratives can be told to people assumed to know or not know the story, although it has been shown that this variable makes little difference for certain linguistic features (Brenneise-Sarshad, et al., 1991).

Some fluent patients progress in a few months to such a high level of linguistic facility that it can be difficult to tell that they have aphasia. They sometimes have to tell us when they are having difficulty finding a word. Verbal expression is a bit hesitant at times. Writing is most revealing, as it may take ten minutes to write two sentences. Patients who thrive on demanding linguistic situations want to get better. Some aphasic people are writers or want to return to work that involves verbal sparring and writing reports. They buy word game books to exercise their language abilities. One patient, KT, had completed gathering data for a dissertation when she suffered a stroke. After a few months of concentrating on recovering from aphasia, she started thinking about finishing her project. Earning her doctorate in mid-life was important to her. However, she had not thought much about her topic since the stroke. Typing a simple paragraph took hours, and she did not have enough confidence in her speaking ability to defend her dissertation.

First, it was determined that KT's doctoral adviser would be supportive of an effort to complete the project. Content for treatment was drawn from the dissertation proposal, and the clinician prepared by determining the tasks ahead. Tasks included interpreting the data, discussing interpretations with the adviser, and putting thoughts into words with a word processor. Treatment eventually would include role-playing meetings with the adviser and the defense itself. Sessions began by having KT explain basic concepts underlying her research, and she practiced retrieving names of authors in the literature associated with these concepts. She discovered that she could do this fairly well, and these successes reduced her fear of trying. The main frustration was her tedious rate of writing. Homework included writing explanations of concepts and recording how long it took. Complexity was increased by having her compose comparisons between concepts. In effect, treatment did not move into writing the dissertation right away, and KT agreed with this pace. Meanwhile, she wanted to meet others with aphasia, and she was introduced to a community support group of aphasic people and their families. Having been active in the politics of her community, she decided that now she wanted to become involved in encouraging others with aphasia who, in turn, inspired her. She is still working toward earning her doctoral degree.

Agrammatic aphasia also occurs in a mild form with good comprehension and occasional omissions or mistakes with grammatical morphemes. Patients reach a ceiling of improvement. We need not follow a "building-block" organization of treatment by waiting for production of complete sentences before eliciting discourse. Attributes of schemas are embedded in semantic memory and are somewhat independent of linguistic details. A patient who produces fragmented sentences can produce functional components and organizational features of routines and narratives. A patient can begin treatment by repeating short stories of three or four sentences. The expected response is a paraphrase with story elements (i.e., beginning, middle, end). Single picture description established earlier can be expanded with pictures in a procedural sequence (e.g., everyday routines) or narrative sequence (e.g., car-

toons). As a vertical context, intact episodic memory is a wealth of input to the storytelling mechanism. Patients tell good stories accompanied by thematic props such as pictures.

Other Cognitive Dysfunctions

In treating discourse dysfunctions, we maximize cues for success and gradually increase difficulty. We want to repair a process and encourage compensatory adaptation with intact processes. One attribute of RHD and mild CHI is that language systems are not damaged directly. Treatment can include fearless instruction and discussion. On the other hand, this attribute is one reason why physicians have tended not to refer these patients to speech-language pathologists who have historically treated "aphasia." It is also why many patients do not seek treatment. With mild CHI, deficits are difficult to detect with standard tests. Individuals may seek help only when they return to work and, like Phineas Gage in Chapter 1, cannot handle the job as before. Some of the problems at home may be related to personality changes and the devastation of unanticipated failure. Psychological counseling is an essential component of rehabilitation (Rollin, 1987). Other challenges for vocational rehabilitation may be related to subtle cognitive deficiencies. Our knowledge of primary deficits (Chapters 6, 7) and paradigms used to study discourse processing (Chapter 8) are clues for constructing a hypothetical treatment paradigm.

Comprehension. Ylvisaker and Szekeres (1986) recommended some discourse-level tasks for working on cognitive deficits with CHI. Some tasks are appropriate for a middle phase of recovery at RLA Levels IV to VI (Table 6–1). For problems with selective attention, they recommended "listening to high interest stories or newspaper articles for specific information, listening to reports of events and then relaying that information to another person, and taking telephone messages" (p. 481). Other suggestions were for a late phase of recovery at RLA Levels VII to

VIII. A patient may practice identifying the structure of scripts or stories and imposing organization on information (also, Ylvisaker and Holland, 1985).

It is not clear that treatment should begin with sentence pairs before moving to longer discourse. Detecting cohesion between sentences entails a backward scanning through information in the buffer, and difficulty with this operation may be based on macrostructural operations, to be discussed shortly. Research provides paradigms for treating pronoun antecedent assignment if it is a problem. One task is to choose between two referents for a pronoun when gender (or another cue) determines the antecedent, as in sentences 4 and 5a in Chapter 8 (p. 178). The task is more difficult with gender ambiguity and assignment based on understanding plausible events in a sentence or in sentence pairs (e.g., 5b, 6a, 6b, p. 178). Thus, access to knowledge of the world is essential in detecting cohesion in discourse. When ability to retain information in the buffer is a concern, a treatment may include increasing the verbal distance between antecedents and pronouns (e.g., Ehrlich and Rayner, 1983). These tasks focus on processes applied to text-level buffering in the comprehension of a full discourse or text.

Impaired selective attention may interfere with comprehending a story. Ignored information is not available in the buffer for antecedent assignment and for broader thematic coherence so that a sequence of propositions makes sense. New information may not be distinguished from given information. Guiding attention may be related to the notion of foregrounding information to be held in the buffer. A patient may practice identifying the most salient or important information in a story while considering the theme. Treatment may start with text and present spoken stories later. Identification of salient parts is related to the ability to use common knowledge of narrative structure. Cues to salient information include questions about the setting, introduction of main characters, initiating event, and so on. A patient should underline these parts of a narrative. Similar questions can be asked of newspaper articles, including immediate recall of the classic information of a news story (e.g., who, what, when, where, and so on).

The likelihood of working with someone with RHD is contingent on whether the individual is motivated based on recognition of a deficit, especially one with a clear impact on everyday life. A peripheral deficit affecting reading is **neglect dyslexia**, which includes ignoring the left side of a page. Basic research has shown that shifts of attention to the left side can be cued. A patient can be trained to "talk to himself" as a reminder to look left (Stanton, Yorkston, Kenyon, and Beukelman, 1981). An internal verbal cueing strategy can be used for navigating a hospital. This is indicative of a "double dissociation" for adaptation. Aphasic people use nonverbal capacities, and people with RHD use their spared language system to compensate for deficits in other systems.

RHD may entail **impaired inferencing,** observed in interpretation of metaphors and proverbs. Patients are not literal for all metaphors and may do better with idioms. The item-comparison strategy can be used to identify a starting point. With items that are understood, we may present contextual cues in discussing differences between literal and nonliteral speaker-meanings. Then difficult items are worked into the discussion. Generating elaborative inferences for sentences like 1 in Chapter 8 (p. 172) pertains to one component in comprehending bridging inferences across sentences (e.g., 8b, p. 179). Brownell (1988) thought that difficulties with jokes and other brief tales are due to impaired "backwards inferences." The other component is to work on finding antecedents through backward scanning through the buffer.

Production. To improve access to episodic memory at RLA Levels IV to VI, Ylvisaker and Szekeres (1986) suggested that patients work on "describing main events in life, significant people and places" and "describing simple sequential tasks (e.g., shaving) or scripts for more complex events (e.g., going to a restaurant)" (p. 481). This idea is based on considering the input to the discourse production mechanism (Figure 8–1). Discourse is observed in a variety of clinical tasks involving different kinds of input, and sometimes our impression of someone's storytelling ability is based on one or two types of tasks. Ylvisaker was concerned about episodic memory as input. With other tasks, pictures are analogous environmental conditions in which a discourse is produced. We may be concerned about an RHD's **impaired complex perception** of objects not in a conventional position. There may be a problem with inferring implications of a scene. Suspicion of an input-specific contribution to unusual storytelling should be tested by comparing storytelling in different conditions, including retelling and reminiscing. One hypothesis is that restored perception improves narration tied to a situation and appropriateness of other behavior with respect to a situation.

Disorganized discourse has been related to **impaired executive control.** Ylvisaker and Holland (1985) identified executive control with a charioteer governing the forces of powerful steeds. "In head injury rehabilitation, we have long recognized the need for patients to employ consciously [a] self-governing or charioteer function to facilitate their recovery" (p. 243). This ability was made evident to patients with a sports analogy of *self-coaching.* Components of treatment included self-awareness, goal setting, and planning, which are similar to Duncan's theory of the executive (Chapter 6). Self-awareness may begin with awareness of the structure of routines and stories produced by others. Procedures include those for improving foregrounding. Stories are presented with implausible or illogical sequences to be recognized (e.g., "the waiter brought the food, and then he took the order"). Logic of event sequences can be discussed with respect to the necessity criterion used in studies of the causal relatedness of stories: would event B have occurred, if event A had not occurred

(Trabasso and Sperry, 1985). We can remove an event and then see if the rest of the story makes sense. Organization is also approached through sequencing pictures for routines and stories, telling stories with the pictures present, recalling the stories with the pictures removed, and facilitating recall by using a picture as a cue (e.g., Yorkston, Stanton, and Beukelman, 1981). Increased awareness of organization is put to use through self-coaching for improving self-monitoring.

AN ESSAY ON COGNITIVE REHABILITATION

Addressing closed head injury is suggestive of cognitive rehabilitation as it has evolved in clinical neuropsychology. One theoretical framework that is prominent in this discipline is Luria's (1966) brilliant insights from the clinical examination of patients. However, this theory is missing from the experimental psychology of normal cognition. "Cognitive rehabilitation" (or cognitive retraining) is associated with attention, perception, memory, and nonverbal systems. It is also associated with particular clinical populations (e.g., CHI). This sense is reflected in the content of the companion journals *Brain and Language* and *Brain and Cognition.* At least one community college offers an associate degree in cognitive retraining without a course title or text addressing aphasia explicitly (Frangicetto, 1989). Yet, graduates of this program may end up working with aphasic patients. This is why talk of a cognitive basis for aphasia is either peculiar or threatening to some clinical aphasiologists.

The absence of a coherent theoretical foundation across disciplines has contributed to some awkward working relationships among rehabilitation specialists. An occupational therapist (OT) may be conducting naming practice for a patient with CHI, calling it cognitive rehabilitation. A speech-language pathologist may be disturbed because it seems that different clinicians are working on the same thing with a patient. Questions are raised at staff meetings. Is the OT doing "aphasia therapy" but disguising it as cognitive retraining? Is the speech-language pathologist not recognizing a treatment of visual agnosia? There may be no conflict when the clinicians are recognizing the difference between cognitive processes and the tasks used to assess and treat them. Assuming that object-naming involves several processes (Chapters 4, 7), a speech-language pathologist would target word-retrieval with a naming task and other tasks involving this process. Someone else would target visual recognition with a naming task and other tasks for recognition.

Treating someone with CHI does not mean that speech-language pathologists must treat visuospatial attention. Treatment of a generalized cognitive function such as executive planning should address all manifestations of the disorder. In principle, services may be coordinated according to primary cognitive impairments and may be distributed among rehabilitation specialists according to the behavioral manifestation of these impairments. Coordinating goals may include improving executive control or mental imagery. One specialist may work on sequencing steps in carrying out a complex activity and topographical orientation, while another specialist works on telling a coherent story. Smith (1983) explained that speech-language pathology has a dual responsibility for "an aphasic patient, regardless of the etiology" and for language as "secondary manifestations of cognitive disorganization." A deviation in this role occurs where speech-language pathologists are the only individuals inclined or trained to conduct any form of cognitive retraining. The manipulative use of "cognition" to define professional boundaries should be replaced by identifying disorders and objectives according to cognitive systems and subprocesses, including those involved in language comprehension and formulation. Speech-language pathologists are the most knowledgeable and best trained professionals in dealing with the cognitive bases of language behavior. We have just not generally labeled our domain in this way.

SUMMARY AND CONCLUSIONS

Treatment of aphasia is based on the general understanding that aphasias are disruptions of processing rather than losses of knowledge. Stimulation of processes is organized according to principles of behavioral programming. Operant procedures, while amenable to experimental study, have a poor record of generalizing beyond stimuli and tasks in the treatment. These procedures are becoming more like stimulation, with loose training that seems more aligned with assumptions about the nature of aphasia. The field of programming lends a discipline to planning pragmatic procedures designed to promote transfer of partially restored processes to functional communicative tasks.

Applied psycholinguistics and related cognitive sciences are devoted to sharpening the specificity of diagnosis so that treatments may be aligned with particular deficits of language processing. Conclusions are conflicting, but implications for clinical realities should be clear, and the research should be encouraged by clinicians. More accurate identification of impairment should lead to more efficient treatment. When a diagnosis is fuzzy (e.g., disorder of syntax, disorder of discourse), a treatment may take aim at all aspects of the diagnosis. Syntactic processing has multiple components and is only partially impaired in people with Broca's aphasia. Efficiency may also be reduced by skirting the edges of a primary disorder when focusing on one behavioral manifestation. There are hundreds of questions in these notions that should motivate applied research for quite a while. The patient is probably the best guide, however. Aphasic people have an uncanny knack of sensing the treatments that are likely to be helpful and the ones that do not fit. After all, it is their processors that we are tinkering with.

Just as strange things happen in an inadequately funded and staffed legal system, strange things happen in an inadequately funded and staffed health care system. This text has alluded to some of these things, such as speech-language pathologists working outside their traditional domain in a desire to do the best for their patients. This text has also been a tale of clinical professionals continually trying to improve their craft. This text has spoken of aphasic people and their families and the progress that they make. This is a tale of intrepid souls and heroic deeds.

BIBLIOGRAPHY

ABBOTT, V., BLACK, J.B., & SMITH, E.E. (1985). The representation of scripts in memory. *Journal of Memory and Language, 24,* 179–199.

ABEYSINGHE, S.C., BAYLES, K.A., & TROSSET, M.W. (1990). Semantic memory deterioration in Alzheimer's subjects: Evidence from word association, definition, and associate ranking tasks. *Journal of Speech and Hearing Research, 33,* 574–582.

ADAMOVICH, B.L., & HENDERSON, J.A. (1984). Can we learn more from word fluency measures with aphasic, right brain injured, and closed head trauma patients? In R.H. Brookshire (Ed.), *Clinical aphasiology conference proceedings* (pp. 124–131). Minneapolis: BRK.

ADAMS, M.L., REICH, A.R., & FLOWERS, C.R. (1989). Verbal-fluency characteristics of normal and aphasic speakers. *Journal of Speech and Hearing Research, 32,* 871–879.

AITCHISON, J. (1987). *Words in the mind: An introduction to the mental lexicon.* Oxford, England: Basil Blackwell.

AKMAJIAN, A., DEMERS, R.A., & HARNISH, R.M. (1984). *Linguistics: An introduction to language and communication* (Second Edition). Cambridge, MA: MIT Press.

ALAJOUANINE, T. (1948). Aphasia and artistic realization. *Brain, 71,* 229–241.

ALAJOUANINE, T. (1956). Verbal realization in aphasia. *Brain, 79,* 1–28.

ALAJOUANINE, T., & LHERMITTE, F. (1964). Non verbal communication in aphasia. In A. DeReuck & M. O'Connor (Eds.), *Disorders of language* (pp. 168–177). London: Churchill.

ALBERT, M.L. (1976). Short-term memory and aphasia. *Brain and Language, 3,* 28–33.

ALBERT, M.L., & BEAR, D. (1974). Time to understand. A case study of word deafness with reference to the role of time in auditory comprehension. *Brain, 97,* 373–384.

ALBERT, M.L., BUTTERS, N., & LEVIN, J. (1979). Temporal gradients in the retrograde amnesia of patients with alcoholic Korsakoff's disease. *Archives of Neurology, 36,* 211–216.

ALBERT, M.L., & MILBERG, W. (1989). Semantic processing in patients with Alzheimer's disease. *Brain and Language, 37,* 163–171.

ALBERT, M.L., & OBLER, L.K. (1978). *The bilingual brain.* New York: Academic Press.

ALBERT, M.L., SPARKS, R., & HELM, N.A. (1973). Melodic intonation therapy. *Archives of Neurology, 29*, 130–131.

ALEXANDER, M.P., NAESER, M.A., & PALUMBO, C.L. (1987). Correlations of subcortical CT lesion sites and aphasia profiles. *Brain, 110*, 961–991.

ALEXANDER, M.P., FISCHETTE, M.R., & FISCHER, R.S. (1989). Crossed aphasias can be mirror image or anomalous: Case reports, review and hypothesis. *Brain, 112*, 953–973.

ALTMAN, G.T.M. (1989). Parsing and interpretation: An introduction. *Language and Cognitive Processes, 4*, SI 1–20.

ANDERSON, D.W., & McLAUREN, R.L. (EDS.) (1980). Report on the national head and spinal cord injury survey conducted by NINCDS. *Journal of Neurosurgery*, Supplement, 1–43.

ANDERSON, J.R. (1983). *The architecture of cognition.* Cambridge, MA: Harvard University Press.

ANDREWS, S. (1986). Morphological influences on lexical access: Lexical or nonlexical effects? *Journal of Memory and Language, 25*, 726–740.

ANSELL, B.J., & FLOWERS, C.R. (1982a). Aphasic adults' understanding of complex adverbial sentences. *Brain and Language, 15*, 82–91.

ANSELL, B.J., & FLOWERS, C.R. (1982b). Aphasic adults' use of heuristic and structural linguistic cues for sentence analysis. *Brain and Language, 16*, 61–72.

APPELL, J., KERTESZ, A., & FISMAN, M. (1982). A study of language functioning in Alzheimer patients. *Brain and Language, 17*, 73–91.

ARMUS, S.R., BROOKSHIRE, R.H., & NICHOLAS, L.E. (1989). Aphasic and non-brain-damaged adults' knowledge of scripts for common situations. *Brain and Language, 36*, 518–528.

ARVEDSON, J.C., McNEIL, M.R., & WEST, T.L. (1985). Prediction of Revised Token Test overall, subtest, and linguistic unit scores by two shortened versions. In R.H. Brookshire (Ed.), *Clinical aphasiology* (Vol. 15) (pp. 57–63). Minneapolis: BRK.

ASHCRAFT, M.H. (1989). *Human memory and cognition.* Gleview, IL: Scott, Foresman.

ATEN, J.L. (1986). Functional communication treatment. In R. Chapey (Ed.), *Language intervention strategies in adult aphasia* (Second Edition) (pp. 266–276). Baltimore: Williams & Wilkins.

ATEN, J.L., & LYON, J.G. (1978). Measures of PICA subtest variance: A preliminary assessment of their value as predictors of language recovery in aphasic patients. In R.H. Brookshire (Ed.), *Clinical aphasiology conference proceedings* (pp. 106–116). Minneapolis: BRK.

ATKINSON, R.C., & SHIFFRIN, R.M. (1971). The control of short-term memory. *Scientific American, 225*, 82–90.

AU, R., ALBERT, M.L., & OBLER, L.K. (1988). The relation of aphasia to dementia. *Aphasiology, 2*, 161–174.

BACHMAN, D.L., & ALBERT, M.L. (1990). The pharmacotherapy of aphasia: Historical perspective and directions for future research. *Aphasiology, 4*, 407–413.

BADDELEY, A.D. (1986). *Working memory.* London: Oxford University Press.

BADECKER, W., & CARAMAZZA, A. (1985). On considerations of method and theory governing the use of clinical categories in neurolinguistics and cognitive neuropsychology: The case against agrammatism, *Cognition, 20*, 97–125.

BADECKER, W., & CARAMAZZA, A. (1991). Morphological composition in the lexical output system. *Cognitive Neuropsychology, 8*, 335–368.

BAHRICK, H.P., BAHRICK, P.C., & WITTLINGER, R.P. (1975). Fifty years of memories for names and faces: A cross-sectional approach. *Journal of Experimental Psychology: General, 104*, 54–75.

BAKER, E., BLUMSTEIN, S.E., & GOODGLASS, H. (1981). Interaction between phonological and semantic factors in auditory comprehension. *Neuropsychologia, 19*, 1–15.

BALOTTA, D.A., & CHUMBLEY, J.I. (1985). The locus of word-frequency effects in the pronunciation task: Lexical access and/or production? *Journal of Memory and Language, 24*, 89–106.

BALOTTA, D.A., & DUCHEK, J.M. (1991). Semantic priming effects, lexical repetition effects, and contextual disambiguation effects in healthy aged individuals and individuals with senile dementia of the Alzheimer type. *Brain and Language, 40*, 181–201.

BAMBER, L. (1980). A retrospective study of language recovery in adult aphasics. Thesis, Memphis State University.

BARBIZET, J. (1970). *Human memory and its pathology.* San Francisco: W.H. Freeman.

BARLOW, D.H., & HERSEN, M. (1984). *Single case experimental designs: Strategies for studying behavior change* (Second Edition). New York: Pergamon.

BARR, J.A. (1988). Group treatment: The logical choice. In B.B. Shadden (Ed.), *Communication behavior and aging: A sourcebook for clinicians* (pp. 329–340). Baltimore: Williams & Wilkins.

BARTON, M.I. (1971). Recall of generic properties of words in aphasic patients. *Cortex, 7*, 73–82.

BARTON, M.I., MARUSZEWSKI, M., & URREA, D. (1969). Variation of stimulus context and its effect on word-finding ability in aphasics. *Cortex, 5*, 351–365.

BASILI, A.G., DIGGS, C.C., & RAO, P. (1980). Auditory comprehension of brain-damaged subjects under competitive listening conditions. *Brain and Language, 9*, 362–371.

BASSO, A. (1978). Aphasia rehabilitation. In Y. Lebrun, & R. Hoops (Eds.), *The management of aphasia* (pp. 9–21). Amsterdam: Swets & Zeitlinger.

BASSO, A. (1989). Spontaneous recovery and language rehabilitation. In X. Seron & G. Deloche (Eds.), *Cog-*

nitive approaches in neuropsychological rehabilitation (pp. 17–37). Hillsdale, NJ: Lawrence Erlbaum.

BASSO, A., CAPITANI, E., & VIGNOLO, L.A. (1979). Influence of rehabilitation on language skills in aphasic patients: A controlled study. *Archives of Neurology*, 36, 190–196.

BASSO, A., CAPITANI, E., & MORASCHINI, S. (1982). Sex differences in recovery from aphasia. *Cortex*, 18, 469–475.

BASSO, A., LECOURS, A.R., MORASCHINI, S., & VANIER, M. (1985). Anatomo-clinical correlations of aphasias as defined through computerized tomography: Exceptions. *Brain and Language*, 26, 201–229.

BASSO, A., RAZZANO, C., FAGLIONI, P., & ZANOBIO, M.E. (1990). Confrontation naming, picture description and action naming in aphasic patients. *Aphasiology*, 4, 185–196.

BASSO, A., TABORELLI, A., & VIGNOLO, L.A. (1978). Dissociated disorders of speaking and writing in aphasia. *Journal of Neurology, Neurosurgery, and Psychiatry*, 41, 556–563.

BATES, E.A., CHEN, S., TZENG, O., LI, P., & OPIE, M. (1991). The noun-verb problem in Chinese aphasia. *Brain and Language*, 41, 203–233.

BATES, E.A., FRIEDERICI, A.D., & WULFECK, B.B. (1987a). Comprehension in aphasia: A cross-linguistic study. *Brain and Language*, 32, 19–67.

BATES, E.A., FRIEDERICI, A.D., & WULFECK, B.B. (1987b). Grammatical morphology in aphasia: Evidence from three languages. *Cortex*, 23, 545–574.

BATES, E.A., FRIEDERICI, A.D., WULFECK, B.B., & JUAREZ, L.A. (1988). On the preservation of word order in aphasia: Cross-linguistic evidence. *Brain and Language*, 33, 323–364.

BATES, E.A., HAMBY, S., & ZURIF, E. (1983). The effects of focal brain damage on pragmatic expression. *Canadian Journal of Psychology*, 37, 59–84.

BATES, E.A., MCDONALD, J., MACWHINNEY, B., & APPLEBAUM, M. (1991). A maximum likelihood procedure for the analysis of group and individual data in aphasia research. *Brain and Language*, 40, 231–265.

BATES, E.A., & WULFECK, B. (1989). Comparative aphasiology: A cross-linguistic approach to language breakdown. *Aphasiology*, 3, 111–142.

BATES, E.A., WULFECK, B., & MACWHINNEY, B. (1991). Cross-linguistic research in aphasia: An overview. *Brain and Language*, 41, 123–148.

BAUER, R.M., & RUBENS, A.B. (1985). Agnosia. In K.M. Heilman & E. Valenstein (Eds.), *Clinical neuropsychology* (Second Edition) (pp. 187–241). New York: Oxford University Press.

BAUM, S.R., (1988). Syntactic processing in agrammatism: Evidence from lexical decision and grammaticality judgment tasks. *Aphasiology*, 2, 117–136.

BAUM, S.R., (1989). On-line sensitivity to local and long-distance syntactic dependencies in Broca's aphasia. *Brain and Language*, 37, 327–338.

BAUM, S.R., DANILOFF, J., DANILOFF, R., & LEWIS, J. (1982). Sentence comprehension by Broca's aphasics: Effects on suprasegmental variables. *Brain and Language*, 17, 261–271.

BAYLES, K.A. (1986). Management of neurogenic communication disorders associated with dementia. In R. Chapey (Ed.), *Language intervention strategies in adult aphasia* (Second Edition) (pp. 462–473). Baltimore: Williams & Wilkins.

BAYLES, K.A., & BOONE, D.R. (1982). The potential of language tasks for identifying senile dementia. *Journal of Speech and Hearing Disorders*, 47, 210–217.

BAYLES, K.A., BOONE, D.R., TOMOEDA, C.K., SLAUSON, T.J., & KASZNIAK, A.W. (1989). Differentiating Alzheimer's patients from the normal elderly and stroke patients with aphasia. *Journal of Speech and Hearing Disorders*, 54, 74–87.

BAYLES, K.A., & KASZNIAK, A.W. (1987). *Communication and cognition in normal aging and dementia*. San Diego: Singular.

BAYLES, K.A., & TOMOEDA, C.K. (1983). Confrontation naming impairment in dementia. *Brain and Language*, 19, 98–114.

BEATON, A. (1985). *Left side right side: A review of laterality research*. New Haven CT: Yale University Press.

BEHRENS, S.J. (1988). The role of the right hemisphere in the production of linguistic stress. *Brain and Language*, 33, 104–127.

BEHRENS, S.J. (1989). Characterizing sentence intonation in a right hemisphere-damaged population. *Brain and Language*, 37, 181–200.

BELMORE, S.M., YATES, J.M., BELLACK, D.R., JONES, S.N., & ROSENQUIST, S.E. (1982). Drawing inferences from concrete and abstract sentences. *Journal of Verbal Learning and Verbal Behavior*, 21, 338–351.

BENOWITZ, L.I., MOYA, K.L., & LEVINE, D.N. (1990). Impaired verbal reasoning and constructional apraxia in subjects with right hemisphere damage. *Neuropsychologia*, 28, 231–241.

BENSON, D.F. (1979a). *Aphasia, Alexia, and Agraphia*. New York: Churchill Livingstone.

BENSON, D.F. (1979b). Aphasia rehabilitation. *Archives of Neurology*, 36, 187–189.

BENSON, D.F. & STUSS, D.T. (1986). *The frontal lobes*. New York: Raven.

BENTON, A.L. (1985). Visuoperceptual, visuospatial, and visuoconstructive disorders. In K.M. Heilman & E. Valenstein (Eds.), *Clinical neurospychology* (Second Edition) (pp. 151–185). New York: Oxford University Press.

BENTON, A.L., HAMSHER, K., VARNEY, N.R., & SPREEN, O. (1983). *Contributions to neuropsychological assessment: A clinical manual*. New York: Oxford University Press.

BENTON, A.L., SMITH, K.C., & LANG, M. (1972). Stimulus

characteristics and object naming in aphasic patients. *Journal of Communication Disorders, 5,* 19–24.

BERLIN, I. (1956). *The age of enlightenment.* New York: Mentor.

BERMAN, M., & PEELLE, L.M. (1967). Self-generated cues: A method for aiding aphasic and apractic patients. *Journal of Speech and Hearing disorders, 32,* 372–376.

BERNDT, R.S. (1987). Symptom co-occurrence and dissociation in the interpretation of agrammatism. In M. Coltheart, G. Sartori, & R. Job (Eds.), *The cognitive neuropsychology of language* (pp. 221–233). London: Erlbaum.

BERNDT, R.S., & CARAMAZZA, A. (1980). A redefinition of the syndrome of Broca's aphasia: Implications for a neuropsychological model of language. *Applied Psycholinguistics, 1,* 225–278.

BERNDT, R.S., SALASOO, A., MITCHUM, C.C., & BLUMSTEIN, S.E. (1988). The role of intonation cues in aphasic patients' performance of the grammaticality judgment task. *Brain and Language, 34,* 65–97.

BERNSTEIN-ELLIS, E., WERTZ, R.T., DRONKERS, N.F., & MILTON, S.B. (1985). PICA performance by traumatically brain injured and left hemisphere CVA patients. In R.H. Brookshire (Ed.), *Clinical aphasiology* (Vol. 15) (pp. 97–106). Minneapolis: BRK.

BERTHEIR, M.L., STARKSTEIN, S.E., LYLYK, P., & LEIGUARDA, R. (1990). Differential recovery of languages in a bilingual patient: A case study using selective amytal test. *Brain and Language, 38,* 449–453.

BIHRLE, A.M., BROWNELL, H.H., POWELSON, J.A., & GARDNER, H. (1986). Comprehension of humorous and nonhumorous materials by left and right brain damaged patients. *Brain and Cognition, 5,* 399–411.

BISIACH, E., & LUZZATTI, C. (1978). Unilateral neglect of representational space. *Cortex, 14,* 129–135.

BLACK, F.W., & STRUB, R.L. (1978). Digit repetition performance in patients with focal brain damage. *Cortex, 14,* 12–21.

BLACK, J.B., & BOWER, G.H. (1980). Story understanding as problem-solving. *Poetics, 9,* 223–250.

BLOCH, M.I., & HELLIGE, J.B. (1989). Stimulus intensity, attentional instructions, and the ear advantage during dichotic listening. *Brain and Cognition, 9,* 136–148.

BLOMERT, L. (1990). What functional assessment can contribute to setting goals for aphasia therapy. *Aphasiology, 4,* 307–320.

BLOMERT, L., KOSTER, C., VAN MIER, H., & KEAN, M-L. (1987). Verbal communication abilities of aphasic patients: The everyday language test. *Aphasiology, 1,* 463–474.

BLOOM, M., & FISCHER, J. (1982). *Evaluating practice: Guidelines for the accountable professional.* Englewood Cliffs, NJ: Prentice-Hall.

BLUMSTEIN, S.E. (1973). *A phonological investigation of aphasic speech.* The Hague, Netherlands: Mouton.

BLUMSTEIN, S.E. (1981). Phonological aspects of aphasia. In M.T. Sarno (Ed.), *Acquired aphasia* (pp. 129–155). New York: Academic Press (1981).

BLUMSTEIN, S.E., BAKER, E., & GOODGLASS, H. (1977). Phonological factors in auditory comprehension in aphasia. *Neuropsychologia, 15,* 19–30.

BLUMSTEIN, S.E., COOPER, W.E., GOODGLASS, H., STATLENDER, S., & GOTTLEIB, J. (1980). Production deficits in aphasia: A voice-onset time analysis. *Brain and Language, 9,* 153–170.

BLUMSTEIN, S.E., & GOODGLASS, H. (1972). The perception of stress as a semantic cue in aphasia. *Journal of Speech and Hearing Research, 15,* 800–806.

BLUMSTEIN, S.E., GOODGLASS, H., STATLENDER, S., & BIBER, C. (1983). Comprehension strategies determining reference in aphasia: A study of reflexivization. *Brain and Language, 18,* 115–127.

BLUMSTEIN, S.E., KATZ, B., GOODGLASS, H., SHRIER, R., & DWORETSKY, B. (1985). The effects of slowed speech on auditory comprehension in aphasia. *Brain and Language, 24,* 246–265.

BLUMSTEIN, S.E., MILBERG, W., DWORETZKY, B., ROSEN, A., & GERSHBERG, F. (1991). Syntactic priming effects in aphasia: An investigation of local syntactic dependencies. *Brain and Language, 40,* 393–421.

BLUMSTEIN, S.E., MILBERG, W., & SHRIER, R. (1982). Semantic processing in aphasia: Evidence from an auditory lexical decision task. *Brain and Language, 17,* 301–315.

BLUMSTEIN, S.E., TARTTER, V.C., NIGRO, G., & STATLENDER, S. (1984). Acoustic cues for the perception of place of articulation in aphasia. *Brain and Language, 22,* 128–149.

BOCK, K. (1987). An effect of the accessibility of word forms on sentence structures. *Journal of Memory and Language, 26,* 119–137.

BOLLER, F. (1968). Latent aphasias: Right and left "non-aphasic" brain-damaged patients compared. *Cortex, 4,* 245–256.

BOLLER, F., & GRAFMAN, J. (1983). Acalculia: Historical development and current significance. *Brain and Cognition, 2,* 205–223.

BOLLER, F., KIM, Y., & MACK, J.L. (1977). Auditory comprehension in aphasia. In H. Whitaker & H. Whitaker (Eds.), *Studies in neurolinguistics* (Vol. 3) (pp. 1–63). New York: Academic Press.

BOLLER, F. & VIGNOLO, L.A. (1966). Latent sensory aphasia in hemisphere-damaged patients: An experimental study with the Token Test. *Brain, 89,* 815–830.

BORKOWSKI, J.G., BENTON, A.L., & SPREEN, O. (1967). Word fluency and brain damage. *Neuropsychologia, 5,* 135–140.

BOROD, J.C., CARPER, J.M., & NAESER, M. (1990). Long-term language recovery in left-handed aphasic patients. *Aphasiology, 4,* 561–572.

BOROD, J.C., FITZPATRICK, P.M., HELM-ESTABROOKS, N.,

& GOODGLASS, H. (1989). The relationship between limb apraxia and the spontaneous use of communicative gesture in aphasia. *Brain and Cognition*, 10, 121–131.

BOROD, J.C., GOODGLASS, H., & KAPLAN, E. (1980). Normative data on the Boston Diagnostic Aphasia Examination, Parietal Lobe Battery, and the Boston Naming Test. *Journal of Clinical Neuropsychology*, 2, 209–215.

BOROD, J.C., KOFF, E., PERLMAN-LORCH, M., & NICHOLAS, M. (1986). The expression and perception of facial emotion in brain-damaged patients. *Neuropsychologia*, 24, 169–180.

BOROD, J.C., ST. CLAIR, J., KOFF, E., & ALPERT, M. (1990). Perceiver and poser asymmetries in processing facial emotion. *Brain and Cognition*, 13, 167–177.

BOTTENBERG, D.E., & LEMME, M.L. (1990). Effect of shared and unshared listener knowledge on narratives of normal and aphasic adults. In T.E. Prescott (Ed.), *Clinical aphasiology* (Vol. 19) (pp. 109–116). Austin, TX: Pro-Ed.

BOTTENBERG, D.E., LEMME, M.L., & HEDBERG, N.L. (1985). Analysis of oral narratives of normal and aphasic adults. In R.H. Brookshire (Ed.), *Clinical aphasiology* (Vol. 15) (p. 241–247). Minneapolis: BRK.

BOTTENBERG, D.E., LEMME, M.L., & HEDBERG, N.L. (1987). Effect of story content on narrative discourse of aphasic adults. In R.H. Brookshire (Ed.), *Clinical aphasiology* (Vol. 17) (pp. 202–209). Minneapolis: BRK.

BOYLE, M. (1989). Reducing phonemic paraphasias in the connected speech of a conduction aphasic subject. In T.E. Prescott (Ed.), *Clinical aphasiology* (Vol. 18) (pp. 379–393). Boston: College-Hill/Little, Brown.

BRADLEY, D.C., GARRETT, M.F., & ZURIF, E.B. (1980). Syntactic deficits in Broca's aphasia. In D. Caplan (Ed.), *Biological studies of mental processes* (pp. 269–286). Cambridge, MA: MIT Press.

BRAMWELL, B. (1906). A series of lectures on aphasia. *Lancet*, 1, 71–78, 351–361, 1671–1674, 1742–1747.

BRANCHEREAU, L., & NESPOULOUS, J-L. (1989). Syntactic parsing and the availability of prepositions in agrammatic patients. *Aphasiology*, 3, 411–422.

BRENNEISE-SARSHAD, R., NICHOLAS, L.E., & BROOKSHIRE, R.H. (1991). Effects of apparent listener knowledge and picture stimuli on aphasic and non-brain-damaged speakers' narrative discourse. *Journal of Speech and Hearing Research*, 34, 168–176.

BROCA, P. (1960). Remarks on the seat of the faculty of articulate language, followed by an observation of aphemia. In G. von Bonin (Trans.), *Some papers on the cerebral cortex*. Springfield, IL: Charles C. Thomas.

BROIDA, H. (1977). Language therapy effects in long term aphasia. *Archives of Physical Medicine and Rehabilitation*, 58, 248–253.

BROIDA, H. (1979). *Coping with stroke*. San Diego: Singular.

BROOKS, D.N. (1976). Wechsler memory scale performance and its relationship to brain damage after severe closed head injury. *Journal of Neurology, Neurosurgery, and Psychiatry*, 1976, 39, 593–601.

BROOKS, D.N., AUGHTON, M.E., BOND, M.R., JONES, P., & RIZVI, S. (1980). Cognitive sequelae in relationship to early indices of severity of brain damage after severe blunt head injury. *Journal of Neurology, Neurosurgery, and Psychiatry*, 43, 529–534.

BROOKSHIRE, R.H. (1967). Speech pathology and the experimental analysis of behavior. *Journal of Speech and Hearing Disorders*, 32, 215–227.

BROOKSHIRE, R.H. (1969). Probability learning by aphasic subjects. *Journal of Speech and Hearing Research*, 12, 857–864.

BROOKSHIRE, R.H. (1972). Effects of task difficulty on naming by aphasic subjects. *Journal of Speech and Hearing Research*, 15, 551–558.

BROOKSHIRE, R.H. (1975). Recognition of auditory sequences by aphasic, right-hemisphere-damaged and non-brain-damaged subjects. *Journal of Communication Disorders*, 8, 51–59.

BROOKSHIRE, R.H. (1978a). *An introduction to aphasia* (Second Edition). Minneapolis: BRK.

BROOKSHIRE, R.H. (1978b). A Token Test battery for testing auditory comprehension in brain-injured adults. *Brain and Language*, 6, 149–157.

BROOKSHIRE, R.H. (1986). *An introduction to aphasia* (Third Edition). Minneapolis: BRK.

BROOKSHIRE, R.H., & NICHOLAS, L.E. (1978). Effects of clinician request and feedback behavior on responses of aphasic individuals in speech and language treatment sessions. In R.H. Brookshire (Ed.), *Clinical aphasiology conference proceedings* (pp. 40–48). Minneapolis: BRK.

BROOKSHIRE, R.H., & NICHOLAS, L.E. (1980). Verification of active and passive sentences by aphasic and nonaphasic subjects. *Journal of Speech and Hearing Disorders*, 43, 437–447.

BROOKSHIRE, R.H., & NICHOLAS, L.E. (1984). Consistency of effects of slow rate and pauses on aphasic listeners' comprehension of spoken sentences. *Journal of Speech and Hearing Research*, 27, 323–328.

BROOKSHIRE, R.H., NICHOLAS, L.S., KRUEGER, K.M., & REDMOND, K.J. (1978). The clinical interaction analysis system: A system for observational recording of aphasia treatment. *Journal of Speech and Hearing Disorders*, 43, 437–447.

BROWN, G., & YULE, G. (1983). *Discourse analysis*. Cambridge, UK: Cambridge University Press.

BROWN, J.R., & SCHUELL, H.M. (1950). A preliminary report of a diagnostic test for aphasia. *Journal of Speech and Hearing Disorders*, 15, 21–28.

BROWN, J.W., & CODE, C. (1987). Aphasia from the wrong (right) hemisphere: Questions for crossed aphasia. *Aphasiology*, 1, 401–402.

BROWN, J.W., & JAFFE, J. (1975). Hypothesis on cerebral dominance. *Neuropsychologia*, 13, 107–110.

BROWN, N.R., RIPS, L.J., & SHEVELL, S.K. (1985). The subjective dates of natural events in very-long-term memory. *Cognitive Psychology*, 17, 139–177.

BROWNELL, H.H. (1988). The neuropsychology of narrative comprehension. *Aphasiology*, 2, 247–250.

BROWNELL, H.H., BIHRLE, A.M., & MICHELOW, D. (1986). Basic and subordinate level naming by agrammatic and fluent aphasic patients. *Brain and Language*, 28, 42–52.

BROWNELL, H.H., MICHEL, D., POWELSON, J.A., & GARDNER, H. (1983). Surprise but not coherence: Sensitivity to verbal humor in right hemisphere patients. *Brain and Language*, 18, 20–27.

BROWNELL, H.H., POTTER, H.H., BIHRLE, A.M., & GARDNER, H. (1986). Inference deficits in right brain-damaged patients. *Brain and Language*, 27, 310–321.

BROWNELL, H.H., POTTER, H.H., MICHELOW, D., & GARDNER, H. (1984). Sensitivity to lexical denotation and connotation in brain-damaged patients: A double dissociation? *Brain and Language*, 22, 253–265.

BROWNELL, H.H., SIMPSON, T.L., BIHRLE, A.M., POTTER, H.H., & GARDNER, H. (1990). Appreciation of metaphoric alternative word meanings by left and right brain-damaged patients. *Neuropsychologia*, 28, 375–383.

BRUCE, C., & HOWARD, D. (1988). Why don't Broca's aphasics cue themselves? An investigation of phonemic cueing and tip of the tongue information. *Neuropsychologia*, 26, 253–264.

BRUCE, V., & YOUNG, A.W. (1986). Understanding face recognition. *British Journal of Psychology*, 77, 305–327.

BRUCKERT, R., GONON, M-A.H., MICHEL, F., & BEZ, M. (1989). The use of a computer driven videodisc for the assessment and rehabilitation of aphasia. *Aphasiology*, 3, 473–478.

BRUNN, J.L., & FARAH, M.J. (1991). The relation between spatial attention and reading: Evidence from the neglect syndrome. *Cognitive Neuropsychology*, 8, 59–75.

BRUYER, R. (1991). Covert face recognition in prosopagnosia: A review. *Brain and Cognition*, 15, 223–235.

BRYAN, K.L. (1988). Assessment of language disorders after right hemisphere damage. *British Journal of Disorders of Communication*, 23, 111–125.

BRYAN, K.L. (1989). Language prosody and the right hemisphere. *Aphasiology*, 3(4), 285–300.

BRYDEN, M.P., LEY, R.G. & SUGARMAN, J.H. (1982). A left ear advantage for identifying the emotional quality of tonal sequences. *Neuropsychologia*, 20, 83–88.

BUCK, M. (1968). *Dysphasia: Professional guidance for family and patient*. Englewood Cliffs, NJ: Prentice-Hall.

BUCK, R., & DUFFY, R.J. (1980). Nonverbal communication of affect in brain-damaged patients. *Cortex*, 16, 351–362.

BUCKINGHAM, H.W. (1981a). Lexical and semantic aspects of aphasia. In M.T. Sarno (Ed.), *Acquired aphasia* (pp. 183–214). New York: Academic Press.

BUCKINGHAM, H.W. (1981b). Where do neologisms come from? In J.W. Brown (Ed.), *Jargonaphasia* (pp. 39–62). New York: Academic Press.

BUCKINGHAM, H.W. (1987). Phonemic paraphasias and pycholinguistic production models for neologistic jargon. *Aphasiology*, 1, 381–401.

BUCKINGHAM, H.W. (1989). Mechanisms underlying aphasic transformations. In A. Ardila & P. Ostrosky-Solis (Eds.), *Brain organization of language and cognitive processes* (pp. 123–145). New York: Plenum.

BUCKINGHAM, H.W., & KERTESZ, A. (1976). *Neologistic jargon aphasia*. Amsterdam: Swets and Zeitlinger.

BUCKINGHAM, H.W., & REKART, D.M. (1979). Semantic paraphasia. *Journal of Communication Disorders*, 12, 197–209.

BUCKINGHAM, H.W., WHITAKER, H., & WHITAKER, H.A. (1979). On linguistic perseveration. In H. Whitaker & H.A. Whitaker (Eds.), *Studies in Neurolinguistics* (Vol. 4) (pp. 329–352). New York: Academic Press.

BURGESS, C., & SIMPSON, G.B. (1988). Cerebral hemispheric mechanisms in the retrieval of ambiguous word meanings. *Brain and Language*, 33, 86–103.

BURKE, D.M., MACKAY, D.G., WORTHLEY, J.A., & WADE, E. (1991). On the tip of the tongue: What causes word finding failures in young and older adults? *Journal of Memory and Language*, 30, 542–579.

BURNS, M.S., HALPER, A.S., & MOGIL, S.I. (1985). *Clinical management of right hemisphere dysfunction*. Rockville, MD: Aspen.

BURTON, E., BURTON, A., & LUCAS, W. (1988). The use of microcomputers with aphasic patients. *Aphasiology*, 2, 479–492.

BUSCH, C.R., BROOKSHIRE, R.H., & NICHOLAS, L.E. (1988). Referential communication by aphasic and nonaphasic adults. *Journal of Speech and Hearing Disorders*, 53, 475–482.

BUTFIELD, E., & ZANGWILL, O.L. (1946). Reeducation in aphasia: A review of 70 cases. *Journal of Neurology, Neurosurgery, and Psychiatry*, 9, 75–79.

BUTLER-HINZ, S., CAPLAN, D., & WATERS, G. (1990). Characteristics of syntactic and semantic comprehension deficits following closed head injury versus left cerebrovascular accident. *Journal of Speech and Hearing Research*, 33, 269–280.

BUTTERWORTH, B. (1979). Hesitation and the production of verbal paraphasias and neologisms in jargon aphasia. *Brain and Language*, 18, 133–161.

BUTTERWORTH, B., HOWARD, D., & MCLOUGHLIN, P. (1984). The semantic deficit in aphasia: The relationship between semantic errors in auditory comprehension and picture naming. *Neuropsychologia, 22,* 409–426.

BYNG, S. (1988). Sentence processing deficits: Theory and therapy. *Cognitive Neuropsychology, 5,* 629–676.

BYNG, S., KAY, J., EDMUNDSON, A., & SCOTT. C. (1990). Aphasia tests reconsidered. *Aphasiology, 4,* 67–92.

CAIRNS, H.S. (1984). Research in language comprehension. In R.C. Naremore (Ed.), *Language science: Recent advances* (pp. 211–242). San Diego: College-Hill.

CALVIN, W.H., & OJEMANN, G.A. (1980). *Inside the brain.* New York: Mentor.

CAMPBELL, K., DEACON-ELLIOTT, D., & PROULX, G. (1986). Electrophysiological monitoring of closed head injury. I: Basic principles and techniques. *Cognitive Rehabilitation, 4*(5), 26–32.

CAMPBELL, T.F., & DOLLAGHAN, C.A. (1990). Expressive language recovery in severely brain-injured children and adolescents. *Journal of Speech and Hearing Disorders, 55,* 567–581.

CANCELLIERE, A.E.B., & KERTESZ, A. (1990). Lesion localization in acquired deficits of emotional expression and comprehension. *Brain and Cognition, 13,* 133–148.

CANTER, G.J. (1988). Apraxia of speech and phonemic paraphasia. *Aphasiology, 2,* 251–254.

CANTER, G.J., TROST, J.E., & BURNS, M.S. (1985). Contrasting speech patterns in apraxia of speech and phonemic paraphasia. *Brain and Language, 24,* 204–222.

CAPLAN, D. (1981). On the cerebral localization of linguistic functions: Logical and empirical issues surrounding deficit analysis and functional localization. *Brain and Language, 14,* 120–137.

CAPLAN, D. (1983). A note on the "word-order problem" in agrammatism. *Brain and Language, 20,* 155–165.

CAPLAN, D. (1984). The mental organ for language. In D. Caplan, A.R. Lecours, & A. Smith (Eds.), *Biological perspectives on language* (pp. 8–30). Cambridge, MA: MIT Press.

CAPLAN, D. (1985). Syntactic and semantic structures in agrammatism. In M-L. Kean (Ed.), *Agrammatism* (pp. 125–151). Orlando, FL: Academic Press.

CAPLAN, D. (1986). In defense of agrammatism. *Cognition, 24,* 263–276.

CAPLAN, D. (1987a). Agrammatism and the coindexation of traces: Comments on Grodzinsky's reply. *Brain and Language, 30,* 191–193.

CAPLAN, D. (1987b). *Neurolinguistics and linguistic aphasiology: An introduction.* Cambridge, UK: Cambridge University Press.

CAPLAN, D. (1988). On the role of group studies in neuropsychological and pathopsychological research. *Cognitive Neuropsychology, 5,* 535–548.

CAPLAN, D. (1991). Agrammatism is a theoretically coher-ent aphasic category. *Brain and Language, 40,* 274–281.

CAPLAN, D., BAKER, C., & DEHAUT, F. (1985). Syntactic determinants of sentence comprehension in aphasia. *Cognition, 21,* 117–175.

CAPLAN, D., & EVANS, K.L. (1990). The effects of syntactic structure on discourse comprehension in patients with parsing impairments. *Brain and Language, 39,* 206–234.

CAPLAN, D., & FUTTER, C. (1986). Assignment of thematic roles to nouns in sentence comprehension by an agrammatic patient. *Brain and Language, 27,* 117–134.

CAPLAN, D., & HILDEBRANDT, N. (1988). Specific deficits in syntactic comprehension. *Aphasiology, 2,* 255–258.

CAPLAN, D., MATTHEI, E., & GIGLEY, H. (1981). Comprehension of gerundive constructions in Broca's aphasia. *Brain and Language, 13,* 145–160.

CAPPA, S.F., CAVALLOTTI, G., & VIGNOLO, L. (1981). Phonemic and lexical errors in fluent aphasia: Correlation with lesion site. *Neuropsychologia, 19,* 171–177.

CAPPA, S.F., PAPAGNO, C., & VALLAR, G. (1990). Language and verbal memory after right hemispheric stroke: A clinical-CT scan study. *Neuropsychologia, 28,* 503–509.

CAPPA, S.F., & VIGNOLO, L.A. (1979). 'Transcortical' features of aphasia following left thalamic hemorrhage. *Cortex, 15,* 121–130.

CAPPA, S.F., & VIGNOLO, L.A. (1988). Sex differences in the site of brain lesions underlying global aphasia. *Aphasiology, 2,* 259–264.

CARAMAZZA, A. (1984). The logic of neuropsychological research and the problem of patient classification in aphasia. *Brain and Language, 21,* 9–20.

CARAMAZZA, A. (1986). On drawing inferences about the structure of normal cognitive systems from the analysis of patterns of impaired performance: The case for single-patient studies. *Brain and Cognition, 5,* 41–66.

CARAMAZZA, A. (1988). Some aspects of language processing revealed through the analysis of acquired aphasia: The lexical system. *Annual Review of Neuroscience, 11,* 395–421.

CARAMAZZA, A. (1989). Cognitive neuropsychology and rehabilitation: An unfulfilled promise? In X. Seron & G. Deloche (Eds.), *Cognitive approaches in neuropsychological rehabilitation* (pp. 383–398). Hillsdale, NJ: Lawrence Erlbaum.

CARAMAZZA, A. (1991). Data, statistics, and theory: A comment on Bates, McDonald, MacWhinney, and Applebaum's "A maximum likelihood procedure for the analysis of group and individual data in aphasia research," *Brain and Language, 41,* 43–51.

CARAMAZZA, A., & BADECKER, W. (1991). Clinical syndromes are not God's gift to cognitive neuropsychology: A reply to a rebuttal to an answer to a response to the case against syndrome-based research. *Brain and Cognition, 16,* 211–227.

CARAMAZZA, A., BASILI, A., KOLLER, J.J., & BERNDT, R.S. (1981). An investigation of repetition and language processing in a case of conduction aphasia. *Brain and Language, 14,* 235–271.

CARAMAZZA, A., & BERNDT, R.S. (1978). Semantic and syntactic processes in aphasia: A review of the literature. *Psychological Bulletin, 85,* 898–918.

CARAMAZZA, A., & BERNDT, R.S. (1985). A multicomponential deficit view of agrammatic Broca's aphasia. In M-L. Kean (Ed.), *Agrammatism* (pp. 27–63). Orlando, FL: Academic Press.

CARAMAZZA, A., GORDON, J., ZURIF, E.G., & DELUCA, D. (1976). Right hemisphere damage and verbal problem-solving behavior. *Brain and Language, 3,* 41–46.

CARAMAZZA, A., & HILLIS, A.E. (1989). The disruption of sentence production: Some dissociations. *Brain and Language, 36,* 625–650.

CARAMAZZA, A., & McCLOSKEY, M. (1988). The case for single-patient studies. *Cognitive Neuropsychology, 5,* 517–528.

CARAMAZZA, A., & ZURIF, E.B. (1976). Dissociation of algorithmic and heuristic processes in language comprehension: Evidence from aphasia. *Brain and Language, 3,* 572–582.

CARLOMAGNO, S., LOSANNO, N., EMANUELLI, S., & CASADIO, P. (1991). Expressive language recovery or improved communicative skills: Effects of P.A.C.E. therapy on aphasics' referential communication and story retelling. *Aphasiology, 5,* 419–424.

CARLOMAGNO, S., & PARLATO, V. (1989). Writing rehabilitation in brain-damaged adult patients: A cognitive approach. In X. Seron, & G. Deloche (Eds.), *Cognitive approaches in neuropsychological rehabilitation* (pp. 175–210). London: Erlbaum.

CARMON, A., & NACHSON, I. (1971). Effect of unilateral brain damage on perception of temporal order. *Cortex, 7,* 410–418.

CARPENTER, R.L., & RUTHERFORD, D.R. (1973). Acoustic cue discrimination in adult aphasia. *Journal of Speech and Hearing Research, 16,* 534–544.

CASEY, M.B., & BRABECK, M.M. (1990). Women who excel on a spatial task: Proposed genetic and environmental factors. *Brain and Cognition, 12,* 73–84.

CASTRO-CALDAS, A., CONFRARIA, A., & POPPE, P. (1987). Non-verbal disturbances in crossed aphasia. *Aphasiology, 1,* 403–414.

CAVALLI, M., DeRENZI, E., FAGLIONI, P., & VITALE, A. (1981). Impairment of right brain-damaged patients on a linguistic cognitive task. *Cortex, 17,* 545–556.

CHANG, F.R. (1980). Active memory processes in visual sentence comprehension: Clause effects and pronominal reference. *Memory and Cognition, 8,* 58–64.

CHAPEY, R., RIGRODSKY, S., & MORRISON, E.G. (1977). Aphasia: A divergent semantic interpretation. *Journal of Speech and Hearing Disorders, 42,* 287–295.

CHAPMAN, S.B., & ULATOWSKA, H.K. (1989). Discourse in aphasia: Integration deficits in processing reference. *Brain and Language, 36,* 651–668.

CHAWLUK, J.B., GROSSMAN, M., CALCANO-PEREZ, J.A., ALAVI, A., HURTIG, H.I., & REIVICH, M. (1990). Positron emission tomographic studies of cerebral metabolism in Alzheimer's disease: A critical review stressing current and future neuropsychological methodology. In M.F. Schwartz (Ed.), *Modular deficits in Alzheimer-type dementia* (pp. 101–142). Cambridge, MA: Bradford/MIT Press.

CHEN, L.Y. (1971). Manual communication by combined alphabet and gestures. *Archives of Physical Medicine and Rehabilitation, 52,* 381–384.

CHENERY, H.J., INGRAM, J.C.L., & MURDOCH, B.B. (1990). Automatic and volitional semantic processing in aphasia. *Brain and Language, 38,* 215–232.

CHERTKOW, H., BUB, D., & SEIDENBERG, M. (1989). Priming and semantic memory loss in Alzheimer's disease. *Brain and Language, 36,* 420–446.

CHIARELLO, C. (1985). Hemisphere dynamics in lexical access: Automatic and controlled priming. *Brain and Language, 26,* 146–172.

CHIARELLO, C., SENEHI, J., & NUDING, S. (1987). Semantic priming with abstract and concrete words: Differential asymmetry may be postlexical. *Brain and Language, 31,* 43–60.

CHOMSKY, N. (1968). *Language and mind.* New York: Harcourt Brace Jovanovich.

CHURCHLAND, P.S. (1986). *Neurophilosophy: Toward a unified science of the mind/brain.* Cambridge, MA: Bradford/MIT Press.

CHUSID, J.G. (1979). *Correlative neuroanatomy and functional neurology* (17th Ed.). Los Altos, CA: Lange Medical Publications.

CICONE, M., WAPNER, W., & GARDNER, H. (1980). Sensitivity to emotional expressions and situations in organic patients. *Cortex, 16,* 145–158.

CLARK, A.E., & FLOWERS, C.R. (1987). The effect of semantic redundancy on auditory comprehension in aphasia. In R.H. Brookshire (Ed.), *Clinical aphasiology* (Vol. 17) (pp. 174–179). Minneapolis, BRK.

CLARK, C., CROCKETT, D.J., & KLONOFF, H. (1979a). Empirically derived groups in the assessment of recovery from aphasia. *Brain and Language, 7,* 240–251.

CLARK, C., CROCKETT, D.J., & KLONOFF, H. (1979b). Factor analysis of the Porch Index of Communication Ability. *Brain and Language, 7,* 1–7.

CLARK, H.H., & CLARK, E.V. (1977). *Psychology and Language.* New York: Harcourt, Brace and Jovanovich.

CLARK, H.H., & GERRIG, R.J. (1983). Understanding old words with new meanings. *Journal of Verbal Learning and Verbal Behavior, 22,* 591–608.

CLEREBAUT, N., COYETTE, F., FEYEREISEN, P., & SERON, X. (1984). Une methode de rééducation fonctionelle des aphasiques: La P.A.C.E. *Rééducation Orthophonique, 22,* 329–345.

CODE, C., & ROWLEY, D. (1987). Age and aphasia type: The interaction of sex, time since onset and handedness. *Aphasiology*, 1, 339–346.

COELHO, C.A. (1987). Sign acquisition and use following traumatic brain injury: A case report. *Archives of Physical Medicine and Rehabilitation*, 68, 229–231.

COELHO, C.A. (1990). Acquisition and generalization of simple manual sign grammars by aphasic subjects. *Journal of Communication Disorders*, 23, 383–400.

COELHO, C.A., & DUFFY, R.J. (1985). Communicative use of signs in aphasia: Is acquisition enough? In R.H. Brookshire (Ed.), *Clinical aphasiology* (Vol. 15). (pp. 222–228). Minneapolis: BRK.

COELHO, C.A., & DUFFY, R.J. (1987). The relationship of the acquisition of manual signs to severity of aphasia: A training study. *Brain and Language*, 31, 328–345.

COELHO, C.A., & DUFFY, R.J. (1990). Sign acquisition in two aphasic subjects with limb apraxia. *Aphasiology*, 4, 1–8.

COHEN, N.J., & SQUIRE, L.R. (1980). Preserved learning and retention of pattern-analyzing skill in amnesia: Dissociation of 'knowing how' and 'knowing that.' *Science*, 210, 207–209.

COHEN, R., KELTER, S., & WOLL, G. (1980). Analytical competence and language impairment in aphasia. *Brain and Language*, 10, 331–347.

COHEN, R., & WOLL, G. (1981). Facets of analytical processing in aphasia: A picture ordering task. *Cortex*, 17, 557–570.

COLBY, K.M., CHRISTINAZ, D., PARKISON, R.C., GRAHAM, S., & KARPF, C. (1981). A word-finding computer program with a dynamic lexical-semantic memory for patients with anomia using an intelligent speech prosthesis. *Brain and Language*, 14, 272–281.

COLLINS, A.M., & LOFTUS, E.F. (1975). A spreading activation theory of semantic processing. *Psychological Review*, 82, 407–428.

COLLINS, M. (1986). *Diagnosis and treatment of global aphasia*. San Diego: Singular.

COLLINS, M., MCNEIL, M.R., LENTZ, S., SHUBITOWSKI, Y., & ROSENBEK, J.C. (1984). Word fluency and aphasia: Some linguistic and not-so-linguistic considerations. In R.H. Brookshire (Ed.), *Clinical aphasiology conference proceedings* (pp. 78–84). Minneapolis; BRK.

COLSHER, P.L., COOPER, W.E., & GRAFF-RADFORD, N. (1987). Intonational variability in the speech of right-hemisphere damaged patients. *Brain and Language*, 32, 379–383.

CONRAD, F.G., & RIPS, L.J. (1986). Conceptual combination and the given/new distinction. *Journal of Memory and Language*, 25, 255–278.

COOPER, P.R. (ED.). (1982). *Head injury*. Baltimore: Williams & Wilkins.

COOPER, W.E., SOARES, C., NICOL, J., MICHELOW, D., & GOLOSKIE, S. (1984). Clausal intonation after unilateral brain damage. *Language and Speech*, 27, 17–24.

COPPENS, P. (1991). Why are Wernicke's aphasia patients older than Broca's? A critical view of the hypotheses. *Aphasiology*, 5, 279–290.

CORBALLIS, M.C. (1986). Fresh fields and postures new: A discussion paper. *Brain and Cognition*, 5, 240–252.

CORLEW, M.M., & NATION, J.E. (1975). Characteristics of visual stimuli and naming performance in aphasic adults. *Cortex*, 11, 186–191.

CORREIA, L., BROOKSHIRE, R.H., & NICHOLAS, L.E. (1989). The effects of picture content on descriptions by aphasic and non-brain-damaged speakers. In T.E. Prescott (Ed.), *Clinical aphasiology* (Vol. 18) (pp. 447–462). Austin, TX: Pro-Ed.

COSLETT; H.B., & SAFFRAN, E.M. (1989). Preserved object recognition and reading comprehension in optic aphasia. *Brain*, 112, 1091–1110.

COTMAN, C.W., & LYNCH, G.S. (1989). The neurobiology of learning and memory. *Cognition*, 33, 201–241.

COUGHLAN, A.K., & WARRINGTON, E.K. (1978). Word-comprehension and word-retrieval in patients with localized cerebral lesions. *Brain*, 101, 163–185.

COWPER, E.A. (1992). *A concise introduction to syntactic theory: The Government-Binding approach*. Chicago: University of Chicago Press.

CRAIK, F.I.M., & LOCKHART, R.S. (1972). Levels of processing: A framework for memory research. *Journal of Verbal Learning and Verbal Behavior*, 11, 671–684.

CRARY, M.A., & GONZALEZ ROTHI, L.J. (1989). Predicting the Western Aphasia Battery aphasia quotient. *Journal of Speech and Hearing Disorders*, 54, 163–166.

CRARY, M.A., HAAK, N.J., & MALINSKY, A.E. (1989). Preliminary psychometric evaluation of an acute aphasia screening protocol. *Aphasiology*, 3, 611–618.

CRARY, M.A., & KERTESZ, A. (1988). Evolving error profiles during aphasia syndrome remission. *Aphasiology*, 2, 67–78.

CRIPE, L.I. (1987). The neuropsychological assessment and management of closed head injury: General guidelines. *Cognitive Rehabilitation*, 5, 18–22.

CRITCHLEY, M. (1960). Jacksonian ideas and the future, with special reference to aphasia. *British Medical Journal*, 6, 6–11.

CROCKETT, D., & PURVES, B. (1988). Don't throw out the Porch with the bathwater: A second look at the future of the PICA. *Aphasiology*, 2, 507–510.

CROSSON, B. (1985). Subcortical functions in language: A working model. *Brain and Language*, 25, 257–292.

CROSSON, B., PARKER, J.C., KIM, A.K., WARREN, R.L., KEPES, J.J., & TULLY, R. (1986). A case of thalamic aphasia with postmortem verification. *Brain and Language*, 29, 301–314.

CRYSTAL, D., FLETCHER P., & GARMAN, M. (1976). *The grammatical analysis of language disability*. New York: Elsevier.

CUBELLI, R., FORESTI, A., & CONSOLINI, T. (1988). Reeducation strategies in conduction aphasia. *Journal of Communication Disorders*, 21, 239–249.

CUBELLI, R., NICHELLI, P., BONITO, V., DE TANTI, A., & INZAGHI, M.G. (1991). Different patterns of dissociation in unilateral spatial neglect. *Brain and Cognition,* 15, 139–159.

CUMMINGS, J.L., & BENSON, D. (1983). *Dementia: A clinical approach.* Boston: Butterworths.

CUMMINGS, J.L., BENSON, D.F., HILL, M., & READ, S. (1985). Aphasia in dementia of the Alzheimer's type. *Neurology,* 34, 394–397.

CURTISS, S., JACKSON, C.A., KEMPLER, D., HANSON, W.R., & METTER, E.J. (1986). Length vs. structural complexity in sentence comprehension in aphasia. In R.H. Brookshire (Ed.), *Clinical aphasiology* (Vol. 16) (pp. 45–55). Minneapolis: BRK.

DAHLBERG, C.C., & JAFFE, J. (1977). *Stroke: A doctor's personal story of his recovery.* New York: Norton.

DAMASIO, A.R., VAN HOESEN, G.W., & HYMAN, B.T. (1990). Reflections on the selectivity of neuropathological changes in Alzheimer's disease. In M.F. Schwartz (Ed.), *Modular deficits in Alzheimer-type dementia* (pp. 83–100). Cambridge, MA: Bradford/MIT Press.

DAMASIO, H.D., & DAMASIO, A.R. (1980). The anatomical basis of conduction aphasia. *Brain,* 103, 337–350.

DANILOFF, J.K., FRITELLI, G., BUCKINGHAM, H.W., HOFFMAN, P.R., & DANILOFF, R.G. (1986). Amer-Ind versus ASL: Recognition and imitation in aphasic subjects. *Brain and Language,* 28, 95–113.

DANILOFF, J.K., LLOYD, L., & FRISTOE, M. (1983). Amer-Ind transparency. *Journal of Speech and Hearing Disorders,* 48, 103–110.

DANILOFF, J.K., NOLL, J.D., FRISTOE, M., & LLOYD, L.L. (1982). Gesture recognition in patients with aphasia. *Journal of Speech and Hearing Disorders,* 47, 43–49.

DANKS, J.H. (1977). Producing ideas and sentences. In S. Rosenberg (Ed.), *Sentence production: Developments in research and theory* (pp. 229–258). Hillsdale, NJ: Erlbaum.

DANNENBAUM, S.E., PARKINSON, S.R., & INMAN, V.W. (1988). Short-term forgetting: Comparisons between patients with dementia of the Alzheimer type, depressed, and normal elderly. *Cognitive Neuropsychology,* 5, 213–234.

DARLEY, F.L. (1982). *Aphasia.* Philadelphia: W.B. Saunders.

DARLEY, F.L. (1983). Aphasia: With and without adjectives. In R.H. Brookshire (Ed.), *Clinical aphasiology conference proceedings* (pp. 281–284). Minneapolis: BRK.

DAVID, R., ENDERBY, P., & BAINTON, D. (1982). Treatment of acquired aphasia: Speech therapists and volunteers compared. *Journal of Neurology, Neurosurgery and Psychiatry,* 45, 957–961.

DAVIS, G.A. (1973). Linguistics and language therapy: The sentence construction board. *Journal of Speech and Hearing Disorders,* 38, 205–214.

DAVIS, G.A. (1983). *A survey of adult aphasia.* Englewood Cliffs, NJ: Prentice-Hall.

DAVIS, G.A. (1986). Questions of efficacy in clinical aphasiology. In R.H. Brookshire (Ed.), *Clinical aphasiology conference proceedings* (pp. 154–162). Minneapolis: BRK.

DAVIS, G.A. (1989). The cognitive cloud and language disorders. *Aphasiology,* 3, 723–734.

DAVIS, G.A., & HESS, C. (1986). A study of imagery in sentence verification with adult aphasic subjects. *Human Communication Canada,* 10, 11–16.

DAVIS, G.A., & HOLLAND, A.L. (1981). Age in understanding and treating aphasia. In D.S. Beasley & G.A. Davis (Eds.), *Aging: Communication processes and disorders* (pp. 207–228). New York: Grune & Stratton.

DAVIS, G.A., & WILCOX, M.J. (1985). *Adult aphasia rehabilitation: Applied pragmatics.* San Diego: Singular.

DEAL, J.L., & DEAL, L.A. (1978). Efficacy of aphasia rehabilitation: Preliminary results. In R.H. Brookshire (Ed.), *Clinical aphasiology conference proceedings* (pp. 66–77). Minneapolis: BRK.

DEAL, J.L., DEAL, L., WERTZ, R.T., KITSELMAN, K., & DWYER, C. (1979a). Right hemisphere PICA percentiles: Some speculations about aphasia. In R.H. Brookshire (Ed.), *Clinical aphasiology conference proceedings* (pp. 30–37). Minneapolis: BRK.

DEAL, L.A., DEAL, J.L., WERTZ, R.T., KITSELMAN, K., & DWYER, C. (1979b). Statistical prediction of change in aphasia: Clinical application of multiple regression analysis. In R.H. Brookshire (Ed.), *Clinical aphasiology conference proceedings* (pp. 95–100). Minneapolis: BRK.

DEKOSKEY, S., HEILMAN, K.M., BOWERS, D., & VALENSTEIN, E. (1980). Recognition and discrimination of emotional faces and pictures. *Brains and Language,* 9, 206–214.

DELIS, D.C., WAPNER, W., GARDNER, H., & MOSES, JR., J.A. (1983). The contribution of the right hemisphere to the organization of paragraphs. *Cortex,* 19, 43–50.

DELL, G.S. (1988). The retrieval of phonological forms in production: Tests of predictions from a connectionist model. *Journal of Memory and Language,* 27, 124–142.

DELL, G.S., MCKOON, G., & RATCLIFF, R. (1983). The activation of antecedent information during the processing of anaphoric reference in reading. *Journal of Verbal Learning and Verbal Behavior,* 22, 121–132.

DELL, G.S., & REICH, P.A. (1981). Stages in sentence production: An analysis of speech error data. *Journal of Verbal Learning and Verbal Behavior,* 20, 611–629.

DELOCHE, G., & SERON, X. (1981). Sentence understanding and knowledge of the world. Evidences from a sentence-picture matching task performed by aphasic patients. *Brain and Language,* 14, 57–69.

DEMEURISSE, G., DEMOL, O., DEROUCK, M., DE BEUCKELAER, R., COEKAERTS, M.-J. & CAPON, A. (1980). Quantitative study of the rate of recovery from aphasia due to ischemic stroke. *Stroke,* 11, 455–458.

DENES, P.B., & PINSON, E.N. (1963). *The speech chain.* Garden City, NY: Anchor.

DENNIS, M. (1980a). Capacity and strategy for syntactic comprehension after left or right hemidecortication. *Brain and Language,* 10, 287–317.

DENNIS, M. (1980b). Language acquisition in a single hemisphere: Semantic organization. In D. Caplan

(Ed.), *Biological studies of mental processes* (pp. 159–185). Cambridge, MA: MIT Press.

DeRenzi, E. (1979). A shortened version of the Token Test. In F. Boller & M. Dennis (Eds.), *Auditory comprehension: Clinical and experimental studies with the Token Test* (pp. 33–44). New York: Academic Press.

DeRenzi, E. (1986). Prosopagnosia in two patients with CT-scan evidence of damage confined to the right hemisphere. *Neuropsychologia, 24,* 385–389.

DeRenzi, E., & Faglioni, P. (1978). Normative data and screening power of a shortened version of the Token Test. *Cortex, 14,* 41–49.

DeRenzi, E., Faglioni, P., & Ferrari, C. (1980). The influence of sex and age on the incidence and type of aphasia. *Cortex, 16,* 627–630.

DeRenzi, E., Faglioni, P., & Previdi (1978). Increased susceptibility of aphasics to a distractor task in the recall of verbal commands. *Brain and Language, 6,* 14–21.

DeRenzi, E., & Ferrari, C. (1978). The Reporter's Test: A sensitive test to detect expressive disturbances in aphasics. *Cortex, 14,* 279–293.

DeRenzi, E., Motti, F., & Nichelli, P. (1980). Imitating gestures: A quantitative approach to ideomotor apraxia. *Archives of Neurology, 37,* 6–10.

DeRenzi, E., & Vignolo, L.A. (1962). The Token Test: A sensitive test to detect receptive disturbances in aphasics. *Brain, 85,* 665–678.

DeVilliers, J. (1974). Quantitative aspects of agrammatism in aphasia. *Cortex, 10,* 36–54.

Diggs, C.C., & Basili, A.G. (1987). Verbal expression of right cerebrovascular accident patients: Convergent and divergent language. *Brain and Language, 30,* 130–146.

Diesdfeldt, H.F.A. (1989). Semantic impairment in senile dementia of the Alzheimer type. *Aphasiology, 3,* 41–54.

DiSimoni, F., Keith, R.L., Holt, D.L., & Darley, F.L. (1975). Practicality of shortening the Porch Index of Communicative Ability. *Journal of Speech and Hearing Research, 18,* 491–497.

DiSimoni, F., Keith, R.L., & Darley, F.L. (1980). Prediction of PICA overall score by short versions of the test. *Journal of Speech and Hearing Research, 23,* 511–516.

Dosher, B.A., & Corbett, A.T. (1982). Instrument inferences and verb schemata. *Memory & Cognition, 10,* 531–539.

Doyle, P.J., & Goldstein, H. (1985). Experimental analysis of acquisition and generalization of syntax in Broca's aphasia. In R.H. Brookshire (Ed.), *Clinical aphasiology* (Vol. 15) (pp. 205–213). Minneapolis: BRK.

Doyle P.J., Goldstein, H., & Bourgeois, M.S. (1987). Experimental analysis of syntax training in Broca's aphasia: A generalization and social validation study. *Journal of Speech and Hearing Disorders, 52,* 143–155.

Duffy, J.R. (1986). Schuell's stimulation approach to rehabilitation. In R. Chapey (Ed.), *Language intervention strategies in adult aphasia* (Second Edition) (pp. 187–214). Baltimore: Williams & Wilkins.

Duffy, J.R., & Dale, B.J. (1977). The PICA scoring scale: Do its statistical shortcomings cause clinical problems? In R.H. Brookshire (Ed.), *Clinical aphasiology conference proceedings* (pp. 290–296). Minneapolis: BRK.

Duffy, J.R., & Duffy, R.J. (1989). The limb apraxia test: An imitative measure of upper limb apraxia. In T.E. Prescott (Ed.), *Clinical aphasiology* (Vol. 18) (pp. 145–160). Boston: College-Hill/Little, Brown.

Duffy, J.R., Duffy, R.J., & Uryase, D. (1989). The limb apraxia test: Development of a short form. In T.E. Prescott (Ed.), *Clinical aphasiology* (Vol. 18) (pp. 161–172). Boston: College-Hill/Little, Brown.

Duffy J.R., Keith R.L., Shane, H., & Podraza, B.L. (1976). Performance of normal (non-brain-injured) adults on the Porch Index of Communicative Ability. In R.H. Brookshire (Ed.), *Clinical aphasiology conference proceedings* (p. 32–42). Minneapolis: BRK.

Duffy, J.R., & Liles, B.Z. (1979). A translation of Finkelnberg's (1870) lecture on aphasia as "asymbolia" with commentary. *Journal of Speech and Hearing Disorders, 44,* 156–168.

Duffy, J.R., & Peterson, R.C. (1992). Primary progressive aphasia. *Aphasiology, 6,* 1–16.

Duffy, R.J., & Buck, R. (1979). A study of the relationship between propositional (pantomime) and subpropositional (facial expression) extraverbal behaviors in aphasics. *Folia Phoniatrica, 31,* 129–136.

Duffy, R.J., & Duffy, J.R. (1981). Three studies of deficits in pantomimic expression and pantomimic recognition in aphasia. *Journal of Speech and Hearing Research, 24,* 70–84.

Duffy, R.J., & Duffy, J.R. (1984). *Assessment of Nonverbal Communication.* Tigard, OR: C.C. Publications.

Duffy, R.J., Duffy, J.R., & Pearson, K. (1975). Pantomime recognition in aphasia. *Journal of Speech and Hearing Research, 18,* 115–132.

Duffy, R.J., & Ulrich, S.R. (1976). A comparison of impairments in verbal comprehension, speech, reading, and writing in adult aphasics. *Journal of Speech and Hearing Disorders, 41,* 110–119.

Dumond, D.L., Hardy, J.C., & Van Demark, A.A. (1978). Presentation by order of difficulty of test tasks to persons with aphasia. *Journal of Speech and Hearing Research, 21,* 350–360.

Duncan, J. (1986). Disorganisation of behaviour after frontal lobe damage. *Cognitive Neuropsychology, 3,* 271–290.

Eddy, J., & Glass, A. (1981). Reading and listening to high and low imagery sentences. *Journal of Verbal Learning and Verbal Behavior, 20,* 333–345.

Edelman, G. (1987). Global aphasia: The case for treatment. *Aphasiology, 1,* 75–80.

EDELSTEIN, B.A., & COUTURE, E.T. (EDS.). (1984). *Behavioral assessment and rehabilitation of the traumatically brain-damaged.* New York: Plenum Press.

EDWARDS, B. (1989). *Drawing on the right side of the brain* (Revised Edition). Lost Angeles: Tarcher.

EHRLICH, J.S. (1988). Selective characteristics of narrative discourse in head-injured and normal adults. *Journal of Communication Disorders,* 21, 1–9.

EHRLICH, K. (1980). Comprehension of pronouns. *Quarterly Journal of Experimental Psychology,* 32, 247–255.

EHRLICH, K., & RAYNER, K. (1983). Pronoun assignment and semantic integration during reading: Eye movements and immediacy of processing. *Journal of Verbal Learning and Verbal Behavior,* 22, 75–87.

EISENSON, J. (1954). *Examining for aphasia.* New York: The Psychological Corporation.

EISENSON, J. (1962). Language and intellectual findings associated with right cerebral damage. *Language and Speech,* 5, 49–53.

EISENSON, J. (1984). *Adult aphasia* (Second Edition). Englewood Cliffs, NJ: Prentice-Hall.

ELLIS, A.W., FLUDE, B.M., & YOUNG, A.W. (1987). "Neglect dyslexia" and the early visual processing of letters in words and nonwords. *Cognitive Neuropsychology,* 4, 439–464.

ELLIS, A.W., MILLER, D., & SIN, G. (1983). Wernicke's aphasia and normal language processing: A case study in cognitive neuropsychology. *Cognition,* 15, 111–114.

ELLIS, A.W., & SHEPHERD, J.W. (1974). Recognition of abstract and concrete words presented in the left and right visual fields. *Journal of Experimental Psychology,* 103, 1035–1036.

ELLIS, A.W., & YOUNG, A.W. (1988). *Human cognitive neuropsychology.* London: Erlbaum.

ELMORE-NICHOLAS, L., & BROOKSHIRE, R.H. (1981). Effects of pictures and picturability on sentence verification by aphasic and nonaphasic subjects. *Journal of Speech and Hearing Research,* 24, 292–297.

EMERICK, L.L., & HATTEN, J.T. (1979). *Diagnosis and evaluation in speech pathology* (Second Edition). Englewood Cliffs, N.J.: Prentice-Hall.

EMMOREY, K.D. (1987). The neurological substrates for prosodic aspects of speech. *Brain and Language,* 30, 305–320.

EMMOREY, K.D. (1989). Auditory morphological priming in the lexicon. *Language and Cognitive Processes,* 4, 73–92.

ENGUM, E.S., PENDERGRASS, T.M., CRON, L., LAMBERT, E.W., & HULSE, C.K. (1988). Cognitive Behavioral Driver's Inventory. *Cognitive Rehabilitation,* 6(5), 34–50.

ERNEST-BARON, C.R., BROOKSHIRE, R.H., & NICHOLAS, L.E. (1987). Story structure and retelling of narratives by aphasic and non-brain-damaged adults. *Journal of Speech and Hearing Research,* 30, 44–49.

EYSENCK, M.W., & KEANE, M.T. (1990). *Cognitive psychology: A student's handbook.* Hove, UK: Erlbaum.

FAGLIONI, P., SPINNLER, H., & VIGNOLO, L. (1969). Contrasting behavior of right and left hemisphere-damaged patients on a discriminative and a semantic task of auditory recognition. *Cortex,* 5, 366–389.

FARAH, M.J. (1988). Is a visual imagery really visual? Overlooked evidence from neuropsychology. *Psychological Review,* 95, 307–317.

FARAH, M.J., GAZZANIGA, M.S., HOLTZMAN, J.D., & KOSSLYN, S.M. (1985). A left hemisphere basis for visual mental imagery? *Neuropsychologia,* 23, 115–118.

FERREIRA, F., & CLIFTON, JR., C. (1986). The independence of syntactic processing. *Journal of Memory and Language,* 25, 348–368.

FERRO, J.M., SANTOS, M.E., CASTRO-CALDAS, A., & MARIANO, G. (1980). Gesture recognition in aphasia. *Journal of Clinical Neuropsychology,* 2, 277–292.

FEYEREISEN, P. (1991). Communicative behaviour in aphasia. *Aphasiology,* 5, 323–334.

FEYEREISEN, P., BARTER, D., GOOSENS, M., & CLEREBAUT, N. (1988). Gestures and speech referential communication by aphasic subjects: Channel use and efficiency. *Aphasiology,* 2, 21–32.

FEYEREISEN, P., & SERON, X. (1982). Nonverbal communication and aphasia: A review. I. Comprehension. *Brain and Language,* 16, 191–212.

FILLENBAUM, S., JONES, L.V., & WEPMAN, J.M. (1961). Some linguistic features of speech from aphasic patients. *Language and Speech,* 4, 91–108.

FINKE, R.A. (1989). *Principles of mental imagery.* Cambridge, MA: MIT Press.

FISCHER, S.C., & PELLEGRINO, J.W. (1988). Hemisphere differences for components of mental rotation. *Brain and Cognition,* 7, 1–15.

FISHER, C.M. (1982). Disorientation for place. *Archives of Neurology,* 39, 33–36.

FISHER, L. (1989). The emergence of microcomputer technology in neuropsychological therapies. In X. Seron, & G. Deloche, (Eds.), *Cognitive approaches in neuropsychological rehabilitation* (pp. 355–382). London: Erlbaum.

FISHMAN, S. (1988). *A bomb in the brain.* New York: Avon.

FITCH, J.L., & CROSS, S.T. (1983). Telecomputer treatment for aphasia. *Journal of Speech and Hearing Disorders,* 48, 335–336.

FITCH-WEST, J. (1983). Heightening visual imagery: A new approach to aphasia therapy. In E. Perecman (Ed.), *Cognitive processing in the right hemisphere* (pp. 215–228). New York: Academic Press.

FITCH-WEST, J., & SANDS, E.S. (1987). *Bedside Evaluation Screening Test.* Rockville, MD: Aspen.

FLEMING, R., HUBBARD, D.J., SCHINSKY, L., & DATTA, K. (1982). Consideration of PICA subtest variability in cases of aphasia secondary to blunt head trauma. In

R.H. Brookshire (Ed.), *Clinical aphasiology conference proceedings* (pp. 85–92). Minneapolis: BRK.

FLETCHER, C.R. (1981). Short-term memory processes in text comprehension. *Journal of Verbal Learning and Verbal Behavior, 20,* 564–574.

FLETCHER, C.R. (1986). Strategies for the allocation of short-term memory during comprehension. *Journal of Memory and Language, 25,* 467–486.

FLETCHER, C.R., & BLOOM, C.P. (1988). Causal reasoning in the comprehension of simple narrative texts. *Journal of Memory and Language, 27,* 235–244.

FLICKER, C., FERRIS, S.H., CROOK, T., & BARTUS, R.T. (1987). Implications of memory and language dysfunction in the naming deficit of senile dementia. *Brain and Language, 31,* 187–200.

FLOWERS, C.R., & DANFORTH, L.C. (1979). A step-wise auditory comprehension improvement program administered to aphasic patients by family members. In R.H. Brookshire (Ed.), *Clinical aphasiology conference proceedings* (pp. 196–202). Minneapolis: BRK.

FLOWERS, C.R., & WYSE, M. (1985). Assessing gestural intelligibility of normal and aphasic subjects. In R.H. Brookshire (Ed.), *Clinical aphasiology* (Vol. 15) (pp. 64–71). Minneapolis: BRK.

FLUDE, B.M., ELLIS, A.W., & KAY, J. (1989). Face processing and name retrieval in an anomic aphasic: Names are stored separately from semantic information about familiar people. *Brain and Cognition, 11,* 60–72.

FODOR, J.A. (1983). *The modularity of mind.* Cambridge, MA: Bradford/MIT Press.

FODOR, J.A., BEVER, T.G., & GARRETT, M.F. (1974). *The psychology of language: An introduction to psycholinguistics and generative grammar.* New York: McGraw-Hill.

FOLDI, N.S. (1987). Appreciation of pragmatic interpretations of indirect commands: Comparison of right and left hemisphere brain-damaged patients. *Brain and Language, 31,* 88–108.

FOLSTEIN, M.F., FOLSTEIN, S.E., & MCHUGH, P.R. (1975). "Mini-mental state": A practical method for grading the mental state of patients for the clinician. *Journal of Psychiatric Research, 12,* 189–198.

FORSTER, K.I., & CHAMBERS, S.M. (1973). Lexical access and naming time. *Journal of Verbal Learning and Verbal Behavior, 12,* 627–635.

FOSS, D.J. (1969). Decision processes during sentence comprehension: Effects of lexical item difficulty and position upon decision times. *Journal of Verbal Learning and Verbal Behavior, 8,* 457–462.

FOSS, D.J. (1970). Some effects of ambiguity on sentence comprehension. *Journal of Verbal Learning and Verbal Behavior, 9,* 699–706.

FOSS, D.J., & HAKES, D.T. (1978). *Psycholinguistics: An introduction to the psychology of language.* Englewood Cliffs, NJ: Prentice-Hall.

FRANCIK, E.P., & CLARK, H.H. (1985). How to make requests that overcome obstacles to compliance. *Journal of Memory and Language, 24,* 560–568.

FRANGICETTO, T. (1989). Northampton Community College: Cognitive retraining program. *Cognitive Rehabilitation, 7*(6), 10–16.

FRANKLIN, S. (1989). Dissociations in auditory word comprehension; evidence from nine fluent aphasic patients. *Aphasiology, 3,* 189–208.

FRATTALI, C.M. (1992). Functional assessment of communication: Merging public policy with clinical views. *Aphasiology, 6,* 63–84.

FRAZIER, L., & FRIEDERICI, A. (1991). On deriving the properties of agrammatic comprehension. *Brain and Language, 40,* 51–66.

FRAZIER, L., & RAYNER, K. (1982). Making and correcting errors during sentence comprehension: Eye movements in the analysis of structurally ambiguous sentences. *Cognitive Psychology, 14,* 178–210.

FREEDMAN, M., & CERMAK, L.S. (1986). Semantic encoding deficits in frontal lobe disease and amnesia. *Brain and Cognition, 5,* 108–114.

FRIEDERICI, A.D. (1982). Syntactic and semantic processes in aphasic deficits: The availability of prepositions. *Brain and Language, 15,* 249–258.

FRIEDERICI, A.D. (1983). Aphasics' perception of words in sentential context: Some real-time processing evidence. *Neuropsychologia, 21,* 351–358.

FRIEDERICI, A.D. (1988). Agrammatic comprehension: Picture of a computational mismatch. *Aphasiology, 2,* 279–284.

FRIEDERICI, A.D., & GRAETZ, P.A.M. (1987). Processing passive sentences in aphasia: Deficits and strategies. *Brain and Language, 30,* 93–105.

FRIEDRICH, F.J., GLENN, C.G., & MARIN, O.S.M. (1984). Interruption of phonological coding in conduction aphasia. *Brain and Language, 22,* 266–291.

FRIEDRICH, F.J., MARTIN, R., & KEMPER, S.J. (1985). Consequences of a phonological coding deficit on sentence processing. *Cognitive Neuropsychology, 2,* 385–412.

FROMKIN, V., & RODMAN, R. (1988). *An introduction to language* (Fourth Edition). New York: Holt, Rinehart and Winston.

FROMM, D., & HOLLAND, A.L. (1989). Functional communication in Alzheimer's disease. *Journal of Speech and Hearing Disorders, 54,* 535–540.

FUNNELL, E., & ALLPORT, A. (1989). Symbolically speaking: Communicating with Blissymbols in Aphasia. *Aphasiology, 3,* 279–300.

GADDIE, A., NAESER, M.A., PALUMBO, C.L., & STIASSNY-EDER, D. (1989). Recovery of auditory comprehension after one year: A computed tomography scan study. In T.E. Prescott (Ed.), *Clinical aphasiology* (Vol. 18) (pp. 463–478). Boston: College-Hill/Little, Brown.

GADO, M.H., COLEMAN, R.E., MERLIS, A.L., ALDERSON,

P.O., & LEE, K.S. (1976). Comparison of CT and RN imaging in "stroke." *Stroke,* 7, 109–113.

GAINOTTI, G. (1972). Emotional behavior and hemispheric side of lesion. *Cortex,* 8, 41–55.

GAINOTTI, G. (1976). The relationship between semantic impairment in comprehension and naming in aphasic patients. *British Journal of Disorders of Communication,* 11, 57–61.

GAINOTTI, G., CALTAGIRONE, C., & IBBA, A. (1975). Semantic and phonemic aspects of auditory language comprehension in aphasia. *Linguistics,* 154/5, 15–29.

GAINOTTI, G., CALTAGIRONE, C., & MICELI, G. (1983). Selective impairment of semantic-lexical discrimination in right-brain-damaged patients. In E. Perecman (Ed.), *Cognitive processing in the right hemisphere* (pp. 149–167). New York: Academic Press.

GAINOTTI, G., CARLOMAGNO, S., CRACA, A., & SILVERI, M.C. (1986). Disorders of classificatory activity in aphasia. *Brain and Language,* 28, 181–195.

GAINOTTI, G., & LEMMO, M.A. (1976). Comprehension of symbolic gestures in aphasia. *Brain and Language,* 3, 451–460.

GALABURDA, A.M. (1984). The anatomy of language: Lessons from comparative anatomy. In D. Caplan, A.R. Lecours, & A. Smith (Eds.), *Biological perspectives on language* (pp. 290–302). Cambridge, MA: MIT Press.

GALIN, D. (1976). The two modes of consciousness and the two halves of the brain. In P.R. Lee, R.E. Ornstein, D. Galin, A. Deikman, & C.T. Tart, *Symposium on consciousness.* New York: Penguin.

GALIN, D., JOHNSTONE, J. & HERRON, J. (1978). Effects of task difficulty on EEG measures of cerebral engagement. *Neuropsychologia,* 16, 461–472.

GALLAHER, A.J. (1979). Temporal reliability of aphasic performance on the Token Test. *Brain and Language,* 7, 34–41.

GALLAHER, A.J. (1981). Syntactic versus semantic performances of agrammatic Broca's aphasics on tests of constituent-element-ordering. *Journal of Speech and Hearing Research,* 24, 217–223.

GALLAHER, A.J., & CANTER, G.J. (1982). Reading and listening comprehension in Broca's aphasia: Lexical versus syntactical errors. *Brain and Language,* 17, 183–192.

GANDOUR, J., & DARDARANANDA, R. (1982). Voice onset time in aphasia: Thai. I. Perception. *Brain and Language,* 17, 24–33.

GANDOUR, J., & DARDARANANDA, R. (1983). Identification of tonal contrasts in Thai aphasic patients. *Brain and Language,* 18, 98–114.

GANDOUR, J., PETTY, S.H., & DARDARANANDA, R. (1988). Perception and production of tone in aphasia. *Brain and Language,* 35, 201–240.

GARDNER, H. (1973). The contribution of operativity to naming capacity in aphasic patients. *Neuropsychologia,* 11, 213–220.

GARDNER, H. (1974). *The shattered mind.* New York: Vintage Books.

GARDNER, H. (1982). *Art, mind, and brain: A cognitive approach to creativity.* New York: Basic Books.

GARDNER, H. (1983). *Frames of mind: The theory of multiple intelligences.* New York: Basic Books.

GARDNER, H. (1985). *The mind's new science: A history of the cognitive revolution.* New York: Basic Books.

GARDNER, H., BROWNELL, H.H. WAPNER, W., & MICHELOW, D. (1983). Missing the point: The role of the right hemisphere in the processing of complex linguistic materials. In E. Perecman (Ed.). (1983), *Cognitive processing in the right hemisphere* (pp. 169–191). New York: Academic Press.

GARDNER, H., & DENES, G. (1973). Connotative judgments by aphasic patients on a pictorial adaptation of the semantic differential. *Cortex,* 9, 183–196.

GARDNER, H., DENES, G., & ZURIF, E.B. (1975). Critical reading at the sentence level in aphasics. *Cortex,* 11, 60–72.

GARDNER, H., LING, P.K., FLAMM, L., & SILVERMAN, J. (1975). Comprehension and appreciation of humorous material following brain damage. *Brain,* 98, 399–412.

GARDNER, H., ZURIF, E.G., BERRY, T., & BAKER, E. (1976). Visual communication in aphasia. *Neuropsychologia,* 14, 275–292.

GARNHAM, A. (1985). *Psycholinguistics: Central Topics.* London: Methuen.

GARRETT, M.F. (1982). Production of speech: Observations from normal and pathological language use. In A.W. Ellis (Ed.), *Normality and pathology in cognitive functions* (pp. 49–68). London: Academic Press.

GARRETT, M.F. (1984). The organization of processing structure for language production: Applications to aphasic speech. In D. Caplan, A.R. Lecours, & A. Smith (Eds.), *Biological perspectives on language* (pp. 172–193). Cambridge, MA: MIT Press.

GARROD, S., & SANFORD, A. (1977). Interpreting anaphoric relations: The integration of semantic information while reading. *Journal of Verbal Learning and Verbal Behavior,* 16, 77–90.

GATES, A., & BRADSHAW, J.L. (1977). The role of the cerebral hemispheres in music. *Brain and Language,* 4, 403–431.

GAZZANIGA, M.S. (1970). *The bisected brain.* New York: Appleton-Century-Crofts.

GAZZANIGA, M.S. (1974). Determinants of cerebral recovery. In D.G. Stein, J.J. Rosen, & N. Butters (Eds.), *Plasticity and recovery of function in the central nervous system* (pp. 203–215). New York: Academic Press.

GAZZANIGA, M.S., & SMYLIE, C.S. (1984). Dissociation of language and cognition. *Brain,* 107, 145–153.

GENTILINI, M., FAGLIONI, P., & DeRENZI, E. (1988). Are body part names selectively disrupted by aphasia? *Aphasiology,* 2, 567–576.

GESCHWIND, N. (1965). Disconnexion syndromes in animals and man. *Brain*, 88, 237–294, 585–644.

GESCHWIND, N. (1967). The varieties of naming errors. *Cortex*, 3, 96–112.

GESCHWIND, N. (1979). Specializations of the human brain. *Scientific American*, 241, 180–199.

GEWIRTH, L.R., SHINDLER, A.G., & HIER, D.B. (1984). Altered patterns of word associations in dementia and aphasia. *Brain and Language*, 21, 307–317.

GIBBS, JR., R.W. (1986). What makes some indirect speech acts conventional? *Journal of Memory and Language*, 25, 181–196.

GIBBS, JR., R.W., NAYAK, N.P., & CUTTING, C. (1989). How to kick the bucket and not decompose: Analyzability and idiom processing. *Journal of Memory and Language*, 28, 576–593.

GLASS, A.L., MILLEN, D.R., BECK, L.G., & EDDY, J.K. (1985). Representation of images in sentence verification. *Journal of Memory and Language*, 24, 442–465.

GLASS, A.V., GAZZANIGA, M.S., & PREMACK, D. (1973). Artificial language training in global aphasia. *Neuropsychologia*, 11, 95–103.

GLASSMAN, R.B. (1978). The logic of the lesion experiment and its role in the neural sciences. In S. Finger (Ed.), *Recovery from brain damage: Research and theory*. New York: Plenum Press.

GLEASON, J.B., GOODGLASS, H., GREEN, E., ACKERMAN, N., & HYDE, M.R. (1975). The retrieval of syntax in Broca's aphasia. *Brain and Language*, 2, 451–471.

GLEASON, J.B., GOODGLASS, H., OBLER, L., GREEN, E., HYDE, M.R., & WEINTRAUB, S. (1980). Narrative strategies of aphasic and normal-speaking subjects. *Journal of Speech and Hearing Research*, 23, 370–382.

GLINDEMANN, R., WILLMES, K., HUBER, W., & SPRINGER, L. (1991). The efficacy of modeling in PACE-therapy. *Aphasiology*, 5, 425–430.

GLONING, K., TRAPPL, R., HEISS, W., & QUATMEMBER, R. (1976). Prognosis and speech therapy in aphasia. In Y. Lebrun & R. Hoops (Eds.), *Recovery in aphasics* (pp. 57–64). Amsterdam: Swets & Zeitlinger.

GLOSSER, G., & DESER, T. (1991). Patterns of discourse production among neurological patients with fluent language disorders. *Brain and Language*, 40, 67–88.

GLOSSER, G., WIENER, M., & KAPLAN, E. (1986). Communicative gestures in aphasia. *Brain and Language*, 27, 345–359.

GLUCKSBERG, S., GILDEA, P., & BOOKIN, H.A. (1982). On understanding nonliteral speech: Can people ignore metaphors? *Journal of Verbal Learning and Verbal Behavior*, 21, 85–98.

GOBBLE, E.M., DUNSON, L., SZEKERES, S.F., & CORNWALL, J. (1987). Avocational programming for the severely impaired head injured individual. In M. Ylvisaker & E.M. Gobble (Eds.), *Community re-entry for head injured adults* (pp. 349–380). Boston: College-Hill/Little, Brown.

GODFREY, C.M., & DOUGLASS, E. (1959). The recovery process in aphasia. *Canadian Medical Association Journal*, 80, 618–624.

GOLDEN, C.J. (1984). Rehabilitation and the Luria-Nebraska Neuropsychological Battery: Introduction to theory and practice. In B.A. Edelstein & E.T. Couture (Eds.), *Behavioral assessment and rehabilitation of the traumatically brain-damaged* (pp. 83–120). New York: Plenum.

GOLDEN, C.J., HEMMEKE, T.A., & PURISCH, A.D. (1980). *The Luria-Nebraska Neuropsychological Battery*. Los Angeles: Western Psychological Services.

GOLDENBERG, G., & ARTNER, C. (1991). Visual imagery and knowledge about the visual appearance of objects in patients with posterior cerebral artery lesions. *Brain and Cognition*, 15, 160–186.

GOLDSTEIN, F.A., & LEVIN, H.S. (1991). Question-asking strategies after severe closed head injury. *Brain and Cognition*, 17, 23–30.

GOLDSTEIN, K. (1942). *Aftereffects of brain injuries in war*. New York: Grune & Stratton.

GOLDSTEIN, K. (1948). *Language and language disturbances*. New York: Grune & Stratton.

GOLPER, L.A.C., RAU, M.T., ERKSINE, B., LANGHANS, J.J., & HOULIHAN, J. (1987). Aphasic patients' performance on a mental status examination. In R.H. Brookshire (Ed.), *Clinical aphasiology* (Vol. 17) (pp. 124–136). Minneapolis: BRK.

GOODENOUGH, C., ZURIF, E.B., WEINTRAUB, S., & VON STOCKERT, T. (1977). Aphasics' attention to grammatical morphemes. *Language and Speech*, 20, 11–19.

GOODGLASS, H. (1976). Agrammatism. In H. Whitaker & H.A. Whitaker (Eds.), *Studies in neurolinguistics* (Vol. 1) (pp. 237–260). New York: Academic Press.

GOODGLASS, H. (1989). Commentary: Cognitive psychology and clinical aphasiology. *Aphasiology*, 4, 93–97.

GOODGLASS, H., & BAKER, E. (1976). Semantic field, naming, and auditory comprehension in aphasia. *Brain and Language*, 3, 359–374.

GOODGLASS, H., BARTON, M.I., & KAPLAN, E.F. (1968). Sensory modality and object-naming in aphasics. *Journal of Speech and Hearing Research*, 11, 488–496.

GOODGLASS, H., & BERKO, J. (1960). Agrammatism and inflectional morphology in English. *Journal of Speech and Hearing Research*, 3, 257–267.

GOODGLASS, H., BLUMSTEIN, S.E., GLEASON, J.B., HYDE, M.R., GREEN, E., & STATLENDER, S. (1979). The effect of syntactic encoding on sentence comprehension in aphasia. *Brain and Language*, 7, 201–209.

GOODGLASS, H., FODOR, I.G., & SCHULHOFF, C. (1967). Prosodic factors in grammar–evidence from aphasia. *Journal of Speech and Hearing Research*, 10, 5–20.

GOODGLASS, H., & GESCHWIND, N. (1976). Language disorders (aphasia). In E.C. Carterette & M.P. Friedman (Eds.), *Handbook of perception* (Vol. VII) (pp. 390–428). New York: Academic Press.

GOODGLASS, H., HYDE, M.R., BLUMSTEIN, S. (1969). Frequency, picturability and availability of nouns in aphasia. *Cortex, 5,* 104–119.

GOODGLASS, H., & KAPLAN, E. (1983). *The assessment of aphasia and related disorders* (Second Edition). Philadelphia: Lea & Febiger.

GOODGLASS, H., KAPLAN, E., WEINTRAUB, S., & ACKERMAN, N. (1976). The "tip-of-the-tongue" phenomenon in aphasia. *Cortex, 12,* 145–153.

GOODGLASS, H., KLEIN, B., CAREY, P.W., & JONES, K.J. (1966). Specific semantic word categories in aphasia. *Cortex, 2,* 74–89.

GOODGLASS, H., & MENN, L. (1985). Is agrammatism a unitary phenomenon? In M-L. Kean (Ed.), *Agrammatism* (pp. 1–26). Orlando, FL: Academic Press.

GOODGLASS, H., QUADFASEL, F.A., & TIMBERLAKE, W.H. (1964). Phrase length and the type and severity of aphasia. *Cortex, 1,* 133–153.

GOODGLASS, H., & STUSS, D.T. (1979). Naming to picture versus description in three aphasic subgroups. *Cortex, 15,* 199–211.

GOODMAN, R.A., & WHITAKER, H.A. (1985). Hemispherectomy: A review (1928–1981) with special reference to the linguistic abilities and disabilities of the residual right hemisphere. In C.T. Best (Ed.), *Hemispheric function and collaboration in the child* (pp. 121–156). Orlando, FL: Academic Press.

GOODSPEED, B.W. (1983). *The Tao Jones averages: A guide to whole-brained investing.* New York: Dutton.

GORDON, B., & CARAMAZZA, A. (1983). Closed- and open-class lexical access in agrammatic and fluent aphasics. *Brain and Language, 19,* 335–345.

GORDON, H.W. (1978). Left hemisphere dominance for rhythmic elements in dichotically-presented melodies. *Cortex, 14,* 58–70.

GORELICK, P.B., HIER, D.B., BENEVENTO, L., LEVITT, S., & TAN, W. (1984). Aphasia after left thalamic infarction. *Archives of Neurology, 41,* 1296–1298.

GRAF, P., & SCHACTER, D. (1985). Implicit and explicit memory for new associations in normal and amnesic subjects. *Journal of Experimental Psychology: Learning, Memory and Cognition, 11,* 501–518.

GRANT, D.A., & BERG, E.A. (1948). A behavioral analysis of degree of reinforcement and ease of shifting to new responses in a Weigl-type card-sorting problem. *Journal of Experimental Psychology, 38,* 404–411.

GRAVES, R., LANDIS, T., & GOODGLASS, H. (1981). Laterality and sex differences for visual recognition of emotional and non-emotional words. *Neuropsychologia, 19,* 95–102.

GREITEMANN, G., & WOLF, E. (1991). Making dynamic use of different modes of expression: The efficacy of the PACE-approach. Paper presented to the Academy of Aphasia, Rome.

GRICE, L.P. (1975). Logic and conversation. In P. Cole & J.L. Morgan (Ed.), *Syntax and semantics: Speech acts* (Vol. 3) (pp. 41–58). New York: Academic Press.

GROBER, E., BUSCHKE, H., KAWAS, C., & FULD, P. (1985).

Impaired ranking of semantic attributes in dementia. *Brain and Language, 26,* 276–286.

GROBER, E., PERECMAN, E., KELLAR, L., & BROWN, J. (1980). Lexical knowledge in anterior and posterior aphasics. *Brain and Language, 10,* 318–330.

GRODZINSKY, Y. (1984). The syntactic characterization of agrammatism. *Cognition, 16,* 99–120.

GRODINSKY, Y. (1986). Language deficits and the theory of syntax. *Brain and Language, 27,* 135–159.

GRODZINSKY, Y. (1989). Agrammatic comprehension of relative clauses. *Brain and Language, 37,* 480–499.

GRODZINSKY, Y. (1991). There is an entity called agrammatic aphasia. *Brain and Language, 41,* 555–564.

GRODZINSKY, Y., & MAREK, A. (1988). Algorithmic and heuristic processes revisited. *Brain and Language, 33,* 216–225.

GRODZINSKY, Y., SWINNEY, D., & ZURIF, E. (1985). Agrammatism: Structural deficits and antecedent processing disruptions. In M-L. Kean (Ed.), *Agrammatism* (pp. 65–81). Orlando, FL: Academic Press.

GROHER, M. (1977). Language and memory disorders following closed head trauma. *Journal of Speech and Hearing Research, 20,* 212–223.

GROSJEAN, F. (1982). *Life with two languages: An introduction to bilingualism.* Cambridge, MA: Harvard University Press.

GROSJEAN, F. (1985). Polyglot aphasics and language mixing: A comment on Perecman (1984). *Brain and Language, 26,* 349–355.

GROSJEAN, F. (1989). Neurolinguists, beware! The bilingual is not two monolinguals in one person. *Brain and Language, 36,* 3–15.

GROSSI, D., ORSINI, A., & MODAFFERI, A. (1986). Visuo-imaginal constructional apraxia: On a case of selective deficit of imagery. *Brain and Cognition, 5,* 255–267.

GROSSMAN, M. (1981). A bird is a bird is a bird: Making reference within and without superordinate categories. *Brain and Language, 12,* 313–331.

GROSSMAN, M. (1988). Drawing deficits in brain-damaged patients' freehand pictures. *Brain and Cognition, 8,* 189–205.

GROSSMAN, M., CAREY, S., ZURIF, E., & DILLER, L. (1986). Proper and common nouns: Form class judgments in Broca's aphasia. *Brain and Language, 28,* 114–125.

GROSSMAN, M., & HABERMAN, S. (1982). Aphasics' selective deficits in appreciating grammatical agreements. *Brain and Language, 16,* 109–120.

GROSSMAN, M., & WILSON, M. (1987). Stimulus categorization by brain-damaged patients. *Brain and Cognition, 6,* 55–71.

GRUBB, R.L., & COXE, W.S. (1978). Central nervous system trauma: Cranial. In S.G. Eliasson, A.L. Prensky, & W.B. Hardin (Eds.), *Neurological pathophysiology* (Second Edition) (pp. 329–347). New York: Oxford University Press.

GRUEN, A.K., FRANKLE, B.C., & SCHWARTZ, R. (1990). Word fluency generation skills of head-injured patients in an acute trauma center. *Journal of Communication Disorders, 23,* 163–170.

GURLAND, G., CHWAT, S., & WOLLNER, S. (1982). Establishing a communication profile in adult aphasia: Analysis of communicative acts and conversational sequences. In R.H. Brookshire (Ed.), *Clinical aphasiology conference proceedings* (pp. 18–27). Minneapolis: BRK.

HAARMANN, H.J., & KOLK, H.H.J. (1991). Syntactic priming in Broca's aphasics: Evidence for slow activation. *Aphasiology, 5,* 247–264.

HABERLANDT, K.F., & GRAESSER, A.C. (1990). Integration and buffering of new information. In A.C. Graesser & G.H. Bower (Eds.), *Inferences and text comprehension* (pp. 71–88). San Diego: Academic Press.

HAGEMAN, C.F., & FOLKESTAD, A. (1986). Performance of aphasic listeners on an expanded Revised Token Test subtest presented verbally and nonverbally. In R.H. Brookshire (Ed.), *Clinical aphasiology* (Vol. 16) (pp. 227–233). Minneapolis: BRK.

HAGEMAN, C.F., & LEWIS, D.L. (1983). The effects of intrastimulus pause on the quality of auditory comprehension in aphasia. In R.H. Brookshire (Ed.), *Clinical aphasiology conference proceedings* (pp. 177–185). Minneapolis, MN: BRK.

HAGEMAN, C.F., MCNEIL, M., RUCCI-ZIMMER, S., & CARISKI, D. (1982). The reliability of patterns of auditory processing deficits: Evidence from the Revised Token Test. In R.H. Brookshire (Ed.), *Clinical aphasiology conference proceedings* (pp. 230–234). Minneapolis: BRK.

HAGEN, C. (1973). Communication abilities in hemiplegia: Effect of speech therapy. *Archives of Physical Medicine and Rehabilitation, 54,* 454–463.

HAGEN, C. (1981). Language disorders secondary to closed head injury: Diagnosis and treatment. *Topics in Language Disorders, 1,* 73–87.

HAGEN, C. (1984). Language disorders in head trauma. In A.L. Holland (Ed.), *Language disorders in adults: Recent advances* (pp. 245–282). San Diego: College-Hill.

HAGIWARA, H., & CAPLAN, D. (1990). Syntactic comprehension in Japanese aphasics: Effects of category and thematic role order. *Brain and Language, 38,* 159–170.

HAGOORT, P. (1989). Processing of lexical ambiguities: A comment on Milberg, Blumstein, and Dworetzky (1987). *Brain and Language, 36,* 335–348.

HAKUTA, K. (1986). *Mirror of language: The debate on bilingualism.* New York: Basic Books.

HALLIDAY, M.A.K. (1985). *An introduction to functional grammar.* London: Edward Arnold.

HALPERN, H., DARLEY, F.L., & BROWN, J.R. (1973). Differential language and neurologic characteristics in cerebral involvement. *Journal of Speech and Hearing Disorders, 38,* 162–173.

HALSEY, J.H., BLAUENSTEIN, U.W., WILSON, E.M., & WILLS, E.L. (1980). Brain activation in the presence of brain damage. *Brain and Language, 9,* 47–60.

HALSTEAD, W.C., & WEPMAN, J.M. (1949). The Halstead-Wepman aphasia screening test. *Journal of Speech and Hearing Disorders, 14,* 9–15.

HANLEY, J.R., YOUNG, A.W., & PEARSON, N.A. (1989). Defective recognition of familiar people. *Cognitive Neuropsychology, 6,* 179–210.

HANLON, R.E., BROWN, J.W., & GERSTMAN, L.J. (1990). Enhancement of naming in nonfluent aphasia through gesture. *Brain and Language, 38,* 298–314.

HANSON, W.R., & CICCIARELLI, A.W. (1978). The time, amount, and pattern of language improvement in adult aphasics. *British Journal of Disorders of Communication, 13,* 59–63.

HANSON, W.R., METTER, E.J., & RIEGE, W.H. (1989). The course of chronic aphasia. *Aphasiology, 3,* 19–30.

HARASYMIW, S.J., HALPER, A., & SUTHERLAND, B. (1981). Sex, age, and aphasia type. *Brain and Language, 12,* 190–198.

HARRIS L.J. (1985). Teaching the right brain: Historical perspective on a contemporary educational fad. In C.T. Best (Ed.), *Hemispheric function and collaboration in the child* (pp. 231–274). Orlando, FL: Academic Press.

HART, J., BERNDT, R.S., & CARAMAZZA, A. (1985). Category-specific naming deficit following cerebral infarction. *Nature, 316,* 439–440.

HART, R.P., KWENTUS, J.A., HARKINS, S.W., & TAYLOR, J.R. (1988). Rate of forgetting in mild Alzheimer's type dementia. *Brain and Cognition, 7,* 31–38.

HARTJE, W., KERSCHENSTEINER, M., POECK, K., & ORGASS, B. (1973). A cross-validation study on the Token Test. *Neuropsychologia, 11,* 119–121.

HARTLEY, L.L., & LEVIN, H.S. (1990). Linguistic deficits after closed head injury: A current appraisal. *Aphasiology, 4,* 353–370.

HARTMAN, J. (1981). Measurement of early spontaneous recovery of aphasia with stroke. *Annals of Neurology, 9,* 89–91.

HATFIELD, F.M., HOWARD, D., BARBER, J., JONES, C., & MORTON, J. (1977). Object naming in aphasics: The lack of effect of context or realism. *Neuropsychologia, 15,* 717–728.

HATFIELD, G. (1988). Neuro-philosophy meets psychology: Reduction, autonomy, and physiological constraints. *Cognitive Neuropsychology, 5,* 723–746.

HAUT, M.W., PETROS, T.V., FRANK, R.G., & HAUT, J.S. (1991). Speed of processing within semantic memory following severe closed head injury. *Brain and Cognition, 17,* 31–41.

HAYNES, W.O., & ORATIO, A.R. (1978). A study of clients' perceptions of therapeutic effectiveness. *Journal of Speech and Hearing Disorders, 43,* 21–33.

HEAD, H. (1920). Aphasia and kindred disorders of speech. *Brain, 43,* 87–165.

HEAD, H. (1926). *Aphasia and kindred disorders of speech* (2 Vols.). London: Cambridge University Press.

HEBB, D.O. (1949). *The organization of behavior.* New York: Wiley.

HEESCHEN, C. (1980). Strategies of decoding actor-object relations by aphasic patients. *Cortex, 16,* 5–19.

HEESCHEN, C. (1985). Agrammatism versus paragrammatism: A fictitious opposition. In M-L. Kean (Ed.), *Agrammatism* (pp. 207–248). Orlando, FL: Academic Press.

HEESCHEN, C., & KOLK, H. (1988). Agrammatism and paragrammatism. *Aphasiology, 2,* 299–302.

HEILMAN, K.M., BOWERS, D., SPEEDIE, L., & COSLETT, H.B. (1984). Comprehension of affective and non-affective prosody. *Neurology, 34,* 917–921.

HEILMAN, K.M., ROTHI, L., CAMPANELLA, D., & WOLFSON, S. (1979). Wernicke's and global aphasia without alexia. *Archives of Neurology, 36,* 129–133.

HEILMAN, K.M., SAFRAN, A., & GESCHWIND, N. (1971). Closed head trauma and aphasia. *Journal of Neurology, Neurosurgery, and Psychiatry, 34,* 265–269.

HEILMAN, K.M., & SCHOLES, R.J. (1976). The nature of comprehension errors in Broca's, conduction and Wernicke's aphasics. *Cortex, 12,* 258–265.

HEILMAN, K.M., SCHWARTZ, H.D., & WATSON, R.T. (1978). Hypoarousal in patients with the neglect syndrome and emotional indifference. *Neurology, 28,* 229–232.

HEILMAN, K.M., & VALENSTEIN, E. (EDS.) (1985). *Clinical neuropsychology* (Second Edition). New York: Oxford University Press.

HIELMAN, K.M., WATSON R.T., & VALENSTEIN, E. (1985). Neglect and related disorders. In K.M. Heilman & E. Valenstein (Eds.), *Clinical neuropsychology* (Second Edition) (pp. 243–293). New York: Oxford University Press.

HELM, N.A., & BARRESI, B. (1980). Voluntary control of involuntary utterances: A treatment approach for severe aphasia. In R.H. Brookshire (Ed.), *Clinical aphasiology conference proceedings* (pp. 308–315). Minneapolis: BRK.

HELM-ESTABROOKS, N. (1981). *Helm Elicited Language Program for Syntax Stimulation (HELPSS).* Chicago: Riverside.

HELM-ESTABROOKS, N. (1983). Exploiting the right hemisphere for language rehabilitation: Melodic intonation therapy. In E. Perecman (Ed.), *Cognitive processing in the right hemisphere* (pp. 229–240). New York: Academic Press.

HELM-ESTABROOKS, N. (1991). *Test of Oral and Limb Apraxia (TOLA).* Chicago: Riverside.

HELM-ESTABROOKS, N., & ALBERT, M.L. (1991). *A manual of aphasia therapy.* Chicago: Riverside.

HELM-ESTABROOKS, N., FITZPATRICK, P.M., & BARRESI, B.N. (1981). Response of an agrammatic patient to a syntax stimulation program for aphasia. *Journal of Speech Hearing Disorders, 46,* 422–427.

HELM-ESTABROOKS, N., FITZPATRICK, P.M., & BARRESI, B.N. (1982). Visual action therapy for global aphasia. *Journal of Speech and Hearing Disorders, 47,* 385–389.

HELM-ESTABROOKS, N., & HOTZ, G. (1990). *Brief Test of Head Injury (BTHI).* Chicago: Riverside.

HELM-ESTABROOKS, N., NICHOLAS, M., & MORGAN, A.R. (1989). *Melodic Intonation Therapy (MIT).* Chicago: Riverside.

HELM-ESTABROOKS, N., & RAMSBERGER, G. (1986). Treatment of agrammatism in long-term Broca's aphasia. *British Journal of Disorders of Communication, 21,* 39–45.

HELM-ESTABROOKS, N., RAMSBERGER, G., MORGAN, A.R., & NICHOLAS, M. (1989). *Boston Assessment of Severe Aphasia (BASA).* Chicago: Riverside.

HENDERSON, V.W., MACK, W., FREED, D.M., KEMPLER, D., & ANDERSEN, E.S. (1990). Naming consistency in Alzheimer's disease. *Brain and Language, 39,* 530–538.

HERRMANN, M., KOCH, U., JOHANNSEN-HORBACH, H., & WALLESCH, C-W. (1989). Communicative skills in chronic and severe nonfluent aphasia. *Brain and language, 37,* 339–352.

HERRMANN, M., & WALLESCH, C.W. (1989). Psychosocial changes and psychosocial adjustment with chronic and severe nonfluent aphasia. *Aphasiology, 3,* 513–526.

HERRMANN, M., & WALLESCH, C.W. (1990). Expectations of psychosocial adjustment in aphasia: A MAUT study with the Code-Muller Scale of Psychosocial Adjustment. *Aphasiology, 4,* 527–538.

HIER, D.B., HAGENLOCKER, K., & SHINDLER, A.G. (1985). Language disintegration in dementia: Effects of etiology and severity. *Brain and Language, 25,* 117–133.

HIER, D.B., & KAPLAN, J. (1980). Verbal comprehension deficits after right hemisphere damage. *Applied Psycholinguistics, 1,* 279–294.

HILDEBRANDT, N., CAPLAN, D., & EVANS, K. (1987). The man. left t. without a trace: A case study of aphasic processing of empty categories. *Cognitive Neuropsychology, 4,* 257–302.

HILLIS, A.E., & CARAMAZZA, A. (1989). The graphemic buffer and attentional mechanisms. *Brain and Language, 36,* 208–235.

HILLIS, A.E., RAPP, B.C., ROMANI, C., & CARAMAZZA, A. (1990). Selective impairment of semantics in lexical processing. *Cognitive Neuropsychology, 7,* 191–244.

HINES, D. (1977). Differences in tachistoscopic recognition between abstract and concrete words as a function of visual half-field and frequency. *Cortex, 13,* 66–74.

HIRST, W., & BRILL, G.A. (1980). Contextual aspects of pronoun assignment. *Journal of Verbal Learning and Verbal Behavior, 19,* 168–175.

HIRST, W., LEDOUX, J., & STEIN, S. (1984). Constraints on the processing of indirect speech acts: Evidence from aphasiology. *Brain and Language, 23,* 26–33.

HOLCOMB, P.J., & NEVILLE, H.J. (1990). Auditory and visual semantic priming in lexical decision: A comparison using event-related brain potentials. *Language and Cognitive Processes,* 5, 281–312.

HOLLAND, A.L. (1970). Case studies in aphasia rehabilitation using programmed instruction. *Journal of Speech and Hearing Disorders,* 35, 377–390.

HOLLAND, A.L. (1975). Aphasics as communicators: A model and its implications. Paper presented to the American Speech and Hearing Association, November, Washington, D.C.

HOLLAND, A.L. (1977). Some practical considerations in aphasia rehabilitation. In M. Sullivan & M.S. Kommers (Eds.), *Rationale for adult aphasia therapy* (pp. 167–180). University of Nebraska Medical Center.

HOLLAND, A.L. (1978). Functional communication in the treatment of aphasia. In L.J. Branford, (Ed.), *Communicative disorders: An audio journal for continuing education.* New York: Grune & Stratton.

HOLLAND, A.L. (1980a). *Communicative abilities in daily living.* Baltimore: University Park Press.

HOLLAND, A.L. (1980b). The usefulness of treatment for aphasia: A serendipitous study. In R.H. Brookshire (Ed.), *Clinical aphasiology conference proceedings* (pp. 240–247). Minneapolis: BRK.

HOLLAND, A.L. (1982a). Observing functional communication of aphasic adults. *Journal of Speech and Hearing Disorders,* 47, 50–56.

HOLLAND, A.L. (1982b). When is aphasia aphasia? The problem of closed head injury. In R.H. Brookshire (Ed.), *Clinical aphasiology conference proceedings* (pp. 345–349). Minneapolis: BRK.

HOLLAND, A.L. (1983). Remarks on the problems of classifying aphasic patients. In R.H. Brookshire (Ed.), *Clinical aphasiology conference proceedings* (pp. 289–291). Minneapolis: BRK.

HOLLAND, A.L. (1991). Functional intervention in aphasia therapy. Presented for the Kessler Institute of Rehabilitation, October, West Orange, New Jersey.

HOLLAND, A.L., GREENHOUSE, J., FROMM, D., & SWINDELL, C.S. (1989). Predictors of language restitution following stroke: A multivariate analysis. *Journal of Speech and Hearing Research,* 32, 232–238.

HOLLAND, A.L., & HARRIS, A. (1968). Aphasia rehabilitation using programmed instruction: An intensive case history. In H.N. Sloane & B.D. Macaulay (Eds.), *Operant procedures in remedial speech and language training* (pp. 197–218). New York: Houghton Mifflin.

HOLLAND, A.L., MILLER, J., REINMUTH, O.M., BARTLETT, C., FROMM, D., PASHEK, G., STEIN, D., & SWINDELL, C. (1985). Rapid recovery from aphasia: A detailed language analysis. *Brain and Language,* 24, 156–173.

HOLLAND, A.L., & SONDERMAN, J.C. (1974). Effects of a program based on the Token Test for teaching comprehension skills to aphasics. *Journal of Speech and Hearing Research,* 17, 589–598.

HOLTZAPPLE, P., POHLMAN, K., LaPOINTE, L.L., & GRAHAM, L.F. (1989). Does SPICA mean PICA? In T.E. Prescott (Ed.), *Clinical aphasiology* (Vol. 18) (pp. 131–144). Boston: College-Hill/Little, Brown.

HOOPER H.W. (1958). *The Hooper visual organization test manual.* Los Angeles: Western Psychological Services.

HORN, J.L., & DONALDSON, G. (1976). On the myth of intellectual decline in adulthood. *American Psychologist,* 31, 701–719.

HORNER, J., & NAILLING, K. (1980). Raven's Coloured Progressive Matrices: Interpreting results through analysis of problem-type and error-type. In R.H. Brookshire (Ed.), *Clinical aphasiology conference proceedings* (pp. 226–239). Minneapolis: BRK.

HOUGH, M.S. (1989). Category concept generation in aphasia: The influence of context. *Aphasiology,* 3, 553–568.

HOUGH, M.S. (1990). Narrative comprehension in adults with right and left hemisphere brain-damage: Theme organization. *Brain and Language,* 38, 253–277.

HOWARD, D., & PATTERSON, K. (1989). Models for therapy. In X. Seron & G. Deloche (Eds.), *Cognitive approaches in neuropsychological rehabilitation* (pp. 39–64). Hillsdale, NJ: Lawrence Erlbaum.

HOWARD, D., PATTERSON, K., FRANKLIN, S., ORCHARD-LISLE, V., & MORTON, J. (1985a). The facilitation of picture naming in aphasia. *Cognitive Neuropsychology,* 2, 49–80.

HOWARD, D., PATTERSON, K., FRANKLIN, S., ORCHARD-LISLE, V., & MORTON, J. (1985b). Treatment of word retrieval deficits in aphasia. *Brain,* 108, 817–829.

HOWES, D.H. (1964). Application of the word-frequency concept to aphasia. In A.V.S. de Reuck & M. O'Connor (Eds.), *Disorders of the language.* London: Churchill.

HOWES, D.H. (1967). Hypotheses concerning the functions of the language mechanism. In K. Salzinger & S. Salzinger (Eds.), *Research in verbal behavior and some neurological implications.* New York: Academic Press.

HUBER, M. (1946). Linguistic problems of brain-injured servicemen. *Journal of Speech and Hearing Disorders,* 11, 143–147.

HUBER, W., & GLEBER, J. (1982). Linguistic and non-linguistic processing of narratives in aphasia. *Brain and Language,* 16, 1–18.

HUBER, W., POECK, K., & WILLMES, K. (1984). The Aachen Aphasia Test. In F.C. Rose (Ed.), *Progress in aphasiology* (pp. 291–303). New York: Raven Press.

HUFF, F.J., CORKIN, S., & GROWDON, J.H. (1986). Semantic impairment and anomia in Alzheimer's disease. *Brain and Language,* 28, 235–249.

HUFF, F.J., MACK, L., MAHLMANN, J. & GREENBERG, S. (1988). A comparison of lexical-semantic impairments in left hemisphere stroke and Alzheimer's disease. *Brain and Language,* 34, 262–279.

HUGHES, D.L. (1985). *Language treatment and generalization.* Boston: College-Hill/Little, Brown.

HUGHES, D.L., CHAN, J.L., & SU, M.S. (1983). Aprosodia in Chinese patients with right cerebral lesions. *Archives of Neurology, 40,* 732–736.

HUMPHREYS, G.W., & RIDDOCH, M.J. (1987). *To see but not to see: A case study of visual agnosia.* London: Erlbaum.

HUMPHREYS, G.W., RIDDOCH, M.J., & QUINLAN, P.T. (1988). Cascade processes in picture identification. *Cognitive Neuropsychology, 5,* 67–104.

HUNTRESS, L.M., LEE, L., CREAGHEAD, N.A., WHEELER, D.D., & BRAVERMAN, K.M. (1990). Aphasic subjects' comprehension of synthetic and natural speech. *Journal of Speech and Hearing Disorders, 55,* 21–27.

ITOH, M., SASANUMA, S., HIROSE, H., YOSHIOKA, H., & SAWASHIMA, M. (1983). Velar movements during speech in two Wernicke aphasic patients. *Brain and Language, 19,* 283–292.

ITOH, M., SASANUMA, S., TATSUMI, I.F., MURAKAMI, S., FUKUSAKO, Y., & SUZUKI, T. (1982). Voice onset time characteristics in apraxia of speech. *Brain and Language, 17,* 193–210.

ITOH, M., TATSUMI, I.F., SASANUMA, S., & FUKUSAKO, Y. (1986). Voice onset time perception in Japanese aphasic patients. *Brain and Language, 28,* 71–85.

JACKENDOFF, R. (1987). *Consciousness and the computational mind.* Cambridge, MA: Bradford, MIT Press.

JACKSON, J.H. (1879). On affections of speech from disease of the brain. *Brain, 1,* 304–330.

JAKOBSON, R. (1971). Two aspects of language and two types of aphasic disturbances. In R. Jakobson & M. Halle (Eds.), *Fundamentals of language* (Second Edition). The Hague, Netherlands: Mouton.

JAREMA, G., & KADZIELAWA, D. (1987). Agrammatism in Polish: A case study. *Aphasiology, 2,* 223–234.

JENKINS, J.J., & SCHUELL, H.M. (1964). Further work on language deficit in aphasia. *Psychological Review, 71,* 87–93.

JENNETT, B., & TEASDALE, G. (1981). *Management of head injuries.* Philadelphia: F.A. Davis.

JOANETTE, Y., & GOULET, P. (1986). Criterion-specific reduction of verbal fluency in right-brain-damaged right-handers. *Neuropsychologia, 24,* 875–879.

JOANETTE, Y., GOULET, P., & LE DORZE, G. (1988). Impaired word naming in right-brain-damaged right-handers: Error types and time-course analyses. *Brain and Language, 34,* 54–64.

JOANETTE, Y., GOULET, P., SKA, B., & NESPOULOUS, J-L. (1986). Informative content of narrative discourse in right-brain-damaged right-handers. *Brain and Language, 29,* 81–105.

JOANETTE, Y., LECOURS, A.R., LEPAGE, Y., & LAMOUREUX, M. (1983). Language in right-handers with right-hemisphere lesions: A preliminary study including anatomical, genetic and social factors. *Brain and Language, 20,* 217–248.

JOHANNSEN-HORBACK, H., CEGLA, B., MAGER, U., SCHEMPP, B., & WALLESCH, C-W (1985). Treatment of chronic global aphasia with a non-verbal communication system. *Brain and Language, 24,* 74–82.

JOHNSON, G. (1991). *In the palaces of memory: How we build the worlds inside our heads.* New York: Knopf.

JOHNSON, J.P., SOMMERS, R.K., & WEIDNER, W.E. (1977). Dichotic ear preference in aphasia. *Journal of Speech and Hearing Research, 20,* 116–129.

JOHNSON-LAIRD, P.N. (1983). *Mental models: Towards a cognitive science of language, inference, and consciousness.* Cambridge, UK: Cambridge University Press.

JONES, L.V., & WEPMAN, J.M. (1961). Dimensions of language performance in aphasia. *Journal of Speech and Hearing Research, 4,* 220–232.

JONES, L.V., & WEPMAN, J.M. (1967). Grammatical indicants of speaking style in normal and aphasic speakers. In K. Salzinger & S. Salzinger (Eds.), *Research in verbal behavior and some neurological implications.* New York: Academic Press.

JONES, R.S. (1982). *Physics as metaphor.* New York: Meridian.

JUNQUE, C., VENDRELL, P., VENDRELL-BRUCET, J.M., & TOBENA, A. (1989). Differential recovery in naming in bilingual aphasics. *Brain and Language, 36,* 16–22.

JUST, M.A., DAVIS, G.A., CARPENTER, P.A. (1977). A comparison of aphasic and normal adults in a sentence-verification task. *Cortex, 13,* 402–423.

KACZMAREK, B.L.J. (1984). Neurolinguistic analysis of verbal utterances in patients with focal lesions of frontal lobes. *Brain and Language, 21,* 52–58.

KAHN, H.J., JOANETTE, Y., SKA, B., & GOULET, P. (1990). Discourse analysis in neuropsychology: Comment on Chapman and Ulatowska. *Brain and Language, 38,* 454–461.

KAPLAN, E. (1988). The process approach to neuropsychological assessment. *Aphasiology, 2,* 309–312.

KAPLAN, E., GOODGLASS, H., & WEINTRAUB, S. (1983). *The Boston Naming Test.* Philadelphia: Lea & Febiger.

KAPLAN, J.A., BROWNELL, H.H., JACOBS, J.R., & GARDNER, H. (1990). The effects of right hemisphere damage on the pragmatic interpretation of conversational remarks. *Brain and Language, 38,* 315–333.

KARANTH, P., & RANGAMANI, G.N. (1988). Crossed aphasia in multilinguals. *Brain and Language, 34,* 169–180.

KATSUKI-NAKAMURA, J., BROOKSHIRE, R.H., & NICHOLAS, L.E. (1988). Comprehension of monologues by aphasic listeners. *Journal of Speech and Hearing Disorders, 53,* 408–415.

KATZ, R.C. (1986). *Aphasia treatment and microcomputers.* Boston: College-Hill/Little, Brown.

KATZ, R.C. (1987). Efficacy of aphasia treatment using microcomputers. *Aphasiology, 1,* 141–150.

KATZ, R.C., & WERTZ, R.T. (1992). Computerized hierarchical reading treatment in aphasia. *Aphasiology, 6,* 165–178.

KATZ, W.F. (1988). An investigation of lexical ambiguity in Broca's aphasics using an auditory lexical priming technique. *Neuropsychologia*, 26, 747–752.

KAZDIN (1982). *Single-case research designs: Methods for clinical and applied settings.* New York: Oxford University Press.

KEARNS, K.P. (1985). Response elaboration training for patient initiated utterances. In R.H. Brookshire (Ed.), *Clinical aphasiology* (Vol. 15) (pp. 196–204). Minneapolis: BRK.

KEARNS, K.P. (1986a). Flexibility of single-subject experimental designs. Part II: Design selection and arrangement of experimental phases. *Journal of Speech and Hearing Disorders*, 51, 204–214.

KEARNS, K.P. (1986b). Group therapy for aphasia: Theoretical and practical considerations. In R. Chapey (Ed.), *Language intervention strategies in adult aphasia* (Second Edition) (pp. 304–319). Baltimore: Williams & Wilkins.

KEARNS, K.P. (1986c). Systematic programming of verbal elaboration skills in chronic Broca's aphasia. In R.C. Marshall (Ed.), *Case studies in aphasia rehabilitation: For clinicians by clinicians* (pp. 225–244). Austin, Tx: Pro-Ed.

KEARNS, K.P., & SALMON, S.J. (1984). An experimental analysis of auxiliary and copula verb generalization in aphasia. *Journal of Speech and Hearing Disorders*, 49, 152–163.

KEARNS, K.P., & SIMMONS, N.N. (1983). A practical procedure for the grammatical analysis of aphasic language impairments: The LARSP. In R.H. Brookshire (Ed.), *Clinical aphasiology conference proceedings* (pp. 4–14). Minneapolis: BRK.

KEENAN, J.S., & BRASSELL, E.G. (1974). A study of factors related to prognosis for individual aphasic patients. *Journal of Speech and Hearing Disorders*, 39, 257–269.

KEENAN, J.S., & BRASSELL, E.G. (1975). *Aphasia Language Performance Scales.* Murfreesboro, TN: Pinnacle Press.

KEMPLER, D., CURTISS, S., & JACKSON, C. (1987). Syntactic preservation in Alzheimer's disease. *Journal of Speech and Hearing Research*, 30, 343–350.

KENNEDY, A., MURRAY, W.S., JENNINGS, F., & REID, C. (1989). Parsing complements: Comments on the generality of the principle of minimal attachment. *Language and Cognitive Processes*, 4, SI 51–76.

KENNEDY, E., & CHARLES, S.C. (1990). *On becoming a counselor: A basic guide for nonprofessional counselors* (New Edition). New York: Continuum.

KENNEDY, M., & MURDOCH, B.E. (1989). Speech and language disorders subsequent to subcortical vascular lesions. *Aphasiology*, 3, 221–248.

KENNEDY, M., & MURDOCH, B.E. (1991). Patterns of speech and language recovery following left striato-capsular hemorrhage. *Aphasiology*, 5, 489–510.

KERSCHENSTEINER, M., POECK, K., & BRUNNER, E.

(1972). The fluency-nonfluency dimension in the classification of aphasic speech. *Cortex*, 8, 233–247.

KERTESZ, A. (1979). *Aphasia and associated disorders: Taxonomy, localization, and recovery.* New York: Grune & Stratton.

KERTESZ, A. (1981). The anatomy of jargon. In J.W. Brown (Ed.), *Jargonaphasia* (pp. 63–112). New York: Academic Press.

KERTESZ, A. (1982). *Western Aphasia Battery.* New York: Grune & Stratton.

KERTESZ, A. (1985). Recovery and treatment. In K.M. Heilman & E. Valenstein (Eds.), *Clinical neuropsychology* (Second Edition) (pp. 481–505). New York: Oxford University Press.

KERTESZ. A. (1990). What should be the core of aphasia tests? (The authors promise but fail to deliver.) *Aphasiology*, 4, 97–102.

KERTESZ, A. (1991). Tutorial review. Language cortex. *Aphasiology*, 5, 207–234.

KERTESZ, A., & BENSON, D.F. (1970). Neologistic jargon—a clinicopathological study. *Cortex*, 6, 362–386.

KERTESZ, A., & McCABE, P. (1975). Intelligence and aphasia: Performance of aphasics on Raven's Coloured Progressive Matrices (RCPM). *Brain and Language*, 2, 387–395.

KERTESZ, A., & McCABE, P. (1977). Recovery patterns and prognosis in aphasia. *Brain*, 100, 1–18.

KERTESZ, A., & PHIPPS, J.B. (1977). Numerical taxonomy of aphasia. *Brain and Language*, 4, 1–10.

KERTESZ, A., & POOLE, E. (1974). The aphasia quotient: The taxonomic approach to measurement of aphasic disability. *Canadian Journal of Neurological Sciences*, 1, 7–16.

KERTESZ, A., & SHEPPARD, A. (1981). The epidemiology of aphasic and cognitive impairment in stroke: Age, sex, aphasia type and laterality differences. *Brain*, 104, 117–128.

KIMURA, D. (1961). Cerebral dominance and the perception of verbal stimuli. *Canadian Journal of Psychology*, 15, 166–171.

KIMURA, D. (1964). Left-right differences in the perception of melodies. *Quarterly Journal of Experimental Psychology*, 16, 355–358.

KIMURA, D. (1983). Sex differences in cerebral organization for speech and praxic functions. *Canadian Journal of Psychology*, 37, 19–35.

KING, F.L., & KIMURA, D. (1972). Left-ear superiority in dichotic perception of vocal nonverbal sounds. *Canadian Journal of Psychology*, 26, 111–116.

KINSBOURNE, M., & HISCOCK, M. (1977). Does cerebral dominance develop? In S.J. Segalowitz & F.A. Gruber (Eds.), *Language development and neurological theory* (pp. 172–193). New York: Academic Press.

KINSELLA, G., & DUFFY, F. (1978). The spouse of the aphasic patient. In Y. Lebrun & R. Hoops (Eds.), *The management of aphasia* (pp. 26–49). Amsterdam: Swets & Zeitlinger.

KINSEY, C. (1990). Analysis of dysphasics' behaviour in computer and conventional therapy environments. *Aphasiology, 4,* 293–296.

KINTSCH, W., & VAN DIJK, T.A. (1978). Toward a model of text comprehension and production. *Psychological Review, 85,* 363–394.

KIRSHNER, H.S., CASEY, P.F., HENSON, J., & HEINRICH, J.J. (1989). Behavioural features and lesion localization in Wernicke's aphasia. *Aphasiology, 3,* 169–176.

KIRSHNER, H.S., TANRIDAG, O., THURMAN, L., & WHETSELL, JR., W.O. (1987). Progressive aphasia without dementia: Two cases with focal spongiform degeneration. *Annals of Neurology, 22,* 527–532.

KIRSHNER, H.S., & WEBB, W.G. (1981). Selective involvement of the auditory-verbal modality in an acquired communication disorder: Benefit from sign language therapy. *Brain and Language, 13,* 161–170.

KIRSHNER, H.S., WEBB, W.G., & DUNCAN, G.W. (1981). Word deafness in Wernicke's aphasia. *Journal of Neurology, Neurosurgery, and Psychiatry, 45,* 197–201.

KLIMA, E.S., BELLUGI, U., & POIZNER, H. (1988). Grammar and space in sign aphasiology. *Aphasiology, 2,* 319–328.

KLOR, B.M., & MICOCH, A.G. (1984). Auditory comprehension in aphasia: Type vs. severity. In R.H. Brookshire (Ed.), *Clinical aphasiology conference proceedings* (pp. 223–226). Minneapolis: BRK.

KNOTEK, P.C., BAYLES, K.A., & KASZNIAK, A.W. (1990). Response consistency on a semantic memory task in persons with dementia of the Alzheimer type. *Brain and Language, 38,* 465–475.

KOEMEDA-LUTZ, M., COHEN, R., & MEIER, E. (1987). Organization of and access to semantic memory in aphasia. *Brain and Language, 30,* 321–337.

KOHLMEYER, K. (1976). Aphasia due to focal disorders of cerebral circulation: Some aspects of localization and of spontaneous recovery. In Y. Lebrun & R. Hoops (Eds.), *Recovery in aphasics* (pp. 79–95). Amsterdam: Swets & Zeitlinger.

KOHN, S.E. (1984). The nature of the phonological disorder in conduction aphasia. *Brain and Language, 23,* 97–115.

KOHN, S.E. (1989). The nature of the phonemic string deficit in conduction aphasia. *Aphasiology, 3,* 209–240.

KOHN, S.E., & FRIEDMAN, R.B. (1986). Word-meaning deafness: A phonological-semantic dissociation. *Cognitive Neuropsychology, 3,* 291–308.

KOHN, S.E., & GOODGLASS, H. (1985). Picture-naming in aphasia. *Brain and Language, 24,* 266–283.

KOHN, S.E., & SMITH, K.L. (1990). Between-word speech errors in conduction aphasia. *Cognitive Neuropsychology, 7,* 133–156.

KOLK, H.H.J., & BLOMERT, L. (1985). On the Bradley hypothesis concerning agrammatism: The nonword-interference effect. *Brain and Language, 26,* 94–105.

KOLK, H.H.J., & FRIEDERICI, A.D. (1985). Strategy and impairment in sentence understanding by Broca's and Wernicke's aphasics. *Cortex, 21,* 47–67.

KOLK, H.H.J., & HEESCHEN, C. (1990). Adaptation symptoms and impairment symptoms in Broca's aphasia. *Aphasiology, 4,* 221–232.

KOLK, H.H.J., & VAN GRUNSVEN, M.M.F. (1985). Agrammatism as a variable phenomenon. *Cognitive Neuropsychology, 2,* 347–384.

KOLK, H.H.J., VAN GRUNSVEN, M.J.F., & KEYSER, A. (1985). On parallelism between production and comprehension in agrammatism. In M-L. Kean (Ed.), *Agrammatism* (pp. 165–205). Orlando, FL: Academic Press.

KOPELMAN, M.D. (1985). Rates of forgetting in Alzheimer-type dementia and Korsakoff's syndrome. *Neuropsychologia, 23,* 623–638.

KOSSLYN, S.M. (1983). *Ghosts in the mind's machine: Creating and using images in the brain.* New York: Norton.

KOSSLYN, S.M. (1987). Seeing and imaging in the cerebral hemispheres: A computational approach. *Psychological Review, 94,* 148–175.

KRAAT, A.W. (1990). Augmentative and alternative communication: Does it have a future in aphasia rehabilitation? *Aphasiology, 4,* 312–338.

KREINDLER, A., GHEORGHITA, N., & VOINESCU, I. (1971). Analysis of verbal reception of a complex order with three elements in aphasics. *Brain, 94,* 375–386.

KUDO, T. (1984). The effect of semantic plausibility on sentence comprehension in aphasia. *Brain and Language, 21,* 208–218.

LACKNER, J.R., & TEUBER, H.L. (1973). Alternation in auditory fusion thresholds after cerebral injury in man. *Neuropsychologia, 11,* 409–415.

LAPOINTE, L.L. (1985). Aphasia therapy: Some principles and strategies for treatment. In D.F. Johns (Eds.), *Clinical management of neurogenic communicative disorders* (pp. 179–241). Boston: Little, Brown.

LAPOINTE, L.L., HOLTZAPPLE, P., & GRAHAM, L.F. (1985). The relationship among two measures of auditory comprehension and daily living communication skills. In R.H. Brookshire (Ed.), *Clinical aphasiology* (Vol. 15) (pp. 38–46). Minneapolis: BRK.

LAPOINTE, L.L., HOLTZAPPLE, P., & GRAHAM, L.F. (1986). Comprehension of three-part commands by aphasic subjects: Analysis of error location. In R.H. Brookshire (Ed.), *Clinical aphasiology* (Vol. 16) (pp. 65–72). Minneapolis: BRK.

LAPOINTE, L.L., & HORNER, J. (1979). *Reading Comprehension Battery for Aphasia.* Chicago: Riverside.

LAPOINTE, L.L., ROTHI, L.J., & CAMPANELLA, D.J. (1978). The effects of repetition of Token Test commands on auditory comprehension. In R.H. Brookshire (Ed.),

Clinical aphasiology conference proceedings (pp. 262–269). Minneapolis: BRK.

LAPOINTE, S.G. (1985). A theory of verb form use in the speech of agrammatic aphasics. *Brain and Language, 24,* 100–155.

LASKY, E.Z., & WEIDNER, W.E., & JOHNSON, J.P. (1976). Influence of linguistic complexity, rate of presentation, and interphrase pause time on auditory-verbal comprehension of adult aphasic patients. *Brain and Language, 3,* 386–395.

LASSEN, N.A., INGVAR, D.H., & SKINHOJ, E. (1978). Brain function and blood flow. *Scientific American, 239,* 62–71.

LAURENCE, S., & STEIN, D.G. (1978). Recovery after brain damage and the concept of localization of function. In S. Finger (Ed.), *Recovery from brain damage: Research and theory* (pp. 369–407). New York: Plenum Press.

LAYMAN, S., & GREENE, E. (1988). The effect of stroke on object recognition. *Brain and Language, 7,* 87–114.

LEBRUN, Y., & HOOPS, R. (1974). *Intelligence and aphasia.* Amsterdam: Swets & Zeitlinger.

LECOURS, A.R. (1982). On neologisms. In J. Mehler, E.C.T. Walker, & M. Garrett (Eds.), *Perspectives on mental representation.* Hillsdale, NJ: Erlbaum.

LECOURS, A.R., & NESPOULOUS, J.-L. (1988). The phonetic-phonemic dichotomy in aphasiology. *Aphasiology, 2,* 329–336.

LECOURS, A.R., & VANIER-CLEMENT, M. (1976). Schizophasia and jargonaphasia. *Brain and Language, 3,* 516–565.

LE DORZE, G., & NESPOULOUS, J.-L. (1989). Anomia in moderate aphasia: Problems in accessing the lexical representation. *Brain and Language, 37,* 381–400.

LEDOUX, J.E., BLUM, C., & HIRST, W. (1983). Inferential processing of context: Studies of cognitively impaired subjects. *Brain and Language, 19,* 216–224.

LEDOUX, J.E., & HIRST, W. (EDS). (1986). *Mind and brain: Dialogues in cognitive neuroscience.* Cambridge, UK: Cambridge University Press.

LEE, G.P., LORING, D.W., MEADER, K.J., & BROOKS, B.B. (1990). Hemispheric specialization for emotional expression: A reexamination of results from intracarotid administration of sodium amobarbital. *Brain and Cognition, 12,* 267–280.

LEE, L. (1971). *Northwestern Syntax Screening Test.* Evanston, IL: Northwestern University Press.

LEITH, W.R. (1984). *Handbook of clinical methods in communication disorders.* Boston: College-Hill/Little, Brown.

LE MAY, A., DAVID, R., & THOMAS, A.P. (1988). The use of spontaneous gesture by aphasic patients. *Aphasiology, 2,* 137–146.

LENDREM, W., & LINCOLN, N.B. (1985). Spontaneous recovery of language in patients with aphasia between 4 and 34 weeks after stroke. *Journal of Neurology, Neurosurgery, and Psychiatry, 48,* 743–748.

LENNEBERG, E. (1967). *Biological foundations of language.* New York: Wiley.

LESSER, R. (1974). Verbal comprehension in aphasia: An English version of three Italian tests. *Cortex, 10,* 247–263.

LESSER, R. (1976). Verbal and non-verbal components of the Token Test. *Neuropsychologia, 14,* 79–85.

LESSER, R. (1979). Turning tokens into things: Linguistic and mnestic aspects of the initial sections of the Token Test. In F. Boller & M. Dennis (Eds.), *Auditory comprehension: Clinical and experimental studies with the Token Test* (pp. 71–88). New York: Academic Press.

LESSER, R. (1986). Disorders of grammar and the lexicon. *Seminars in Speech and Language, 7,* 147–158.

LESSER, R. (1987). Cognitive neuropsychological influences on aphasia therapy. *Aphasiology, 1,* 189–200.

LEVELT, W.J.M. (1989). *Speaking: From intention to articulation.* Cambridge, MA: MIT Press.

LEVIN, H.S. (1981). Aphasia in closed head injury. In M.T. Sarno (Ed.), *Acquired aphasia* (pp. 427–463). New York: Academic Press.

LEVIN, H.S., GROSSMAN, R.G., & KELLY, P.J. (1976). Aphasic disorders in patients with closed head injury. *Journal of Neurology, Neurosurgery, and Psychiatry, 39,* 1062–1070.

LEVIN, H.S., GROSSMAN. R.G., SARWAR, M., & MEYERS, C.A. (1981). Linguistic recovery after closed head injury. *Brain and Language, 12,* 360–374.

LEVIN, H.S., O'DONNELL, V.M., & GROSSMAN, R.G. (1979). The Galveston orientation and amnesia test: A practical scale to assess cognition after head injury. *Journal of Nervous and Mental Disease, 167,* 675–684.

LEVINE, S.C., BANICH, M.T., & KOCH-WESER, M.P. (1988). Face recognition: A general or specific right hemisphere capacity? *Brain and Cognition, 8,* 303–325.

LEVINSON, S.C. (1983). *Pragmatics.* Cambridge, UK: Cambridge University Press.

LEVY, J., TREVARTHEN, C., & SPERRY, R.W. (1972). Perception of bilateral chimeric figures following hemispheric deconnexion. *Brain, 95,* 61–78.

LEY, R.G., & BRYDEN, M.P. (1979). Hemispheric differences in recognizing faces and emotions. *Brain and Language, 7,* 127–138.

LEZAK, M.D. (1979). Recovery of memory and learning functions following traumatic brain injury. *Cortex, 15,* 63–72.

LEZAK, M.D. (1983). *Neuropsychological assessment* (2nd Ed.). New York: Oxford University Press.

LI, E.C., & WILLIAMS, S.E. (1989). The efficacy of two types of cues in aphasic patients. *Aphasiology, 3,* 619–626.

LI, E.C., & WILLIAMS, S.E. (1990). The effects of grammatic class and cue type on cueing responsiveness in aphasia. *Brain and Language, 38,* 48–60.

LICHTHEIM, L. (1885). On aphasia. *Brain*, 7, 433–484.

LIEBERMAN, R.J., & MICHAEL, A. (1986). Content relevance and content coverage in tests of grammatical ability. *Journal of Speech and Hearing Disorders*, 51, 71–81.

LIGHT, L.L., & CAPPS, J.L. (1986). Comprehension of pronouns in young and older adults. *Developmental Psychology*, 22, 580–585.

LILES, B.Z., & BROOKSHIRE, R.H. (1975). The effects of pause time on auditory comprehension of aphasic subjects. *Journal of Communication Disorders*, 8, 221–236.

LILES, B.Z., COELHO, C.A., DUFFY, R.J., & ZALAGENS, M.R. (1989). Effects of elicitation procedures on the narratives of normal and closed head-injured adults. *Journal of Speech and Hearing Disorders*, 54, 356–366.

LIMA, S.D., & POLLATSEK, A. (1983). Lexical access via an orthographic Code? The Basic Orthographic Syllabic Structure (BOSS) reconsidered. *Journal of Verbal Learning and Verbal Behavior*, 22, 310–332.

LINCOLN, N.B. (1988). Using the PICA in clinical practice: Are we flogging a dead horse? *Aphasiology*, 2, 501–506.

LINCOLN, N.B., & ELLS, P. (1980). A shortened version of the PICA. *British Journal of Disorders of Communication*, 15, 183–187.

LINCOLN, N.B., & McGUIRK, E. (1987). Letter to the editor. *Aphasiology*, 1, 442–443.

LINCOLN, N.B., McGUIRK, E., MULLY, G.P., LENDREM, W., JONES, A.C., & MITCHELL, J.R.A. (1984). The effectiveness of speech therapy for aphasic stroke patients: A randomized controlled trial. *Lancet*, 1, 1197–1200.

LINEBARGER, M., SCHWARTZ, M.F., & SAFFRAN, E.M. (1983). Sensitivity to grammatical structure in so-called agrammatic aphasics. *Cognition*, 13, 361–392.

LINEBAUGH, C.W. (1983). Treatment of anomic aphasia. In W.H. Perkins (Ed.), *Language handicaps in adults* (pp. 35–44). New York: Thieme-Stratton.

LOFTUS, G.R., & LOFTUS, E.F. (1974). The influence of one memory retrieval on a subsequent memory retrieval. *Memory and Cognition*, 2, 467–471.

LOHMAN, T., ZIGGAS, D., & PIERCE, R.S. (1989). Word fluency performance on common categories by subjects with closed head injuries. *Aphasiology*, 3, 685–694.

LOHMANN, L., & PRESCOTT, T.E. (1978). The effects of substituting "objects" for "forms" on the Revised Token Test (RTT) performance of aphasic subjects. In R.H. Brookshire (Ed.), *Clinical aphasiology conference proceedings* (pp. 138–146). Minneapolis: BRK.

LOMAS, J., & KERTESZ, A. (1978). Patterns of spontaneous recovery in aphasic groups: A study of adult stroke patients. *Brain and Language*, 5, 388–401.

LOMAS, J., PICKARD, L., BESTER, S., ELBARD, H., FINLAYSON, A., & ZOGHAIB, C. (1989). The Communicative Effectiveness Index: Development and psycho-metric evaluation of a functional communication measure for adult aphasia. *Journal of Speech and Hearing Disorders*, 54, 113–124.

LONZI, L., & ZANOBIO, M.E. (1983). Syntactic component in language responsible cognitive structure: Neurological evidence. *Brain and Language*, 18, 177–191.

LOVE, R.J., & WEBB, W.G. (1977). The efficacy of cueing techniques in Broca's aphasia. *Journal of Speech and Hearing Disorders*, 42, 170–178.

LOVERSO, F.L. (1987). Unfounded expectations: Computers in rehabilitation. *Aphasiology*, 1, 157–160.

LOVERSO, F.L., PRESCOTT, T.E., & SELINGER, M. (1988). Cueing verbs: A treatment strategy for aphasic adults. *Journal of Rehabilitation Research*, 25, 47–60.

LOVERSO, F.L., PRESCOTT, T.E., & SELINGER, M. (1992). Microcomputer treatment applications in aphasiology. *Aphasiology*, 6, 155–164.

LOVERSO, F.L., PRESCOTT, T.E., SELINGER, M., & RILEY, L. (1989). Comparison of two modes of aphasia treatment: Clinician and computer-clinician assisted. In T.E. Prescott (Ed.), *Clinical aphasiology* (Vol. 18). (pp. 297–320). Boston: College-Hill/Little, Brown.

LOVERSO, F.L., PRESCOTT, T.E., SELINGER, M., WHEELER, K.M., & SMITH, R.D. (1985). The application of microcomputers for the treatment of aphasic adults. In R.H. Brookshire (Ed.), *Clinical aphasiology* (Vol. 15) (pp. 189–195). Minneapolis: BRK.

LOVERSO, F.L., SELINGER, M., & PRESCOTT, T.E. (1979). Application of verbing strategies to aphasia treatment. In R.H. Brookshire (Ed.), *Clinical aphasiology conference proceedings* (pp. 229–238). Minneapolis: BRK.

LUBINSKI, R. (1981). Environmental language intervention. In R. Chapey (Ed.), *Language intervention strategies in adult aphasia* (First Edition) (pp. 223–248). Baltimore: Williams & Wilkins.

LUBINSKI, R. (1988). A model for intervention: Communication skills, effectiveness, and opportunity. In B.B. Shadden (Ed.), *Communication behavior and aging: A sourcebook for clinicians* (pp. 295–308). Baltimore: Williams & Wilkins.

LUBINSKI, R., DUCHAN, J., & WEITNER-LIN, B. (1980). Analysis of breakdowns and repairs in aphasic adult communication. In R.H. Brookshire (Ed.), *Clinical aphasiology conference proceedings* (pp. 111–116). Minneapolis: BRK.

LUDLOW, C.L. (1977). Recovery from aphasia: A foundation for treatment. In M. Sullivan & M.S. Kommers (Eds.), *Rational for adult aphasia therapy* (pp. 97–134). University of Nebraska Medical Center.

LUKATELA, K., CRAIN, S., & SHANKWEILER, D. (1988). Sensitivity to inflectional morphology in agrammatism: Investigation of a highly inflected language. *Brain and Language*, 33, 1–15.

LURIA, A.R. (1966). *Higher cortical functions in man.* New York: Basic Books.

LURIA, A.R. (1970a). The functional organization of the brain. *Scientific American*, 222(3), 66–78.

LURIA, A.R. (1970b). *Traumatic aphasia*. The Hague, Netherlands: Mouton.

LURIA, A.R., & TSVETKOVA, L.S. (1968). The mechanism of "dynamic aphasia." *Foundations of Language*, 4, 296–307.

LUZZATTI, C., WILLMES, K., TARICCO, M., COLOMBO, C., & CHIESA, G. (1989). Language disturbances after severe head injury: Do neurological or other associated cognitive disorders influence type, severity and evolution of the verbal impairment? A preliminary report. *Aphasiology*, 3, 643–654.

LYON, J.G. (1989). Communicative partners: Their value in reestablishing communication with aphasic adults. In T.E. Prescott (Ed.), *Clinical aphasiology* (Vol. 18) (pp. 11–17). Austin, TX: Pro-Ed.

LYON, J.G., & HELM-ESTABROOKS, N. (1987). Drawing: Its communicative significance for expressively restricted aphasic adults. *Topics in Language Disorders*, 8, 61–71.

LYON, J.G., & SIMS, E. (1989). Drawing: Its use as a communicative aid with aphasic and normal adults. In T.E. Prescott (Ed.), *Clinical aphasiology* (Vol. 18) (pp. 339–355). Austin, TX: Pro-Ed.

MACK, J.L., & BOLLER, F. (1979). Components of auditory comprehension: Analysis of errors in a revised Token Test. In F. Boller & M. Dennis (Eds.), *Auditory comprehension: Clinical and experimental studies with the Token Test* (pp. 45–70). New York: Academic Press.

MACMILLAN, M.B. (1986). A wonderful journey through skull and brains: The travels of Mr. Gage's tamping iron. *Brain and Cognition*, 5, 67–107.

MACWHINNEY, B., BATES, E., & KLIEGL, R. (1984). Cue validity and sentence interpretation in English, German, and Italian. *Journal of Verbal Learning and Verbal Behavior*, 23, 127–150.

MACWHINNEY, B., & OSMAN-SAGI, J. (1991). Inflectional marking in Hungarian aphasics. *Brain and Language*, 41, 165–183.

MACWHINNEY, B., OSMAN-SAGI, J., & SLOBIN, D.I. (1991). Sentence comprehension in aphasia in two clear case-marking languages. *Brain and Language*, 41, 234–249.

MALT, B.C. (1985). The role of discourse structure in understanding anaphora. *Journal of Memory and Language*, 24, 271–289.

MANDLER, J.M. (1987). On the psychological reality of story structure. *Discourse Processes*, 10, 1–29.

MARKS, M.M., TAYLOR, M., & RUSK, H.A. (1957). Rehabilitation of the aphasic patient: A survey of three years' experience in a rehabilitation setting. *Neurology*, 7, 837–843.

MARR, D. (1982). *Vision: A computational investigation into the human representation and processing of visual information*. San Francisco: W.H. Freeman.

MARSHALL, R.C. (1976). Word retrieval behavior of aphasic adults. *Journal of Speech and Hearing Disorders*, 41, 444–451.

MARSHALL, R.C. (1986). Treatment of auditory comprehension deficits. In R. Chapey (Ed.), *Language intervention strategies in adult aphasia* (2nd ed.) (pp. 370–393). Baltimore: Williams & Wilkins.

MARSHALL, R.C. (1987). Reapportioning time for aphasia rehabilitation: A point of view. *Aphasiology*, 1, 59–74.

MARSHALL, R.C., NEUBURGER, S.I., & STARCH, S.A. (1985). Aphasic confrontation naming elaboration. In R.H. Brookshire (Ed.), *Clinical aphasiology* (Vol. 15) (p. 295–300). Minneapolis: BRK.

MARSHALL, R.C., & PHILLIPS, D.S. (1983). Prognosis for improved verbal communication in aphasic stroke patients. *Archives of Physical Medicine and Rehabilitation*, 64, 597–600.

MARSHALL, R.C., & TOMPKINS, C.A. (1982). Verbal self-correction behaviors of fluent and nonfluent aphasic subjects. *Brain and Language*, 15, 292–306.

MARSHALL, R.C., WERTZ, R.G., WEISS, D.G., ATEN, J.L., BROOKSHIRE, R.H., GARCIA-BUNUEL, L., HOLLAND, A.L., KURTZKE, J.F., LaPOINTE, L.L., MILIANTI, F.J., BRANNEGAN, R., GREENBAUM, H., VOGEL, D., CARTER, J., BARNES, N.S., & GOODMAN, R. (1989). Home treatment for aphasic patients by trained nonprofessionals. *Journal of Speech and Hearing Disorders*, 54, 462–470.

MARSLEN-WILSON, W., & TYLER, L.K. (1980). The temporal structure of spoken language understanding. *Cognition*, 8, 1–71.

MARTIN, A., BROUWERS, P., COX, C., & FEDIO, P. (1985). On the nature of the verbal memory deficit in Alzheimer's disease. *Brain and Language*, 25, 323–341.

MARTIN, A., & FEDIO, P. (1983). Word production and comprehension in Alzheimer's disease: The breakdown of semantic knowledge. *Brain and Language*, 19, 124–141.

MARTIN. A.D. (1981). Therapy with the jargonaphasic. In J.W. Brown (Ed.), *Jargonaphasia* (pp. 305–326). New York: Academic Press.

MARTIN, R.C. (1987). Articulatory and phonological deficits in short-term memory and their relation to syntactic processing. *Brain and Language*, 32, 159–192.

MARTIN, R.C., & BLOSSOM-STACH, C. (1986). Evidence of syntactic deficits in a fluent aphasic. *Brain and Language*, 28, 196–234.

MARTIN, R.C., & FEHER, E. (1990). The consequences of reduced memory span for the comprehension of semantic versus syntactic information. *Brain and Language*, 38, 1–20.

MARTINO, A.A., PIZZAMIGLIO, L., & RAZZANO, C. (1976). A new version of the "Token Test" for aphasics: A concrete objects form. *Journal of Communication Disorders*, 9, 1–5.

MARZI, C.A. (1986). Transfer of visual information after

unilateral input to the brain. *Brain and Cognition, 5*, 163–173.

MATTHEI, E.H., & KEAN, M-L. (1989). Postaccess processes in the open vs. closed class distinction. *Brain and Language, 36*, 163–180.

MATTIS, S. (1976). Mental status examination for organic mental syndrome in the elderly patient. In R. Bellack & B. Karasu (Eds.), *Geriatric psychiatry* (pp. 77–121). New York: Grune & Stratton.

MATTSON, A., & LEVIN, H.S. (1990). Frontal lobe dysfunction following closed head injury. *Journal of Nervous and Mental Disease, 178*, 282–291.

MAZZIOTTA, J.C., PHELPS, M.E., CARSON, R.E., & KUHL, D.E. (1982). Tomographic mapping of human cerebral metabolism: Auditory stimulation. *Neurology, 32*, 921–937.

MAZZOCCHI, F., & VIGNOLO, L.A. (1978). Computer assisted tomography in neuropsychological research: A simple procedure for lesion mapping. *Cortex, 14*, 136–144.

MAZZOCCHI, F., & VIGNOLO, L.A. (1979). Localization of lesions in aphasia: Clinical-CT scan correlations in stroke patients. *Cortex, 15*, 627–654.

MCCARTHY, R., & WARRINGTON, E.K. (1985). Category-specificity in an agrammatic patient: The relative impairment of verb retrieval and comprehension. *Neuropsychologia, 23*, 709–727.

MCCLEARY, C. (1988). The semantic organization and classification of fourteen words by aphasic patients. *Brain and Language, 34*, 183–202.

MCCLEARY, C., & HIRST, W. (1986). Semantic classification in aphasia: A study of basic, superordinate, and function relations. *Brain and Language, 27*, 199–209.

MCCLELLAND, J.L., & RUMELHART, D.E. (1985). Distributed memory and the representation of general and specific information. *Journal of Experimental Psychology: General, 114*, 159–188.

MCCLOSKEY, M., & CARAMAZZA, A. (1988). Theory and methodology in cognitive neuropsychology: A response to our critics. *Cognitive Neuropsychology, 5*, 583–623.

MCDONALD, J.L. (1987). Assigning linguistic roles: The influence of conflicting cues. *Journal of Memory and Language, 26*, 100–117.

MCDONALD, S., & WALES, R. (1986). An investigation of the ability to process inferences in language following right hemisphere brain damage. *Brain and Language, 29*, 68–80.

MCFARLING, D., ROTHI, L.J., & HEILMAN, K.M. (1982). Transcortical aphasia from ischemic infarcts of the thalamus: A report of two cases. *Journal of Neurology, Neurosurgery, and Psychiatry, 45*, 107–112.

MCFIE, J. (1975). *Assessment of organic intellectual impairment.* New York: Academic Press.

MCGLONE, J. (1977). Sex differences in the cerebral organization of verbal functions in patients with unilateral cerebral lesions. *Brain, 100*, 775–793.

MCKEE, G., HUMPHREY, B., & MCADAM, D.W. (1973). Scaled lateralization of alpha activity during linguistic and musical tasks. *Psychophysiology, 10*, 441–443.

MCKHANN, G., DRACHMAN, D., FOLSTEIN, M., KATZMAN, R., PRICE, D., & STADLIN, E.M. (1984). Clinical diagnosis of Alzheimer's disease: Report of the NINCDS-ADRDA work group under the auspices of the Department of Health and Human Services Task Force on Alzheimer's disease. *Neurology, 34*, 939–944.

MCMULLEN, P.A., & BRYDEN, M.P. (1987). The effects of word imageability and frequency on hemispheric asymmetry in lexical decisions. *Brain and Language, 31*, 11–25.

MCNEIL, M.R., DIONIGI, C.M., LANGLOIS, A., & PRESCOTT, T.E. (1989). A measure of Revised Token Test ordinality and intervality. *Aphasiology, 3*, 31–40.

MCNEIL, M.R., & HAGEMAN, C.F. (1979). Auditory processing deficits in aphasia evidenced on the Revised Token Test: Incidence and prediction of across subtest and across item within subtest patterns. In R.H. Brookshire (Ed.), *Clinical aphasiology conference proceedings* (pp. 47–69). Minneapolis: BRK.

MCNEIL, M.R., & KIMELMAN, M.D.Z. (1986). Toward an integrative information-processing structure of auditory comprehension and processing in adult aphasia. *Seminars in Speech and Language, 7*, 123–146.

MCNEIL, M.R., & PRESCOTT, T.E. (1978). *Revised Token Test.* Baltimore, MD: University Park Press.

MCNEIL, M.R., PRESCOTT, T.E., & CHANG, E.C. (1978). A measure of PICA ordinality. In R.H. Brookshire (Ed.), *Clinical aphasiology collected proceedings 1972–1976* (pp. 185–195). Minneapolis: BRK.

MCRAE, K., JARED, D., & SEIDENBERG, M.S. (1990). On the roles of frequency and lexical access in word naming. *Journal of Memory and Language, 29*, 43–65.

MCREYNOLDS, L.V., & KEARNS, K.P. (1983). *Single-subject experimental designs in communicative disorders.* Baltimore: University Park Press.

MEHLER, J., MORTON, J., & JUSCZYK, P.W. (1984). On reducing language to biology. *Cognitive Neuropsychology, 1*, 83–116.

MEIKLE, M., WECHSLER, E., TUPPER, A., BENENSON, M., BUTLER, J., MULHALL, D., & STERN, G. (1979). Comparative trial of volunteer and professional treatments of dysphasia after stroke. *British Medical Journal, 2*, 87–89.

MENDELSOHN, S. (1988). Language lateralization in bilinguals: Facts and fantasy. *Journal of Neurolinguistics, 3*, 261–292.

MENDEZ, M.F., & BENSON, D.F. (1985). Atypical conduction aphasia: A disconnection syndrome. *Archives of Neurology, 42*, 886–891.

MENTIS, M. & PRUTTING, C.A. (1987). Cohesion in the discourse of normal and head-injured adults. *Journal of Speech and Hearing Research, 30*, 88–98.

METTER, E.J. (1985). Feature: Letter. *Asha, 27*, 43.

METTER, E.J. (1986). Medical aspects of stroke rehabilitation. In R. Chapey (Ed.), *Language intervention strategies in adult aphasia* (Second Edition) (pp. 141–159). Baltimore: Williams & Wilkins.

METTER, E.J. (1987). Neuroanatomy and physiology of aphasia: Evidence from positron emission tomography. *Aphasiology*, 1, 3–33.

METTER, E.J., RIEGE, W.H., HANSON, W.R., CAMRAS, L., KUHL, D.E., & PHELPS, M.E. (1984). Correlations of cerebral glucose metabolism and structural damage to language function in aphasia. *Brain and Language*, 21, 187–207.

METTER, E.J., RIEGE, W.H., HANSON, W.R., KUHL, D.E., & PHELPS, M.E. (1984). Commonality and differences in aphasia: Evidence from the BDAE and PICA. In R.H. Brookshire (Ed.), *Clinical aphasiology conference proceedings* (pp. 70–77). Minneapolis: BRK.

METTER, E.J., RIEGE, W.H., HANSON, W.R., KUHL, D.E., PHELPS, M.E., SQUIRE, L.R., WASTERLAIN, C.G., & BENSON, D.F. (1983). Comparison of metabolic rates, language, and memory in subcortical aphasias. *Brain and Language*, 19, 33–47.

MEYER, D.E., & SCHVANEVELDT, R.W. (1971). Facilitation in recognizing pairs of words: Evidence of a dependence between retrieval operations. *Journal of Experimental Psychology*, 90 227–234.

MEYER, J.S., SHINOHARA, Y., KANDA, T., FUKUUCHI, Y., ERICSSON, A.D., & KOK, N.K. (1970). Diaschisis resulting from acute unilateral cerebral infarction. *Archives of Neurology*, 23, 241–247.

MICELI, G., CALTAGIRONE, C., GAINOTTI, G., & PAYER-RIGO, P. (1978). Discrimination of voice versus place consonants in aphasia. *Brain and Language*, 6, 47–51.

MICELI, G., GAINOTTI, G., CALTAGIRONE, C., & MASULLO, C. (1980). Some aspects of phonological impairment in aphasia. *Brain and Language*, 11, 159–170.

MICELI, G., MAZZUCCHI, A., MENN, L., & GOODGLASS, H. (1983). Contrasting cases of Italian agrammatic aphasia without comprehension disorder. *Brain and Language*, 19, 65–97.

MICELI, G., SILVERI, M.C., NOCENTINI, U., & CARAMAZZA, A. (1988). Patterns of dissociation in comprehension and production of nouns and verbs. *Aphasiology*, 2, 351–358.

MICELI, G., SILVERI, M.C., ROMANI, C., & CARAMAZZA, A. (1989). Variation in the pattern of omissions and substitutions of grammatical morphemes in the spontaneous speech of so-called agrammatic patients. *Brain and Language*, 36, 447–492.

MICELI, G., SILVERI, M.C., VILLA, G., & CARAMAZZA, A. (1984). On the basis for the agrammatic's difficulty in producing main verbs. *Cortex*, 20, 207–220.

MILBERG, W., & BLUMSTEIN, S.E. (1981). Lexical decision and aphasia: Evidence for semantic processing. *Brain and Language*, 14, 371–385.

MILBERG, W., & BLUMSTEIN, S.E. (1989). Reaction time methodology and the aphasic patient: A reply to Hagoort. *Brain and Language*, 36, 349–353.

MILBERG, W., BLUMSTEIN, S.E., & DWORETZKY, B. (1987). Processing of lexical ambiguities in aphasia. *Brain and Language*, 31, 151–170.

MILLER, D., & ELLIS, A.W. (1987). Speech and writing errors in "neologistic jargonaphasia": A lexical activation hypothesis. In M. Coltheart, G., Sartori, & R. Job (Eds.), *The cognitive neuropsychology of language* (pp. 253–272). London: Erlbaum.

MILLS, R.H. (1977). The effects of environmental sound on the naming performance of aphasic subjects. In R.H. Brookshire (Ed.), *Clinical aphasiology conference proceedings* (pp. 68–79). Minneapolis: BRK.

MILLS, R.H. (1982). A microcomputerized treatment system for chronic aphasic patients. In R.H. Brookshire (Ed.), *Clinical aphasiology conference proceedings* (pp. 147–152). Minneapolis: BRK.

MILLS, R.H. (1986). Computerized management of aphasia. In R. Chapey (Ed.), *Language intervention strategies in adult aphasia* (Second Edition) (pp. 333–344). Baltimore: Williams & Wilkins.

MILNER, B. (1967). Brain mechanisms suggested by studies of temporal lobes. In C.H. Milikan & F.L. Darley (Eds.), *Brain mechanisms underlying speech and language* (pp. 122–145). New York: Grune & Stratton.

MILTON, S.B., WERTZ, R.T., KATZ, R.C., & PRUTTING, C.A. (1981). Stimulus saliency in the sorting behavior of aphasic adults. In R.H. Brookshire (Ed.), *Clinical aphasiology conference proceedings* (pp. 46–54). Minneapolis: BRK.

MITCHELL, D.C. (1989). Verb-guidance and other lexical effects in parsing. *Language and Cognitive Processes*, 4, SI 123–155.

MOHR, J.P., PESSIN, M., FINKELSTEIN, S., FUNKENSTEIN, H., DUNCAN, G., & DAVIS, K. (1978). Broca's aphasia: pathologic and clinical. *Neurology*, 28, 311–324.

MOHR, J.P., WEISS, G., CAVENESS, W.F., DILLON, J.D., KISTLER, J.P., MEIROWSKY, A.M., & RISH, B.L. (1980). Language and motor deficits following penetrating head injury in Vietnam. *Neurology*, 30, 1273–1279.

MOLFESE, D.L. (1977). Infant cerebral asymmetry. In S.J. Segalowitz & F.A. Gruber (Eds.), *Language development and neurological theory* (pp. 22–33). London: Academic Press.

MOLFESE, V.J., MOLFESE, D.L., & PARSONS, C. (1983). Hemisphere processing of phonological information. In S.J. Segalowitz (Ed.), *Language functions and brain organization* (pp. 29–49). New York: Academic Press.

MONOI, H., FUKUSAKO, Y., ITOH, M., & SASANUMA, S. (1983). Speech sound errors in patients with conduction and Broca's aphasia. *Brain and Language*, 20, 175–194.

MOORE, JR., W.H. (1989). Language recovery in aphasia: A right hemisphere perspective. *Aphasiology*, 3, 101–110.

MORGAN, A.L.R., & HELM-ESTABROOKS, N. (1987). Back to the drawing board: A treatment program for nonverbal aphasic patients. In R.H. Brookshire (Ed.), *Clinical aphasiology* (Vol. 17) (pp. 64–72). Minneapolis: BRK.

MORLEY, G.K., LUNDGREN, S., & HAXBY, J. (1979). Comparison and clinical applicability of auditory comprehension scores on the Behavioral Neurology Deficit Examination, Boston Diagnostic Aphasia Examination, Porch Index of Communicative Ability and Token Test. *Journal of Clinical Neuropsychology, 1,* 249–258.

MORRIS. R.G. (1986). Short-term forgetting in senile dementia of the Alzheimer's type. *Cognitive Neuropsychology, 3,* 77–97.

MORRIS, R.G. (1987). Articulatory rehearsal in Alzheimer type dementia. *Brain and Language, 30,* 351–362.

MORROW, L., RATCLIFF, G., & JOHNSTON, S. (1985). Externalizing spatial knowledge in patients with right hemisphere lesions. *Cognitive Neuropsychology, 2,* 265–274.

MORROW, L., VRTUNSKI, P.B., KIM, Y., & BOLLER, F. (1981). Arousal responses to emotional stimuli and laterality of lesion. *Neuropsychologia, 19,* 65–71.

MORTON, J. (1970). A functional model for memory. In D.A. Norman (Ed.), *Models of human memory* (pp. 203–254). New York: Academic Press.

MORTON, J. (1985). The problem with amnesia: The problem with human memory. *Cognitive Neuropsychology, 2,* 281–290.

MOSCOVITCH, M., & OLDS, J. (1982). Asymmetries in spontaneous facial expressions and their possible relation to hemispheric specialization. *Neuropsychologia, 20,* 71–82.

MOSS, C.S. (1972). *Recovery with aphasia: The aftermath of my stroke.* Urbana, IL: University of Illinois Press.

MOWRER, D.E. (1982). *Methods of modifying speech behaviors: Learning theory in speech pathology* (Second Edition). Prospect Heights, IL: Waveland Press.

MURDOCH, B.E. (1988). Computerized tomographic scanning: Its contributions to the understanding of the neuroanatomical basis of aphasia. *Aphasiology, 2,* 437–462.

MURDOCH, B.E., AFFORD, R.J., LING, A.R., & GANGULEY, B. (1986). Acute computerized tomographic scans: Their value in the localization of lesions and as prognostic indicators in aphasia. *Journal of Communication Disorders, 19,* 311–345.

MURDOCH, B.E., CHENERY, H.J., WILKS, V., & BOYLE, R.S. (1987). Language disorders in dementia of the Alzheimer type. *Brain and Language, 31,* 122–137.

MUTTER, S.A., HOWARD, D.V., HOWARD, JR., J.H., & WIGGS, C.L. (1990). Performance on direct and indirect tests of memory after closed head injury. *Cognitive Neuropsychology, 7,* 329–346.

MYERS, P.S. (1979). Profiles of communication deficits in patients with right cerebral hemisphere damage. In R.H. Brookshire (Ed.), *Clinical aphasiology conference proceedings* (pp. 38–46). Minneapolis: BRK.

MYERS, P.S. (1986). Right hemisphere communication impairment. In R. Chapey (Ed.), *Language intervention strategies in adult aphasia* (Second Edition) (pp. 444–461). Baltimore: Williams & Wilkins.

MYERS, P.S., LINEBAUGH, C.W., & MACKISACK-MORIN, L. (1985). Extracting implicit meaning: Right versus left hemisphere damage. In R.H. Brookshire (Ed.), *Clinical aphasiology* (Vol. 15) (pp. 72–82). Minneapolis: BRK.

MYERS, P.S., & MACKISACK, E.L. (1986). Defining single versus dual definition idioms: The performance of right hemisphere and non-brain-damaged adults. In R.H. Brookshire (Ed.), *Clinical aphasiology* (Vol. 16) (pp. 267–274). Minneapolis: BRK.

MYERSON, R., & GOODGLASS, H. (1972). Transformational grammars of aphasic patients. *Language and Speech, 15,* 40–50.

NAESER, M.A. (1988). Some effects of subcortical white matter lesions on language behavior in aphasia. *Aphasiology, 2,* 363–368.

NAESER, M.A., & HAYWARD, R.W. (1978). Lesion localization in aphasia with cranial computed tomography and the Boston Diagnostic Aphasia Exam. *Neurology, 28,* 545–551.

NAESER, M.A., HAYWARD, R.W., LAUGHLIN, S.A., & ZATZ, L.M. (1981). Quantitative CT scan studies in aphasia. I. Infarct size and CT numbers. *Brain and Language, 12,* 140–164.

NAESER, M.A., PALUMBO, C.L., HELM-ESTABROOKS, N., STIASSNY-EDER, D., & ALBERT, M.L. (1989). Severe nonfluency in aphasia. Role of the medial subcallosal fasciculus and other white matter pathways in recovery of spontaneous speech. *Brain, 112,* 1–38.

NASS, R., DECOUDRES PETERSON, H., & KOCH, D. (1989). Differential effects of congenital left and right brain injury on intelligence. *Brain and Cognition, 9,* 258–266.

NAVIA, B.A., JORDAN, B.D., & PRICE, R.W (1986). The AIDS dementia complex: I. Clinical features. *Annals of Neurology, 19,* 517–524.

NEBES, R.D. (1985). Preservation of semantic structure in dementia. In H.K. Ulatowska (Ed.), *The aging brain: Communication in the elderly* (pp. 109–122). San Diego, CA: College-Hill.

NEBES, R.D., BOLLER, F., & HOLLAND, A.L. (1986). Use of semantic context by patients with Alzheimer's disease. *Psychology and Aging, 1,* 261–269.

NEEDHAM, L.S., & SWISHER, L.P. (1972). A comparison of three tests of auditory comprehension for adult aphasics. *Journal of Speech and Hearing Disorders, 37,* 123–131.

NEELY, J.H. (1976). Semantic priming and retrieval from lexical memory: Evidence for facilitatory and inhibitory processes. *Memory & Cognition, 13,* 140–144.

NEELY, J.H. (1977). Semantic priming and retrieval from lexical memory: Roles of inhibitionless spreading activation and limited-capacity attention. *Journal of Experimental Psychology: General, 106,* 226–254.

NEISSER, U. (1967). *Cognitive psychology*. New York: Appleton-Century-Crofts.

NESPOULOUS, J., DORDAIN, M., PERRON, C., SKA, B., BUB, D., CAPLAN, D., MEHLER, J., & LECOURS, A.R. (1988). Agrammatism in sentence production without comprehension deficits: Reduced availability of syntactic structures and/or of grammatical morphemes? A case study. *Brain and Language, 33,* 273-295.

NEVILLE, H.J., KUTAS, M., CHESNEY, G., & SCHMIDT, A.L. (1986). Event-related brain potentials during initial encoding and recognition memory of congruous and incongruous words. *Journal of Memory and Language, 25,* 75-92.

NEWCOMBE, F. (1969). *Missile wounds to the brain: A study of psychological deficits*. Oxford: Clarendon Press.

NEWHOFF, M.N., & DAVIS, G.A. (1978). A spouse intervention program: Planning, implementation and problems of evaluation. In H. Brookshire (Ed.), *Clinical aphasiology conference proceedings* (pp. 318-326). Minneapolis: BRK.

NEWMEYER (1986). *Linguistic theory in America* (Second Edition). Orlando, FL: Academic Press.

NICHELLI, P., RINALDI, M., & CUBELLI, R. (1989). Selective spatial attention and length representation in normal subjects and in patients with unilateral spatial neglect. *Brain and Cognition, 9,* 57-70.

NICHOLAS, L.E., & BROOKSHIRE, R.H. (1979). An analysis of how clinicians respond to unacceptable patient responses in aphasia treatment sessions. In R.H. Brookshire (Ed.), *Clinical aphasiology conference proceedings* (pp. 131-138). Minneapolis: BRK.

NICHOLAS, L.E., & BROOKSHIRE, R.H. (1986). Consistency of the effects of rate of speech on brain-damaged adults' comprehension of narrative discourse. *Journal of Speech and Hearing Research, 29,* 462-470.

NICHOLAS, L.E., BROOKSHIRE, R.H., MacLENNAN, D.L., SCHUMACHER, J.G., & PORRAZZO, S.A. (1989). Revised administration and scoring procedures for the Boston Naming Test and norms for non-brain-damaged adults. *Aphasiology, 3,* 569-580.

NICHOLAS, L.E., MacLENNAN, D.L., & BROOKSHIRE, R.H. (1986). Validity of multiple-sentence reading comprehension tests for aphasic adults. *Journal of Speech and Hearing Disorders, 51,* 82-87.

NICHOLAS, M., OBLER, L.K., ALBERT, M.L., & HELM-ESTABROOKS, N. (1985). Empty speech in Alzheimer's disease and fluent aphasia. *Journal of Speech and Hearing Research, 28,* 405-410.

NILIPOUR, R., & ASHAYERI, H. (1989). Alternating antagonism between two languages with successive recovery of a third in a trilingual aphasic patient. *Brain and Language, 36,* 23-48.

NOLL, J.D., & RANDOLF, S.R. (1978). Auditory semantic, syntactic, and retention errors made by aphasic subjects on the Token Test. *Journal of Communication Disorders, 11,* 543-553.

NORTHEN, B., HOPCUTT, B., & GRIFFITHS, H. (1990). Progressive aphasia without generalized dementia. *Aphasiology, 4,* 55-66.

NOVOA, O.P., & ARDILA, A. (1987). Linguistic abilities in patients with prefrontal damage. *Brain and Language, 30,* 206-225.

OBER, B.A., DRONKERS, N.F., KOSS, E., DELIS, D.C., & FRIEDLAND, R.P. (1986). Retrieval from semantic memory in Alzheimer-type dementia. *Journal of Clinical and Experimental Neuropsychology, 8,* 75-92.

OBLER, L.K., & ALBERT, M.L. (1977). Influence of aging on recovery from aphasia in polyglots. *Brain and Language, 4,* 460-463.

OBLER, L.K., & ALBERT, M.L. (1981). Language in the elderly aphasic and the dementing patient. In M.T. Sarno (Ed.), *Acquired aphasia* (pp. 385-398). New York: Academic Press.

OBLER, L.K., ALBERT, M.L., GOODGLASS, H., & BENSON, D.F. (1978). Aging and aphasia type. *Brain and Language, 6,* 318-322.

OBLER, L.K., ZATORRE, R.J., GALLOWAY, L., & VAID, J. (1982). Cerebral lateralization in bilinguals: Methodological issues. *Brain and Language, 15,* 40-54.

OJEMANN, G.A. (1983). Brain organization for language from the perspective of electrical stimulation mapping. *Behavioral and Brain Sciences, 6,* 189-230.

OJEMANN, G.A., & WHITAKER, H.A. (1978). Language lateralization and variability. *Brain and Language, 6,* 239-260.

OLDENDORF, W.H. (1978). The quest for an image of brain: A brief historical and technical review of brain imaging techniques. *Neurology, 28,* 517-533.

OLSEN, S.T., BRUHN, P., & OBERG, R.G.E. (1986). Cortical hypoperfusion as a possible cause of subcortical aphasia. *Brain, 109,* 393-410.

ORGASS, B., & POECK, K. (1969). Assessment of aphasia by psychometric methods. *Cortex, 5,* 317-330.

ORNSTEIN, R., JOHNSTONE, J., HERRON, J., & SWENCIONIS, C. (1980). Differential right hemisphere engagement in visuospatial tasks. *Neuropsychologia, 18,* 49-64.

ORTONY, A., SCHALLERT, D.L., REYNOLDS, R.E., & ANTOS, S.J. (1978). Interpreting metaphors and idioms: Some effects of context on comprehension. *Journal of Verbal Learning and Verbal Behavior, 17,* 465-477.

OSTRIN, R.K., & SCHWARTZ, M.F. (1986). Reconstructing from a degraded trace: A study of sentence repetition in agrammatism. *Brain and Language, 28,* 328-345.

PAIVIO, A. (1986). *Mental representations: A dual coding approach*. Oxford, UK: Oxford University Press.

PARADIS, M. (1977). Bilingualism and aphasia. In H. Whitaker & H.A. Whitaker (Eds.), *Studies in neurolinguistics* (Vol. 3) (pp. 65-122). New York: Academic Press.

PARADIS, M. (1990). Language lateralization in biluals: Enough already! *Brain and Language, 39,* 576-586.

PARADIS, M., & GOLDBLUM, M-C. (1989). Selective crossed aphasia in a trilingual aphasic patient followed by reciprocal antagonism. *Brain and Language,* 36, 62–75.

PARADIS, M., GOLDBLUM, M-C., & ABIDI, R. (1982). Alternate antagonism with paradoxical translation behavior in two bilingual aphasic patients. *Brain and Language,* 15, 55–69.

PARISI, D., & PIZZAMIGLIO, L. (1971). Syntactic comprehension in aphasia. *Cortex,* 6, 204–215.

PARSONS, C.L. (1987a). Call me irresponsible, but don't try to mislead me. *Aphasiology,* 1, 443–444.

PARSONS, C.L. (1987b). Is there support for assumptions underlying 'Reapportioning time for aphasia rehabilitation: A point of view'? *Aphasiology,* 1, 81–86.

PARSONS. C.L., LAMBIER, J.D., & MILLER, A. (1988). Phonological processes and phonemic paraphasias. *Aphasiology,* 2, 45–54.

PATE, D.S., SAFFRAN, E.M., & MARTIN, N. (1987). Specifying the nature of the production impairment in a conduction aphasic: A case study. *Language and Cognitive Processes,* 2, 43–84.

PATRONAS, N.J., DEVEIKIS, J.P., & SCHELLINGER, D. (1987). The use of computed tomography in studying the brain. In H.G. Mueller & V.C. Geoffrey (Eds.), *Communication disorders in aging: Assessment and management* (pp. 107–134). Washington, DC: Gallaudet University Press.

PATTERSON, K., PURELL C., & MORTON, J. (1983). The facilitation of word retrieval in aphasia. In C. Code & D.J. Muller (Eds.), *Aphasia therapy* (pp. 76–87). London: Edward Arnold.

PATTERSON, K., & WILSON, B. (1990). A ROSE is a ROSE or a NOSE: A deficit in initial letter identification. *Cognitive Neuropsychology,* 7, 447–478.

PEACH, R.K. (1987). A short-term memory treatment approach to the repetition deficit in conduction aphasia. In R.H. Brookshire (Ed.), *Clinical aphasiology* (Vol. 17) (pp. 35–45). Minneapolis: BRK.

PEACH, R.K., CANTER, G.J., & GALLAHER, A.J. (1988). Comprehension of sentence structure in anomic and conduction aphasia. *Brain and Language,* 35, 119–137.

PEASE, D.M., & GOODGLASS, H. (1978). The effects of cuing on picture naming in aphasia. *Cortex,* 14, 178–189.

PENFIELD, W., & PEROT, P. (1963). The brain's record of visual and auditory experience: A final summary and discussion. *Brain,* 86, 595–696.

PENFIELD, W., & ROBERTS, L. (1959). *Speech and brain mechanisms.* Princeton, NJ: Princeton University Press.

PERECMAN, E. (1984). Spontaneous translation and language mixing in a polyglot aphasic. *Brain and Language,* 23, 43–63.

PERFETTI, C.A., BELL, L.C., & DELANEY, S.M. (1988). Automatic (prelexical) phonetic activation in silent word reading: Evidence from backward masking. *Journal of Memory and Language,* 27, 59–70.

PETERSON, S.E., FOX, P.T., POSNER, M.I., MINTUN, M.A., & RAICHLE, M.E. (1988). PET studies of the cortical anatomy of single-word processing. *Nature,* 331, 585–589.

PETTIT, J.M., McNEIL, M.R., & KEITH, R.L. (1989). The use of novel and real-word stimuli in the assessment of English morphology in adults with aphasia. *Aphasiology,* 3, 655–666.

PETTIT, J.M., & NOLL, J.D. (1979). Cerebral dominance in aphasia recovery. *Brain and Language,* 7, 191–200.

PEUSER, G., & SCHRIEFERS, H. (1980). Sentence comprehension in aphasics: Results of administration the "Three-Figures-Test" (TFT). *British Journal of Disorders of Communication,* 15, 157–173.

PFEIFFER, E. (1975). A short portable mental status questionnaire for the assessment of organic brain deficit in elderly patients. *Journal of the American Geriatrics Society,* 23, 433–441.

PIAZZA, D.M. (1980). The influence of sex and handedness in the hemispheric specialization of verbal and nonverbal tasks. *Neuropsychologia,* 18, 163–176.

PICKERSGILL, M.J., & LINCOLN, N.B. (1983). Prognostic indicators and the pattern of recovery of communication in aphasic stroke patients. *Journal of Neurology, Neurosurgery, and Psychiatry,* 46, 130–139.

PICTON, T.W., & STUSS, D.T. (1984). Event-related potentials in the study of speech and language: A critical review. In D. Caplan, A.R. Lecours, & A. Smith (Eds.), *Biological perspectives on language* (pp. 303–360). Cambridge, MA: MIT Press.

PIEHLER, M.F., & HOLLAND, A.L. (1984). Cohesion in aphasic language. In R.H. Brookshire (Ed.), *Clinical aphasiology: conference proceedings* (pp. 208–214). Minneapolis: BRK.

PIERCE, R.S. (1982). Facilitating the comprehension of syntax in aphasia. *Journal of Speech and Hearing Research,* 25, 408–413.

PIERCE, R.S. (1988). Influence of prior and subsequent context on comprehension in aphasia. *Aphasiology,* 2, 577–582.

PIERCE, R.S., & BEEKMAN, L.A. (1985). Effects of linguistic and extralinguistic context on semantic and syntactic processing in aphasia. *Journal of Speech and Hearing Research,* 28, 250–254.

PIERCE, R.S., JARECKI, J., & CANNITO, M. (1990). Single word comprehension in aphasia: Influence of array size, picture relatedness and situational context. *Aphasiology,* 4, 155–166.

PIZZAMIGLIO, L., & APPICCIAFUOCO, A. (1971). Semantic comprehension in aphasia. *Journal of Communication Disorders,* 3, 280–288.

PIZZAMIGLIO, L., MAMMUCARI, A., & RAZZANO, C. (1985). Evidence for sex differences in brain organization in recovery in aphasia. *Brain and Language,* 25, 213–223.

PODRAZA, B.L., & DARLEY, F.L. (1977). Effect of auditory

prestimulation on naming in aphasia. *Journal of Speech and Hearing Research, 20,* 669–683.

POECK, K., & HARTJE, W. (1979). Performance of aphasic patients in visual versus auditory presentation of the Token Test: Demonstration of a supramodal deficit. In F. Boller & M. Dennis (Eds.), *Auditory comprehension: Clinical and experimental studies with the Token Test* (pp. 107–116). New York: Academic Press.

POECK, K., HUBER, W., & WILLMES, K. (1989). Outcome of intensive language treatment in aphasia. *Journal of Speech and Hearing Disorders, 54,* 471–478.

POECK, K., KERSCHENSTEINER, M., & HARTJE, W. (1972). A quantitative study on language understanding in fluent and nonfluent aphasia. *Cortex, 8,* 299–304.

POECK, K., ORGASS, B., KERSCHENSTEINER, M., & HARTJE, W. (1974). A qualitative study on Token Test performance in aphasic and non-aphasic brain damaged patients. *Neuropsychologia, 12,* 49–54.

POECK, K., & PIETRON, H. (1981). The influence of stretched speech presentation on Token Test performance of aphasic and right brain damaged patients. *Neuropsychologia, 19,* 133–136.

POIZNER, H., KLIMA, E.S., & BELLUGI, U. (1987). *What the hands reveal about the brain.* Cambridge, MA: MIT Press.

POLLIO, H.R., SMITH, M.K., & POLLIO, M.R. (1990). Figurative language and cognitive psychology. *Language and Cognitive Processes, 5,* 141–167.

PORCH, B.E. (1967). *Porch Index of Communicative Ability, Volume I: Theory and development.* Palo Alto, CA: Consulting Psychologists Press.

PORCH, B.E. (1971). *Porch Index of Communicative Ability: Volume II: Administration, scoring, and interpretation* (Second Edition). Palo Alto, CA: Consulting Psychologists Press.

PORCH, B.E. (1974). Comments on Silverman's "Psychometric problem." *Journal of Speech and Hearing Disorders, 39,* 226–227.

PORCH, B.E. (1978). Profiles of aphasia: Test interpretation regarding the localization of lesions. In R.H. Brookshire (Ed.), *Clinical aphasiology conference proceedings* (pp. 78–92). Minneapolis: BRK.

PORCH, B.E. (1981). *Porch Index of Communicative Ability, Volume II: Administration, scoring, and interpretation* (Third Edition). Palo Alto, CA: Consulting Psychologists Press.

PORCH, B.E. (1986). Therapy subsequent to the Porch Index of Communicative Ability (PICA). In R. Chapey (Ed.), *Language intervention strategies in adult aphasia* (Second Edition) (pp. 295–303). Baltimore: Williams & Wilkins.

PORCH, B.E., & CALLAGHAN, S. (1981). Making predictions about recovery: Is there HOAP? In R.H. Brookshire (Ed.), *Clinical aphasiology conference proceedings* (pp. 187–200). Minneapolis: BRK.

PORCH, B.E., COLLINS, M., WERTZ, R.T., & FRIDEN, T.P.

(1980). Statistical prediction of change in aphasia. *Journal of Speech and Hearing Research, 23,* 312–321.

PORCH, B.E., & DE BERKELEY-WYKES, J. (1985). Bilingual aphasia and its implications for cerebral organization and recovery. In R.H. Brookshire (Ed.), *Clinical aphasiology* (Vol. 15) (pp. 107–112). Minneapolis: BRK.

PORCH, B.E., & PALMER, P.M. (1986). Right hemisphere PICA percentiles revised. In R.H. Brookshire (Ed.), *Clinical aphasiology* (Vol. 16) (pp. 275–280). Minneapolis: BRK.

PORCH, B.E., & POREC, J.P. (1977). Medical-legal application of PICA results. In R.H. Brookshire (Ed.), *Clinical aphasiology conference proceedings* (pp. 302–309). Minneapolis: BRK.

POREC, J.P., & PORCH, B.E. (1977). The behavioral characteristics of "simulated" aphasia. In R.H. Brookshire (Ed.), *Clinical aphasiology conference proceedings* (pp. 207–301). Minneapolis: BRK.

PORTER, J.L., & DABUL, B. (1977). The application of transactional analysis to therapy with wives of adult aphasic patients. *Asha, 19,* 244–248.

POSNER, J.D., GORMAN, K.M., & WOLDOW, A. (1984). Stroke in the elderly: I. Epidemiology. *Journal of the American Geriatrics Society, 32,* 95–102.

POSNER, M.I., WALKER, J.A., FRIEDRICH, F.J., & RAFAL, R.D. (1987). How do the parietal lobes direct covert attention? *Neuropsychologia, 25,* 135–146.

POWELL, G.E., BAILEY, S., & CLARK, E. (1980). A very short form of the Minnesota Aphasia Test. *British Journal of Social and Clinical Psychology, 19,* 189–194.

POWELL, G.E., CLARK, E., & BAILEY, S. (1979). Categories of aphasia: A cluster-analysis of Schuell test profiles. *British Journal of Disorders of Communication, 14,* 111–122.

PRESCOTT, T.E., GRUBER, J.L., OLSON, M., & FULLER, K.C. (1987). Hanoi revisited. In R.H. Brookshire (Ed.), *Clinical aphasiology* (Vol. 17) (pp. 249–259). Minneapolis: BRK.

PRESCOTT, T.E., LOVERSO, F.L., & SELINGER, M. (1984). Differences between normal and left brain damaged (aphasic) subjects in a nonverbal problem solving task. In R.H. Brookshire (Ed.), *Clinical aphasiology conference proceedings* (pp. 235–240). Minneapolis: BRK.

PRIGATANO, G.P. (1987). Recovery and cognitive retraining after craniocerebral trauma. *Journal of Learning Disabilities, 20,* 603–613.

PRINS, R.S., SNOW, C.E., & WAGENAAR, E. (1978). Recovery from aphasia: Spontaneous speech versus language comprehension. *Brain and Language, 6,* 192–211.

PRUTTING, C.A., & KIRCHNER, D.M. (1987). A clinical appraisal of the pragmatic aspects of language. *Journal of Speech and Hearing Disorders, 52,* 105–119.

QUINTEROS, B., WILLIAMS D.R.R., WHITE, C.A.M., & PICKERING, M. (1984). The costs of using trained and supervised volunteers as part of a speech therapy service for dysphasic patients. *British Journal of Disorders of Communication,* 19, 205–212.

RAPPORT, R.L., TAN, C.T., & WHITAKER, H.A. (1983). Language function and dysfunction among Chinese- and English-speaking polyglots: Cortical stimulation, Wada testing, and clinical studies. *Brain and Language,* 18, 342–366.

RAVEN, J.C., COURT, J.H., & RAVEN, J. (1976). *Manual for Raven's Progressive Matrices and Vocabulary Scales, Section I: General overview.* London: H.K. Lewis.

RAYNER, K., CARLSON, M., & FRAZIER, L. (1983). The interaction of syntax and semantics during sentence processing: Eye movements in the analysis of semantically biased sentences. *Journal of Verbal Learning and Verbal Behavior,* 22, 358–374.

RAYNER, K., & POLLATSEK, A. (1989). *The psychology of reading.* Englewood Cliffs, NJ: Prentice-Hall.

RAYNER, K., SERENO, S.C., MORRIS, R.K., SCHMAUDER, A.R., & CLIFTON, C. (1989). Eye movements and on-line language comprehension processes. *Language and Cognitive Processes,* 4, SI 21–50.

READ, D.E. (1981). Solving deductive reasoning problems after unilateral temporal lobectomy. *Brain and Language,* 12, 116–127.

REED, S.K. (1992). *Cognition* (Third Edition). Pacific Grove, CA: Brooks/Cole.

REITAN, R.M., & TARSHES, E.L. (1959). Differential effects of lateralized brain lesions on the Trail Making Test. *Journal of Nervous and Mental Disease,* 129, 257–262.

REITAN, R.M., & WOLFSON, D. 1985). *The Halstead-Reitan Neuropsychological Test Battery: Theory and clinical interpretation.* Tucson, AZ: Neuropsychology Press.

RICE, B., PAULL, A., & MULLER, D.J. (1987). An evaluation of a social support group for spouses of aphasic partners. *Aphasiology,* 1, 247–256.

RIDDOCH, M.J. (1990). Loss of visual imagery: A generation deficit. *Cognitive Neuropsychology,* 7, 249–274.

RIDDOCH, M.J., HUMPHREYS, G.W., CLETON, P., & FERRY, P. (1990). Interaction of attentional and lexical processes in neglect dyslexia. *Cognitive Neuropsychology,* 7, 479–518.

RIDDOCH, M.J., HUMPHREYS, G.W., COLTHEART, M., & FUNNELL, E. (1988). Semantic systems or system? Neuropsychological evidence re-examined. *Cognitive Neuropsychology,* 5, 3–26.

RIEDEL, K., & STUDDERT-KENNEDY, M. (1985). Extending formant transitions may not improve aphasics' perception of stop consonant place of articulation. *Brain and Language,* 24, 223–232.

RIEGE, W.H., METTER, E.J., & HANSON, W.R. (1980). Verbal and nonverbal recognition memory in aphasic and nonaphasic stroke patients. *Brain and Language,* 10, 60–70.

RIMEL, R.W., & JANE, J.A. (1983). Characteristics of the head-injured patient. In M. Rosenthal, E.R. Griffith, M.R. Bond, & J.D. Miller (Eds.), *Rehabilitation of the head injured adult* (pp. 9–22). Philadelphia: F.A. Davis.

RINNERT, C., & WHITAKER, H.A. (1973). Semantic confusions by aphasic patients. *Cortex,* 9, 56–81.

RIPICH, D.N., & TERRELL, B.Y. (1988). Patterns of discourse cohesion and coherence in Alzheimer's disease. *Journal of Speech and Hearing Disorders,* 53, 8–15.

RIVERS, D.L., & LOVE, R.J. (1980). Language performance on visual processing tasks in right hemisphere lesion cases. *Brain and Language,* 10, 348–366.

ROBERTS, J.A., & WERTZ, R.T. (1989). Comparison of spontaneous and elicited oral-expressive language in aphasia. In T.E. Prescott (Ed.), *Clinical aphasiology* (Vol. 18) (pp. 479–488). Boston: College-Hill/Little, Brown.

ROBERTSON, I. (1990). Does computerized cognitive rehabilitation work? *Aphasiology,* 4, 381–405.

ROBIN, D.A., & SCHIENBERG, S. (1990). Subcortical lesions and aphasia. *Journal of Speech and Hearing Disorders,* 55, 90–100.

ROBINSON, R.G., KUBOS, K.L., STARR, L.B., RAO, K., & PRICE, T.R. (1984). Mood disorders in stroke patients: Importance of location of lesion. *Brain,* 107, 81–93.

ROCHFORD, G., & WILLIAMS, M. (1965). Studies in the development and breakdown of the use of names, IV: The effects of word frequency. *Journal of Neurology, Neurosurgery, and Psychiatry,* 28, 407–413.

ROGERS, C.R. (1951). *Client-centered therapy.* Boston: Houghton Mifflin.

ROGERS, C.R. (1961). *On becoming a person.* Boston: Houghton Mifflin.

ROLLIN, W.J. (1987). *The psychology of communication disorders in individuals and their families.* Englewood Cliffs, NJ: Prentice-Hall.

ROMAN, M., BROWNELL, H.H., POTTER, H.H., SEIBOLD, M.S., & GARDNER, H. (1987). Script knowledge in right hemisphere-damaged and in normal elderly adults. *Brain and Language,* 31, 151–170.

ROSCH, E., & MERVIS, C.B. (1975). Family resemblances: Studies in the internal structure of categories. *Cognitive Psychology,* 7, 573–605.

ROSE, S. (1989). *The conscious brain* (Revised Edition). New York: Paragon.

ROSENBEK, J.C. (1982). When is aphasia aphasia? In R.H. Brookshire (Ed.), *Clinical aphasiology conference proceedings* (pp. 360–366). Minneapolis: BRK.

ROSENBEK, J.C., LaPOINTE, L.L., & WERTZ, R.T. (1989). *Aphasia: A clinical approach.* San Diego: Singular.

ROSENBERG, B., ZURIF, E., BROWNELL, H., GARRETT, M., & BRADLEY, D. (1985). Grammatical class effects in relation to normal and aphasic sentence processing. *Brain and Language,* 26, 287–303.

Ross, E.D. (1981). The aprosodias: Functional-anatomic organization of the affective components of language in the right hemisphere. *Archives of Neurology, 38,* 561–569.

Ross, E.D., & Mesulam, M. (1979). Dominant language functions of the right hemisphere? Prosody and emotional gesturing. *Archives of Neurology, 36,* 144–148.

Ross, G.W., Cummings, J.L., & Benson, D.F. (1990). Speech and language alterations in dementia syndromes: Characteristics and treatment. *Aphasiology, 4,* 339–352.

Rothi, L.J., & Hutchinson, E.C. (1981). Retention of verbal information by rehearsal in relation to the fluency of verbal output in aphasia. *Brain and Language, 12,* 347–359.

Rubens, A.B. (1977a). The role of changes within the central nervous system during recovery from aphasia. In M. Sullivan & M.S. Kommers (Eds.), *Rationale for adult aphasia therapy* (pp. 28–43). University of Nebraska Medical Center.

Rubens, A.B. (1977b). What neurologists expect of clinical aphasiologists. In R.H. Brookshire (Ed.), *Clinical aphasiology conference proceedings* (pp. 1–4). Minneapolis: BRK.

Russell, W.R., & Espir, M.L.E. (1961). *Traumatic aphasia.* London: Oxford University Press.

Ryalls, J.H. (1986). What constitutes a primary disturbance of speech prosody? A reply to Shapiro and Danly. *Brain and Language, 29,* 183–187

Ryalls, J.H., & Behrens, S.J. (1988). An overview of changes in fundamental frequency associated with cortical insult. *Aphasiology, 2,* 107–116.

Sackheim, H.A., Greenberg, M.S, Weiman, A.L., Gur, R.C., Hungerbuhler, J.P., & Geschwind, N. (1982). Hemisphere asymmetry in the expression of positive and negative emotion. *Archives of Neurology, 39,* 210–218.

Sacks, O. (1985). *The man who mistook his wife for a hat and other clinical tales.* New York: Summit.

Saffran, E.M., & Marin, O.S.M. (1975). Immediate memory for word lists and sentences in a patient with deficient auditory-verbal short-term memory. *Brain and Language, 2,* 420–433.

Saffran, E.M., & Schwartz, M.F. (1988). "Agrammatic" comprehension it's not: Alternatives and implications. *Aphasiology, 2,* 389–394.

Saffran, E.M., Schwartz, M.F., & Marin, O.S.M. (1980). The word order problem in agrammatism. II. Production. *Brain and Language, 10,* 263–280.

Salvatore, A.P. (1985). Experimental analysis of acquisition and generalization of syntax in Broca's aphasia. In R.H. Brookshire (Ed.), *Clinical aphasiology* (Vol. 15) (pp. 214–221). Minneapolis: BRK.

Salvatore, A.P., & Thompson C.K. (1986). Intervention for global aphasia. In R. Chapey (Ed.), *Language intervention strategies in adult aphasia* (Second Edition) (pp. 402–418). Baltimore: Williams & Wilkins.

Salvatore, A.P., Trunzo, M.J., Holtzapple, P., & Graham, L. (1983). Investigation of the sentence hierarchy of the Helm Elicited Language Program for Syntax Stimulation. In R.H. Brookshire (Ed.), *Clinical aphasiology conference proceedings* (pp. 73–84). Minneapolis: BRK.

Samuels, J.A., & Benson, D.F. (1979). Some aspects of language comprehension in anterior aphasia. *Brain and Language, 8,* 275–286.

Sanders, S.B. (1986). Maximum recovery: By what definition? In R.C. Marshall (Ed.), *Case studies in aphasia rehabilitation: For clinicians by clinicians* (pp. 89–104). Austin, Tx: Pro-Ed.

Sanders, S.B., & Davis, G.A. (1978). A comparison of the Porch Index of Communicative Ability and the Western Aphasia Battery. In R.H. Brookshire (Ed.), *Clinical aphasiology conference proceedings* (pp. 117–126). Minneapolis: BRK.

Sanders, S.B., Davis, G.A., & Wells, R. (1981). Influence of the preposition in language comprehension subtests of the PICA. In R.H. Brookshire (Ed.), *Clinical aphasiology conference proceedings* (pp. 115–119). Minneapolis: BRK.

Sanders, S.B., Hamby, E.I., & Nelson, M. (1984). *You are not alone: Organizing your local stroke club.* Nashville: Tennessee Affiliate of the American Heart Association.

Sands, E., Sarno, M.T., & Shankweiler, D. (1969). Long-term assessment of language function in aphasia due to stroke. *Archives of Physical Medicine and Rehabilitation, 50,* 202–207.

Santo Pietro, M.J., & Goldfarb, R. (1985). Characteristic patterns of word association responses in institutionalized elderly with and without senile dementia. *Brain and Language, 26,* 230–243.

Sarno, J.E., Sarno, M.T., & Levita, E. (1971). Evaluating language improvement after completed stroke. *Archives of Physical Medicine and Rehabilitation, 52,* 73–78.

Sarno, M.T. (1969). *The functional communication profile manual of directions.* Rehabilitation Monograph 42, New York University Medical Center.

Sarno, M.T. (1980). The nature of verbal impairment after closed head injury. *Journal of Nervous and Mental Disease, 168,* 685–692.

Sarno, M.T. (1981). Recovery and rehabilitation in aphasia. In M.T. Sarno (Ed.), *Acquired aphasia* (pp. 485–529). New York: Academic Press.

Sarno, M.T., Buonaguro, A., & Levita, E. (1987). Aphasia in closed head injury and stroke. *Aphasiology, 1,* 331–338.

Sarno, M.T., & Levita, E. (1971). Natural course of recovery in severe aphasia. *Archives of Physical Medicine and Rehabilitation, 52,* 175–178.

Sarno, M.T., & Levita, E. (1979). Recovery in treated aphasia during the first year post-stroke. *Stroke, 10,* 663–670.

Sarno, M.T., & Levita, E. (1981). Some observations on

the nature of recovery in global aphasia after stroke. *Brain and Language, 13,* 1–12.

SARNO, M.T., SILVERMAN, M., & SANDS, E. (1970). Speech therapy and language recovery in severe aphasia. *Journal of Speech and Hearing Research, 13,* 607–623.

SCHACTER, D.L. (1987). Implicit memory: History and current status. *Journal of Experimental Psychology: Learning, Memory, and Cognition, 13,* 501–518.

SCHERER, N.J., & OLSWANG, L.B. (1989). Using structured discourse as a language intervention technique with autistic children. *Journal of Speech and Hearing Disorders, 54,* 383–394.

SCHIENBERG, S., & HOLLAND, A. (1980). Conversational turn-taking in Wernicke's aphasia. In R. Brookshire (Ed.), *Clinical aphasiology conference proceedings* (pp. 106–110). Minneapolis: BRK.

SCHLANGER, B.B., SCHLANGER, P.H., & GERSTMAN, L.J. (1976). The perception of emotionally toned sentences by right hemisphere-damaged and aphasic subjects. *Brain and Language, 3,* 396–403.

SCHLANGER, P.H., & SCHLANGER, B.B. (1970). Adapting role playing activities with aphasic patients. *Journal of Speech and Hearing Disorders, 35,* 229–235.

SCHNEIDERMAN, E.I., & SADDY, J.D. (1988). A linguistic deficit resulting from right-hemisphere damage. *Brain and Language, 34,* 38–54.

SCHNITZER, M.L. (1978). Toward a neurolinguistic theory of language. *Brain and Language, 6,* 342–361.

SCHONLE, P.W. (1988). Compound noun stimulation: An intensive treatment approach for severe aphasia. *Aphasiology, 2,* 401–404.

SCHUELL, H.M. (1957). A short examination for aphasia. *Neurology, 7,* 625–634.

SCHUELL, H.M. (1966). A re-evaluation of the short examination for aphasia. *Journal of Speech and Hearing Disorders, 31,* 137–147.

SCHUELL, H.M. (1969). Aphasia in adults. In *Human communication and its disorders—an overview.* Bethesda, MD: U.S. Department of Health, Education, and Welfare.

SCHUELL. H.M. (1973). *Differential diagnosis of aphasia with the Minnesota test* (Second Edition, revised by Sefer, J.W.). Minneapolis: University of Minnesota Press.

SCHUELL, H.M., & JENKINS, J.J. (1959). The nature of language deficit in aphasia. *Psychological Review, 66,* 45–67.

SCHUELL H.M., & JENKINS, J.J. (1961a). Comment on "Dimensions of language performance in aphasia." *Journal of Speech and Hearing Research, 4,* 295–299.

SCHUELL, H.M., & JENKINS, J.J. (1961b). Reduction of vocabulary in aphasia. *Brain, 84,* 243–261.

SCHUELL, H.M., JENKINS, J.J., & CARROLL, J.B. (1962). A factor analysis of the Minnesota Test for the Differential Diagnosis of Aphasia. *Journal of Speech and Hearing Research, 5,* 349–369.

SCHUELL, H.H., JENKINS, J.J., & JIMENEZ-PABON, E. (1964). *Aphasia in adults.* New York: Harper and Row.

SCHUELL, H.M., JENKINS, J.J., & LANDIS, L. (1961). Relationships between auditory comprehension and word frequency in aphasia. *Journal of Speech and Hearing Research, 4,* 30–36.

SCHULTE, E. (1986). Effects of imposed delay of response and item complexity on auditory comprehension by aphasics. *Brain and Language, 29,* 358–371.

SCHUSTACK, M.W., EHRLICH, S.F., & RAYNER, K. (1987). Local and global sources of contextual facilitation in reading. *Journal of Memory and Language, 26,* 322–340.

SCHWARTZ, M.F. (1984). What the classical aphasia categories can't do for us, and why. *Brain and Language, 21,* 3–9.

SCHWARTZ, M.F. (1987). Patterns of speech production deficit within and across aphasia syndromes: Application of a psycholinguistic model. In M. Coltheart, G. Sartori, & R. Job (Eds.), *The cognitive neuropsychology of language* (pp. 163–199). London: Erlbaum.

SCHWARTZ, M.F., LINEBARGER, M.C., & SAFFRAN, E.M. (1985). The status of the syntactic deficit theory of agrammatism. In M-L. Kean (Ed.), *Agrammatism* (pp. 83–124). Orlando, FL: Academic Press.

SCHWARTZ, M.F., LINEBARGER, M.C., SAFFRAN, E.M., & PATE, D.S. (1987). Syntactic transparency and sentence interpretation in aphasia. *Language and Cognitive Processes, 2,* 85–114.

SCHWARTZ, M.F., SAFFRAN, E.M., & MARIN, O.S.M. (1980). The word order problem in agrammatism. I. Comprehension. *Brain and Language, 10,* 249–262.

SCHWARTZ, S., MONTAGNER, S., & KIRSNER, K. (1987). Are there different methods of lexical access for words presented in the left and right visual fields? *Brain and Language, 31,* 301–307.

SCHWARTZ-COWLEY, R., & STEPHANIK, M.J. (1989). Communication disorders and treatment in the acute trauma center setting. *Topics in language disorders, 9,* 1–14.

SCHWEIZER, A., WECHSLER, A.F., & MAZZIOTTA, J.C. (1987). Metabolic correlates of linguistic functions in a patient with crossed aphasia: A case study. *Aphasiology, 1,* 415–422.

SCOTT, C., & BYNG, S. (1989). Computer assisted remediation of a homophone comprehension disorder in surface dyslexia. *Aphasiology, 3,* 301–320.

SEARLE, J.R. (1969). *Speech acts.* London: Cambridge University Press.

SEARLE, J.R. (Ed.). (1979). *Expression and meaning.* Cambridge, UK: Cambridge University Press.

SEIDENBERG, M.S., & McCLELLAND, J.L. (1989). A distributed, developmental model of word recognition and naming. *Psychological Review, 96,* 523–568.

SEIDENBERG, M.S., TANENHAUS, M.K., LEIMAN, J.M., & BIENKOWSKI, M. (1982). Automatic access of the meanings of ambiguous words in context: Some limitations of knowledge-based processing. *Cognitive Psychology, 14,* 489–537.

SEIDENBERG, M.S., WATERS, G.S., BARNES, M., & TANENHAUS, M.K. (1984). When does irregular spelling or pronunciation influence word recognition? *Journal of Verbal Learning and Verbal Behavior, 23,* 383–404.

SELINGER, M., PRESCOTT, T.E., & KATZ, R.C. (1987). Handwritten vs computer responses on Porch Index of Communicative Ability Graphic subtests. In R.H. Brookshire (Ed.), *Clinical aphasiology* (Vol. 17) (pp. 136–142). Minneapolis: BRK.

SELINGER, M., PRESCOTT, T.E., LOVERSO, F., & FULLER, K. (1987). Below the 50th percentile: Application of the verb as core model. In R.H. Brookshire (Ed.), *Clinical aphasiology* (Vol. 17) (pp. 55–63). Minneapolis: BRK.

SEMENZA, C., DENES, G., LUCCHESE, D., & BISIACCHI, P. (1980). Selective deficit of conceptual structures in aphasia: Class versus thematic relations. *Brain and Language, 10,* 243–248.

SERGENT, J. (1982). Theoretical and methodological consequences of variations in exposure duration in visual laterality studies. *Perception & Psychophysics, 31,* 451–461.

SERGENT, J. (1990). The neuropsychology of visual image generation: Data, method, and theory. *Brain and Cognition, 13,* 98–129.

SERGENT, J., & HELLIGE, J.B. (1986). Role of input factors in visual-field asymmetries. *Brain and Cognition, 5,* 174–199.

SERON, X. (1987). Cognition first, microprocessor second. *Aphasiology, 1,* 161–163.

SERON, X., & DELOCHE, G. (1981). Processing of locatives "in," "on," and "under" by aphasic patients: An analysis of the regression hypothesis. *Brain and Language, 14,* 70–80.

SERON, X., & DELOCHE, G. (Eds). (1989). *Cognitive approaches in neuropsychological rehabilitation.* Hillsdale, NJ: Lawrence Erlbaum.

SERON, X., DELOCHE, G., MOULARD, G., & ROUSELLE, M. (1980). A computer-based therapy for the treatment of aphasic subjects with writing disorders. *Journal of Speech and Hearing Disorders, 45,* 45–58.

SERON, X., VAN DER KAA, M., REMITZ, A., & VAN DER LINDEN, M. (1979). Pantomime interpretation and aphasia. *Neuropsychologia, 17,* 661–668.

SERON, X., VAN DER KAA, M., VAN DER LINDEN, M., REMITZ, A., & FEYEREISEN, P. (1982). Decoding paralinguistic signals: Effect of semantic and prosodic cues on aphasics' comprehension. *Journal of Communication Disorders, 15,* 223–231.

SHADDEN, B.B. (1988). Education, counseling, and support for significant others. In B.B. Shadden (Ed.), *Communication behavior and aging: A sourcebook for clinicians* (pp. 309–328). Baltimore: Williams & Wilkins.

SHALLICE, T. (1987). Impairments of semantic processing: Multiple dissociations. In M. Coltheart, G.

Sartori, & R. Job (Eds.), *The cognitive neuropsychology of language* (pp. 111–127). London: Erlbaum.

SHALLICE, T. (1988). *From neuropsychology to mental structure.* Cambridge, UK: Cambridge University Press.

SHALLICE, T., & WARRINGTON, E.K. (1977). Auditory-verbal short-term memory impairment and spontaneous speech. *Brain and Language, 4,* 479–491.

SHANKWEILER, D., CRAIN, S., GORRELL, P., & TULLER, B. (1989). Reception of language in Broca's aphasia. *Language and Cognitive Processes, 4,* 1–34.

SHAPIRO, B.E., & DANLY, M. (1985). The role of the right hemisphere in the control of speech prosody in propositional and affective contexts. *Brain and Language, 25,* 19–36.

SHAPIRO, B.E., GROSSMAN, M., & GARDNER, H. (1981). Selective musical processing deficits in brain damaged populations. *Neuropsychologia, 19,* 161–169.

SHAPIRO, L.P., & LEVINE, B.A. (1990). Verb processing during sentence comprehension in aphasia. *Brain and Language, 38,* 21–47.

SHATTUCK-HUFNAGEL, S. (1979). Speech errors as evidence for a serial ordering mechanism in speech production. In W.E. Cooper & E.C.T. Walker (Eds.), *Sentence processing: Psycholinguistic studies presented to Merrill Garrett* (pp. 295–342). Hillsdale, NJ: Erlbaum.

SHEEHAN, V.M. (1946). Rehabilitation of aphasics in an army hospital. *Journal of Speech and Hearing Disorders, 11,* 149–157.

SHEPARD, R.N., & METZLER, J. (1971). Mental rotation of three-dimensional objects. *Science, 171,* 701–703.

SHERMAN, J.C., & SCHWEICKERT, J. (1989). Syntactic and semantic contributions to sentence comprehension in agrammatism. *Brain and Language, 37,* 419–439.

SHEWAN, C.M. (1976). Error patterns in auditory comprehension of adult aphasics. *Cortex, 12,* 325–336.

SHEWAN, C.M. (1979). *Auditory Comprehension Test for Sentences.* Chicago: Biolinguistics Clinical Institutes.

SHEWAN, C.M. (1982). To hear is not to understand: Auditory processing deficits and factors influencing performance in aphasic individuals. In N.J. Lass (Ed.), *Speech and language: Advances in basic research and practice* (Vol. 7) (pp. 1–70). New York: Academic Press.

SHEWAN, C.M. (1988a). Expressive language recovery in aphasia using the *Shewan Spontaneous Language Analysis* (SSLA) system. *Journal of Communication Disorders, 21,* 155–169.

SHEWAN, C.M. (1988b). The *Shewan Spontaneous Language Analysis* (SSLA) system for aphasic adults: Description, reliability, and validity. *Journal of Communication Disorders, 21,* 103–138.

SHEWAN, C.M., & BANDUR, D.L. (1986). *Treatment of aphasia: A language-oriented approach.* San Diego: Singular.

SHEWAN, C.M., & CANTER, G.J. (1971). Effects of vocabulary, syntax, and sentence length on auditory comprehension in aphasic patients. *Cortex, 7,* 209–226.

SHEWAN, C.M. & KERTESZ, A. (1980). Reliability and validity characteristics of the Western Aphasia Battery (WAB). *Journal of Speech and Hearing Disorders*, 45, 308-324.

SHEWAN, C.M., & KERTESZ, A. (1984). Effects of speech and language treatment on recovery from aphasia. *Brain and Language*, 23, 272-299.

SHIMBERG, E.F. (1990). *Strokes: What families should know*. New York: Ballantine.

SHUTTLEWORTH, E.C., & HUBER, S.J. (1988). The naming disorder of dementia of Alzheimer type. *Brain and Language*, 34, 222-234.

SIDTIS, J.J., & VOLPE, B.T. (1988). Selective loss of complex-pitch or speech discrimination after unilateral lesion. *Brain and Language*, 34, 235-245.

SIEROFF, E. (1990). Focusing on/in visual/verbal stimuli in patients with parietal lesions. *Cognitive Neuropsychology*, 7, 519-554.

SIEROFF, E., POLLATSEK, A., & POSNER, M.I. (1988). Recognition of visual letter strings following injury to the posterior visual spatial attention system. *Cognitive Neuropsychology*, 5, 427-450.

SIES, L.F. (Ed.). (1974). *Aphasia theory and therapy: Selected lectures and papers of Hildred Schuell*. Baltimore: University Park Press.

SILBERMAN, E.K., & WEINGARTNER, H. (1986). Hemispheric lateralization of functions related to emotion. *Brain and Cognition*, 5, 322-354.

SILVERMAN, F.H. (1974). PICA: A psychometric problem and its solution. *Journal of Speech and Hearing Disorders*, 39, 225-226.

SILVERMAN, F.H. (1989). *Communication for the speechless* (Second Edition). Englewood Cliffs, NJ: Prentice-Hall.

SIMMONS, N.N. (1989). A trip down Easy Street. In T.E. Prescott (Ed.), *Clinical aphasiology* (Vol. 18) (pp. 19-30). Austin, TX: Pro-Ed.

SIMPSON, G.B. (1984). Lexical ambiguity and its role in models of word recognition. *Psychological Bulletin*, 96, 316-340.

SIMPSON, G.B., & BURGESS, C. (1985). Activation and selection processes in the recognition of ambiguous words. *Journal of Experimental Psychology: Human Perception and Performance*, 11, 28-39.

SKELLY, M. (1975). Aphasic patients talk back. *American Journal of Nursing*, 75, 1140-1142.

SKELLY, M. (1979). *Amer-Ind gestural code based on universal American Indian hand talk*. New York: Elsevier.

SKILBECK, C.E., WADE, D.T., HEWER, R.L., & WOOD, V.A. (1983). Recovery after stroke. *Journal of Neurology, Neurosurgery, and Psychiatry*, 46, 5-8.

SKILBECK, S.J. (1984). Computer assistance in the management of memory and cognitive impairment. In B.A. Wilson & N. Moffat (Eds.), *Clinical management of memory problems* (pp. 112-131). Rockville, MD: Aspen.

SKLAR, M. (1973). *Sklar Aphasia Scale* (Revised Edition). Los Angeles: Western Psychological Services.

SLOANE, H.N., & MACAULAY, B.D. (Eds.). (1968). *Operant procedures in remedial speech and language training*. Boston: Houghton Mifflin.

SMITH, A. (1971). Objective indices of severity of chronic aphasia in stroke patients. *Journal of Speech and Hearing Disorders*, 36, 167-207.

SMITH, A. (1973). *Symbol Digit Modalities Test*. Los Angeles: Western Psychological Services.

SMITH, A.D., & FULLERTON, A.M. (1981). Age differences in episodic and semantic memory: Implications for language and cognition. In D.S. Beasley & G.A. Davis (Eds.), *Aging: Communication processes and disorders* (pp. 139-158). New York: Grune & Stratton.

SMITH, E.E. (1988). Concepts and thought. In R.J. Sternberg & E.E. Smith (Eds.), *The psychology of human thought* (pp. 19-49). Cambridge, UK: Cambridge University Press.

SMITH, E.E., SHOBEN, E.J., & RIPS, L.J. (1974). Structure and process in semantic memory: A featural model for semantic decisions. *Psychological Review*, 81, 214-241.

SMITH, F. (1982). *Understanding reading: A psycholinguistic analysis of reading and learning to read* (Third Edition). New York: Holt, Rinehart and Winston.

SMITH, R.M. (1983). Treatment of communication disorders. In M. Rosenthal, E.R. Griffith, M.R. Bond, & J.D. Miller (Eds.), *Rehabilitation of the head injured adult* (pp. 355-366). Philadelphia: F.A. Davis.

SMITH, S.D. & BATES, E. (1987). Accessibility of case and gender contrasts for agent-object assignment in Broca's aphasics and fluent anomics. *Brain and Language*, 30, 8-32.

SMITH, S.R., CHENERY, H.J., & MURDOCH, B.E. (1989). Semantic abilities in dementia of the Alzheimer type. II. Grammatical semantics. *Brain and Language*, 36, 533-542.

SOLIN, D. (1989). The systematic misrepresentation of bilingual-crossed aphasia data and its consequences. *Brain and Language*, 36, 92-116.

SOLSO, R.L. (1991). *Cognitive psychology* (Third Edition). Boston: Allyn and Bacon.

SPARKS, R.W. (1978). Parastandardized examination guidelines for adult aphasia. *British Journal of Disorders of Communication*, 13, 135-146.

SPARKS, R.W., & DECK, J.W. (1986). Melodic intonation therapy. In R. Chapey (Ed.), *Language intervention strategies in adult aphasia* (Second Edition) (pp. 320-333). Baltimore: Williams & Wilkins.

SPARKS, R.W., HELM, N.A., & ALBERT, M.L. (1974). Aphasia rehabilitation resulting from melodic intonation therapy. *Cortex*, 10, 303-316.

SPARKS, R.W., & HOLLAND, A.L. (1976). Method: Melodic intonation therapy for aphasia. *Journal of Speech and Hearing Disorders*, 41, 287-297.

SPELLACY, F.J., & SPREEN, O. (1969). A short form of the Token Test. *Cortex*, 5, 390–397.

SPERBER, D., & WILSON, D. (1986). *Relevance: Communication and cognition*. Cambridge, MA: Harvard University Press.

SPIERS, P.A. (1981). Have they come to praise Luria or to bury him? The Luria-Nebraska Battery controversy. *Journal of Consulting and Clinical Psychology*, 49, 331–341.

SPINNLER, H., DELLA SALLA, S., BANDERA, R., & BADDELEY, A. (1988). Dementia, aging, and the structure of human memory. *Cognitive Neuropsychology*, 5, 193–212.

SPINNLER, H., & VIGNOLO, L. (1966). Impaired recognition of meaningful sounds in aphasia. *Cortex*, 2, 337–348.

SPREEN, O., & BENTON, A.L. (1977). *Neurosensory center comprehensive examination for aphasia (NCCEA)* (Revised). Victoria, British Columbia: Neuropsychology Laboratory, University of Victoria.

SPREEN, O., & WACHAL, R.S. (1973). Psycholinguistic analysis of aphasic language: Theoretical formulations and procedures. *Language and Speech*, 16, 130–146.

SPRINGER, L., GLINDEMANN, R., HUBER, W., & WILLMES K. (1991). How efficacious is PACE-therapy when "Language Systematic Training" is incorporated? *Aphasiology*, 5, 391–399.

SPRINGER, S.P., & DEUTSCH, G. (1989). *Left brain, right brain* (Third Edition). New York: W.H. Freeman.

SQUIRE, L.R. (1987). *Memory and brain*. New York: Oxford University Press.

STACHOWIAK, F., HUBER, W., POECK, K., & KERSCHENSTEINER, M. (1977). Text comprehension in aphasia. *Brain and Language*, 4, 177–195.

STANTON, K., YORKSTON, K.M. KENYON, V.T., & BEUKELMAN, D.R. (1981). Language utilization in teaching reading to left neglect patients. In R.H. Brookshire (Ed.), *Clinical aphasiology conference proceedings* (pp. 262–271). Minneapolis: BRK.

STARCH, S., & FALLTRICK, E. (1990). The importance of a home evaluation for brain injured clients: A team approach. *Cognitive Rehabilitation*, 8(6), 28–32.

STARKSTEIN, S.E., & ROBINSON, R.G. (1988). Aphasia and depression. *Aphasiology*, 2, 1–20.

STATE UNIVERSITY OF NEW YORK AT BUFFALO (1990). *Guide for use of the uniform data set for medical rehabilitation*. Buffalo, NY: Research Foundation.

STEELE, R.D., WEINRICH, M., WERTZ, R.T., KLECZEWSKA, M., & CARLSON, G.S. (1989). Computer-based visual communication in aphasia. *Neuropsychologia*, 27, 409–426.

STEIN, N.L., & GLENN, C.G. (1979). An analysis of story comprehension in elementary school children. In R.O. Freedle (Ed.), *New directions in discourse processes* (pp. 53–120). Norwood, NJ: Ablex.

STEMBERGER, J.P. (1984). Structural errors in normal and agrammatic speech. *Cognitive Neuropsychology*, 1, 281–314.

STERNBERG, R.J. (1985). *Beyond IQ: A theory of human intelligence*. Cambridge, UK: Cambridge University Press.

STILLINGS, N.A., FEINSTEIN, M.H., GARFIELD, J.L., RISSLAND, E.L., ROSENBAUM, D.A., WEISLER, S.E., & BAKER-WARD, L. (1987). *Cognitive science: An introduction*. Cambridge, MA: Bradford/MIT Press.

STIMLEY, M.A., & NOLL, J.D. (1991). The effects of semantic and phonemic prestimulation cues on picture naming in aphasia. *Brain and Language*, 41, 496–509.

STOKES, T., & BAER, D. (1977). An implicit technology of generalization. *Journal of Applied Behavior Analysis*, 10, 349–367.

STRAUSS, E., & MOSCOVITCH, M. (1981). Perception of facial expressions. *Brain and Language*, 13, 308–332.

STROHNER, H., COHEN, R., KELTER, S., & WOLL, G. (1978). "Semantic" and "acoustic" errors of aphasic and schizophrenic patients in a sound-picture matching task. *Cortex*, 14, 391–403.

STUBBS, M. (1983). *Discourse analysis: The sociolinguistic analysis of natural language*. Chicago, IL: University of Chicago Press

STUMP, D.A., & WILLIAMS, R. (1980). The noninvasive measurement of regional cerebral circulation. *Brain and Language*, 9, 35–46.

SULLIVAN, M.P., & BROOKSHIRE, R.H. (1989). Can generalization differentiate whether learning or facilitation of a process occurred? In T.E. Prescott (Ed.), *Clinical aphasiology* (Vol. 18) (pp. 247–256). Boston: College-Hill/Little, Brown.

SULLIVAN, M.P., FISHER, B., & MARSHALL, R.C. (1986). Treating the repetition deficit in conduction aphasia. In R.H. Brookshire (Ed.), *Clinical aphasiology* (Vol. 16) (pp. 172–180). Minneapolis: BRK.

SWINDELL, C.S., BOLLER, F., & HOLLAND, A.L. (1988). Expressive language characteristics in probable Alzheimer's disease. *Aphasiology*, 2, 411–416.

SWINDELL, C.S., HOLLAND, A.L., & FROMM, D. (1984). Classification of aphasia: WAB type versus clinical impression. In R.H. Brookshire (Ed.), *Clinical aphasiology conference proceedings* (pp. 48–54). Minneapolis: BRK.

SWINDELL, C.S., HOLLAND, A.L., FROMM, D., & GREENHOUSE, J.B., (1988). Characteristics of recovery of drawing ability in left and right brain-damaged subjects. *Brain and Cognition*, 7, 16–30.

SWINNEY, D.A. (1979). Lexical access during sentence comprehension: (Re)consideration of context effects. *Journal of Verbal Learning and Verbal Behavior*, 20, 645–660.

SWINNEY, D.A., & HAKES, D.T. (1976). Effects of prior context upon lexical access during sentence comprehension. *Journal of Verbal Learning and Verbal Behavior*, 15, 681–689.

SWINNEY, D.A., ZURIF, E., & NICOL, J. (1989). The effects of focal brain damage on sentence processing: An examination of the neurological organization of a mental module. *Journal of Cognitive Neuroscience,* 1, 25–37.

SWISHER, L., & HIRSH, I.J. (1972). Brain damage and the ordering of two temporally successive stimuli. *Neuropsychologia,* 10, 137–152.

SWISHER, L.P., & SARNO, M.T. (1969). Token Test scores of three matched patient groups: Left brain-damaged with aphasia; right brain-damaged without aphasia, non-brain damaged. *Cortex,* 5, 264–273.

TAFT, M. (1979). Lexical access via an orthographic code: The Basic Orthographic Syllable Structure (BOSS). *Journal of Verbal Learning and Verbal Behavior,* 18, 21–40.

TAFT, M. (1990). Lexical processing of functionally constrained words. *Journal of Memory and Language,* 29, 245–257.

TALLAL, P., & NEWCOMBE, F. (1978). Impairment of auditory perception and language comprehension in dysphasia. *Brain and Language,* 5, 13–24.

TANENHAUS, M.K., LEIMAN, J.M., & SEIDENBERG, M.S. (1979). Evidence for multiple stages in the processing of ambiguous words in syntactic contexts. *Journal of Verbal Learning and Verbal Behavior,* 18, 427–440.

TANNEN, D. (1986). *That's not what I meant! How conversational style makes or breaks relationships.* New York: Ballantine.

TANNER, D.C., & GERSTENBERGER, D.L. (1988). The grief response in neuropathologies of speech and language. *Aphasiology,* 2, 79–84.

TANRIDAG, O., & KIRSHNER, H.S. (1987). Language disorders in stroke syndromes of the dominant capsulostriatum—a clinical review. *Aphasiology,* 1, 107–118.

TANRIDAG, O., KIRSHNER, H.S., & CASEY, P.F. (1987). Memory functions in aphasic and non-aphasic stroke patients. *Aphasiology,* 1, 201–214.

TAYLOR, M.L., & MARKS, M.M. (1959). *Aphasia rehabilitation manual and therapy kit.* New York: McGraw-Hill.

THAL, L.J. (1988). Treatment strategies: Present and future. In M.K. Aronson (Ed.), *Understanding Alzheimer's disease* (pp. 50–66). New York: Scribners.

THOMPSON, C.K. (1989). Generalization research in aphasia: A review of the literature. In T.E. Prescott (Ed.), *Clinical aphasiology* (Vol. 18) (pp. 195–222). Austin, TX: Pro-ed.

THOMPSON, C.K. & BYRNE, M.E. (1984). Across setting generalization of social conventions in aphasia: An experimental analysis of "loose training." In R.H. Brookshire (Ed.), *Clinical aphasiology conference proceedings* (pp. 132–144). Minneapolis: BRK.

THOMPSON, C.K., HALL, H.R., & SISON, C.E. (1985). Effects of hypnosis and imagery training on naming in aphasia. In R.H. Brookshire (Ed.), *Clinical aphasiol-*

ogy conference proceedings (pp. 301–310). Minneapolis: BRK.

THOMPSON, C.K., & KEARNS, K.P. (1981). An experimental analysis of acquisition, generalization, and maintenance of naming behavior in a patient with anomia. In R.H. Brookshire (Ed.), *Clinical aphasiology conference proceedings* (pp. 35–45.) Minneapolis: BRK.

THOMPSON, C.K., & MCREYNOLDS, L.V. (1986). Wh-interrogative production in agrammatic aphasia: An experimental analysis of auditory-visual stimulation and direct-production treatment. *Journal of Speech and Hearing Research,* 29, 193–206.

THOMPSON, C.K., MCREYNOLDS, L.V., AND VANCE, C.E. (1982). Generative use of locatives in multiword utterances in agrammatism: A matrix-training approach. In R.H. Brookshire (Ed.), *Clinical aphasiology conference proceedings* (pp. 289–297). Minneapolis: BRK.

THOMPSON, J., & ENDERBY, P. (1979). Is all your Schuell really necessary? *British Journal of Disorders of Communication,* 14, 195–201.

THOMPSON, R.F. (1985). *The brain: An introduction to neuroscience.* New York: W.H. Freeman.

THOMPSON, R.F., & DONEGAN, N.H. (1986). The search for the engram. In J.L. Martinez & R.P. Kesner (Eds.), *Learning and memory: A biological view* (pp. 3–52). Orlando, FL: Academic Press.

THOMSEN, I.V. (1975). Evaluation and outcome of aphasia in patients with severe closed head trauma. *Journal of Neurology, Neurosurgery, and Psychiatry,* 38, 713–718.

THOMSEN, I.V. (1984). Late outcome of very severe blunt head trauma: A 10–15 year second followup. *Journal of Neurology, Neurosurgery, and Psychiatry,* 47, 260–268.

THORNDYKE, P.W. (1977). Cognitive structures in comprehension and memory of narrative discourse. *Cognitive Psychology,* 9, 77–110.

TOMPKINS, C.A. (1990). Knowledge and strategies for processing lexical metaphor after right or left hemisphere brain damage. *Journal of Speech and Hearing Research,* 33, 307–316.

TOMPKINS, C.A., & FLOWERS, C.R. (1985). Perception of emotional intonation by brain-damaged adults: The influence of task processing levels. *Journal of Speech and Hearing Research,* 28, 527–538.

TOMPKINS, C.A., & FLOWERS, C.R. (1987). Contextual mood priming following left and right hemisphere damage. *Brain and Cognition,* 6, 361–376.

TOMPKINS, C.A., HOLLAND, A.L., RATCLIFF, G., COSTELLO, A., LEAHY, L.F., & COWELL, V. (1990). Predicting cognitive recovery from closed head-injury in children and adolescents. *Brain and Cognition,* 13, 86–97.

TOMPKINS, C.A., JACKSON, S.T., & SCHULZ, R. (1990). On prognostic research in adult neurologic disorders. *Journal of Speech and Hearing Research,* 33, 398–401.

TOMPKINS, C.A., RAU, M.T., MARSHALL, R.C.,

LAMBRECHT, K.J., GOLPER, L.A.C., & PHILLIPS, D.S. (1980). Analysis of a battery assessing mild auditory comprehension involvement in aphasia. In R.H. Brookshire (Ed.), *Clinical aphasiology conference proceedings* (pp. 209–216). Minneapolis: BRK.

TONKOVICH, J.D. AND LOVERSO, F.L. (1982). A training matrix approach for gestural acquisition by the agrammatic patient. In R.H. Brookshire (Ed.), *Clinical aphasiology conference proceedings* (pp. 283–288). Minneapolis: BRK.

TONKOVICH, J.D., & PEACH, R.K. (1989). What to treat: Apraxia of speech, aphasia or both. In P. Square-Storer (Ed.), *Acquired apraxia of speech in aphasic adults: Theoretical and clinical issues* (pp. 115–144). London: Taylor & Francis.

TOPPIN, C.J. & BROOKSHIRE, R.H. (1978). Effects of response delay and token relocation on Token Test performance of aphasic subjects. *Journal of Communication Disorders, 11,* 65–78.

TRABASSO, T., & SPERRY, L.L. (1985). Causal relatedness and importance of stort events. *Journal of Memory and Language, 24,* 595–611.

TREXLER, L.E., & ZAPPALA, G. (1988). Neuropathological determinants of acquired attention disorders in traumatic brain injury. *Brain and Cognition, 8,* 291–302.

TROSTER, A.I., SALMON, D.P., MCCULLOUGH, D., & BUTTERS, N. (1989). A comparison of the category fluency deficits associated with Alzheimer's and Huntington's disease. *Brain and Language, 37,* 500–513.

TRUPE, E.H. (1984). Reliability of rating spontaneous speech in the Western Aphasia Battery: Implications for classification. In R.H. Brookshire (Ed.), *Clinical aphasiology conference proceedings* (pp. 55–69). Minneapolis: BRK.

TRUPE, E.H., & HILLIS, A. (1985). Paucity vs. verbosity: Another analysis of right hemisphere communication deficits. In R.H. Brookshire (Ed.), *Clinical aphasiology* (Vol. 15) (pp. 83–96). Minneapolis: BRK.

TULVING, E. (1972). Episodic and semantic memory. In E. Tulving & W. Donaldson (Eds.), *Organization of memory* (pp. 382–403). New York: Academic Press.

TULVING, E., SCHACTER, D.L., MCLACHLAN, D.R., & MOSCOVITCH, M. (1988). Priming of semantic autobiographical knowledge: A case study of retrograde amnesia. *Brain and Cognition, 8,* 3–20.

TYLER, L.K. (1987). Spoken language comprehension in aphasia: A real-time processing perspective. In M. Coltheart, G. Sartori, & R. Job (Eds.), *The cognitive neuropsychology of language* (pp. 145–162). London: Erlbaum.

TYLER, L.K. (1988). Spoken language comprehension in a fluent aphasic patient. *Cognitive Neuropsychology, 5,* 375–400.

TYLER, L.K., & COBB, H. (1987). Processing bound grammatical morphemes in context: The case of an aphasic patient. *Language and Cognitive Processes, 2,* 245–262.

TYLER, L.K., & MARSLEN-WILSON, W. (1986). The effects of context on the recognition of polymorphemic words. *Journal of Memory and Language, 25,* 741–752.

TYLER, L.K., MARSLEN-WILSON, W., RENTOUL, J., & HANNEY, P. (1988). Continuous and discontinuous access in spoken word-recognition: The role of derivational prefixes. *Journal of Memory and Language, 27,* 368–381.

UDELL R., SULLIVAN, R.A., & SCHLANGER, P.H. (1980). Legal competency of aphasic patients: Role of speech-language pathologists. *Archives of Physical Medicine and Rehabilitation, 61,* 374–375.

ULATOWSKA, H.K., CANNITO, M.P., HAYASHI, M.M., & FLEMING, S.G. (1985). Language abilities in the elderly. In H.K. Ulatowska (Ed.), *The aging brain: Communication in the elderly* (pp. 125–140). San Diego: Singular.

ULATOWSKA, H.K., DOYEL, A.W., STERN, R.F., HAYNES, S.M., & NORTH, A.J. (1983). Production of procedural discourse in aphasia. *Brain and Language, 18,* 315–341.

ULATOWSKA, H.K., FREEDMAN-STERN, R., DOYEL, A.W., MACALUSO-HAYNES, S., & NORTH, A.J. (1983). Production of narrative discourse in aphasia. *Brain and Language, 19,* 317–334.

ULATOWSKA, H.K., MACALUSO-HAYNES, S., & MENDEL-RICHARDSON, S. (1976). The assessment of communicative competence in aphasia. In R.H. Brookshire (Ed.), *Clinical aphasiology conference proceedings* (pp. 22–31). Minneapolis: BRK.

URYASE, D., DUFFY, R.J., & LILES, B.Z. (1990). Analysis and description of narrative discourse in right-hemisphere-damaged adults: A comparison to neurologically normal and left-hemisphere-damaged aphasic adults. In T.E. Prescott (Ed.), *Clinical aphasiology* (Vol. 19) (pp. 125–138). Austin, TX: Pro-Ed.

UZELL, B.P., DOLINSKAS, C.A., WISER, R.F., & LANGFITT, T.W. (1987). Influence of lesions detected by computed tomography on outcome and neuropsychological recovery after severe head injury. *Neurosurgery, 20,* 396–402.

VAID, J. (1983). Bilingualism and brain lateralization. In S. Segalowitz (Ed.), *Language functions and brain organization* (pp. 315–339). New York: Academic Press.

VALLAR, G., & BADDELEY, A.D. (1984a). Fractionation of working memory: Neuropsychological evidence for a phonological short-term store. *Journal of Verbal Learning and Verbal Behavior, 23,* 151–161.

VALLAR, G., & BADDELEY, A.D. (1984b). Phonological short-term store, phonological processing and sentence comprehension: A neuropsychological case study. *Cognitive Neuropsychology, 1,* 121–142.

VALLAR, G., & BADDELEY, A.D. (1987). Phonological short-term store and sentence processing. *Cognitive Neuropsychology, 4,* 417–438.

VAN DEMARK, A.A. (1974). Comment on PICA interpretation. *Journal of Speech and Hearing Disorders, 39,* 510–511.

VAN DEMARK, A.A., LEMMER, E.C., & DRAKE, M.L.

(1982). Measurement of reading comprehension in aphasia with the RCBA. *Journal of Speech and Hearing Disorders*, 47, 288–291.

VAN DIJK, T.A., & KINTSCH, W. (1983). *Strategies of discourse comprehension.* New York: Academic Press.

VAN LANCKER, D., & KREIMAN, J. (1986). Preservation of familiar speaker recognition but not unfamiliar speaker discrimination in aphasic patients. In R.H. Brookshire (Ed.), *Clinical aphasiology* (Vol. 16) (pp. 234–240). Minneapolis: BRK.

VAN LANCKER, D.R., & KEMPLER, D. (1987). Comprehension of familiar phrases by left- but not by right-hemisphere damaged patients. *Brain and Language*, 32, 265–277.

VAN RIPER, C., & EMERICK, L. (1990). *Speech correction: An introduction to speech pathology and audiology* (Eighth Edition). Englewood Cliffs, NJ: Prentice-Hall.

VAN STREIN, J.W., LICHT, R., BUOMA, A., & BAKKER, D.J. (1989). Event-related potentials during word-reading and figure-matching in left-handed and right-handed males and females. *Brain and Language*, 37, 525–547.

VARNEY, N.R. (1982). Pantomime recognition defect in aphasia: Implications for the concept of asymbolia. *Brain and Language*, 15, 32–39.

VARNEY, N.R. (1984). Phonemic imperception in aphasia. *Brain and Language*, 21, 85–94.

VARNEY, N.R., & BENTON, A.L. (1978). *Pantomime Recognition Test.* Iowa City: Benton Laboratory of Neuropsychology.

VARNEY, N.R., & BENTON, A.L. (1979). Phonemic discrimination and aural comprehension among aphasic patients. *Journal of Clinical Neuropsychology*, 1, 65–73.

VARNEY, N.R., & BENTON, A.L. (1982). Qualitative aspects of pantomime recognition defect in aphasia. *Brain and Cognition*, 1, 132–139.

VERFAELLIE, M., BOWERS, D., & HEILMAN, K.M. (1988). Hemispheric asymmetries in mediating inattention, but not selective attention. *Neuropsychologia*, 26, 521–532.

VIGNOLO, L.A., BOCCARDI, E., & CAVERNI, L. (1986). Unexpected CT-scan findings in global aphasia. *Cortex*, 22, 55–69.

VOGEL, D., & COSTELLO, R.M. (1986). Bilingual aphasic adults: Measures of word retrieval. In R.H. Brookshire (Ed.). *Clinical aphasiology* (Vol. 16) (pp. 80–86). Minneapolis: BRK.

VON STOCKERT, T.R., & BADER, L. (1976). Some relations of grammar and lexicon in aphasia. *Cortex*, 12, 49–60.

VOYER, D., & BRYDEN, M.P. (1990). Level of spatial ability, and lateralization of mental rotation. *Brain and Cognition*, 13, 18–29.

WADE, D.T., HEWER, R.L., DAVID, R.M., & ENDERBY, P.M. (1986). Aphasia after stroke: Natural history and associated deficits. *Journal of Neurology, Neurosurgery, and Psychiatry*, 49, 11–16.

WAHRBORG, P. (1991). *Assessment and management of* emotional reactions to brain damage and aphasia. San Diego: Singular.

WALKER, C.H., & YEKOVICH, F.R. (1987). Activation and use of script-based antecedents in anaphoric reference. *Journal of Memory and Language*, 26, 673–691.

WALKER-BATSON, D., BARTON, M.M., WENDT, J.S., & REYNOLDS, S. (1987). Symbolic and affective nonverbal deficits in left- and right-hemisphere injured adults. *Aphasiology*, 1, 257–262.

WALLACE, G.L., & CANTER, G.J. (1985). Effects of personally relevant language materials on the performance of severely aphasic individuals. *Journal of Speech and Hearing Disorders*, 50, 385–390.

WALLESCH, C-W. (1985). Two syndromes of aphasia occurring with ischemic lesions involving the left basal ganglia. *Brain and Language*, 25, 357–361.

WAMBAUGH, J.L., & THOMPSON, C.K. (1989). Training and generalization of agrammatic aphasic adults' *wh*-interrogative productions. *Journal of Speech and Hearing Disorders*, 54, 509–525.

WARRINGTON, E.K. (1975). The selective impairment of semantic memory. *Quarterly Journal of Experimental Psychology*, 27, 635–657.

WARRINGTON, E.K. (1991). Right neglect dyslexia: A single case study. *Cognitive Neuropsychology*, 8, 193–212.

WARRINGTON, E.K., & McCARTHY, R. (1983). Category-specific access dysphasia. *Brain*, 106, 859–878.

WARRINGTON, E.K., & McCARTHY, R. (1987). Categories of knowledge: Further fractionations and an attempted integration. *Brain*, 110, 1273–1296.

WARRINGTON, E.K., & SHALLICE, T. (1969). The selective impairment of auditory verbal short-term memory. *Brain*, 92, 885–896.

WARRINGTON, E.K., & SHALLICE, T. (1984). Category-specific semantic impairments. *Brain*, 107, 829–854.

WARRINGTON, E.K., & TAYLOR, A.M. (1978). Two categorical stages of object recognition. *Perception*, 7, 695–705.

WASSERSTEIN, J., ZAPPULLA, R., ROSEN, J., GERSTMAN, L., & ROCK, D. (1987). In search of closure: Subjective contour illusions, gestalt completion tests, and implications. *Brain and Cognition*, 6, 1–14.

WATERS, G., CAPLAN, D., & HILDEBRANDT, N. (1991). On the structure of verbal short-term memory and its functional role in sentence comprehension: Evidence from neuropsychology. *Cognitive Neuropsychology*, 8, 81–126.

WATSON, J.M., & RECORDS, L.E. (1978). The effectiveness of the Porch Index of Communicative Ability as a diagnostic tool in assessing specific behaviors of senile dementia. In R.H. Brookshire (Ed.), *Clinical aphasiology conference proceedings* (pp. 93–105). Minneapolis: BRK.

WATZLAWICK, P. (1978). *The language of change: Elements of therapeutic communication.* New York: Basic Books.

WEBB, D-M. (1991). Increasing carryover and independent use of compensatory strategies in brain injured patients. *Cognitive Rehabilitation, 9*(3), 28–35.

WEBB, W.G., & LOVE, R.J. (1983). Reading problems in chronic aphasia. *Journal of Speech and Hearing Disorders, 48,* 164–171.

WEBSTER, E.J., & NEWHOFF, M. (1981). Intervention with families of communicatively impaired adults. In D.S. Beasley & G.A. Davis (Eds.), *Aging: Communication processes and disorders* (pp. 229–240). New York: Grune & Stratton.

WECHSLER, D. (1945). A standardized memory scale for clinical use. *Journal of Psychology, 19,* 87–95.

WECHSLER, D. (1981). *Wechsler Adult Intelligence Scale-Revised.* New York: Psychological Corporation.

WEDDELL, R.A. (1989). Recognition memory for emotional facial expressions in patients with focal cerebral lesions. *Brain and Cognition, 11,* 1–17.

WEIDNER, W.E., & JINKS, A.F. (1983). The effects of single versus combined cue presentations on picture naming by aphasic adults. *Journal of Speech and Hearing Disorders, 16,* 111–121.

WEIDNER, W.E., & LASKY, E.Z. (1976). The interaction of rate and complexity of stimulus on the performance of adult aphasic subjects. *Brain and Language, 3,* 34–40.

WEIGL, E. (1970). Neuropsychological studies of structure and dynamics of semantic fields with the deblocking method. In A.J. Greimas, R. Jakobson, M.R. Mayenowa, S.K. Saumjan, W. Steinitz, & S. Zolkiewski (Eds.), *Sign, language, culture* (pp. 287–290). The Hague, Netherlands: Mouton.

WEIGL, E., & BIERWISCH, M. (1970). Neuropsychology and linguistics: Topics of common research. *Foundations of Language, 6,* 1–18.

WEINBERG, R.M., AUERBACH, S.H., & MOORE, S. (1987). Pharmacologic treatment of cognitive deficits: A case study. *Brain Injury, 1,* 57–59.

WEINRICH, M., STEELE, R.D., CARLSON, G.S., KLECZEWSKA, M., WERTZ, R.T., & BAKER, E. (1989). Processing of visual syntax in a globally aphasic patient. *Brain and Language, 36,* 391–405.

WEINTRAUB, S., MESULAM, M., & KRAMER, L. (1981). Disturbances in prosody: A right-hemisphere contribution to language. *Archives of Neurology, 38,* 742–744.

WEISENBURG, T.H., & McBRIDE, K.E. (1935). *Aphasia.* New York: Commonwealth Fund.

WEISS, H.D. (1982). Neoplasms. In M.A. Samuels (Ed.), *Manual of neurologic therapeutics with essentials of diagnosis* (Second Edition). Boston: Little, Brown.

WEPMAN, J.M. (1951). *Recovery from aphasia.* New York: Ronald Press.

WEPMAN, J.M. (1953). A conceptual model for the processes involved in recovery from aphasia. *Journal of Speech and Hearing Disorders, 18,* 4–13.

WEPMAN, J.M. (1968). Aphasia therapy: Some "relative" comments and some purely personal prejudices. In J.W. Black & E.G. Jancosek (Eds.), *Proceedings of the conference on language retraining for aphasics* (pp. 95–107). Columbus, OH: Ohio State University.

WEPMAN, J.M. (1972). Aphasia therapy: A new look. *Journal of Speech and Hearing Disorders, 37,* 203–214.

WEPMAN, J.M., & JONES, L.V. (1961). *Studies in aphasia: A approach to testing.* Chicago: Education-Industry Service.

WEPMAN, J.M., & JONES, L.V. (1964). Five aphasias: A commentary on aphasia as a regressive linguistic phenomenon. In D. Rioch & E. Weinstein (Eds.), *Disorders of communication.* Baltimore: Williams & Wilkins.

WEPMAN, J.M., & JONES, L.V. (1966). Studies in aphasia: Classification of aphasic speech by the noun-pronoun ratio. *British Journal of Disorders of Communication, 1,* 46–54.

WEPMAN, J.M., JONES, L.V., BOCK, R.D., & VAN PELT, D. (1960). Studies in aphasia: Background and theoretical formulations. *Journal of Speech and Hearing Disorders, 25,* 323–332.

WEPMAN, J.M., & VAN PELT, D. (1955). A theory of cerebral language disorders based on therapy. *Folia Phoniatrica, 7,* 223–235.

WERNICKE, C. (1977). The aphasia symptom complex: A psychological study on an anatomic basis. In G.H. Eggert (Trans.), *Wernicke's works on aphasia: A sourcebook and review.* The Hague, Netherlands: Mouton.

WERTZ, R.T. (1983). Classifying the aphasias: Commodious or chimerical? In R.H. Brookshire (Ed.), *Clinical aphasiology conference proceedings* (pp. 296–303). Minneapolis: BRK.

WERTZ, R.T. (1985). Neuropathologies of speech and language: An introduction to patient management. In D.F. Johns (Ed.), *Clinical management of neurogenic communicative disorders* (Second Edition) (pp. 1–96). Boston: Little, Brown.

WERTZ, R.T. (1987). Language treatment for aphasia is efficacious, but for whom? *Topics in Language Disorders, 8*(1), 1–10.

WERTZ, R.T., BERNSTEIN-ELLIS, E.G., & ROBERTS, J.A. (1989). A case of conduction aphasia or apraxia of speech. In N. Helm-Estabrooks & J.L. Aten (Eds). *Difficult diagnoses in adult communication disorders* (pp. 135–145). San Diego: Singular.

WERTZ, R.T., COLLINS, M.J., WEISS, D.G., KURTZKE, J.F., FRIDEN, R., BROOKSHIRE, R.H., PIERCE, J., HOLZAPPLE, P., HUBBARD, D.J., PORCH, B.E., WEST, J.A., DAVIS, L., MATOVICH, V., MORLEY, G.K., & RESURRECCION, E. (1981). Veterans Administration cooperative study on aphasia: A comparison of individual and group treatment. *Journal of Speech and Hearing Research, 24,* 580–594.

WERTZ, R.T., DEAL, J.L., HOLLAND, A.L., KURTZKE, J.F.,

& WEISS, D.G. (1986). Comments on an uncontrolled aphasia no treatment trial. *Asha, 28,* 31.

WERTZ, R.T., DEAL, J.L., & ROBINSON, A.J. (1984). Classifying the aphasias: A comparison of the Boston Diagnostic Aphasia Examination and the Western Aphasia Battery. In R.H. Brookshire (Ed.), *Clinical aphasiology conference proceedings* (pp. 40–47). Minneapolis: BRK.

WERTZ, R.T., DEAL, L.M., & DEAL, J.L. (1980). Prognosis in aphasia: Investigation of the High-Overall Prediction (HOAP) method and the Short-Direct or HOAP-Slope method to predict change in PICA performance. In R.H. Brookshire (Ed.), *Clinical aphasiology conference proceedings* (pp. 164–173). Minneapolis: BRK.

WERTZ, R.T., DRONKERS, N.F., & SHUBITOWSKI, Y. (1986). Discriminant function analysis of performance by normals and left hemisphere, right hemisphere, and bilaterally brain damaged patients on a word fluency measure. In R.H. Brookshire (Ed.), *Clinical aphasiology* (Vol. 16) (pp. 257–266). Minneapolis: BRK.

WERTZ, R.T., LaPOINTE, L.L., & ROSENBEK, J.C. (1984). *Apraxia of speech in adults: The disorder and its management.* Orlando, FL: Grune & Stratton.

WERTZ, R.T., WEISS, D.G., ATEN, J.L., BROOKSHIRE, R.H., GARCIA-BUNUEL, L., HOLLAND, A.L., KURTZKE, J.F., LaPOINTE, L.L., MILIANTI, F.J., BRANNEGAN, R., GREENBAUM, H., MARSHALL, R.C., VOGEL, D., CARTER, J., BARNES, N.S., & GOODMAN, R. (1986). Comparison of clinic, home, and deferred language treatment for aphasia: A Veterans Administration cooperative study. *Archives of Neurology, 43,* 653–658.

WESSELLS, M.G. (1982). *Cognitive psychology.* New York: Harper & Row.

WEYLMAN, S.T., BROWNELL, H.H., ROMAN, M., & GARDNER, H. (1989). Appreciation of indirect requests by left- and right-brain-damaged patients: The effects of verbal context and conventionality of wording. *Brain and Language, 36,* 580–591.

WHEELER, L., & REITAN, R.M. (1962). Presence and laterality of brain damage predicted from responses to a short aphasia screening test. *Perceptual and Motor Skills, 15,* 783–799.

WHITAKER, H.A., & NOLL, J.D. (1972). Some linguistic parameters of the Token Test. *Neuropsychologia, 10,* 395–404.

WHURR, R. (1974). *An aphasia screening test.* Reading, UK: University of Reading.

WIEGEL-CRUMP, C., & KOENIGSKNECHT, R.A. (1973). Tapping the lexical store of the adult aphasic: Analysis of the improvement made in word retrieval skills. *Cortex, 9,* 411–418.

WILCOX, M.J., DAVIS, G.A., & LEONARD, L.L. (1978). Aphasics' comprehension of contextually conveyed meaning. *Brain and Language, 6,* 362–377.

WILLIAMS, S.E., & CANTER, G.J. (1982). The influence of situational context on naming performance in aphasic syndromes. *Brain and Language, 17,* 92–106.

WILLIAMS, S.E., & CANTER, G.J. (1987). Action-naming performance in four syndromes of aphasia. *Brain and Language, 32,* 124–136.

WILLIAMS, S.E., & SEAVER, E.J. (1986). A comparison of speech sound durations in three syndromes of aphasia. *Brain and Language, 29,* 171–182.

WILSON, B.A., COCKBURN, J., & BADDELEY, A. (1985). *The Rivermead Behavioural Memory Test.* Hants, ENG: Thames Valley Test Company.

WILSON, B.A., & MOFFAT, N. (1984). Running a memory group. In B.A. Wilson & N. Moffat (Eds.), *Clinical management of memory problems* (pp. 171–198). Rockville, MD: Aspen.

WILSON, R.S., KASZNIAK, A.W., & FOX, J.H. (1981). Remote memory in senile dementia. *Cortex, 17,* 41–48.

WINNER, E., & GARDNER, H. (1977). Comprehension of metaphor in brain damaged patients. *Brain, 100,* 717–729.

WOLFE, G.R. (1987). Microcomputers and treatment of aphasia. *Aphasiology, 1,* 165–170.

WONDER, J., & DONOVAN, P. (1984). *Whole-brain thinking: Working from both sides of the brain to achieve peak job performance.* New York: Morrow.

WOOD, R.L. (1986). Rehabilitation of patients with disorders of attention. *Journal of Head Trauma Rehabilitation, 1,* 43–53.

WOODCOCK, R.W., & JOHNSON, M.B. (1989). *Woodcock-Johnson Psycho-Educational Battery.* Allen, TX: DLM.

WOODWARD, S.H., OWENS, J., & THOMPSON, L.W. (1990). Word-to-word variation in ERP component latencies: Spoken words. *Brain and Language, 38,* 488–503.

WULF, H.H. (1979). *My world alone.* Detroit: Wayne State University Press.

WULFECK, B.B. (1988). Grammaticality judgments and sentence comprehension in agrammatic aphasia. *Journal of Speech and Hearing Research, 31,* 72–80.

WULFECK, B.B., BATES, E.A., & CAPASSO, R. (1991). A cross-linguistic study of grammaticality judgments in Broca's aphasia. *Brain and Language, 41,* 311–336.

YARNELL, P., MONROE, M.A., & SOBEL, M.A. (1986). Aphasia outcome in stroke: A clinical neuroradiological correlation. *Stroke, 7,* 516–522.

YLVISAKER, M., & HOLLAND, A.L. (1985). Coaching, self-coaching, and rehabilitation of head injury. In D.F. Johns (Ed.), *Clinical management of neurogenic communicative disorders* (Second Edition) (pp. 243–257). Boston: Little, Brown.

YLVISAKER, M., & SZEKERES, S.F. (1986). Management of the patient with closed head injury. In R. Chapey (Ed.), *Language intervention strategies in adult aphasia* (Second Edition) (pp. 474–490). Baltimore: Williams & Wilkins.

YORKSTON, K.M., & BEUKELMAN, D.R. (1980). An analysis of connected speech samples of aphasic and normal speakers. *Journal of Speech and Hearing Disorders, 45,* 27–36.

YORKSTON, K.M., BEUKELMAN, D.R., & BELL, K.R. (1988). *Clinical management of dysarthric speakers.* San Diego: Singular.

YORKSTON, K.M., MARSHALL, R.C., & BUTLER, M. (1977). Imposed delay of response: Effects on aphasics' auditory comprehension of visually and nonvisually cued material. *Perceptual and Motor Skills, 44,* 647–655.

YORKSTON, K.M., STANTON, K.M., & BEUKELMAN, D.R. (1981). Language-based compensatory training for closed-head-injured patients. In R.H. Brookshire (Ed.), *Clinical aphasiology conference proceedings* (pp. 293–300). Minneapolis: BRK.

YOUNG, A.W., & DE HAAN, E.H.F. (1988). Boundaries of covert recognition in prosopagnosia. *Cognitive Neuropsychology, 5,* 317–336.

YOUNG, A.W., NEWCOMBE, F., & ELLIS, A.W. (1991). Different impairments contribute to neglect dyslexia. *Cognitive Neuropsychology, 8,* 177–192.

YOUNG, J.Z. (1986). What's in a brain? In C. Coen (Ed.), *Functions of the brain* (pp. 1–10). Oxford, UK: Clarendon.

ZAIDEL, E. (1975). A technique for presenting lateralized visual input with prolonged exposure. *Vision Research, 15,* 283–289.

ZANGWILL, O. (1946). Intelligence in aphasia. In A. De Reuck & M. O'Conner (Eds.), *Disorders of language* (pp. 261–274). London: Churchill.

ZATORRE, R.J. (1989). On the representation of multiple languages in the brain: Old problems and new directions. *Brain and Language, 36,* 127–147.

ZDENEK, M. (1983). *The right-brain experience: An intimate program to free the powers of your imagination.* New York: McGraw-Hill.

ZINGESER, L.B., & BERNDT, R.S. (1988). Grammatical class and context effects in a case of pure anomia: Implications for models of lexical processing. *Cognitive Neuropsychology, 5,* 473–516.

ZINGESER, L.B., & BERNDT, R.S. (1990). Retrieval of nouns and verbs in agrammatism and anomia. *Brain and Language, 39,* 14–32.

ZOCCOLOTTI, P., SCABINI, D., & VIOLANI, C. (1982). Electrodermal responses in patients with unilateral brain damage. *Journal of Clinical Neuropsychology, 4,* 143–150.

ZURIF, E.B., CARAMAZZA, A., & MYERSON, R. (1972). Grammatical judgments of agrammatic patients. *Neuropsychologia, 10,* 405–417.

ZURIF, E.B., GARDNER, H., & BROWNELL, H.H. (1989). The case against the case against group studies. *Brain and Cognition, 10,* 237–255.

ZURIF, E.B., GREEN, E., CARAMAZZA, A., & GOODENOUGH, C. (1976). Grammatical intuitions of aphasic patients: Sensitivity to functors. *Cortex, 12,* 183–186.

ZURIF, E.B., & GRODZINSKY, Y. (1983). Sensitivity to grammatical structure in agrammatic aphasics: A reply to Linebarger, Schwartz, and Saffran. *Cognition, 15,* 207–213.

ZURIF, E.B., SWINNEY, D., & FODOR, J.A. (1991). An evaluation of assumptions underlying the single-patient-only position in neuropsychological research: A reply. *Brain and Cognition, 16,* 198–210.

NAME INDEX

SUBJECT INDEX

Attention, 14, 55, 89, 133, 136, 153–54, 165, 293, 318
Auditory agnosia, 13, 83, 161, 169
Auditory Comprehension Test for Sentences (ACTS), 219, 253
Auditory processing, 83–84, 87–89
Augmentative communication, 283–84
Automatic processing, 10, 54–55, 62
Autonomy (also Modularity assumption), 70, 72
Automized speech, 12
Awareness, 134, 136, 153

Backward scanning, 178, 179, 318
Baselines (also Multiple baseline design), 256–57
BDAE (see Boston Diagnostic Aphasia Examination)
Bedside Evaluation Screening Test (BEST), 215
Behaviorism, 2–3, 8
Behavior modification, 3, 269–71
Bilateral disorders, 83, 156, 157, 158, 160, 169, 210
Bilateral signs in PICA, 199–200
Bilingualism, 10–11, 37–38, 97–98, 210–11, 242–43
Bilingual mode, 11, 211
Blissymbols, 284, 296
Borderline region, 246
Borrowing, 98, 211
Boston Assessment of Severe Aphasia (BASA), 232
Boston Diagnostic Aphasia Examination (BDAE), 202–7, 211–12, 220
  as validation, 209, 217, 229
  in research, 104, 117, 250
Boston Naming Test (BNT), 222, 246
Bottom-up processing, 54, 68
Brain scan, 29
Bridging inference, 179, 180, 318
Brief Test of Head Injury (BTHI), 215
Broca's aphasia, 18, 19, 37, 40–41, 42, 103–4, 108–15
  assessment, 108, 129, 204, 209–10, 230, 231
  other research, 117–18, 119, 120–21, 123, 125, 126–27, 129, 141, 168, 174, 175, 188, 247, 273, 283
  treatment, 131, 283, 296–303
Broca's area (area 44), 24, 40–41
Buffer(s) in working memory, 54, 178–80

CADL (see Communicative Abilities in Daily Living)
Canonical word order, 86, 90, 97, 105, 106, 110, 115, 117, 121, 221
Capsulostriatum, 43, 246
Carotid arteries, 22, 23
Carrier phrase (also Completion tasks), 273, 298
Case studies, 102–3
  AE (conduction aphasia), 124–25
  CM (conduction aphasia), 127
  EST (anomic aphasia), 130
  HN (Wernicke's aphasia), 117

JB (neglect dyslexia), 165
KC (amnesia), 137
KF, 53–54
MC (conduction aphasia), 125
PV (conduction aphasia), 124, 125
RH (Wernicke's aphasia), 118
SP (neglect dyslexia), 165
VB (neglect dyslexia), 165
WC (neglect dyslexia), 165
WS (paragrammatism), 121–23
Categorical word fluency, 92, 96, 123, 140, 145, 163, 241, 260
Category-specific deficits, 84, 91, 147
Centrality of disorder, 13–14, 108, 111, 115, 123, 125
Cerebral arteries, 22–24
Cerebrovascular accident (CVA), 21
Certification, 291
Change score, 200, 237–38
CHI (see Closed head injury)
Chinese (see Languages)
Chronic phase, 25–26
Circle of Willis, 22, 23, 26, 281
Circumlocution, 15, 19, 20, 92, 129, 130, 283, 316
Clinical-functional gap, 284, 306, 307, 309
Clinical neuropsychology, 8, 51–52, 78–79, 132–33, 154, 319
Clinical syndrome, 100
Closed class words, 16, 59, 74–75, 104–5, 112, 114
Closed head injury (CHI), 134–42, 186–89, 259–61, 309
  language assessment, 139–40, 212, 215
  language treatment, 150, 317–19, 320
Code-switching, 98, 211
Cognition, defined, 5–6, 9–10, 14
Cognitive neuropsychology, 8, 51–52, 279–80
Cognitive psychology, 5, 8, 51
Cognitive rehabilitation, 262, 277, 319–20
Cognitive science, 8
Cognitive stimulation (see Stimulation treatment)
Coherence, defined, 176
Cohesion, defined, 177
Cohesive tie, 185, 186, 187
Cohort theory, 63
Coindexing, 86
Collateral circulation, 281
Coma, 14, 134–36, 259
Communicative Abilities in Daily Living (CADL), 228–30
  in research, 217, 250, 255
  as validation, 198, 203
Communicative Effectiveness Index (CETI), 230–31
Competence (linguistic), 6, 82–83, 111, 278–79
Competition model, 73, 107
Completed stroke, 23
Completion:
  of objects, 79
  of sentences, 91, 271, 273, 299

Computer-assisted symbol system, 284, 296
Computer-assisted treatment, 274, 277–78, 283, 288, 302–3
Computerized tomography (CT Scan), 29–30, 40–42
Computers in assessment, 133, 196, 199, 224
Concept, 56–58
Concept comparison task, 57, 72
Concept-driven (see Top-down processing)
Conciseness index, 145
Concrete words, 65–66, 165–66
Concretism, 285
Concurrent task (see Dual task)
Conduction aphasia, 19, 41, 124–28
  assessment, 119, 209–10
  other research, 108, 109, 119, 122, 129, 144, 182, 248, 273
  treatment, 305–6
Conduction theory, 119–20
Confrontation naming, 90–91, 93–95
Connectionist models, 62
Constructional apraxia, 80, 158–59, 169, 203
Constructional skills, 46, 133, 181
Content analysis, 93, 140, 145, 163
Content words (see Open-class words)
Context (nonverbal), 172, 285–87, 307–8
Context analysis, 307–8
Context management, 311
Context effects (linguistic), 70, 72–73, 112
Controlled processes (see Optional processes, Strategic processing)
Convergent behavior, 91
Conversational discourse, 92–93, 96, 145, 172, 176, 186, 187, 223, 230, 231–32, 285, 312–15
Conversational coaching, 310, 314–15
Cookie Theft picture, 104, 202
  in research, 93, 104, 188, 223
Cooperative principle, 172, 231
Coping strategies, 134, 285, 292
Coreference, 86, 185
Coreference Battery, 221
Core language processes, 68, 163
Corpus callosum, 5, 33
Cortical quotient (CQ), 208, 253
Counseling, 286, 287, 288, 317
Covert attention, 154
Convert recognition, 137, 158
Criterion (response, task), 276–77, 300
Critical period, 36
Crossed aphasia, 35–36, 37
Cross-linguistic research (also Languages), 11–12, 90, 96–97, 104–5, 109, 110, 111, 121
Cross-modal priming, 70, 72, 112–13
CT scan (see Computerized tomography)
Cue cost, 107
Cue redundancy, 110, 298
Cue validity, 107
Cueing, 271–74, 298, 303, 316
Cueing-verb-treatment, 302